A SMILE
WHERE THERE WAS NONE

Christian Yaste, DDS

A SMILE
WHERE THERE WAS NONE

A PRACTICAL APPROACH TO
FIXED FULL-ARCH IMPLANT DENTISTRY

edra
PUBLISHING

This edition first published 2024

ISBN 9781957260532
eISBN 9781957260570

Editor: Paola Sammaritano, Edra S.p.A.

edra
PUBLISHING

Edra Publishing US LLC
3309 Northlake Boulevard,
Suite 203,
Palm Beach Gardens,
FL 33403
EIN: 844113980

info@edrapublishing.com
www.edrapublishing.com

Printed in Italy in January 2024 by "Printer Trento" S.r.l., Trento

DEDICATION

This book is dedicated to the talented group of women I have the pleasure of working with in my private practice, Ballantyne Dentistry. This team, which I have the honor of leading, plays a crucial role in my ability to restore our patients' smiles, function, health, confidence, and often the essence of their personality. With their support, I have been able to create and fine tune my process, become more efficient, and deliver life-changing results and experiences to our patients. I am humbled to be surrounded by a group of people who are so dedicated to our patients and supportive of one another. Their commitment to our mission and vision has allowed me to bring this book to you. It brings me great joy and pride to recognize and dedicate this work to them.

Director of Operations: Jackie Krinc
Clinical Director: Stephanie Deen
Business Team Leader: Kristina Neely
Treatment Plan Coordinator Team Leader: Jennifer Woods
Practice Consultant: Carla Stack (retired)
Business Team: Allie Plyler, Alyssa Nuhfer, Angela Johnson, Brittney Daniels, Leah Fernandez, Madison Gibson
Clinical Team: Alyssa Harkey, Amber Parks, Cindy Gil, Codi Crocker, Jenni Guerra, Jess Thomas, Kari Licata, Mayce Bowles, Summer Mullinax
Hospitality Coordinator: Gabriela Yaste
Hygiene Team: Bethany Rutledge, Heather Miles, Olivia Holman, Marcia Stewart, Sheena Hinson, Taira Dotson
Treatment Plan Coordinator Team: Ashley Lehman, Jamie Wageman, Jordan Timmons

TABLE OF CONTENTS

SECTION I
INTRODUCTION TO FULL-ARCH IMPLANT DENTISTRY

SECTION IV

THE FIXED FULL-ARCH GUIDED IMPLANT SURGICAL PROCESS

SECTION V
THE PROSTHETIC WORKFLOW

SECTION VI
FIXED FULL-ARCH DENTISTRY MAINTENANCE AND HYGIENE

PREFACE

As a young dentist, early in my career, I observed that many of my patients with failing dentitions had struggled for years, sometimes decades, after spending small fortunes on restorative and periodontal care. They came to me seeking a more predictable solution. Some of these patients told me they were ready to "throw in the towel," so to speak. I believed at the time that helping these patients keep their teeth was the best option. However, for many that meant continuing to battle against dental caries, erosion, periodontal issues, and occlusal disease. The treatment alternatives to saving their teeth, such as dentures and removable appliances, seemed disabling for many of them. Dental implant rehabilitation was incredibly expensive, an enormous time commitment, and somewhat unpredictable. These patients were trapped in a perpetual cycle of dental discouragement. I knew there had to be a better way to help them, but I didn't know what it was. How could I provide a better option that created ideal function, esthetics, and oral health?

My journey to finding the answers started in 2003 when I was introduced to the All-on-4® treatment concept. I had been practicing dentistry for 8 years and was eager to see this new procedure. The room was filled with oral surgeons, periodontists, and prosthodontists . . . and my business partner and me. (I think we may have been the only general dentists in attendance.) After 2 or 3 hours of watching slide after slide of implant surgeons removing teeth and immediately loading four dental implants with a fixed denture, I became fascinated with the concept. My dental implant experience at the time was limited to single-tooth implant placement and restoration. Although the idea of the All-on-4 technique was captivating, it seemed far beyond my reach.

For several years, I referred patients who were interested in fixed full-arch implant rehabilitation to local surgical specialists, and I partnered with them to complete the prosthetic phase of these cases. However, some of these patients had mediocre experiences and outcomes. I became increasingly frustrated with my inability to predict what type of results my patients would receive. Finally, I resorted to referring the entire process out to a large dental franchise that could do the surgical and prosthetic procedure all in one facility. For a time, this seemed acceptable. Yet often I would see new patients who had negative experiences and felt like all they got was a sales pitch. These patients reported little or no empathy expressed by the dental professionals there. It was just not a good fit for them.

Eventually, a local oral surgeon with a significant amount of experience with the All-on-4 technique convinced me to work with him. Once again, I became active in helping my patients get fixed full-arch prosthetics on dental implants. I attended courses and would frequently take part in the surgeries and learn by observing over the surgeon's shoulder. But I was not convinced that estimating bone removal, manually placing multiple dental implants and multiunit abutments, and converting a set of dentures in addition to all of that was the best approach. The analog process of the All-on-4, although interesting, was inefficient, unpredictable, complicated, and unprofitable. It got to the point that I was having a hard time justifying why I was doing it, and my business began to suffer the consequences.

Finally, in 2016, I began using digital technology and software that I was already working with to create a more pragmatic workflow for fixed full-arch rehabilitation. I started investigating and employing stackable surgical guides to perform full-arch implant surgery. The sequential workflow made sense to me. The fact that I could use the technology and software that I had already invested in to accomplish most of the process was exciting. And so, I embarked with a new purpose: to provide the entire rehabilitative process, both surgical and prosthetic, all under one roof, in my own practice. I became empowered to provide fixed full-arch implant dentistry from start to finish and to give my patients a smile where there was none. ■

A NOTE TO MY READERS

When I started the journey of writing down my experience with full-arch implant dentistry, I had to do something very important: I had to make a commitment. I knew this endeavor would take at least 2 years and require many hours of research and writing, taking photos, talking to experts, and recalling my experiences.

Commitment was something I had not given much conscious thought to until 2008, when I reached a breaking point in my life and career. Serendipitously, a friend, Michael York, gave me a copy of a book that he had written entitled *The Ten Commitments* (One Shoe Press, 2005). After reading this book, I gained a new perspective on my life and my career in dentistry. Over time, I developed my own personal set of commitments from the advice and wisdom of my mentors and coaches.

I have shared these commitments with my associates, audiences of my peers, and other dentists who I mentor. This book gives me the opportunity to share them with you as well. You will find the first one in my introduction and others at the beginning of each chapter. The development of these commitments has been a process and a journey. It is my hope that you will find useful concepts in these commitments that help improve your own life. ■

DISCLAIMER

The chapters of this book present an overview of the manner in which I currently provide fixed full-arch implant dentistry to my patients. This book is not intended to educate you in every aspect of fixed full-arch implant rehabilitation, the fundamentals of dental implantology, oral surgery, prosthetics, or occlusion. Understanding these important principles and concepts is essential for getting the most out of this book. This text is a guide to a pragmatic workflow and process that I have helped develop and test with several laboratories and implant companies. If you are a novice dentist with little or no experience in dental implantology and the concepts mentioned above, I encourage you to consider additional training and education. ■

INTRODUCTION

Commitment: Be coachable and teachable.
Everyone needs a coach. I have several coaches, and each one provides value to me and has helped me grow as a dentist and a person.

At the time of this writing, my team and I have completed more than 450 fixed full-arch guided implant cases using the procedures and techniques laid out in this book. We have utilized a wide variety of implant systems, stackable surgical guide designs, guide and prosthetic materials, intraoral scanners and software, and digital workflows. Our dental practice has grown dramatically as patients in our community have become more aware of fixed full-arch implant dentistry, and it has become increasingly popular and in demand.

Some clinicians would argue that guided full-arch implant surgery is unnecessary, inefficient, and costly for clinicians, and that traditional unguided techniques are "good enough." I believe that for the vast majority of general practitioners, digitally planned, prosthetically driven, and guided full-arch implant dentistry is easier, safer, and more reliable than manual placement and analog workflows.

Gaining foundational experience and knowledge in unguided implant surgery is helpful and desirable for clinicians first attempting complex full-arch implant dentistry. Knowing the fundamentals of oral surgery is a must. However, if you are a dentist beginning your journey into this space, consider the advantages of providing full-arch dentistry using stackable surgical guide systems compared with unguided full-arch treatment. It is easier to learn, does not require purchasing additional expensive technology, is duplicable, creates less risk, and provides precise anticipated outcomes for patients.

This book is for general dentists who are interested in providing predictable, full-arch guided dental implant surgery, with an immediate-loaded conversion prosthesis. It also outlines a pragmatic, fixed, implant-supported prosthetic rehabilitation method. The reader is introduced to a method of leveraging technology and software to make the process of fixed full-arch implant dentistry easier and less stressful than it would otherwise be. In addition, it offers guidance in creating positive patient and team experiences. This book can also be used as a teaching tool for your dental auxiliaries, a clinical reference manual for dental laboratories, and an educational digest for those patients who can stomach the photographs.

Over the past several years, I have developed a passion for and an obsession with fixed full-arch implant dentistry. I have spent many hours reading, researching, photographing, attending courses online and in person, observing and having discussions with brilliant dental implantologists and dental laboratory personnel, speaking to the CEOs of leading companies within the dental industry, and working on creating a practical method of providing fixed full-arch dental implant rehabilitation for my patients. This is the most fascinating and rewarding therapeutic care I have ever been able to provide for my patients. Fixed full-arch implant dentistry has created thrilling patient experiences, opened doors to unlikely opportunities, helped me scale my business for sustainability, and kept me up at night.

A close friend and mentor refers to this process as a “smile transplant,” and that is exactly what full-arch implant dentistry is. It restores a person’s life and true personality and can bring enormous pleasure, not only to your patients but to you and your team as well. Do you see patients who have suffered for years from tooth decay, periodontal disease, erosion, worn dentitions, and other debilitating and terminal dental conditions? Of course you do. These patients are desperate for help, and most of them only want four things: to have confidence in their smile, to be able to eat the foods they love, to not suffer with pain, and finally, to be healthy. My hope is that the following pages will help you achieve these four objectives for your patients, give you clarity, competency, and bring a new perspective on a life-changing procedure that you can be a part of. ■

INTRODUCTION TO FULL-ARCH IMPLANT DENTISTRY

SECTION I

WHAT IS FIXED FULL-ARCH IMPLANT DENTISTRY?

CHAPTER **1**

Commitment: Don't overlook opportunity, and take calculated risks.

Keep your eyes open. There are opportunities everywhere; don't be afraid to risk taking one if it aligns with your goals and purpose.

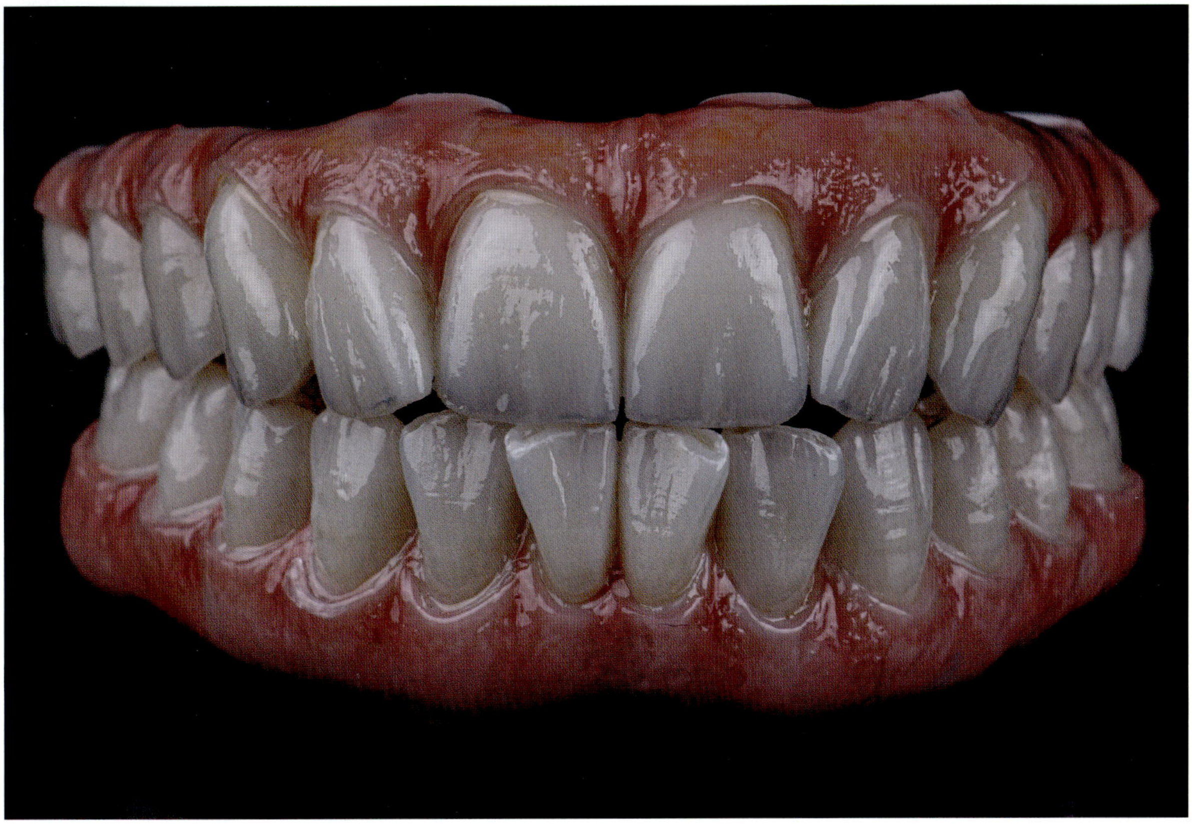

FIXED FULL-ARCH IMPLANT DENTISTRY DEFINED

I have observed and participated in the fixed full-arch dental implant space since my introduction to the All-on-4® concept in 2003. The way it is being explained, discussed, and taught among clinicians today is changing.

The term *fixed full-arch implant dentistry* encompasses a treatment modality that provides full-arch rehabilitation for a patient utilizing dental implants and a fixed dental prosthesis.

This prosthesis can only be removed by a dental clinician. There is a surgical phase in which four or more dental implants are placed and a prosthetic phase where these implants are used to fully support a fixed dental prosthesis. This fixed prosthesis can occupy a defect that includes missing teeth as well as lost bone and tissue. It is designed for rehabilitating patients that are edentulous, partially edentulous, or in a failing dentition.

In the past, fixed full-arch implant dentistry was perceived by many general dentists, including myself, as confusing, time consuming, nonprofitable, and tedious. It was an analog process, generally involving multiple clinicians and laboratory technicians. At present, many dentists placing and/or restoring full-arch dental implants are interested in a more pragmatic approach to fixed full-arch implant dentistry that is simpler, profitable, more efficient, systematic, and rewarding.

> There are five stages to a practical approach for fixed full-arch implant dentistry. This book reviews each stage and its corresponding parts in a step-by-step manner. The five stages are:
> 1. Patient Selection and Data Collection
> 2. Prosthetically Driven Case Engineering and Design
> 3. The Surgical Process Utilizing a Stackable Surgical Guide System
> 4. A Simplified Prosthetic Workflow
> 5. Hygiene and Maintenance

BACKGROUND AND HISTORY OF FIXED FULL-ARCH IMPLANT DENTISTRY

Fixed full-arch implant dentistry did not make its entry into dentistry overnight like some other procedures and technologies that have appeared recently. Fixed full-arch implant dentistry has evolved over time and is rapidly becoming very popular among dentists who practice and promote dental implant therapy.

The evolution of full-arch dental implant therapy has been in progress for over 50 years. It began when Per-Ingvar Brånemark—considered by most in our profession as the patriarch of dental implants—placed the first titanium dental implant into a human volunteer in 1965. He coined the term *osseointegration*. In the years that followed, the "root-form" type of implant made of titanium was developed. Implants were adopted by our profession as the standard of care for replacing a tooth or several teeth. Prof. Brånemark made the following statement that has always resonated with me and has become part of my own philosophy:

> A decisive factor in patient care is simplification of treatment, which should be based on identifying and utilizing the enormous capacity of existing original anchoring tissues. When possible, one should avoid unnecessary advanced and complicated major grafting procedures[1].

In the mid to late 1980s, Dr. Carl Misch developed a classification for dental implant prostheses (abbreviated as FP1, FP2, FP3, RP4, and RP5) that remains in use today[2]. The All-on-4® technique itself was developed in the early 1990s by Dr. Paulo Maló to provide a set of fixed teeth that were immediately loaded for elderly patients who were not good candidates for bone grafting. The term *All-on-4* was later coined by Dr. Maló after he and others performed a series of studies funded by Nobel Biocare to determine the efficiency and cost effectiveness of the approach. It was formally introduced in 2003 and All-on-4 become commonly recognized by dentists and the public alike.

In the years since then, advances in treatment planning software and digital design and engineering have been made. CAD/CAM milling, 3D printing, and the introduction of new materials have all helped shape fixed full-arch implant dentistry. Digital diagnostic data can be collected, uploaded, and merged into software. Interim prostheses, as well as dental implant type, size, and positioning, can be digitally planned. Some surgeons have begun to switch from manual surgery to a guided approach. Once a patient is ready to transition to their definitive prosthesis, the case can be completed with digital technology that is making analog processes obsolete. Dental companies, laboratories, and clinicians have started to collaborate to create an even more predictable way to integrate cutting-edge technology within the dental industry into this space.

DEFINITIONS AND CLASSIFICATIONS OF FIXED FULL-ARCH IMPLANT-SUPPORTED PROSTHETICS

In order for the reader to understand the prosthetics used in fixed full-arch implant-supported dentistry, I will review some classifications that have become widely accepted by dentists throughout the world. Please note, however, that the lines between the different types of fixed prostheses have become blurred over the past several years. This is due to advances in implant and restorative technology. Moreover, some clinicians have recently proposed new categories for classifying patients and determining which prosthesis is most appropriate. To date, however, none has been widely adopted within the industry.

Most dentists today recognize the three types of fixed full-arch implant-supported prostheses described below.

Fixed prosthesis 1 (FP1) (Fig. 1.1)

The FP1 is the most complex and formidable type of full-arch implant surgery and fixed prosthetic dentistry. It is not for the weak of heart, it requires both extraordinary skill and extensive knowledge of bone and soft tissue manipulation on the part of the surgeon, and the associated laboratory costs can be astronomical. Historically, the FP1 was typically surgically sequenced in stages: In qualified patients, teeth were serially extracted, implants were placed in a submerged fashion, and the remaining dentition was used to support temporary fixed partial dentures. Once the implants osseointegrated, the remaining teeth would be extracted, additional implants would be placed, and the osseointegrated implants would support new temporary bridges. Finally, the case could be restored with a more definitive prosthesis. Today, it is more common to do this type of procedure without having to extract the teeth in stages if primary stability of the implants can be achieved. The introduction of multiunit abutments (MUAs), stronger temporary materials, implants designed for immediate placement and loading, and more reliable grafting techniques have made this possible.

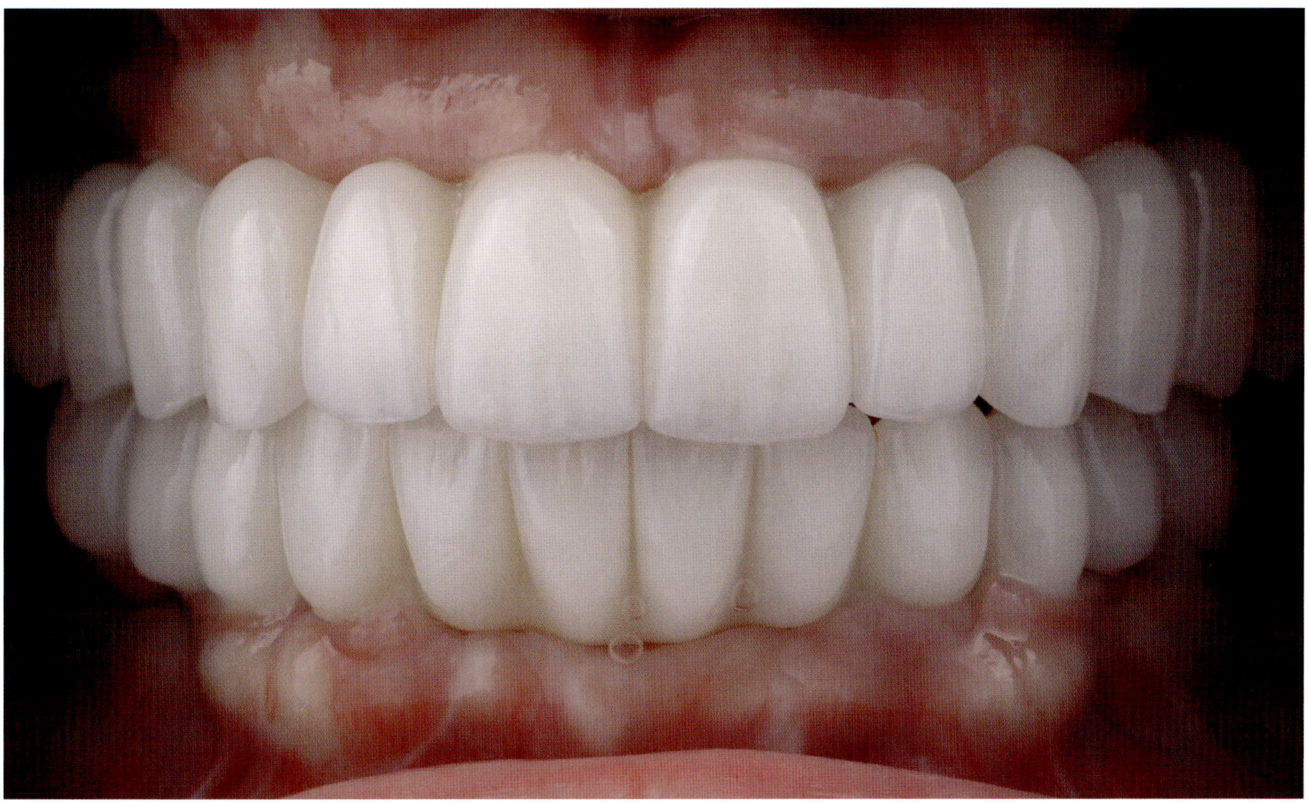

Figure 1.1 **An example of a maxillary FP1 prosthesis except with significant gingival scalloping and contours.**

The **FP1**:

- Can be used in patients with minimal loss of hard and soft tissue
- Replaces only the teeth or crowns and generally includes no pink porcelain
- Is most often desirable in the maxillary anterior region for esthetics
- Is typically supported by six to eight dental implants (or more) often positioned similarly to the roots of the natural teeth
- May require complex bone grafting and augmentation in patients with deficient crestal bone
- May require the patient to undergo gingivoplasty and soft tissue grafting to improve gingival contours in order to address esthetic concerns
- Has required restorative material that was traditionally porcelain-fused-to-metal, but full monolithic and multilayer zirconia is becoming more popular
- Restorations were traditionally built direct to implant and utilized crowns and/or fixed partial dentures on custom implant abutments. Today, many clinicians are using MUAs and designing the definitive prosthesis with either multiple-section or full-arch style bridges
- May involve several dental implant procedures and can take between 6 months and a year or more to complete.

Fixed prosthesis 2 (FP2) (Fig. 1.2)

To me, the FP2 is a kind of crossbreed of the FP1 and FP3. It can have similar complexity, cost, and implant design as the FP1. It is only esthetically acceptable in patients who do not expose gingival tissue with an exaggerated smile. The FP2 allows the clinician to preserve more bone (when appropriate) than the FP3.

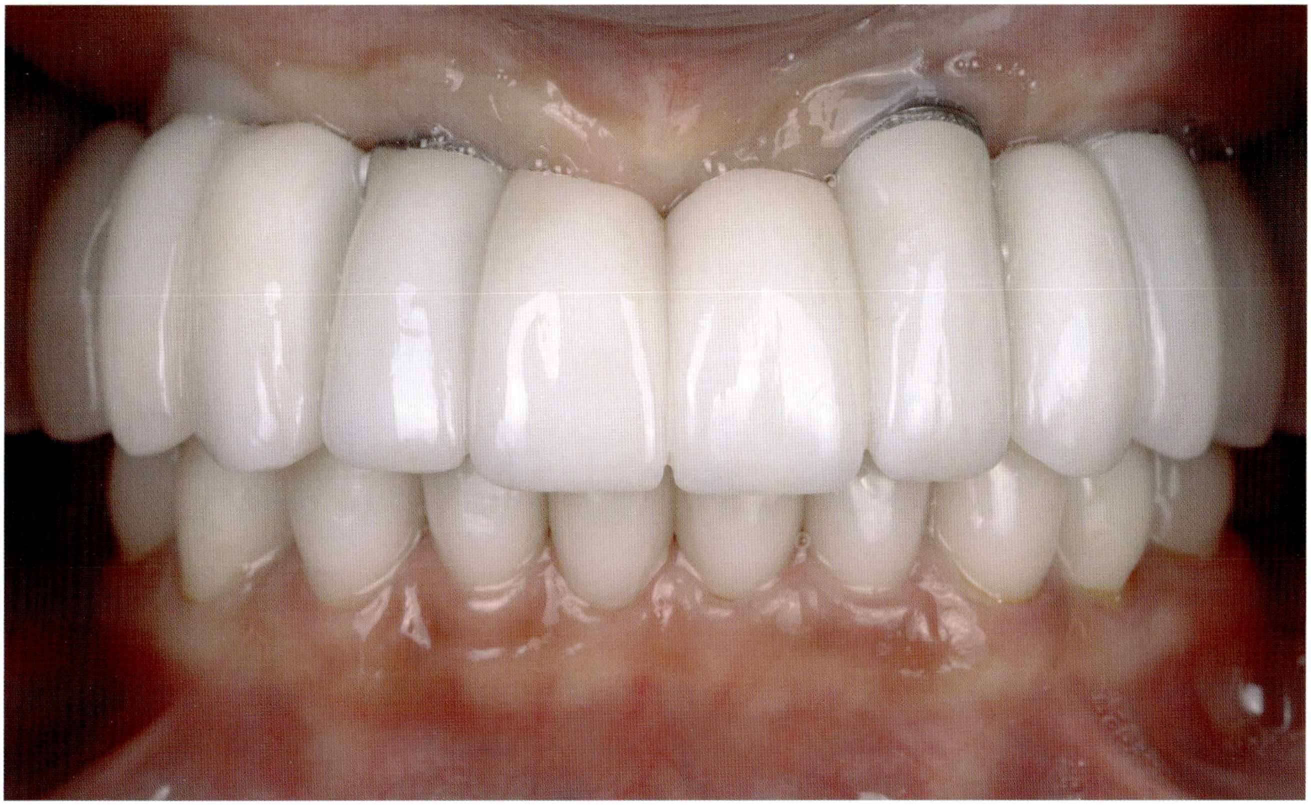

Figure 1.2 **An example of a maxillary FP2 prosthesis built on custom abutments using traditional crown and bridge restorations. This photo was taken 5 years postoperative. Note that the teeth are elongated with a complete lack of papillae.**

The **FP2**:

- Can be used in cases with limited bone loss and with slight gingival recession
- Replaces teeth or crowns and a portion of the root but features little or no pink porcelain
- Has a gingival one-third of the crown that is overextended
- Requires implant placement that is less prescriptive than the FP1 prosthesis, and papillae may or may not be present
- Allows for six to eight (or more) implants to be utilized to support the definitive prosthesis, like the FP1
- Creates an impression of longer teeth in the definitive prosthesis than in an FP1
- Traditionally was fabricated with porcelain-fused-to-metal alloy, like the FP1, but today is often made with full monolithic and multilayer zirconia
- Like the FP1, was often built on custom implant abutments with traditional crown and bridge designs and a direct interface with the dental implants. Today, clinicians are using MUAs as an alternative and designing their FP2 cases much like the FP1s
- Shares a similar timeline to complete as the FP1.

Fixed prosthesis 3 (FP3) (Fig. 1.3)

The FP3 design is what many commonly refer to as the All-on-4 or All-on-X. This design has become increasingly popular among dentists and patients alike. Compared with other options, the cost of the FP3 can be more affordable, there are fewer surgical concerns, and it takes less time to reach completion. Is it the best choice for every patient needing a full arch of dental implants? No, but planned properly, keeping bone reduction in consideration, and maximizing implant support throughout the ridge, this can be a very acceptable prosthesis. I find that many of the patients I serve who have failing dentitions or are fully or almost fully edentulous are good candidates for the FP3 design.

The **FP3**:

- Is a good option when natural resorption has reduced bone height, or bone reduction is required for restorative factors (discussed later in chapter)
- Replaces the missing teeth, gingival architecture, and a portion of the edentulous ridges
- Closely resembles natural dentition and soft tissues when visible during function, speaking, and smiling
- Allows implant placement that is less restrictive compared with the FP1 and FP2
- Requires four to six dental implants
- Offers more options for restorative materials. Substructures have been fabricated from titanium, polyether ether ketone (PEEK), zirconia, and cobalt-chrome, and teeth and gingival architecture may be acrylic, milled, or printed polymethylmethacrylate (PMMA), zirconia, resin composite, or other restorative materials. In addition, new options for substructures, teeth, and gingiva are being developed at a rapid pace.
- Can be completed in as little as 3 to 6 months.

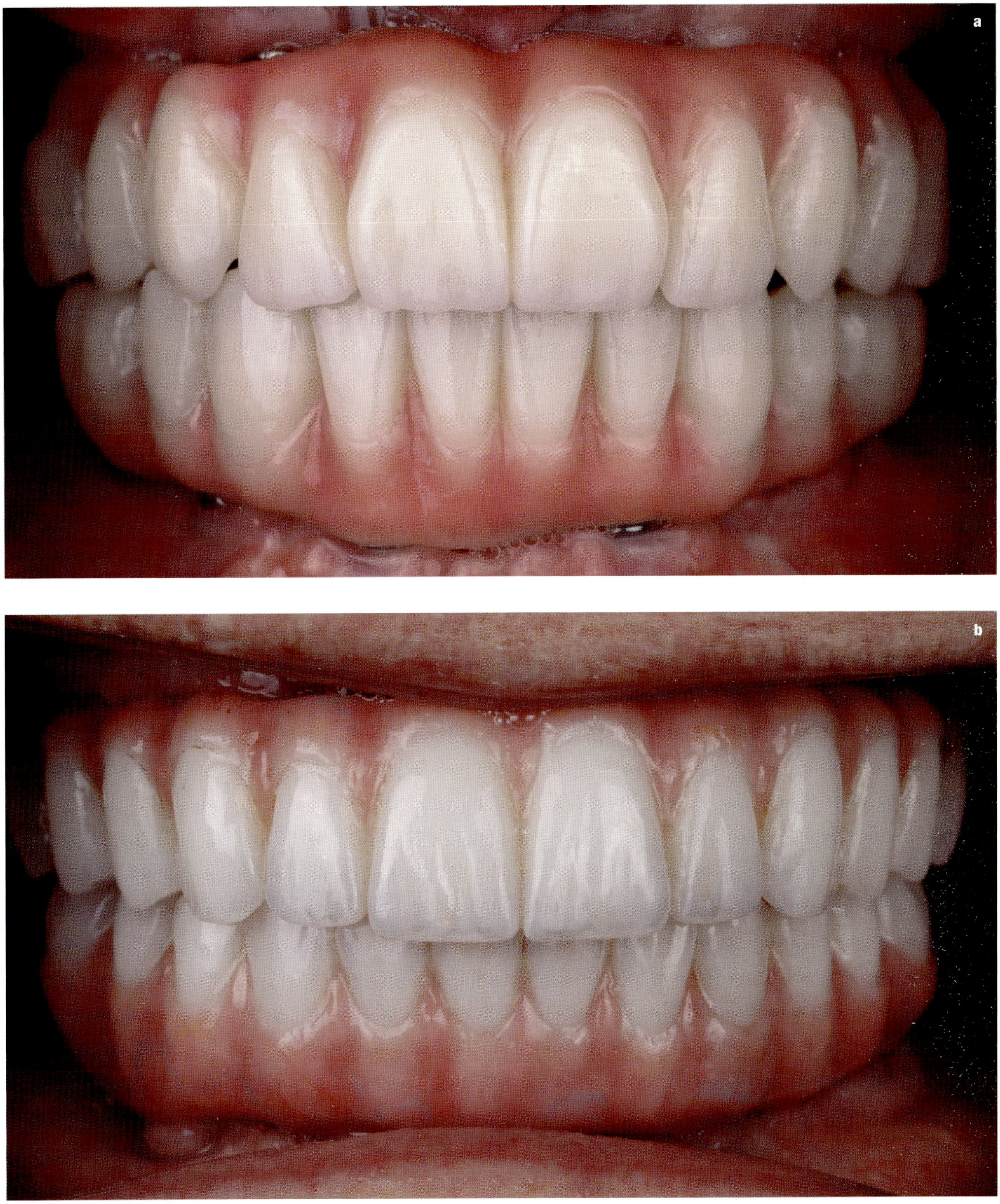

Figure 1.3 (a, b) Two examples of FP3 prostheses in both the maxillary and mandibular arches. Note the presence of gingiva as well as teeth within the prostheses.

THE RIGHT PROCESS AND DESIGN FOR YOUR PATIENT

Each of these prosthetic designs can be accomplished utilizing prosthetically driven case engineering and design, a stackable surgical guide system, and the simplified prosthetic workflow. The surgical process I follow for providing fixed full-arch dentistry to my patients is to extract all remaining dentition, place the dental implants with a stackable surgical guide system, and deliver and immediately load the interim prosthesis all in one visit. The case examples presented in this book will be representative of that. The FP3 design is what I most commonly use in my practice. This is due to many patients failing to meet the requirements for other designs or not being able to afford a more expensive option.

An argument made by some clinicians, mostly academics, is that the design of a case should be based solely on objective physical factors. In the world of academia, practical matters such as the financial and time commitment to the patient and other elements affecting a private practitioner are often overlooked. I would suggest that before settling on a particular design, whether it be FP1, FP2, or FP3, the clinician should consider the patient's desires and expectations as well as their corporeal attributes.

The advantages and disadvantages of the various fixed full-arch implant prosthesis designs should be discussed with patients no less thoroughly than those considering a removable prosthesis. During the initial planning phase, it is important to determine which designs your patients are candidates for and then go through the process of settling on which of those is most appropriate for them.

THE OSTEOPLASTY DEBATE

The need to reduce a considerable amount of bone that sometimes occurs in fixed full-arch implant dentistry has become a source of contention over the years. There are clinicians and academics on both sides. Critics argue that bone reduction is not good for patients. Excessive bone reduction can lead to disability in the event of a catastrophic failure of the implants. Such patients would have to consider additional and more expensive procedures such as sinus elevation and (additional) bone grafting. Dental implants placed in the zygoma and pterygoid regions of the maxilla, and possibly nerve repositioning in the mandible, might also be necessary. However, bone reduction is needed in some cases to avoid esthetic complications. One example in an FP3 type of design is where the transition line between the prosthesis and the patient's maxillary gingival anatomy becomes exposed during smiling. In addition, a certain amount of restorative space must be available to create a prosthesis with strength and longevity. As yet, no standard of care has been established to determine what is appropriate when it comes to bone reduction. Using a prosthetically driven workflow and logical principles to safeguard as much bone as possible are becoming expected concepts when it comes to fixed full-arch implant dentistry. Fortunately, with careful planning, design, and engineering, appropriate bone levels can be preserved.

OBJECTIVES FOR FIXED FULL-ARCH DENTAL IMPLANT REHABILITATION

Clinicians must continually remind themselves of the goals of full-arch implant rehabilitation. Without understanding your own goals as well as those of your patients, you may not succeed in meeting anyone's expectations.

What matters most to patients

Over the years, I have learned that most patients want four things (not necessarily in the order presented).

Function

Patients who have failing dentitions or are edentulous want to be able to eat the foods they love again. Overlooking a patient's masticatory ability and desires is a recipe for disaster. Your objective should be to enable the patient to eat anything on the menu at their favorite restaurant. Of course, there are things that even people in perfectly healthy natural dentitions should not chew. However, if you can give your patients the ability to eat most foods, they will be delighted.

Phonetics is also a part of function. Even though most patients have acceptable speech when you first meet them, those who do not use a fixed or removable appliance or do not have their natural front teeth may struggle to be understood. It should be our goal to give the patient understandable speech that is as good as or better than what they already have.

Confidence

Having confidence in one's smile means being able to interact with others without having to hide one's teeth.

Patients want to be able to speak, smile, and laugh without conscious or subconscious thoughts about what others might be thinking about their teeth. This is paramount to an individual's self-esteem. Patients will sometimes minimize the importance of esthetics to their dentist because of shame and the fear of being judged as vain. In my experience, all patients who go through a rehabilitative dental procedure are interested in improving their appearance to some degree. If the eyes are the window to one's soul, the smile is the front door.

Freedom from pain and discomfort

Patients with missing, broken, or decayed teeth may or may not be in any pain. Many of the dentally disabled patients I visit with have somehow adapted to their situation. However, a certain percentage of patients suffer daily from odontogenic pain. By treating and resolving infection and other sources of pain, we can provide healthier outcomes to our patients both physically and emotionally.

Health

This is usually most important to us as dentists but not always at the top of a patient's list of priorities. In recent years, however, I have noticed that more people have become familiar with the oral-systemic relationship, probably because of the growing attention it has been given in the media, on the internet and social media platforms, as well as by dental health care professionals. Some patients appreciate the link that their mouths have to the rest of their body and are interested in living a healthier lifestyle and extending their lifespan.

My case-planning goals

A fixed interim prosthesis within 48 hours of surgery: *Gratification*

I am a strong believer in loading implants immediately or shortly after surgery with a fixed interim prosthesis. Patients coming to me for rehabilitative implant dentistry are tired of wearing removable appliances or are generally not interested in having teeth removed and being tethered to a denture for even a few months. Although we cannot always promise a patient that they will have a fixed prosthesis after surgery, it is my goal to create value right from the beginning. We can do this by improving their smile and confidence with an immediate fixed prosthesis.

Stability with long-term function and esthetics: *Predictability*

Patients who accept complex restorative implant dentistry are not interested in having the procedure done repeatedly. Unlike much of the restorative dentistry we do, dental implants are considered by our patients to be "permanent." We are very careful to explain to patients that nothing that is in function lasts forever. But our goal is to create an implant foundation that satisfies our patients with long-term service, provided appropriate maintenance is carried out.

A pragmatic surgical and prosthetic protocol: *Efficiency and Profitability*

As a clinician, I am interested in being efficient whenever possible. Efficiency increases profitability, which then allows me to create success for my team as well as our practice. Patients are concerned with efficiency as well. Most people value their time and will appreciate your efforts to streamline a process for them. Using a guided surgical protocol and a simplified prosthetic workflow, we have been able to reduce the amount of time and appointments for patients.

Cont'd ▶

Hygiene and maintenance:
Maintainability

Without the means to maintain their new teeth and implants, patients may eventually have issues that lead to catastrophic failure. It is important to have a support plan in place for patients to help them manage their dental implants and prosthetics. Many patients assume that after a fixed full-arch dental implant procedure, they are free of the dentist at last. "Completely the opposite" is the message I give to my patients, and I like to use analogies about automobiles: "Would you buy a Mercedes and never take it in for an oil change?" Dentists and patients should understand that there are prosthetic forces and loading conditions, as well as biologic factors, that can create significant complications if hygiene and maintenance are not addressed.

Avoidance of unnecessary bone grafting, multiple complex surgeries, and other case complexities:
Affordability

One of the great benefits of fixed full-arch dentistry is that the surgery can frequently be performed without additional complicated forms of bone augmentation and soft tissue grafting. In addition, there is generally one surgical visit vs. multiple surgeries when the traditional serial extraction method is employed in the FP1 and FP2 approach. With advancements over the years, particularly with the introduction of the All-on-4, we know that fewer dental implants are necessary for prosthetic stabilization. All these elements factor into a more cost-effective option for my patients. Granted, the expense of undergoing fixed full-arch implant rehabilitation can be significant, but our goal is to give patients an affordable alternative to more expensive procedures.

OPTIONS FOR EDENTULOUS AND PARTIALLY EDENTULOUS PATIENTS

Fixed full-arch implant-supported prostheses are not the only option for patients who are edentulous, partially edentulous, or have failing dentitions. Although I will be addressing fixed full-arch dentistry throughout this book, it is important to have an overview of what else is out there and what other options are available to patients. This not only gives us a better idea of what the advantages and disadvantages are but also a deeper understanding of why a fixed full-arch rehabilitation may or may not be a good treatment plan for the patients we serve.

Traditional dentures

Complete maxillary and mandibular dentures have been an option for patients who are fully edentulous since the beginning of dentistry (Fig. 1.4). Humans have been replacing their own teeth with teeth from animals or other humans, stones, ivory, and shells since as early as the seventh century BC. People have never wanted to be without teeth, but until the last several decades, the options for fully edentulous patients were limited.

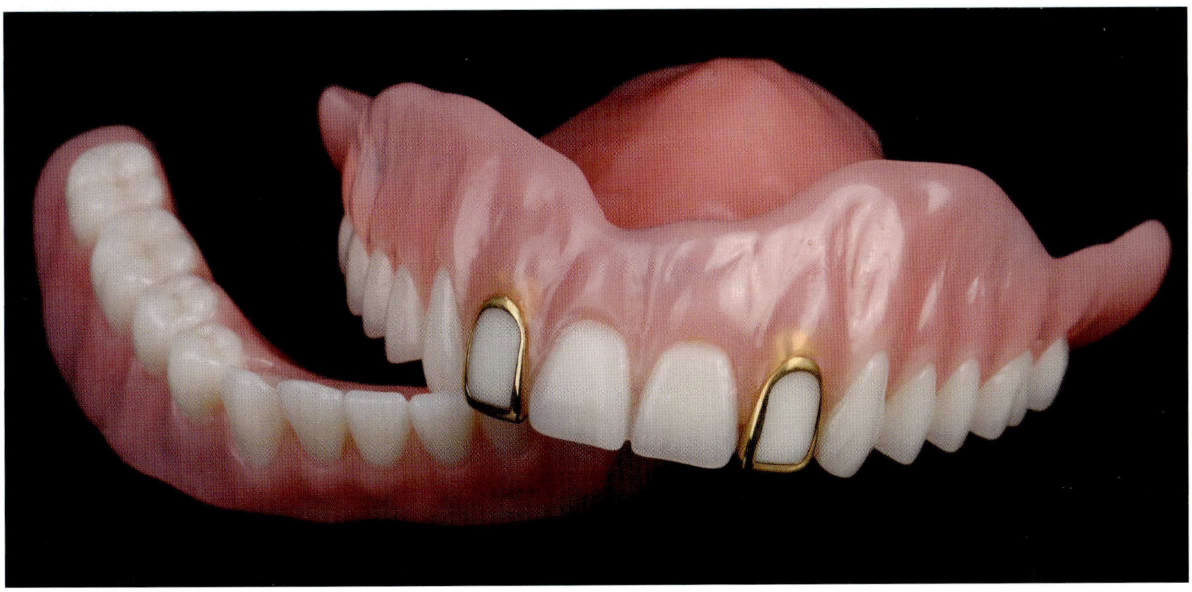

Figure 1.4 **Maxillary and mandibular complete dentures with open-face gold crowns on the maxillary lateral incisors.**

For patients, the modern denture offers both advantages and disadvantages.

Advantages

Cost

The most cost-effective of all options, dentures can vary from hundreds of dollars when provided by a so-called denture mill to thousands of dollars when provided by a general dentist or prosthodontist.

Time

Dentures can be fabricated quite easily due to the advent of scanning technology. A set of "digital" dentures can be completed in as few as two visits.

Removability/ease

The fact that these appliances are removable by the patient with little or no effort may be seen as an advantage as well as a disadvantage. For some patients that may be a benefit, but for others it may be a drawback.

Low maintenance

Denture wearers need to visit the dentist less frequently than individuals with natural dentitions or dental implants. An annual visit for an oral exam and cancer screening as well as evaluation of their appliances is considered acceptable within the industry. Dentures are easy to keep clean and maintain.

Elimination of disease

If a patient is in a failing dentition where there is infection present, removing the teeth creates a healthier overall situation. Dental caries, periodontal disease, and tooth abscesses can be eliminated by removing teeth.

Esthetics

Typically, a patient in an edentulous or failing partially edentulous situation can gain pronounced cosmetic improvement with dentures. There are also ways to be creative with dentures to provide realistic-looking teeth.

Mastication

Chewing may improve for patients with a well-fitting denture compared to a fully edentulous or partially edentulous situation.

Disadvantages

Removability

Though it may be an advantage for some patients, a removable option may not be advantageous for most people. One of the most common complaints I receive from patients with dentures is that they dislike having teeth that are removable.

Bone loss

Most patients do not understand the fact that their bone resorbs as soon as they lose a tooth or teeth. Fear of losing additional bone is a strong motivation for patients to pursue implant options. Bone loss leads to loosening of the dentures over time and in turn creates poor fit of the dentures and collapse of the facial vertical dimension, among other problems.

Phonetic challenges

Many patients report that they experience phonetic challenges when wearing dentures. Up to 88% of patients who are fully edentulous complain of some difficulty with speech[3].

Decreased masticatory ability and stability

Compared with patients in implant-retained/supported prostheses, patients in dentures are significantly more challenged in their chewing. Removable appliances move and shift, creating a considerable struggle which many patients have difficulty adapting to. Although these appliances may feel somewhat stable to a clinician, function, motion, and sometimes speech can cause them to dislodge or become loose. This is why denture adhesive is a multi-billion-dollar industry.

Loss of muscle tone

In patients who are edentulous, the muscles of facial expression lose tone, and ptosis of the buccinator and mentalis muscle attachments occur[3].

Taste impairment and possible gagging

In a traditional denture, the palate is covered. Most patients wearing dentures report significant impairment in their ability to taste, and for those with an active gag reflex, adapting to a removable appliance may be difficult or impossible.

Emotionally disabling

Wearing a denture was considered somewhat socially acceptable for the Silent Generation (those born in the years 1925-1945), where-

Cont'd ▶

as the Baby Boomer generation and beyond seem to be much less satisfied with the idea of wearing traditional dentures. For many, there is a stigma attached to dentures that triggers embarrassment and shame. These individuals find dentures less socially acceptable and are less satisfied with a denture option.

Adaptability

Younger patients tend to adapt more quickly to wearing dentures than older patients. The high level of neuroplasticity that is required by denture wearers is less available as patients get older. Therefore, as people age, they are less likely to cope with wearing dentures.

Overdentures

Overdentures are relatively new compared to traditional dentures. Although they may look similar to traditional dentures when they are in place, overdentures can be retained or supported by dental implants and, in some cases, with natural teeth equipped with anchoring devices. A large variety of designs and types of overdentures are available. Many different types of dental implant designs have been used to support or retain overdentures. These vary from mini and small-diameter implants to traditional and even subperiosteal implants. Attachments for overdentures abound. Moreover, in addition to bars and other underlying supports, overdentures can be designed to fit directly on implants.

Overdenture designs that derive support and retention from dental implants, often using cast and/or milled bars attached to the implants, are referred to as *RP4* appliances, or implant-supported overdentures. Overdentures that use dental implants primarily for retention and rest on the soft tissues for support are referred to as *RP5* designs, or implant-assisted overdentures (Figs. 1.5-1.10).

Overdenture designs have changed and new designs and configurations have proliferated over the years. Consensus about what the standard of care should be is lacking. There is some agreement among clinicians that overdentures offer advantages over traditional removable dentures,

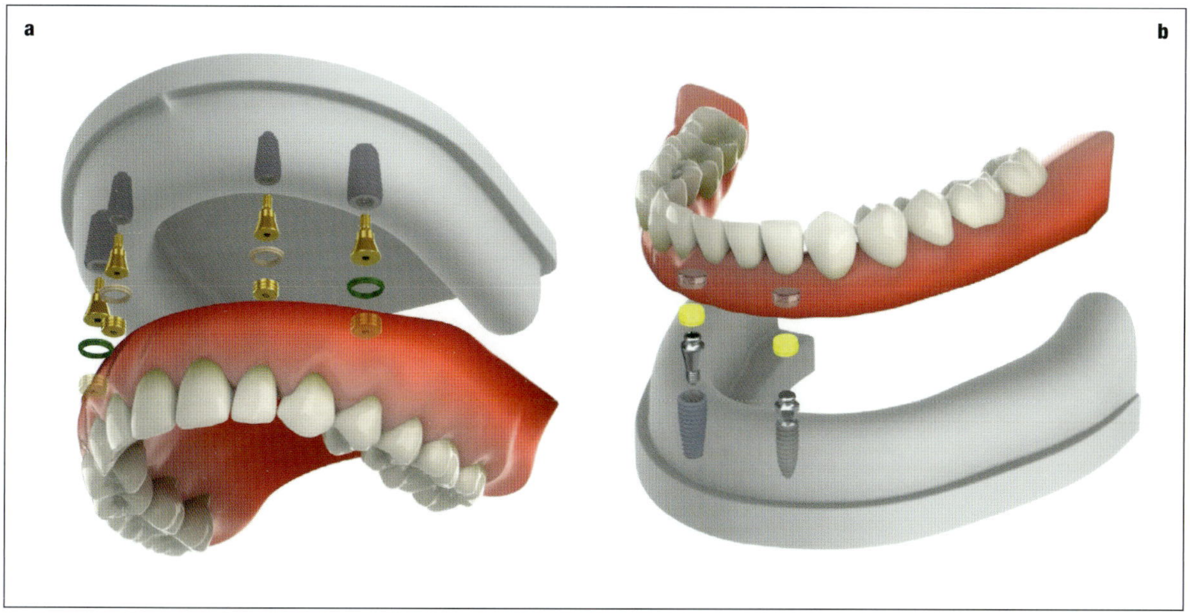

Figure 1.5 Illustrations of RP5 overdentures. (a) An RP5 design that uses four implants to retain a maxillary overdenture. (b) An RP5 design that uses two implants to retain a mandibular overdenture. Both examples use implants for retention and the soft tissues for support. *Source: Courtesy of MegaGen America.*

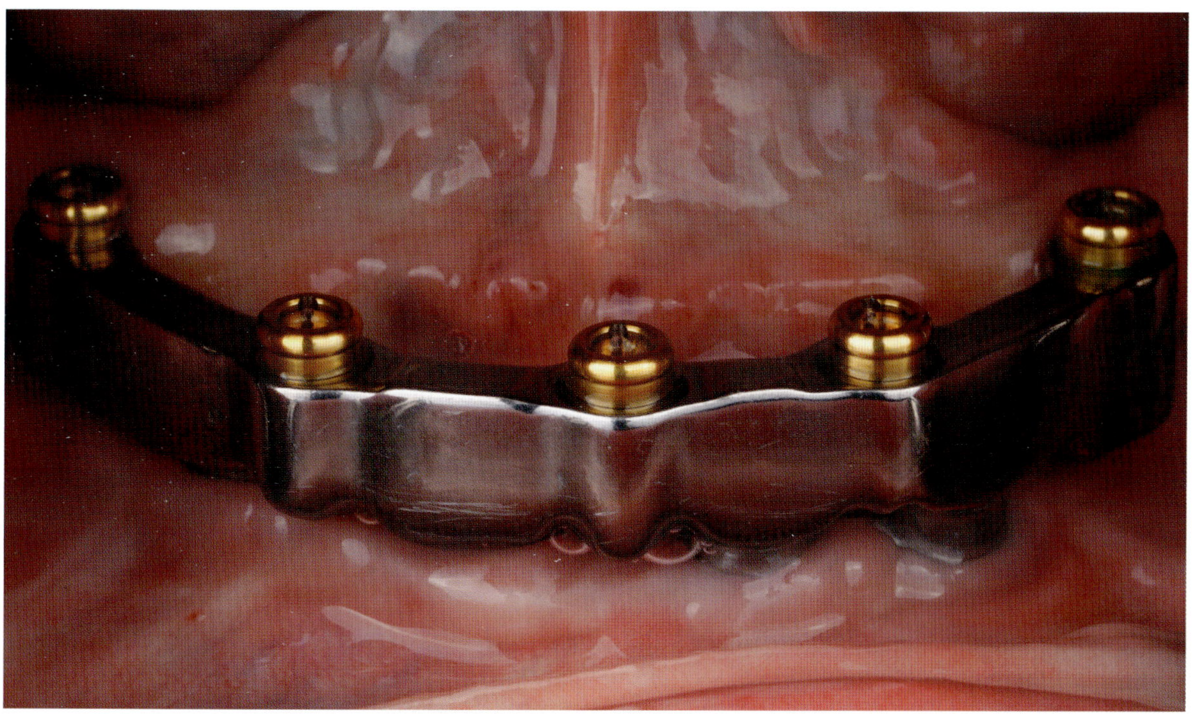

Figure 1.6 Example of a mandibular RP4 overdenture bar fabricated from milled titanium and five Zest Locator® abutments.

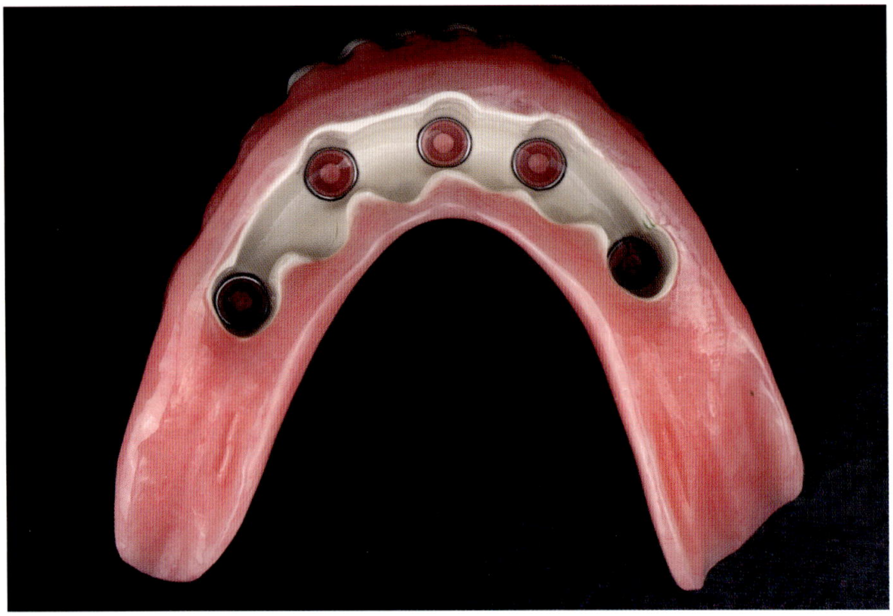

Figure 1.7 Printed overdenture (RP4 design) with polyether ether ketone (PEEK) thermoplastic polymer embedded into the intaglio surface holding Locator housings and nylon inserts.

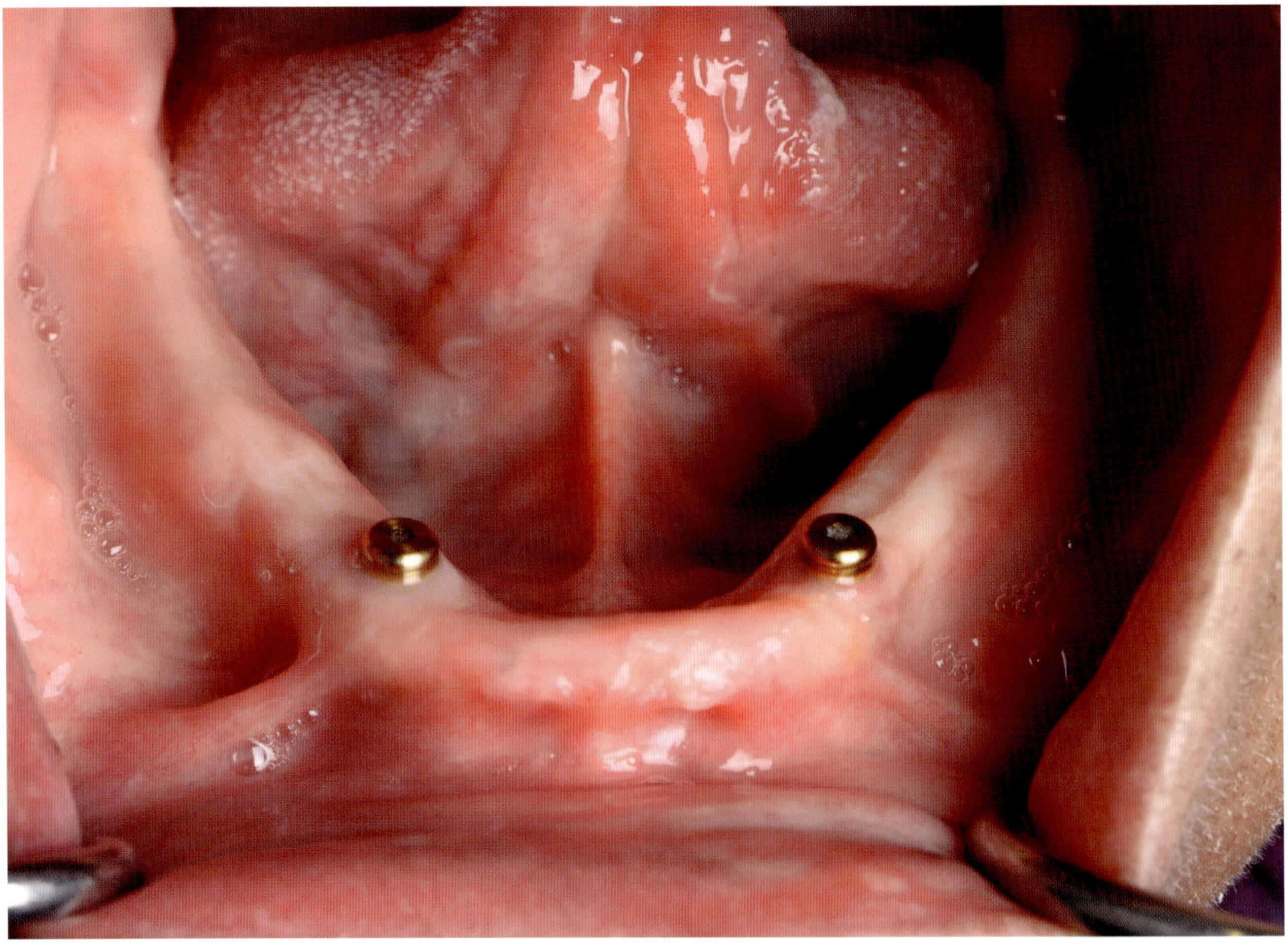

Figure 1.8 Implants placed in the mandibular arch with abutment fixtures designed to retain an overdenture. This is an RP5 design.

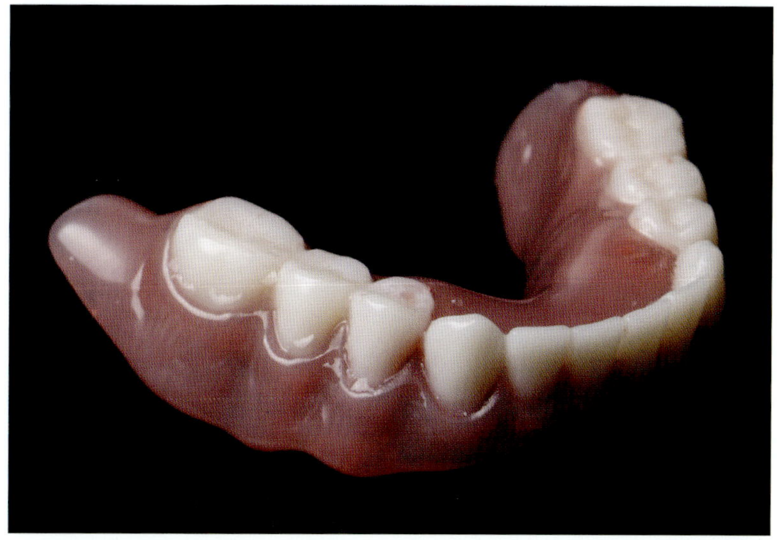

Figure 1.9 Printed mandibular overdenture.

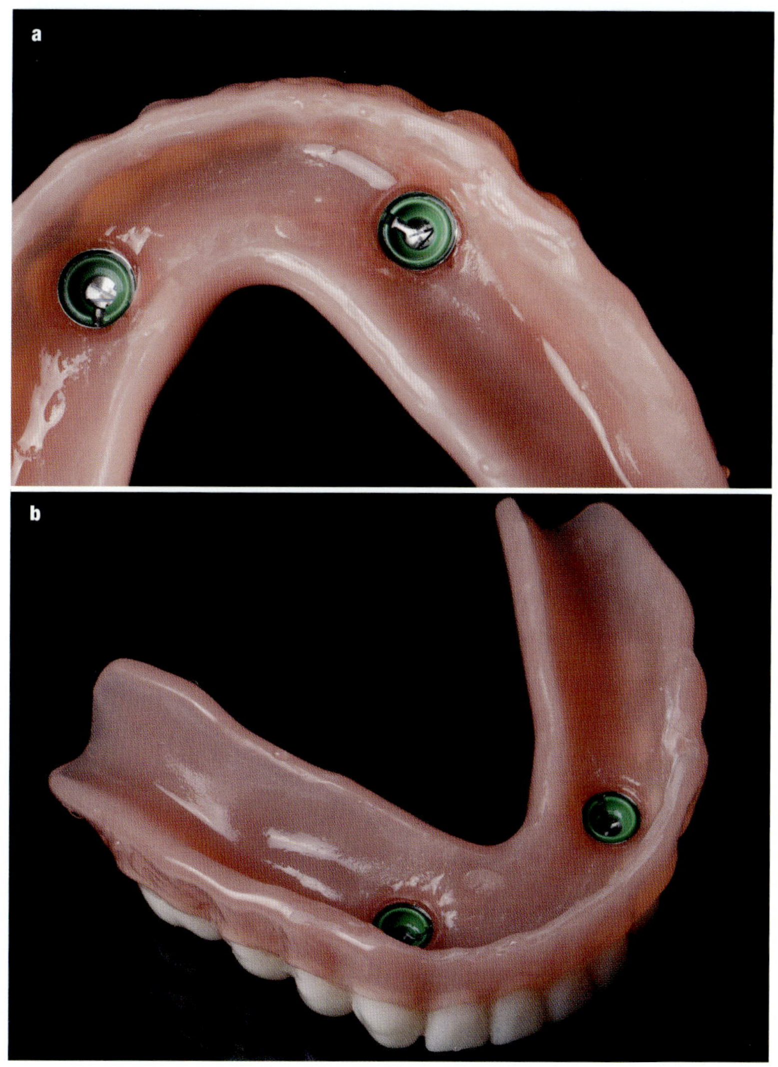

Figure 1.10 (a, b) Printed mandibular overdenture in an RP5 design. This is a Neodent Novaloc® (Straumann) case with titanium matrix housings and retention inserts.

especially when the appropriate number of implants and distance between implants is ideal. However, the failure rate of dental implants is higher in cases where the overdenture is retained or assisted by implants vs. supported by them[4,5].

For clarity and simplicity (and because of its current popularity in dentistry), the discussion of advantages and disadvantages below is based on a maxillary overdenture using four individual, nonsplinted, traditional dental implants with an abutment that has a retention design. This appliance, referred to as an *RP5*, can be described as an overdenture that takes advantage of dental implants as retention fixtures and for assistance, mostly supported by the edentulous ridges.

Advantages

Removability/ease, low maintenance, elimination of disease, esthetics

(See advantages of traditional dentures, above).

Prevention of bone loss

Implants spaced appropriately in the mandible and maxilla can prevent much of the typical bone loss associated with full edentulism. This ridge preservation, although often limited to the anterior regions, reduces patients' chances of losing excessive facial vertical dimension and provides better long-term support.

Improved phonetics and taste (compared with traditional dentures)

In a maxillary overdenture supported by four implants, the palate can often be exposed to some degree, which allows better phonetics for some patients. In addition, it gives patients the ability to taste food as they would with a natural dentition. Although the palate is not entirely open, simply having the center removed is very freeing for most if not all the patients for whom I have provided this service.

Stability

Patients are most aware of the stability of their overdenture during chewing/function and speaking. An edentulous patient will rave about how stable overdentures feel compared to traditional dentures. Overdentures do not require the use of denture adhesives, which is important to many of my patients.

Disadvantages

Removability

Like dentures, overdentures are removable, which is a feature that may be seen as a benefit to some. For the vast majority, especially younger patients or those who have never worn dentures, however, it can be disabling both physically and emotionally.

Not socially acceptable

Patients who are opposed to wearing dentures because of a social stigma of wearing a removable appliance are likely to feel the same about overdentures. As a general rule, overdentures are a significant upgrade for patients already wearing dentures but much harder to adapt to for those with a full or even partial dentition that is failing and may not offer the confidence they are yearning for.

Cost

While a maxillary overdenture tends to be more affordable than a full-arch fixed prosthetic implant option, it can cost considerably more than a traditional denture, especially when four or more traditional implants are used under a reinforced or high-quality prosthesis. Because this option often lands between the two in terms of cost, there are patients who choose to "settle" for this. I usually try to encourage patients to consider a fixed option first. However, if a fixed prosthesis does not fit in their budget and they are good candidates for an overdenture, then an overdenture might be the appropriate choice. Also, if there is enough prosthetic space and appropriate distance between the implants, the possibility of upgrading to a fixed prosthesis may be open to them in the future.

Increased maintenance (compared with traditional dentures)

Implant options will always require more work on the part of the patient. Not only will they need to take care of their implants at home, but I encourage patients with implants to attend a recall appointment no less than once every 6 months. There is some debate over what implant maintenance for fixed and removable implant options are, but very few clinicians would agree that an implant should be placed and then forgotten by the dentist or hygienist. Both the literature and anecdotal evidence show that dental implants are susceptible to peri-mucositis as well as peri-implantitis. Hygiene maintenance should be reviewed with patients before treatment. (See Chapter 10 for more on this topic.)

Replacement parts

Nothing lasts forever, including dental implant abutments and attachments. After several thousand cycles of denture seating and re-

Cont'd ▶

moval, the abutments and attachments wear out. The attachments, many of which are made of plastic or elastomeric material, tend to wear out first and are easily replaced at an insignificant cost. However, the abutments can also begin to wear and gradually provide less retention of the attachment regardless of how much resistance is applied. Like attachments, abutments are quite simple to replace, but the cost to the patient is more significant.

Retention but not support

Overdentures derive most of their stability from the support of the edentulous arch; implants are only designed to provide retention. It is important to make sure patients understand this, so they know even overdentures need to be relined over time. If an RP5 type of overdenture starts to depend on the implants for support, patients are at more risk of implant failure issues as well as lack of retention.

Fixed full-arch implant-supported prosthesis (Fig. 1.11)

A fixed prosthesis, whether an FP1, FP2, or FP3, is typically the option most clinicians would choose for themselves or a family member. So why would we not want this to be the first option we present to people seeking our help? Let us now consider the advantages and disadvantages of the fixed full-arch implant-supported prosthesis.

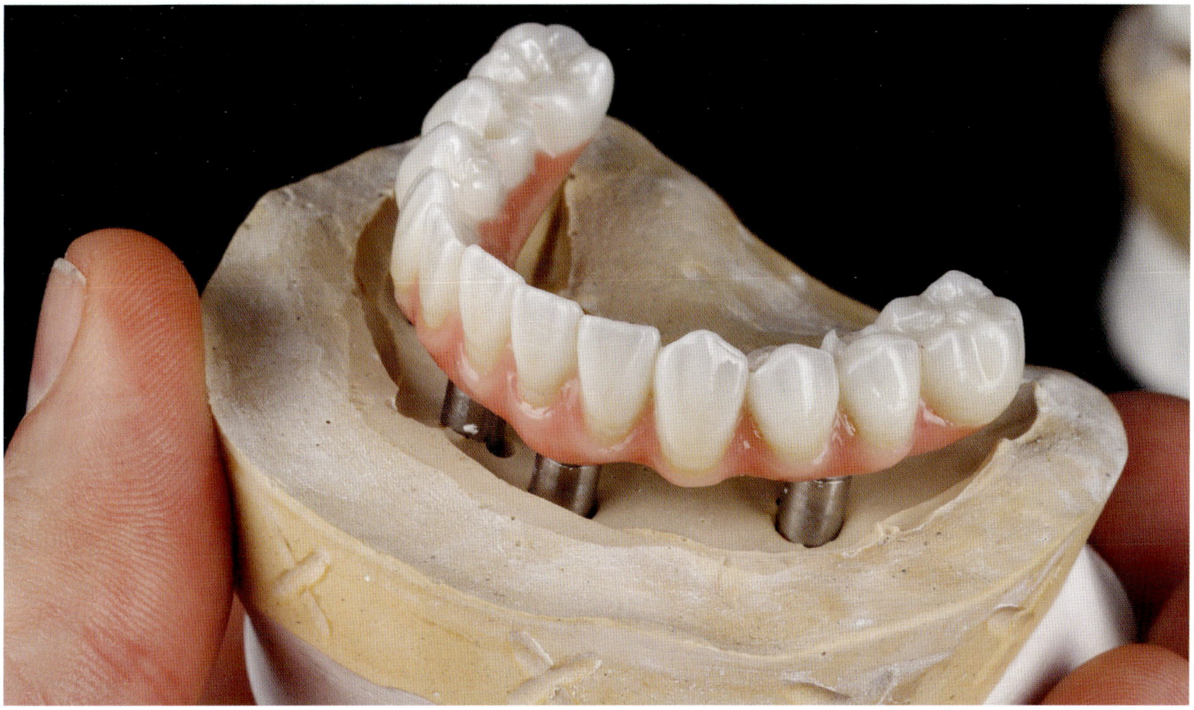

Figure 1.11 **A mandibular fixed full-arch implant-supported prosthesis on a master cast or model.**

Advantages

Elimination of disease

Like the previous two options, this option removes odontogenic and periodontal disease and can reduce occlusal and muscular dysfunction.

Prevention of bone loss

By placing enough implants throughout the arch in appropriate, equidistant locations, bone loss in the jaw can be almost entirely prevented in these areas.

Cross-arch stabilization and primary implant stability

Because of the engineering and design of this prosthesis, cross-arch stabilization and primary implant stability can be achieved, and the prosthesis can be immediately loaded.

Efficiency

Fixed full-arch implant-supported dentistry can be quite efficient. Dentists and patients alike are attracted to this process because it

Cont'd ▶

allows patients to avoid wearing a removable appliance. It also gives patients the ability to be in a fixed prosthesis immediately after surgery in most cases. Efficient workflows help patients avoid additional surgical visits and procedures as well.

Hygiene

Not having to remove dentures or overdentures from their mouth for cleaning is seen as a benefit by most patients. Maintaining these prostheses is straightforward, and most patients are not opposed to brushing and using water flossers around their prosthesis at home.

Unimpaired taste

This prosthetic device has even less palatal coverage than the overdenture and allows patients to experience the normal taste of food as they would with a natural dentition.

Masticatory function

Improved chewing and a more natural-feeling bite can be developed into these prostheses. Most patients report that they chew as well as, or nearly as well as they did with a full natural dentition.

Stability

A fixed prosthesis is far more stable than either dentures or overdentures. Because the prosthesis is supported by the implants and not the edentulous ridges, there is no movement within the system. By eliminating instability, patients acquire a new sense of confidence.

Improved phonetics

Phonetics can be a challenge with all types of dental prosthetics, but with careful planning and custom engineering, the fixed prostheses you create for your patients have a greater chance of allowing them to maintain acceptable speech and to speak without stumbling over their words.

Socially acceptable

In a world where removable teeth are considered a handicap and disabling, the fixed prosthesis is a solution rather than a problem. When made right, a fixed full-arch prosthesis is virtually undetectable by the average nonclinician, and very few patients ever find themselves in situations that make them feel embarrassed or uncomfortable. In fact, patients who have successfully gone through this process in my practice find themselves inspired with confidence, emotionally enabled, and possessed of an improved sense of well-being and self-esteem.

Esthetics

Early in its development, the fixed full-arch prosthesis design and materials were limiting factors in the esthetics of a case. More recently, due to the development of more lifelike materials and the option to digitally plan and design these cases, very few patients complain about their cosmetic transformation. As with any cosmetic dental procedure, esthetics can be less than satisfactory if done incorrectly. However, by following the proper process and paying attention to detail, it is possible to achieve amazing and lifelike, natural esthetics with a fixed full-arch implant restoration (as outlined in the principles of design in Chapter 5).

Reduced risk of damage/loss

Compared to a removable appliance, there is less risk of damage for most patients because the fixed full-arch prosthesis cannot be removed by the patient. And the fact that it is fixed obviously makes it impossible for the patient to lose or misplace it. Making the right material choice and providing protective recommendations to your patients can allow them years of useful benefit with these prostheses.

Disadvantages

Cost

Compared with other teeth replacement options, the cost of a fixed full-arch prosthesis is considerable. In our practice, patients typically spend between US$20,000–$30,000 (or more) per arch, and they will have different expectations of you and your practice when they pay anywhere near that much for treatment. Presenting this option to patients requires a different approach than other options. It is important to spend more time developing a trusting relationship and creating value. Patients who are investing in full-arch implant dentistry are often interested in financing options and/or long-term payment plans.

Along with the initial investment, it is important to consider what a fixed full-arch implant prosthesis will cost a patient over time—for hygiene maintenance visits, for example, or to replace prosthetic screws (and potentially other parts), and possibly to repair or replace their prosthesis at some point in the future. One must also remember the costs associated with potential replacement of one or more failed dental implants or tissue grafting and augmentation procedures that may be needed.

Cont'd ▶

Maintenance

Patients with fixed full-arch prostheses may have the misguided idea that this process is a "one and done," and that is not the case. Patients should be prepared for semi-annual hygiene visits as well as a home care regimen that is more demanding than soaking their dentures at night. Although this may not be considered a disadvantage by most patients, some will choose dentures or removable appliances over a fixed prosthesis because they are less complicated to maintain.

Bone reduction

Denture and overdenture options often require little or no alveolar ridge reduction after teeth are extracted. The prosthetic space requirements are less for most of the removable appliance designs than for a fixed FP3-type prosthesis. Some fixed full-arch implant cases may require a considerable amount of additional bone reduction to create adequate space for the prosthesis. The amount of bone reduction necessary should be thought through carefully to avoid dentally disabling a patient if implant failures were to occur.

FEATURES OF FIXED FULL-ARCH IMPLANT REHABILITATION

The following pages will help you to understand some of the specific attributes of fixed full-arch implant dentistry and why you might consider this option for a patient. The features discussed are more specific to the FP3, or what might be commonly referred to as All-on-X by some practitioners.

Characteristics of the ideal patient

Typically, the ideal patient for a fixed full-arch prosthesis has lost bone volume via natural resorption as a result of full or partial edentulism, particularly in the posterior areas. Patients who lose bone secondary to periodontal infection or disuse atrophy may begin to show signs of a collapsing occlusion, which can reduce the vertical dimension of the face. Patients with gross decay in much of their dentition in addition to periodontal disease, tooth mobility, or edentulism are also candidates for fixed full-arch implant dentistry. In Chapter 2, I discuss the term *terminal dentition*: understanding what this term means and how to classify it will help you determine whether a patient might be ideal for a fixed full-arch prosthesis.

Implants and engineering options

The classic or early All-on-4 fixed full-arch designs used four implants placed in the anterior maxilla and anterior mandible to provide support for prostheses. As time goes on, more implant configurations are being used and have become widely accepted in fixed full-arch implant dentistry.

Maxilla

To make things simpler to explain and understand, we can divide the maxilla into four zones (Fig. 1.12):

- **Zone 1** consists of the anterior maxilla from canine to canine (also referred to as the *premaxilla*).
- **Zone 2** is the area of the premolars.
- **Zone 3** is the molar area.
- **Zone 4** consists of the pterygoid and zygoma regions.

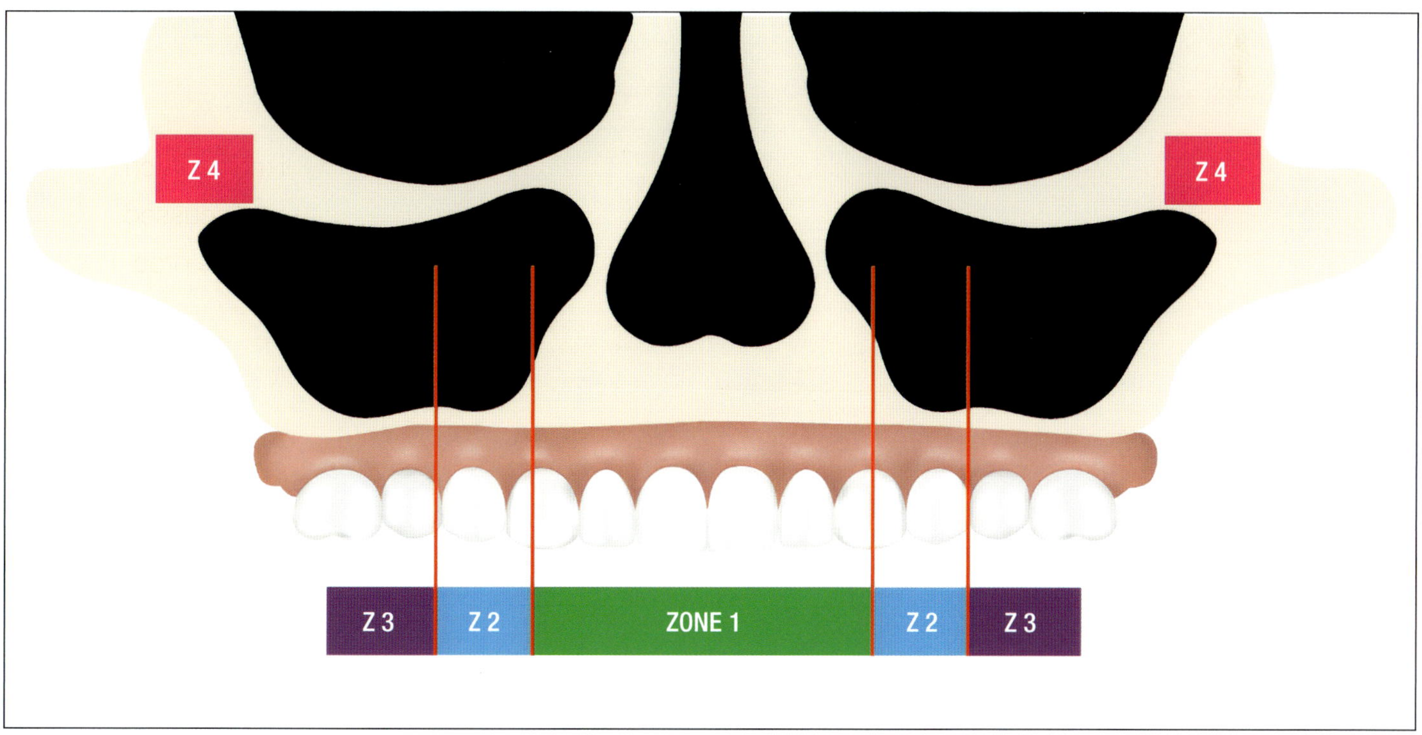

Figure 1.12 Four zones in the maxillary arch.

One of the most common implant engineering designs in fixed full-arch dentistry consists of four to six implants placed anterior to the maxillary sinuses in Zone 1 (Fig. 1.13). The most posterior or terminal implants flank the sinuses, taking advantage of dense bone along the anterior sinus wall, and they are usually tilted somewhere around 30 degrees. (In cases where there is adequate bone to provide the appropriate posterior support for a prosthesis, the terminal implants may or may not be tilted.) The other implants are spaced as equidistant as possible in the remaining area of the anterior maxilla. This design most closely follows the one developed by Dr. Paulo Maló in the 1990s.

The size and position of the maxillary sinuses, the width and height of the alveolar ridge, and the density of the maxillary bone are the primary considerations when it comes to implant choice in the maxilla. In patients with large, pneumatized sinuses, Zone 1 may not have enough bone available for the most common implant engineering, and a fixed full-arch prosthesis may not be possible in such patients without sinus elevation and/or extensive grafting. To address this lim-

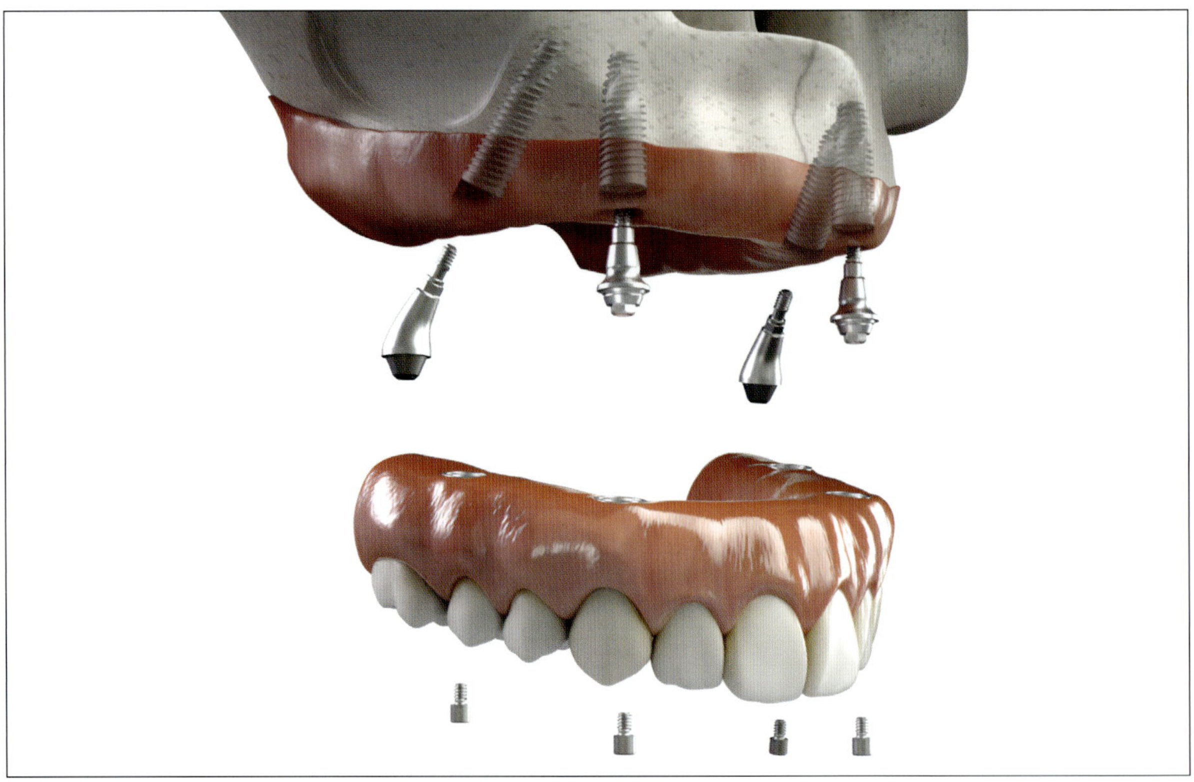

Figure 1.13 **A popular engineering design for a fixed dental implant prosthesis utilizing four dental implants in Zone 1 of the maxillary arch. The terminal implants are tilted 30 degrees and the anterior implants are straight.** ***Illustration used by permission of Straumann Group.***

itation, specially made zygomatic implants have been designed to utilize bone in the zygomatic arch and can be placed (*a*) unilaterally, (*b*) in a dual (×2) design, or (*c*) in a quad (×4) design. These implants get apical support from the zygomatic arch in Zone 4 and generally terminate in Zone 2, which allows for posterior support of a prosthesis and a more appropriate distance between the anterior and posterior implant connections (A-P spread). Implants designed to be stabilized within the zygomatic arch may be placed through the maxillary sinus as well as in an extramaxillary fashion (Fig. 1.14).

Another implant engineering option that is gaining popularity among clinicians involves the use of longer implants in the pterygoid region. This design is also appropriate for patients who do not have adequate bone in Zone 1, to avoid sinus elevation and grafting procedures. In some cases, this implant engineering concept will be used alongside zygomatic implants and in others as an alternative to them. Implants placed in the pterygoid region are good at supporting the posterior areas of the prosthesis and can help clinicians avoid cantilevers in their design. If there is a particular disadvantage to using implants in the pterygoid region, it is that they are placed so far posteriorly that restoring them with the prosthesis can be difficult. This is especially true in patients with limited jaw opening.

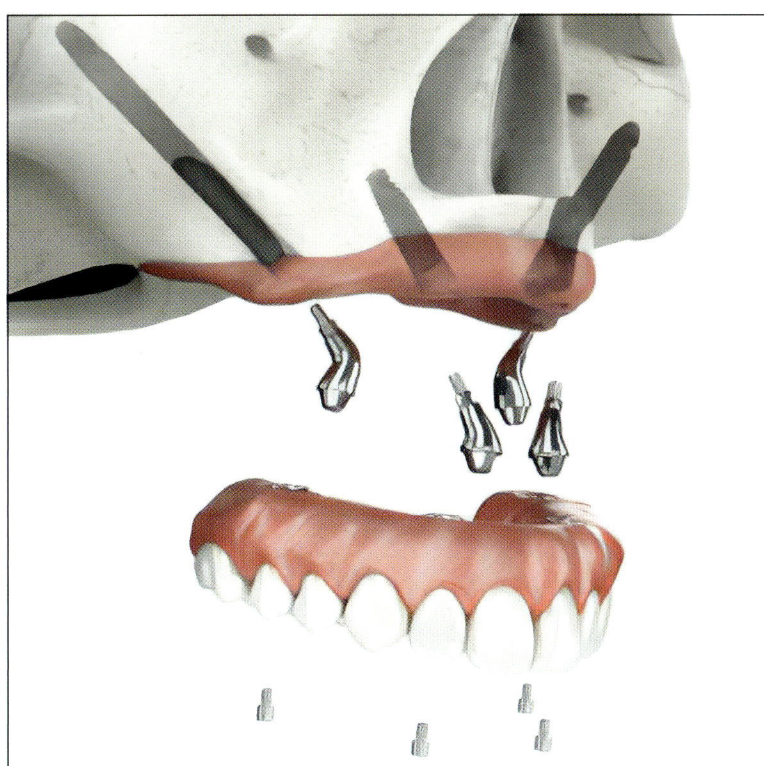

Figure 1.14 **A fixed full-arch prosthesis utilizing dental implants in the anterior maxillary zone 1 as well as in the zygomatic process. Note that the anterior implants are tilted to a similar degree as the terminal implants.** ***Illustration used by permission of Straumann Group.***

Each of these designs is considered acceptable in fixed full-arch implant dentistry. However, zygomatic and pterygoid implants require advanced surgical implant experience on the part of the clinician. Currently, they are not easy to place in conjunction with a stackable surgical guide system and are typically placed manually. Implants placed in the zygoma and pterygoid regions might be considered as alternatives to more traditional implant engineering when:

- Sinus elevation and other grafting procedures are not an option and anteroposterior (A-P) spread is inadequate for support of the fixed full-arch prosthesis.
- In an implant revision case where the dental implants and/or the prosthesis has failed. Implants in the pterygoid or zygomatic regions can be used to salvage a patient's chances of continuing to wear a fixed full-arch prosthesis.

Mandible

Fixed full-arch engineering in the mandible has not changed significantly since the inception of the All-on-4 concept was developed. Clinicians still tend to use the bone in the mandible anterior to the mental foramina for placing implants to support the prosthesis. The primary considerations for engineering implant placement to support prosthetics in the mandible are the location of the alveolar nerves and the height and width of the mandibular bone. It is not uncommon for several implants to be placed vertically in the most anterior region of the mandibular arch and then for the terminal implants to be longer and tilted distally to avoid the inferior alveolar nerves. Because the bone in the mandible is typically more dense, concerns about not having adequate initial stability for an immediate-load prosthesis are not as common as in the maxilla **(Fig. 1.15)**.

There is another implant arrangement I have seen used, which some clinicians seem to prefer. This option uses short implants in a parallel fashion, placed vertically, without terminal implants that are angled. Placing shorter nonangled implants is technically easier and eliminates the need to use corrective angled MUAs to achieve parallelism. However, more implants may be necessary to achieve an adequate A-P spread for biomechanical stability of the prosthesis[6]. Adequate bone height and width in the posterior regions of the mandible are also necessary for this design to be successful **(Fig. 1.16)**.

In the posterior mandible of patients who are dentate, the ridge can be considerably wider than in patients who have become edentulous over time. In these cases, clinicians have used implants posterior to the mental foramen with success. This technique could also be used in conjunction with the more traditional designs, particularly to reduce the amount of cantilever that would be present in the definitive prosthesis when implants in the anterior mandible will not provide as

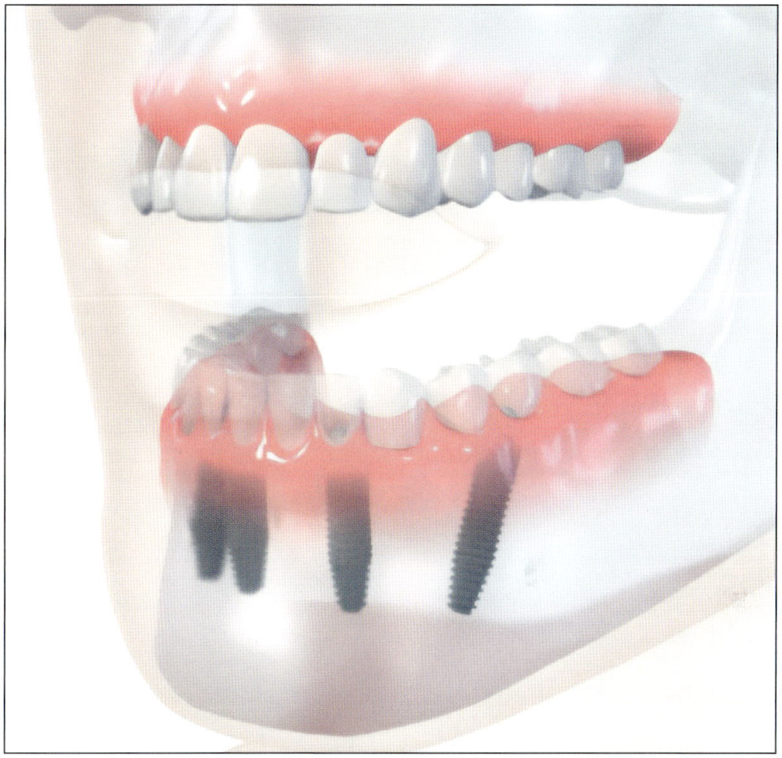

Figure 1.15 Mandibular fixed full-arch prosthesis utilizing tilted implants just anterior to the mental foramina. *Source: Courtesy of the Straumann Group.*

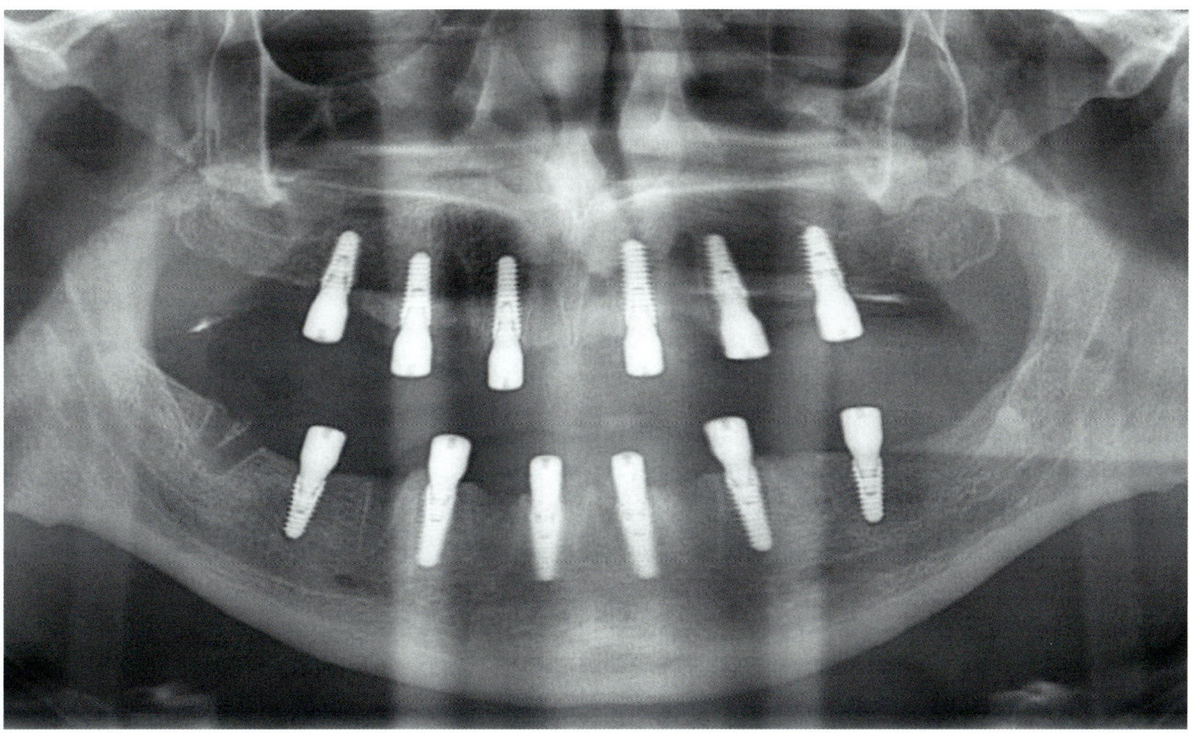

Figure 1.16 Orthopantomogram (OPG) of a full-arch implant design in the maxilla and mandible, where short, straight implants with straight MUAs were utilized in the posterior regions. *Source: Courtesy of MegaGen America.*

much A-P spread for support. Straight and shorter implants can also be used in the maxillary arch in Zones 2 and 3 if bone height and width permit.

When considering alternative placement of the implants within your planning, always keep in mind prosthetic and surgical success variables that will come into play. These may include the amount of bone reduction that will be necessary for adequate thickness of the prosthesis, anatomical landmarks, quality and quantity of bone available, loading forces, and implant locations. Design patterns for implant placement in the maxilla and mandible have been studied carefully over the last two decades. Traditional implant engineering has provided success for many patients, and there is wisdom in the phrase "if it ain't broke, don't fix it." However, there is also a place for deliberate holistic innovation, and I believe we will see more changes and nontraditional designs (and acceptance of them) as research and development continues.

Other implant design considerations

Implant sizes in both maxillary and mandibular fixed full-arch cases can vary in diameter based on the width of the bone present. It is acceptable to use the largest-diameter implants that will fit in the space, as long as respect is paid to the amount of bone present on the buccal or facial aspect. Most dentists I speak to are using 3.5- to 5.0-mm-diameter implants and larger 6- to 7-mm-diameter implants in the posterior maxilla and mandible when the bone permits (Fig. 1.17). Stress created by loading forces may vary based on the diameter of the implant. The use of smaller-diameter implants can create higher stress on the cortical bone, implants, and framework of a prosthesis, whereas the use of larger-diameter implants creates higher stress in the trabecular bone, abutments, and crowns of the prosthesis[7]. For the most predictable outcomes, 2 mm of buccal and lingual bone should be present after placement of the implants, and 3 mm of space should be present between the implants. Implants should have enough space not to be touching at their apices.

The length of implants used in traditionally engineered cases also varies. Clinicians may use implants as short as 8-10 mm in length in the anterior maxilla and mandible. Terminal tilted implants with a length of up to 16 mm are commonly found in the maxilla and mandible. Clinicians place implants frequently along the anterior maxillary sinus wall in Zone 1 and anchor more anterior implants into the anterior nasal sinus floor. In the mandible, they may reach into the inferior cortex for initial and apical stabilization.

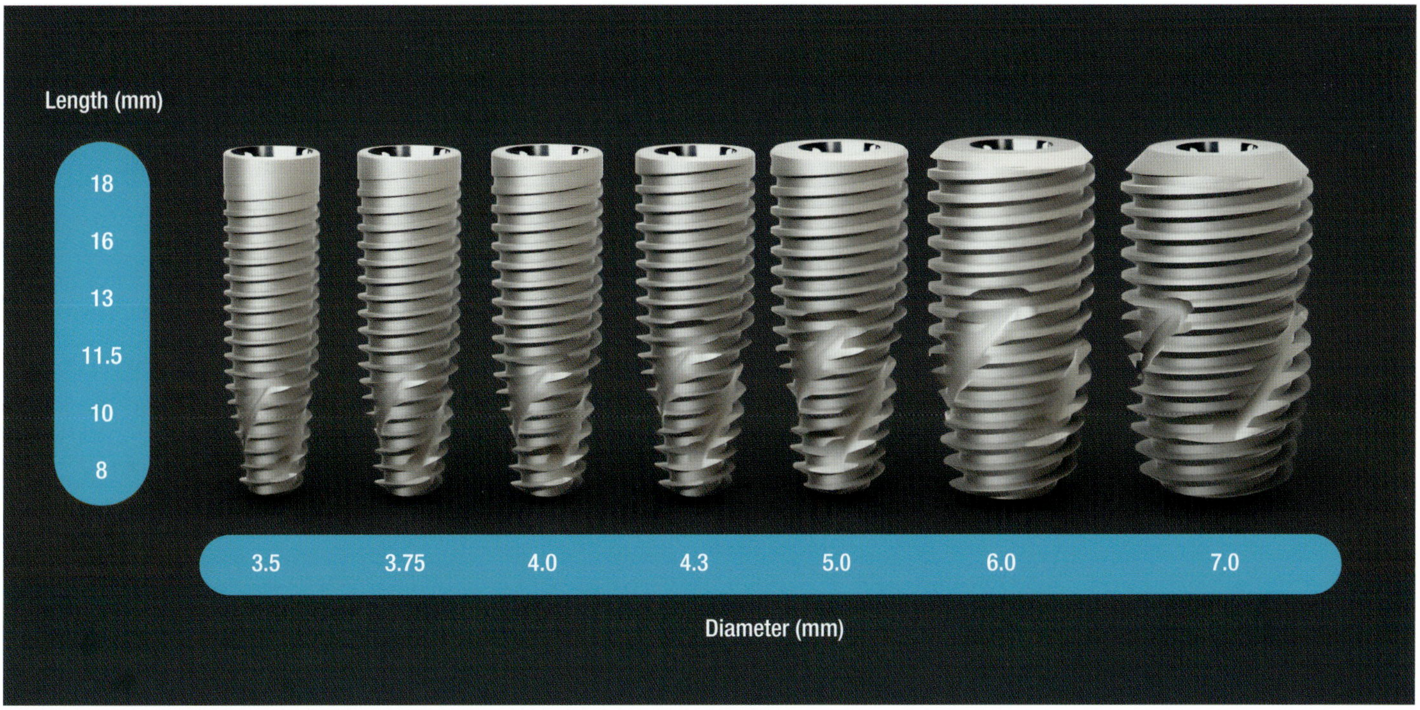

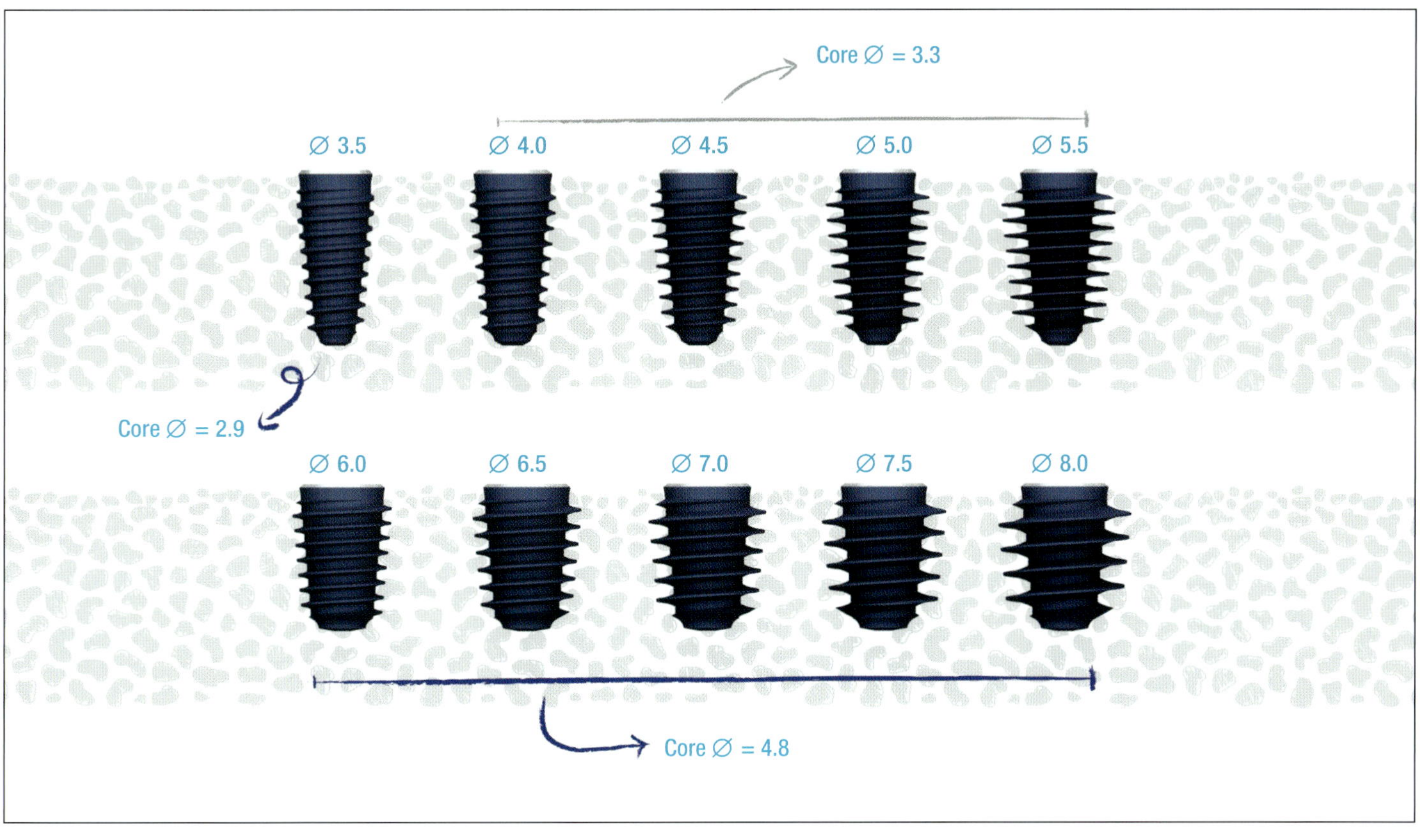

Figure 1.17 Various diameters of implants that can be utilized in fixed full-arch cases. *Source: Courtesy of the Straumann Group and MegaGen America.*

Prosthetic design

At this time the prosthesis most commonly used in fixed full-arch implant dentistry is a single unit one piece design and is referred to by many as "All-on-X". We usually refer to prosthetics that replace partial areas of the arch using more traditional terminology, such as *bridges* or *partials*, although some components of the fixed full-arch process, such as MUAs, can also be used in partial reconstruction circumstances. Fixed full-arch prostheses replace the missing teeth and (in FP3 designs) the gingiva as well as a portion of the edentulous ridge (Fig. 1.18). They are often fabricated from zirconia, printed or milled polymethyl methacrylate (PMMA), or acrylic resins and may be supported by frameworks made of metal, PEEK, or some other reinforcement material. The teeth on the prosthesis typically extend from first molar to contralateral first molar including 10 to 12 teeth. A fixed full-arch prosthesis will often have posterior cantilevers if dental implants cannot feasibly be placed in the most posterior areas of the maxilla and/or mandible.

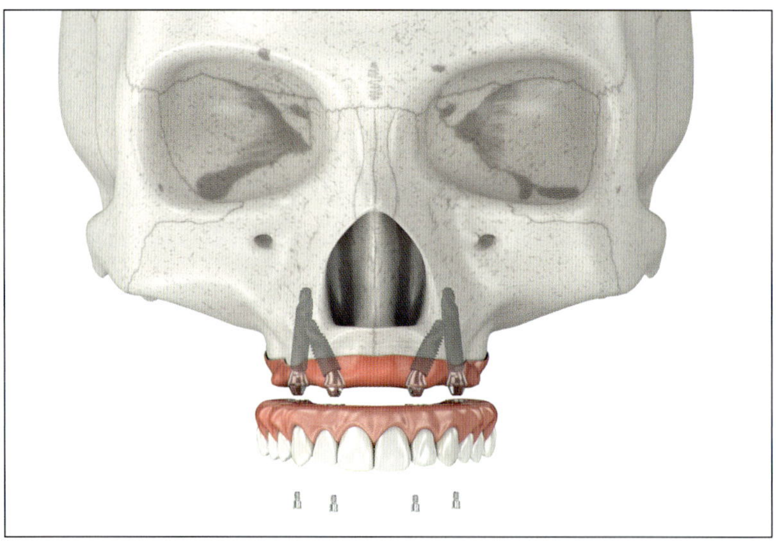

Figure 1.18 A typical maxillary FP3 type of fixed full-arch prosthesis. *Source: Courtesy of the Straumann Group.*

Multiunit abutments (MUAs)

Today, fixed full-arch dental implant cases are typically built on MUAs. These specialized abutments allow the prosthesis to fit passively on the implants by correcting the path of insertion and the screw-access channels to be optimally positioned in the definitive prosthesis. MUAs are also advantageous in leveling out the platform for the prosthesis and allowing for a predictable connection of the prosthesis to the implant at the appropriate height in the gingiva (Fig. 1.19).

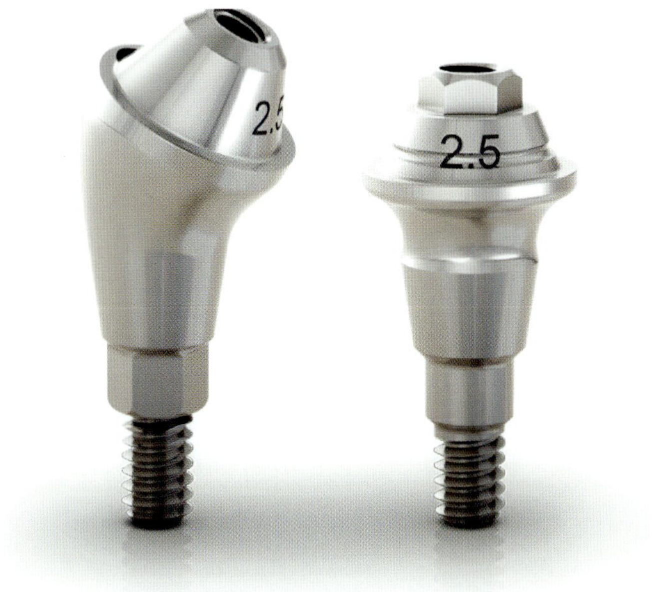

Figure 1.19 **Angled (left) and straight (right) multiunit abutments (MUAs).** ***Source: Courtesy of the Straumann Group.***

MUAs look similar across implant brands but may have varying platform sizing and screw diameters. It is imperative to know which implant brand was used as well as the internal diameter of the implant on some systems. This information is necessary when restoring inherited cases where changes should be considered.

MUAs are available in varying heights and degrees of angulation. Typically, angulations range from 0 to 45 degrees, but manufacturers are developing MUAs with even greater angulation for more clinical flexibility. The heights of the MUAs can vary as well but generally range from 1 to 5 mm. In most cases we aim for placing the implant connection with the MUA at or just below the bone, and the collar of the MUA at or just below the gingiva.

Immediate placement and loading

A fixed full-arch implant prosthesis can generally be immediately loaded on the day of surgery. There are some dentists who will place implants and keep their patients in dentures for 3 to 4 months before loading and placing an interim prosthesis. I have found most patients are looking for a solution that allows them to avoid wearing removable appliances. Placing and loading a full-arch interim prosthesis on the day of surgery is widely accepted and even encouraged by most practicing clinicians. There are, however, some exceptions. I base my decision to load an interim prosthesis at the time of surgery on the current literature, the teachings of well-respected, experienced clinicians and my own personal experience. We know that loading a fixed prosthesis with cross-arch stabilization immediately after surgery, when ideal conditions exist, does not significantly decrease the survival rate of implants, and possibly even decreases marginal bone loss[8-12].

There are several factors that might be considered when deciding whether to load a fixed full-arch prosthesis immediately after surgery: the total torque value of the implants, implant stability quotient (ISQ), a patient's compliance, the presence of extreme bruxism and/or parafunctional habits, and others. However, being able to help patients avoid wearing dentures after surgery is almost always preferred in my practice.

Another reason for seating and loading an interim prosthesis on the day of surgery—besides avoiding the need for the patient to wear a denture or dentures—is avoiding the necessity of a second surgical visit to uncover dental implants. In fixed full-arch implant rehabilitation, I have found that efficiency is a critical component. Having to manage a second surgical visit adds time to the case and appointments for the clinician and patient. This potential loss of efficiency should be taken into consideration during the initial planning phase of any case.

SHOULD YOU CONSIDER ADDING FIXED FULL-ARCH DENTISTRY INTO YOUR PRACTICE?

Fixed full-arch implant dentistry has gained wide acceptance and popularity in the dental community and with patients in recent years. Oral surgeons, prosthodontists, periodontists, as well as general dentists have become more interested in this technique and are embracing it. Dentists are flocking to courses that teach fixed full-arch implant techniques because they see the need for their patients to have alternative options to removable appliances. General dentists are gaining confidence and are more willing to take on these cases themselves without referring to specialists. But is it something you should add to your repertoire? Consider some of the following points.

Profitability

One powerfully attractive feature of fixed full-arch implant dentistry is the high case dollar value associated with this procedure. At first glance it may appear to many dentists that these cases are incredibly profitable, but this can be deceiving. To be profitable, the procedure must be done efficiently and without mistakes: one wrong move in a fixed full-arch implant rehabilitation case can create negative to catastrophic loss to a patient, all considerations of profitability aside.

Determining the profitability of this in your office is important before committing to making it a big part of your practice. Variable expenses such as dental implants and parts, anesthesia and medications, laboratory fees, planning and guide costs, biologics, and other details should be taken into consideration. Technology and equipment expenses are important too. For those starting without the required equipment to provide fixed full-arch implant dentistry, there is a sizable investment to be made.

Time is money, as the saying goes. Contemplate how much your time is worth and figure that into the equation as well. Then you will have to determine what the fee in your practice should be. The number of appointments and the amount of doctor time per appointment are two factors that significantly impact the profitability of these cases.

Another important factor in the equation is knowing what your marketplace will tolerate as an acceptable cost for this procedure, which can vary nationally and internationally by thousands of dollars. For an investment of this magnitude, many patients will investigate what other doctors and practices are charging. While it is not the most important thing for you to consider, keep in mind that patients are cost conscious and will often compare your fees to those of other providers.

Simplicity

Just because someone tells you something is easy, that does not make it simple. Unfortunately, the dental industry is filled with weekend courses promising to make you an overnight expert and assuring you that full-arch dentistry is not complicated. Becoming proficient at anything, including fixed full-arch implant rehabilitation, takes knowledge as well as practice. Make no mistake, this is a complex procedure, but with the appropriate training, education, and time put in, you can master it.

Though it may appear daunting, you can choose to follow an established, systematic method and set of guidelines that can be duplicated time and again. The sequential method and workflow I employ are presented in this book. By utilizing technology and guided surgery, getting textbook results is much simpler than it has been in the past. I often use the analogy that performing fixed full-arch dentistry, with a prosthetically driven approach and stackable surgical guide system, is like coloring by numbers. Nevertheless, there is no single book or course that can make you an expert over a weekend.

Efficiency

In the method I use for fixed full-arch implant dentistry cases, much of the work can be delegated. This frees up a practitioner's time to do other things. As noted above, time is money, and efficiency and time go hand in hand. A dentist's assisting team can be trained to perform many of the tasks necessary to complete the case. Dental auxiliaries can be responsible for much of the data collection, surgical setup, and prosthetic process as well as managing patient expectations and lab communications. I believe case planning and engineering should always be reviewed and approved by the restoring dentist as well as the surgeon (who may be one and the same). In addition, working with a digital treatment planner can really save time. The duties they can perform include the new smile simulation and segmentation of the CBCT. Digital treatment planners can also merge digital impressions, digital proposal, and photographs in planning software, as well as preliminary planning of dental implant placement. Partnering with a trained technician working in a laboratory or implant-planning service allows a dentist to cut a significant amount of time from the process. That said, some of the emerging technology in software that is becoming available is very interesting and could save digital treatment planners and dentists an enormous amount of time. One such software solution I have had the opportunity to test in my practice is Diagnocat™. This software can provide radiology reports, segmentation of CBCT, integration of multiple data sources, cloud storage and viewing, as well as a collaborative tool for multiple clinicians and technicians. Diagnocat uses artificial intelligence (AI) to streamline processes and make things more efficient.

In the last several years, 3D printing and milling machines have become widely available for use in the dental office. Some dentists are under the impression that if they print or mill their own guides and prosthetics, they may save money. I would argue that one must consider the expense of the equipment as well as the time needed to use it and evaluate whether it produces a more- or a less-efficient workflow. As dentists, we are more profitable doing dentistry than just about anything else. Delegate procedures and processes that create unnecessary work for you. Unless you have a well-trained laboratory assistant and/or you are doing a large volume of cases, you may consider outsourcing some of these tasks.

Avoiding extensive grafting and augmentation

Clinicians who follow the principles of the All-on-4 concept and choose their cases discriminatingly often can avoid additional bone grafting and augmentation procedures such as sinus elevation, lateral ridge splitting, vertical ridge augmentation, and so forth. While I do advocate socket preservation and the use of platelet-rich fibrin (PRF) and other biologics when appropriate, more expensive and advanced augmentation procedures are not always necessary for many cases. If you can do this, you will minimize the time and financial burden for yourself and your patient.

Good biomechanics

The term *biomechanics* is generally used in implant dentistry to define how dental implants and prosthesis relate to different forces and stresses. Fixed full-arch implant prostheses can perform very well over time with major biomechanical advantages over alternative therapies, such as dentures and implant-retained overdentures. For this reason, more patients and doctors are drawn toward fixed full-arch dentistry as a viable and even preferred treatment.

Hygiene and maintenance

There has historically been a bit of controversy or at least a lack of agreement and consistency on the topic of how hygiene and maintenance should be handled in fixed full-arch implant dentistry. This can be straightforward and acceptable to both clinician and patients, especially when expectations are laid out clearly prior to surgery.

In my practice, we provide patients with a hygiene and maintenance contract that clearly spells out our recommendations so patients understand what is expected of them and what they can expect from our practice. Most patients are happy to visit our office at least two times a year to have their prosthesis and implants examined and cared for. Some of our patients have exquisite home care and can keep their prostheses clean and the tissue surrounding the implants healthy. Other patients need a little more help. In Chapter 10, I review the specifics of hygiene and maintenance for the fixed full-arch dental implant patient.

Predictable clinical outcomes with high success rates

For almost 20 years, fixed full-arch implant dentistry using All-on-4 type concepts has been completed successfully for hundreds of thousands of individuals with predictable long-term outcomes. Nevertheless, there have been challenges over time, such as:

- Lack of an established, systematic method for doing the surgical procedure
- Lack of consistent and accurate communication between multiple providers and laboratories
- Small numbers of skilled and qualified clinicians and training programs
- A dearth of scientific evidence-based studies, clinical research as well as follow-up with patients in the early stages of its development
- Inadequate analog prosthetic workflows and the use of acrylic denture materials for prosthetics that were less durable than those available today
- The frequent absence of following a prosthetically driven protocol by the dental surgeon.

Recently, however, clinicians and others involved in the development of this treatment modality have been instrumental in advancing the process. Online and in-person training programs have been established throughout the world. Laboratories and manufacturers have developed better materials and methods. Research has been conducted and books have been written to support fixed full-arch implant dentistry. Industry leaders have taken steps to steer what was once a strictly analog procedure into the digital realm using hardware and software solutions.

As dental technology has evolved, this procedure has become easier to provide to patients and has facilitated better results. Following a systematic approach is more reliable with fewer errors and less stress, and it is more rewarding for both patients and clinicians. Technology has brought us into the mindset of a prosthetically driven process. By planning cases with the end in mind, starting with smile simulations and planning software, a dentist can provide more predictable results.

It is and will continue to be important for clinicians, dental laboratories, digital treatment planners, dental companies, and others to work together to get even better and more predictable outcomes for patients. Collaboration within our industry is necessary to provide improved solutions in fixed full-arch dentistry. This will in turn allow us to provide more patients with consistent quality and excellent results.

References

1. Brånemark PI. Foreword. In: Bedrossian E. Implant Treatment Planning for the Edentulous Patient: A Graftless Approach to Immediate Loading. St. Louis, MO: Mosby, 2011: vii.
2. Misch CE. Contemporary Implant Dentistry. 3rd edition. St. Louis, MO: Mosby; 2007.
3. Pikos MA, Miron RJ. Bone Augmentation in Implant Dentistry: A Step-by-Step Guide to Predictable Alveolar Ridge and Sinus Grafting. Chicago: Quintessence, 2019.
4. Pan YH, Chen K-W, Lin T-M, Chang Y-M. Investigation of the implant-supported overdentures in completely edentulous mandibles. J Dent Sci 2015;10:444-449.
5. Seo YH, Bae EB, Kim JW, et al. Clinical evaluation of mandibular implant overdentures via Locator implant attachment and Locator bar attachment. J Adv Prosthodont 2016;8:313-320.
6. Jain N, Gulati M, Garg M, Pathak C. Short implants: New horizon in implant dentistry. J Clin Diagn Res 2016;10:ZE14-ZE17.
7. Sezer T, Kilic K, Esim E. Effect of implant diameter and bruxism on biomechanical performance in maxillary All-on-4 treatment: A 3D finite element analysis. Int J Oral Maxillofac Implants 2022;37:709-721.
8. Velasco-Ortega E, Cracel-Lopes JL, Matos-Garrido N, et al. Immediate functional loading with full-arch fixed implant-retained rehabilitation in periodontal patients: Clinical study. Int J Environ Res Public Health 2022;19(20):13162.
9. Drago C. Frequency and type of prosthetic complications associated with interim, immediately loaded full-arch prostheses: A 2-year retrospective chart review. J Prosthodont 2016;25(6):433-439.
10. Agliardi EL, Pozzi A, Stappert CF, Benzi R, Romeo D, Gherlone E. Immediate fixed rehabilitation of the edentulous maxilla: A prospective clinical and radiological study after 3 years of loading. Clin Implant Dent Relat Res 2014;16(2):292-302.
11. Weinstein R, Agliardi E, Fabbro MD, Romeo D, Francetti L. Immediate rehabilitation of the extremely atrophic mandible with fixed full-prosthesis supported by four implants. Clin Implant Dent Relat Res 2012;14(3):434-441.
12. Agliardi E, Clericò M, Ciancio P, Massironi D. Immediate loading of full-arch fixed prostheses supported by axial and tilted implants for the treatment of edentulous atrophic mandibles. Quintessence Int 2010;41(4):285-293.

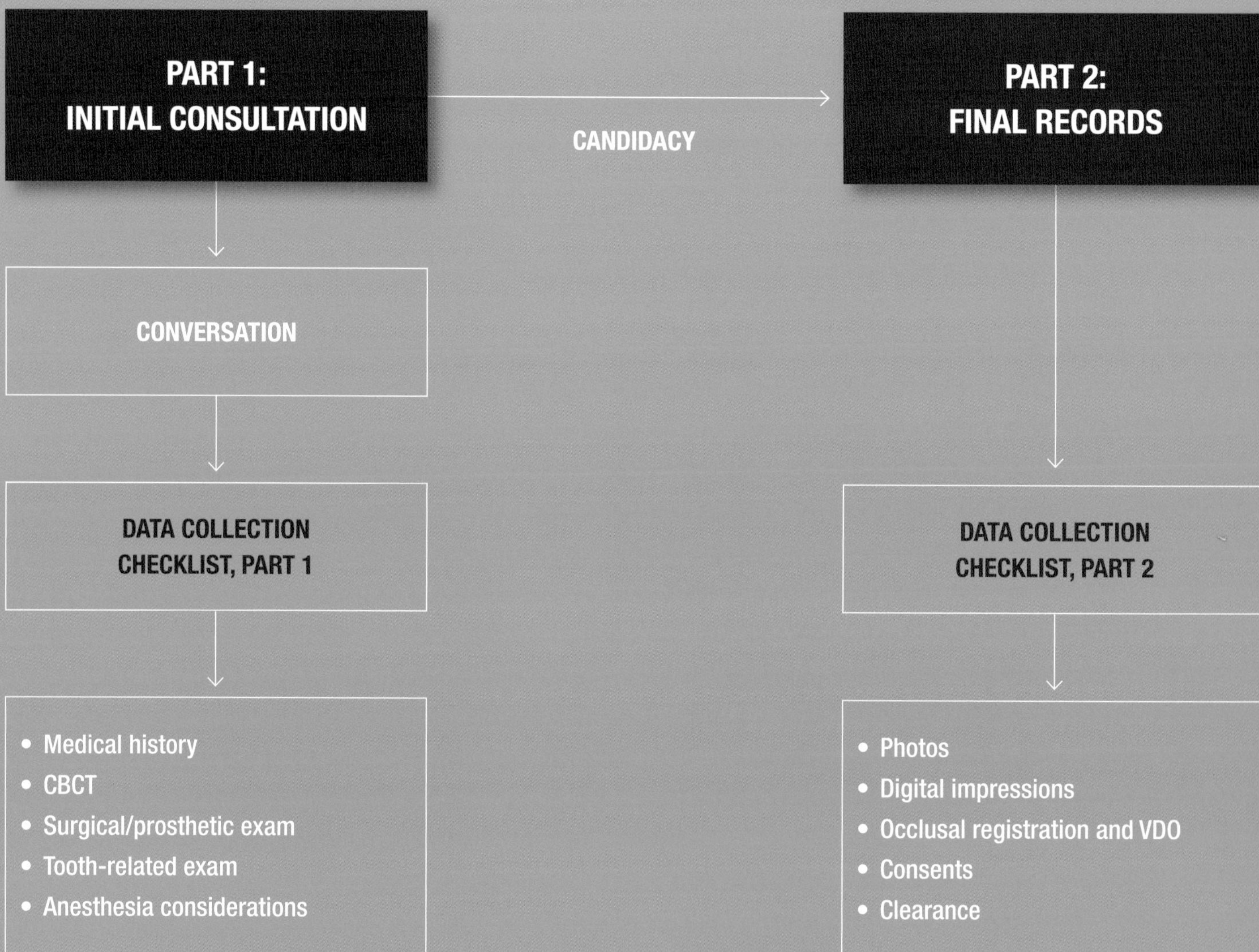
PART 1:
INITIAL CONSULTATION
CANDIDACY
PART 2:
FINAL RECORDS
CONVERSATION
DATA COLLECTION CHECKLIST, PART 1
DATA COLLECTION CHECKLIST, PART 2
• Medical history
• CBCT
• Surgical/prosthetic exam
• Tooth-related exam
• Anesthesia considerations
• Photos
• Digital impressions
• Occlusal registration and VDO
• Consents
• Clearance

PATIENT SELECTION AND DATA COLLECTION

SECTION II

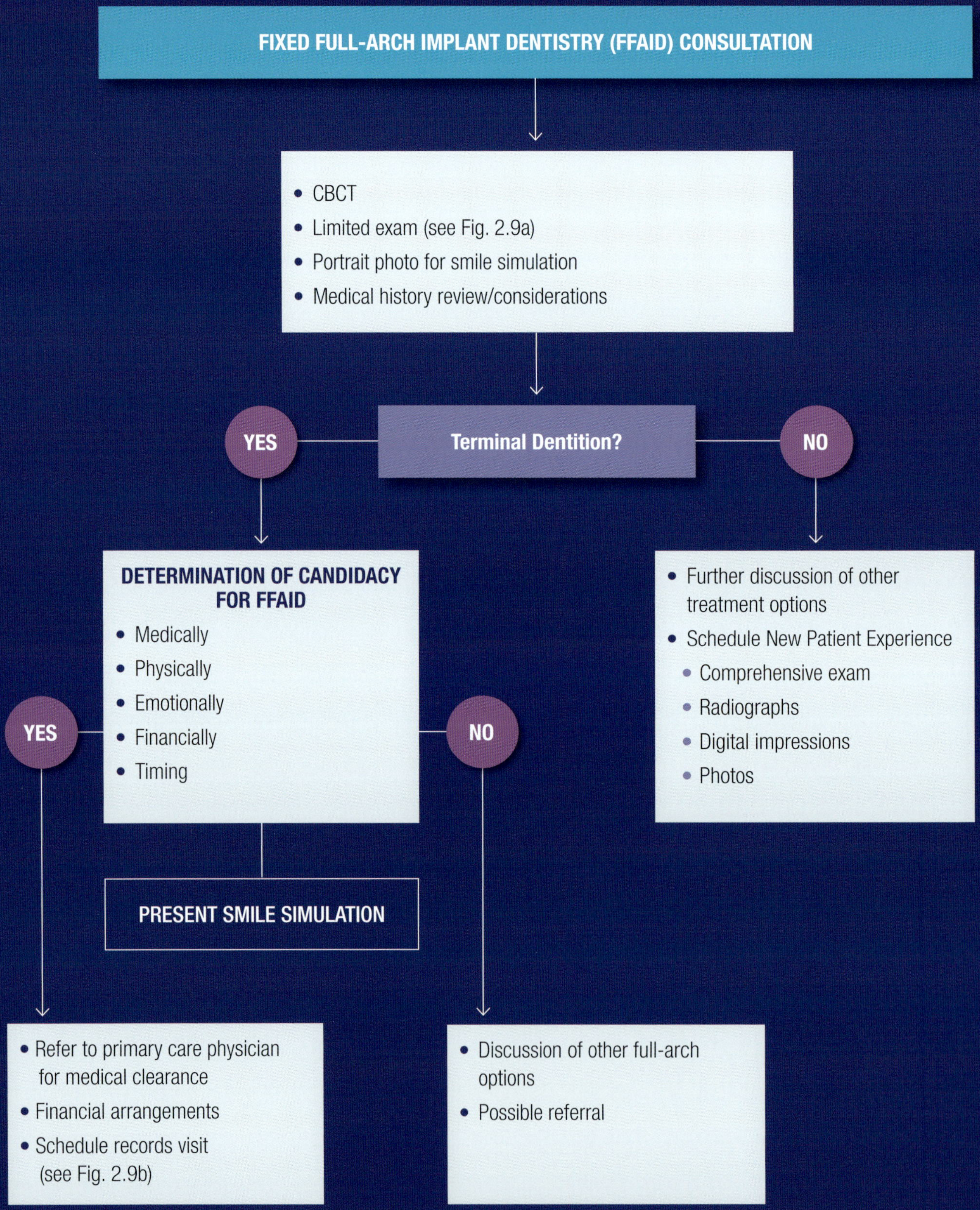

FIXED FULL-ARCH IMPLANT DENTISTRY (FFAID) CONSULTATION
• CBCT
• Limited exam (see Fig. 2.9a)
• Portrait photo for smile simulation
• Medical history review/considerations
YES
Terminal Dentition?
NO
DETERMINATION OF CANDIDACY FOR FFAID
• Medically
• Physically
• Emotionally
• Financially
• Timing
• Further discussion of other treatment options
• Schedule New Patient Experience
• Comprehensive exam
• Radiographs
• Digital impressions
• Photos
YES
NO
PRESENT SMILE SIMULATION
• Refer to primary care physician for medical clearance
• Financial arrangements
• Schedule records visit (see Fig. 2.9b)
• Discussion of other full-arch options
• Possible referral

DATA COLLECTION, PART 1. THE CONSULTATION

CHAPTER **2**

Commitment: Be Humble.

Humility is often easy to forget when you begin to achieve success.
To practice servant leadership, however, you must be humble.
Pride goes before destruction and arrogance before a fall.

A plethora of new digital technology has recently become available to assist dental implant clinicians in the process of fixed full-arch implant dentistry: digital facebows, photogrammetry, facial scanners, 3D printers, milling units, planning software, and even guided robotic surgery. When beginning a journey into fixed full-arch implant dentistry, it is important to think about how much one must “pay to play.” Before investing in unnecessary and expensive equipment, clinicians who are new to fixed full-arch should consider the following. There are only three pieces of technology that are necessary to complete the guided surgery and simplified prosthetic process outlined in this book: a CBCT machine, a camera, and an intraoral scanner. Throughout this text, I identify other optional technology accessories that I highly recommend, but they are not specific to the method I use (although they can be beneficial in other procedures and parts of a dental practice). The devices I review are practical to use, widely accepted, and readily available. As we look to the future, I am certain that new developments in this space will become more cost effective, easier to implement, and make fixed full-arch implant dentistry workflows more efficient and favorable for patients.

Collection of patient data is the first phase of the method I perform and teach. There are several parts to this stage. The first thing is to quickly determine whether a patient is a candidate based on a review of systems, their medical and dental history, and their mental readiness. Then I continue by having a relationship-building conversation and discussing the patient's overall expectations. If we check all the boxes there, I will perform a cursory examination and prescribe a CBCT. Once I have reviewed the CBCT and my clinical findings, I can usually determine whether the patient is a potential candidate for fixed full-arch implant dentistry. This process can take as little as 20 minutes or as long as 1 hour, depending on how much time is spent in discussion with the patient.

THE INITIAL APPOINTMENT

Patient candidacy and readiness evaluation

Having an initial conversation with the patient is where the process really begins. During this discussion, we are trying to develop a trusting relationship and also determine if there are any red flags for the patient pursuing full-arch implant dentistry. Having a clear understanding of why the patient is interested or may want to learn more about having their teeth replaced with an implant-supported prosthesis is important. What are the patient's chief concerns? What is their prior experience with dentistry? What fears do they have? Do they have financial restrictions or time constraints? What expectations do they have after the process has been completed? What is most important to them?

In my practice, we use a form developed by Dr. Paul Homoly called the Discovery Guide™ (www.paulhomoly.com). This tool has become an invaluable part of my relationship development process. It has helped me and my team become better communicators and listeners.

Medical history review and considerations

A thorough medical history and review of systems should be conducted for every new patient. (Before you begin, make sure your medical history intake form is sufficiently comprehensive based on guidelines and recommendations available from your licensing board, certified consultants, or industry associations.) The following information may be helpful to you in determining your patients' candidacy.

General overall health. Consider using the ASA Physical Status Classification System (Tab. 2.1)

Table 2.1 **American Society of Anesthesiologists Physical Status Classification System**[1]

ASA Class	Preoperative Health Status
I	Normal healthy patient
II	Patients with mild systemic disease
III	Patients with severe systemic disease
IV	Patients with severe systemic disease that is a constant threat to life
V	Moribund patients who are not expected to survive without the operation
VI	A declared brain-dead patient whose organs are being removed for donor purposes

Risk factors for dental implants, including

- Nicotine use and smoke inhalation
- Bruxism and parafunctional habits
- Recreational drug use (including illegal substances)
- Uncontrolled diabetes
- Periodontal disease
- Current medications, such as bisphosphonates, proton pump inhibitors, selective serotonin reuptake inhibitors, etc.
- Vitamin D deficiency
- History of chemotherapy or head/neck radiation
- Active autoimmune disorder with symptoms or causing decline in health
- Other disorders and systemic diseases that reduce blood supply to the jaws

Clearance for surgery by the patient's primary care physician or specialists

History of mental illness and/or medications related to mental health disorders

Undiagnosed myofascial or temporomandibular joint (TMJ) pain

A personal or family history of anesthesia complications

Radiographs and preliminary examination

If you are placing dental implants in your practice already, you probably have a CBCT or CT machine in your office. The CBCT is the most cost effective and widely accepted imaging modality for dentists who wish to obtain a 3D view of a patient's jaws. A CBCT is currently considered the standard of care for providing fixed full-arch implant dentistry and an absolute necessity in the workflow. A CBCT scan is necessary during the patient data collection for diagnostic accuracy, assessing bone volume and density, and identifying landmarks, anatomical features, and pathology. A CBCT scan will also be needed during digital case planning and engineering, and for baseline confirmation after the guided surgery.

CBCT scans generally deliver lower amounts of radiation than CT exams but do have higher radiation doses than conventional digital dental radiographs. At present, the American Dental Association and the Food and Drug Administration (FDA) recommend that dentists perform CBCT scans only when necessary for the diagnosis or treatment of disease. The FDA website states that "The clinical benefit of a medically appropriate x-ray imaging exam outweighs the small radiation risk. However, efforts should be made to help minimize this risk"[2]. The rationale for taking CBCT scans should be discussed between you and your patient. Also, the settings on the machine should be optimized for the lowest radiation dose that yields a quality image adequate for diagnosis. Laws about patient radiation exposure vary in different states and countries, and it is up to you to use your best judgment and follow guidelines set forth by your licensing agencies.

The minimal anatomy to capture in a CBCT, or the field of view (FOV), for full-arch dental implant rehabilitation comprises the inferior border of the mandible up to and including the sinus cavities. This can be achieved in most patients by having a CBCT scan that is between 100 × 80 mm and 150 × 80 mm. Scans that meet this requirement will allow you to visualize anatomy that will be critical for diagnosis as well as provide enough information for your dental implant planning.

Patients with dentition

Taking a CBCT is straightforward in most patients. For patients with dentition, a traditional CBCT scan can be taken by placing a bite fork and/or cotton rolls between any posterior teeth. Occasionally you may have a patient with a highly restored dentition with fixed metal in their mouth, such as amalgam fillings, porcelain-fused-to-metal crowns, gold work, or multiple endodontically treated teeth with metal posts. You may also find dental implants with titanium components or even metal plating from previous orthognathic or trauma surgeries. Sometimes in such patients you may observe a phenomenon on the CBCT known as *scatter* or *image artifacts*, which can compromise their accuracy. Fortunately, there are a couple of ways to reduce these artifacts.

For most patients, the easiest method is to place some cotton rolls in the buccal vestibules and between the teeth during the scan. Another more predictable method, if your patient is amenable, involves a dual-scanning process. In this method, polyvinyl siloxane (PVS) impression material is added to a plastic tray sized for the patient's dentition, and four to six radiopaque fiducial markers are placed on the buccal and lingual surfaces of the tray before it is inserted in the patient's mouth. (Have the patient use the chinrest in place of a bite fork, if possible.) A scan is taken with the tray in the patient's mouth, and then a separate CBCT scan of the impression tray is taken with the markers on it (Fig. 2.1). This technique will provide a more accurate way to merge CBCT information in software during the engineering and planning phase of the fixed full-arch process.

Patients who are fully edentulous

The workflow for obtaining a CBCT differs for patients who are fully edentulous in at least one arch. Also, in complex cases—particularly when the patient's vertical dimension of occlusion (VDO) is not in the correct position—more than one CBCT scan may be needed to get to the digital treatment-planning phase. This is discussed in detail in Chapter 3.

When a patient is fully edentulous in at least one arch and has a current denture at the correct VDO, a dual-scan approach can be used (Figs. 2.2-2.4). The dual-scan approach uses fiducial markers attached to the denture in various locations. First, however, you should make sure the denture is well fitting. To check stability, have the patient comfortably bite down and see if the denture (or dentures) shifts or moves. If the denture is loose or does not seat well on the ridge, do a quick PVS wash impression in it or use a chairside hard liner material to perform a reline of the denture. (Many patients appreciate being able to leave the office with a better-fitting denture.) I prefer to use a fast-setting hard reline material.

Once the denture is stable, remove it from the patient's mouth and place four to six radiopaque fiducial markers on it around the buccal/labial and lingual/palatal flanges. Next, take a CBCT scan with the patient biting down with the dentures together in occlusion or one denture against the opposing dentition. While obtaining the scan, have the patient use the chinrest or cotton rolls for this technique instead of the bite fork. Once you have obtained the CBCT of your patient, carefully remove the denture and use a scanning table or foam platform to take a second CBCT scan of it with the fiducial markers in place.

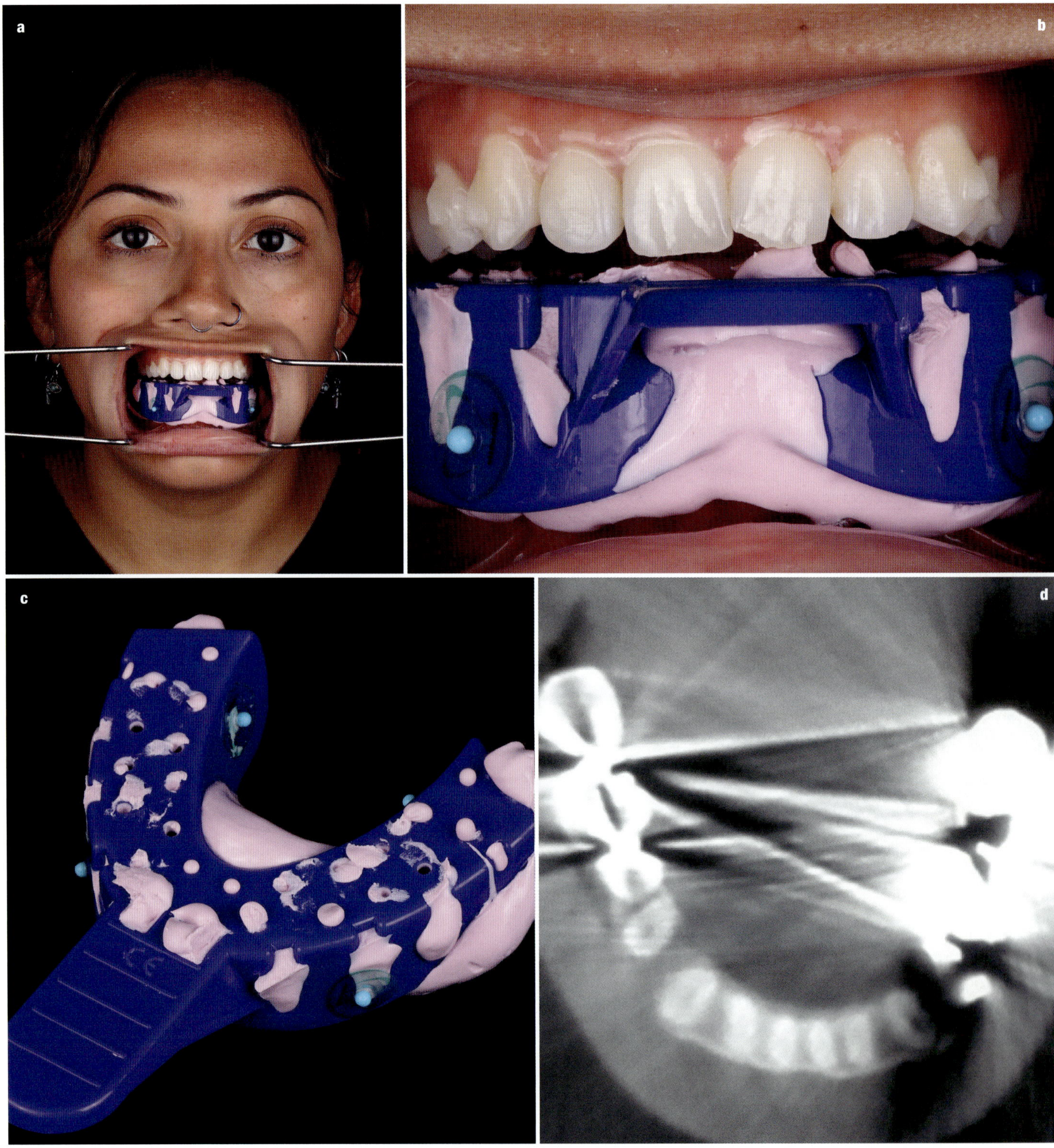

Figure 2.1 (a-c) Demonstration of a technique to reduce scatter artifact in CBCT using polyvinyl siloxane (PVS) in a member of the author's team; (d) Unrelated CBCT scan showing an example of scatter artifact in an axial view of a mandible.

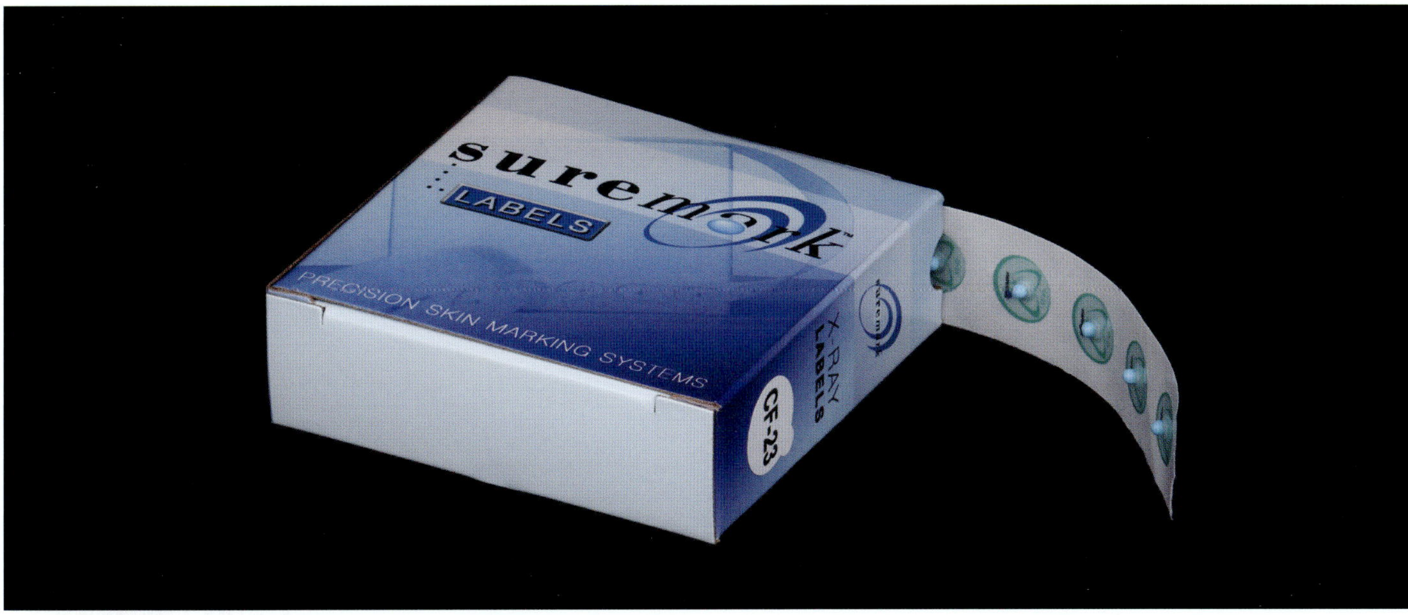

Figure 2.2 Suremark® stickers or labels act as fiducial markers on dentures and other removable appliances during a dual-scan CBCT.

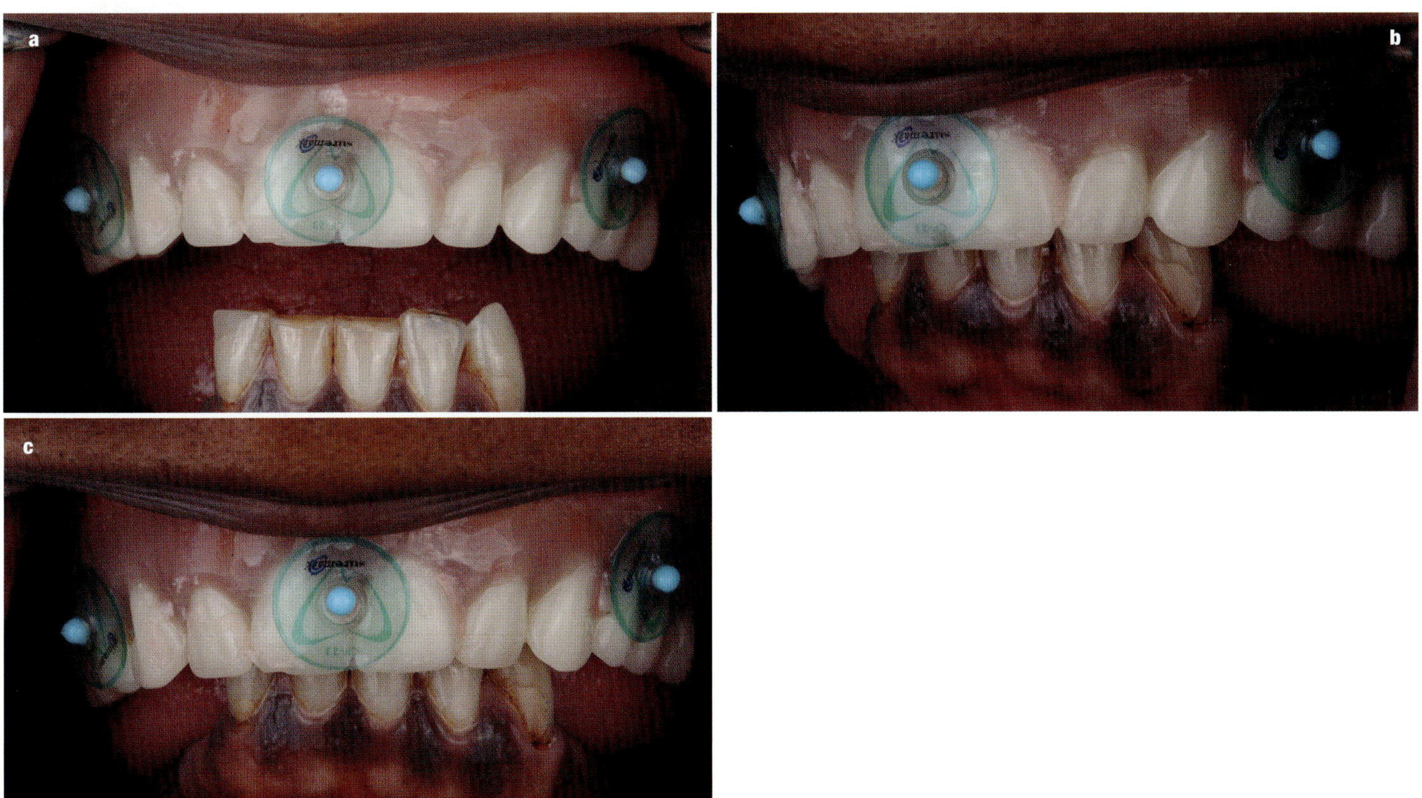

Figure 2.3 (a-c) Dual-scan technique for maxillary denture using fiducial markers (Suremark Labels). Patient should be biting comfortably into maximal intercuspal position (MIP) during the CBCT scan.

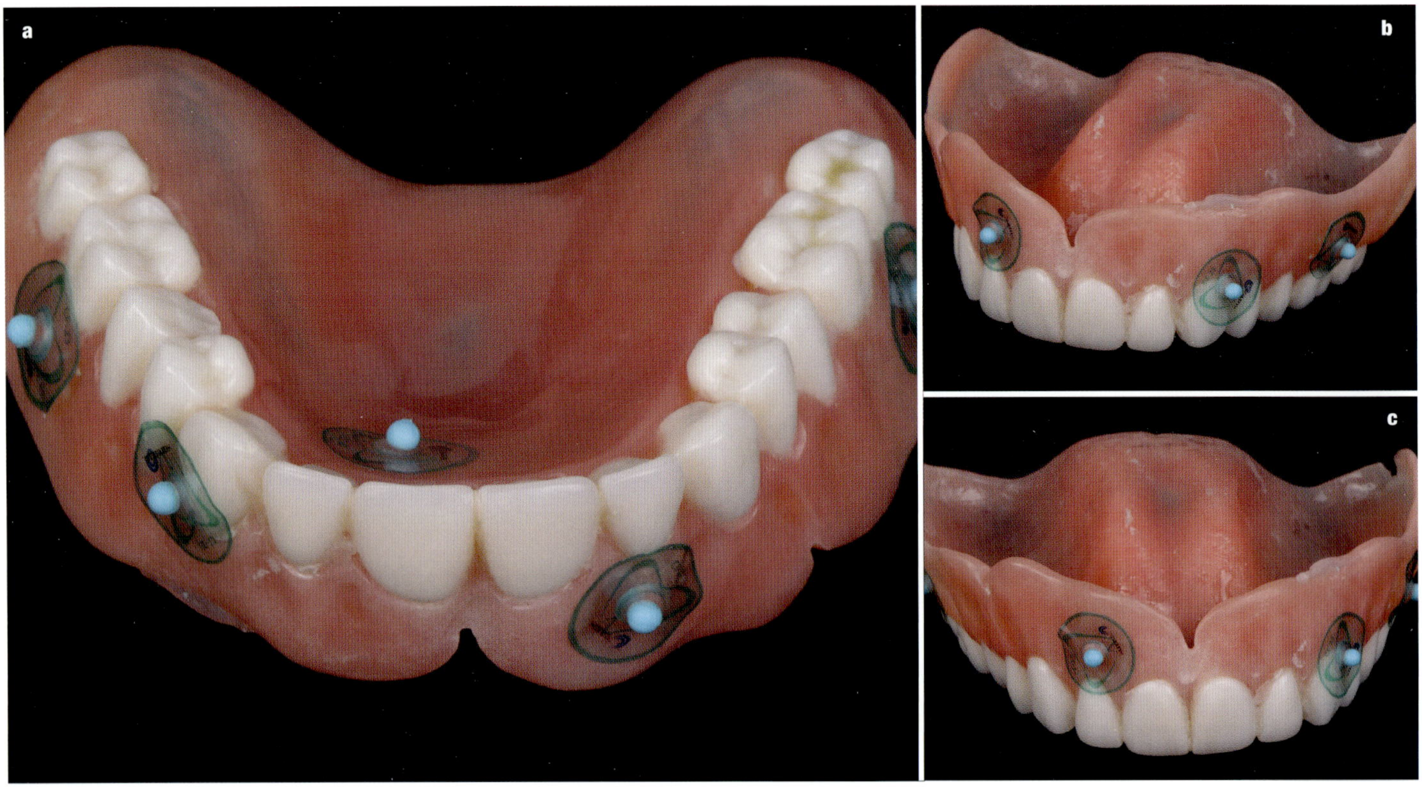

Figure 2.4 (a-c) **Maxillary denture showing placement of Suremark Labels in preparation for dual-scan CBCT.**

If you are working with a patient who is edentulous and does not have a denture or requires a considerable number of changes to establish the new VDO, tooth position, biting position, and so forth, you can have your laboratory technician create a prototype denture, which will allow you to obtain more accurate records and have a more predictable outcome in your future interim prosthesis. This is discussed in more detail in Chapter 3.

Determination of the terminal dentition

During your dental history and examination, you may need to determine whether your patient's dentition is "terminal." We occasionally see patients with a considerable number of teeth who are interested in fixed full-arch implant dentistry for questionable reasons. Some of these reasons honestly do not make sense, like "I read on the internet that if I get dental implants, I won't ever have to have my teeth cleaned again," or "My jaws hurt all the time and my dentist told me that if my teeth were removed and implants were placed, this would stop." However, there are many individuals with a fair number of healthy teeth that would require what I refer to as "hero-dontics" to restore them to complete function without fully edentulating them. For best practices, you should always have proper diagnoses to reach the conclusion of terminal dentition and be able to stand behind that before removing compromised teeth or sacrificing healthy teeth. I remind patients that they may have the choice of rehabilitation without complete edentulation and that there are other options besides fixed full-arch implant dentistry. We educate them on the pros and cons, as well as the risks and benefits of alternative therapies.

To help you reach (or reject) a determination of terminal dentition, consider each of the following:

- Number and distribution of remaining teeth
- Esthetic challenges and/or cosmetic deficiencies
- Functional challenges: Bruxism, clenching, parafunctional habits, temporomandibular joint disorder (TMJD)
- Neurological challenges and pain issues
- Systemic challenges: Medical conditions that limit predictability of dentition such as diabetes and dry mouth that require medication
- Structural considerations: Tooth wear and/or inability to support alternative toothborne prosthetics
- Biologic considerations: Erosion, caries, periodontal disease, congenital tooth defects
- Phonetic issues
- Physical challenges that affect the ability to practice at-home oral care and hygiene
- Access to care after treatment
- Patient wants, time and financial concerns, and emotional state

Edentulism and partial edentulism, which are better described as *adult tooth loss*, are a significant problem worldwide. According to a recent review of the literature, the rate of edentulism is growing, and the number of individuals suffering from it will probably continue to rise as people live longer[3]. Unfortunately, edentulism affects the most vulnerable populations, namely the aging and those who are economically challenged. The consequences of edentulism are significant; it has been linked to nutritional changes, diabetes, obesity, hypertension, obstructive sleep apnea, coronary artery disease, dementia, and some forms of cancer. Full or partial edentulism is commonly a byproduct of trauma, tooth decay, periodontal disease, occlusal parafunction, acid erosion, and access to care, among several other factors[4,5].

The term *terminal dentition* can be described as a dentition that is destined for failure. It has been defined in dentistry as "a condition in which there are insufficient teeth to maintain function and the arch, as a whole, will transition to the edentulous state"[6]. However, the term itself is not well studied or understood. The causes of a patient's terminal dentition are the same as they are for edentulism, but as far as the literature is concerned, there are few if any evidence-based protocols for how to determine terminal dentition.

Terminal Dentition: "A dentition destined for failure"

It is not always easy to assess when a dentition will fail, but we can use guidelines that will create understanding for our patients and help us describe expectations. The number of our patients suffering from terminal dentition is immense, and because of advances in technology and increasing access to care, patients are diagnosed with terminal dentition earlier than they have been in the past. In his article "Terminal dentition: Where do we draw the line?" Dr. Ricardo Mitrani suggests that this made-up dental term is problematic because dentists generally name their own criteria, clinical experience, and personal beliefs in determining whether a patient is in a terminal dentition[7]. He presents a decision tree and algorithm that he developed to help clinicians understand when a patient has reached the point of no return with their teeth. Dr. Maurice Salama, another well-respected clinician and educator, has also developed and teaches a decision tree for diagnosis and determining a treatment plan for patients who may be in a terminal dentition. He has used his classifications successfully in his practice and encourages other clinicians to consider using them as well (Tab. 2.2).

Advanced and irreversible structural and periodontal damage are widely accepted by most clinicians as the most undisputable evidence for classifying a patient's dentition as terminal. However, there are other factors responsible for terminal dentition. These should be considered during a dental history intake. Beyond objective clinical findings, a patient's subjective concerns and wishes should ultimately be reviewed and play some part in the decision-making process. We must continually remind ourselves that we are treating the "whole" and not just the "hole." This means listening to the patient, understanding their values, and letting them be part of the process of deciding what is right for them.

Figures 2.5 to 2.8 are photographs of patients I evaluated and determined to be in terminal dentitions.

Table 2.2 Prosthetic treatment-planning guidelines based on diagnosis or etiology of tooth loss, developed by Dr. Maurice Salama*

Diagnosis/ Reason for Tooth Loss	Periodontal	Tooth Caries	Fracture/Wear	Edentulism
Considerations	Bone and Tissue Loss Considerable: Consider FP2/FP3 design	Bone and Tissue Good: Consider FP1/FP2 design	Bone and Tissue Good: Consider FP1/FP2 design	Bone and Tissue Loss Severe: Consider FP3 design/zygoma and pterygoid implants
	HIGHER RISK Perio Susceptible	**LOW RISK** Moderate Bone Quality	**HIGHER RISK** Dense Bone Quality but High Occlusal Load	**MODERATE RISK** Functional Load
Treatment plan based on reason for tooth loss	• Re-establish keratinized tissue • Remove muscle attachments • Hygienic prosthetic design • Short recall maintenance	**BEST SITUATION** • Minimal implants necessary • Good AP spread • Scalloped design (FP1/ FP2) • Minimal bone reduction	• Maximum number of implants • Overengineer • Consider direct to implant vs. MUA • Occlusion critical • Nightguard appliance a MUST	• Place more implants • Longer time in temporary prosthesis • Evaluate bone quality carefully • FP3 design critical

**(Lecture DentalXP Summit NYC October 2021 Financial District NYC.)*

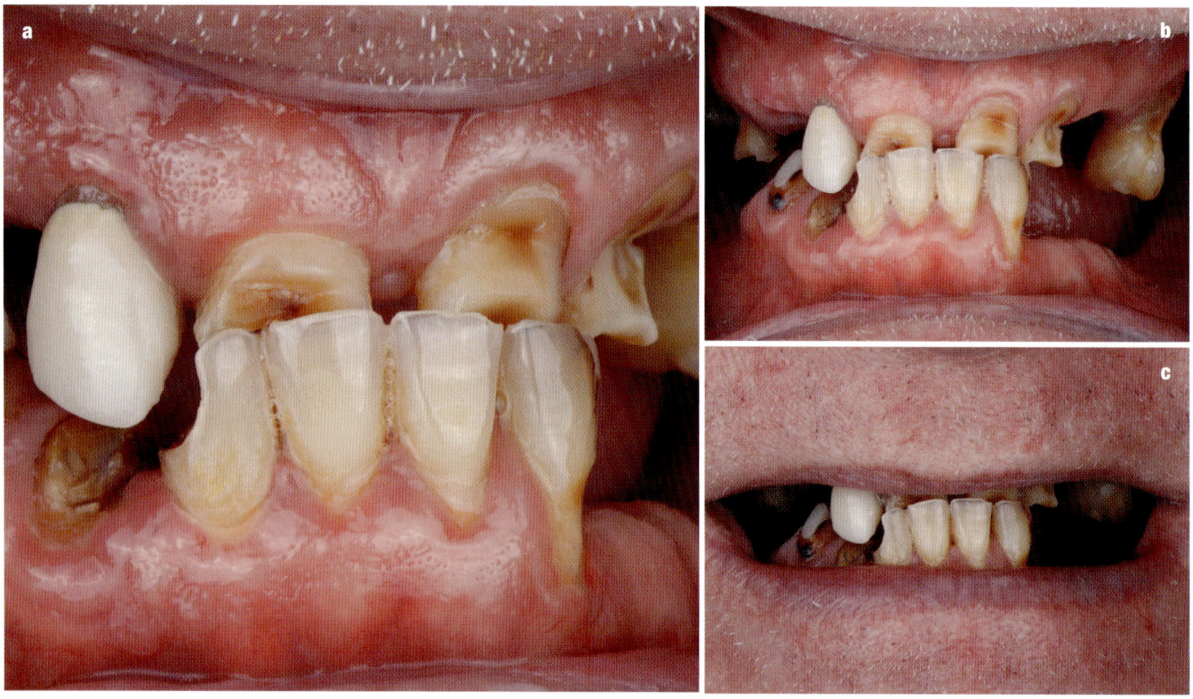

Figure 2.5 (a-c) Severe wear and erosion, dental caries, periodontal disease, malocclusion, and loss of vertical dimension of occlusion (VDO) in both arches in a patient diagnosed with terminal dentition.

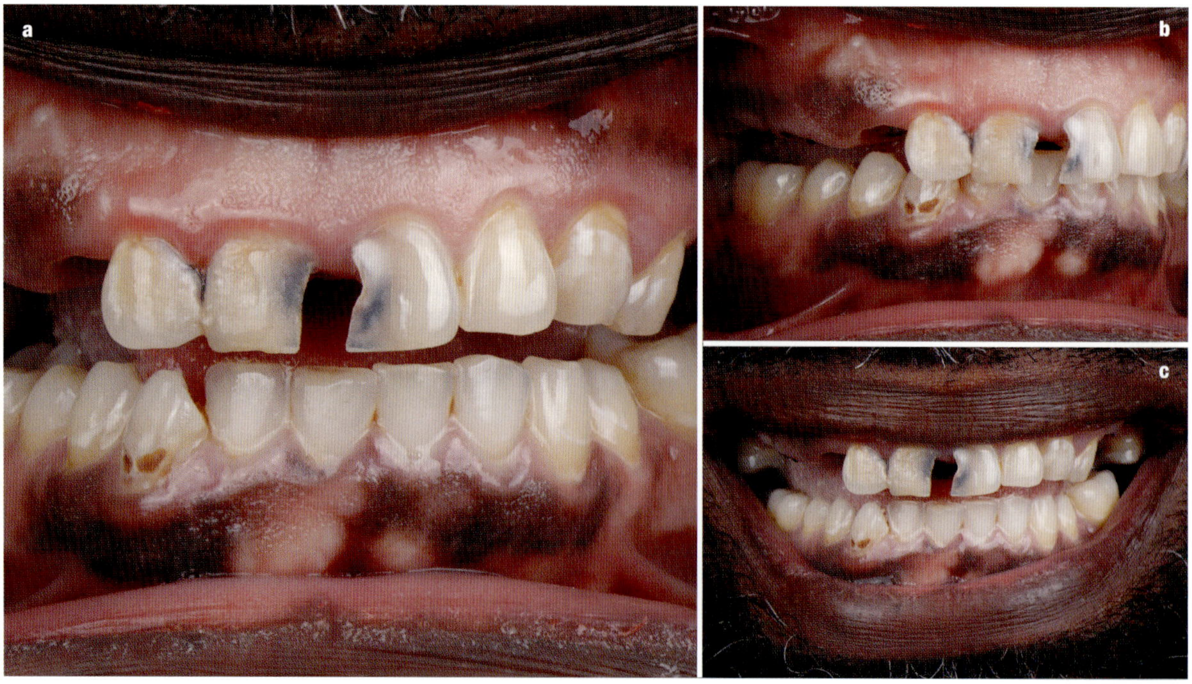

Figure 2.6 (a-c) Dental caries in the maxilla in a patient diagnosed with terminal dentition (maxilla only).

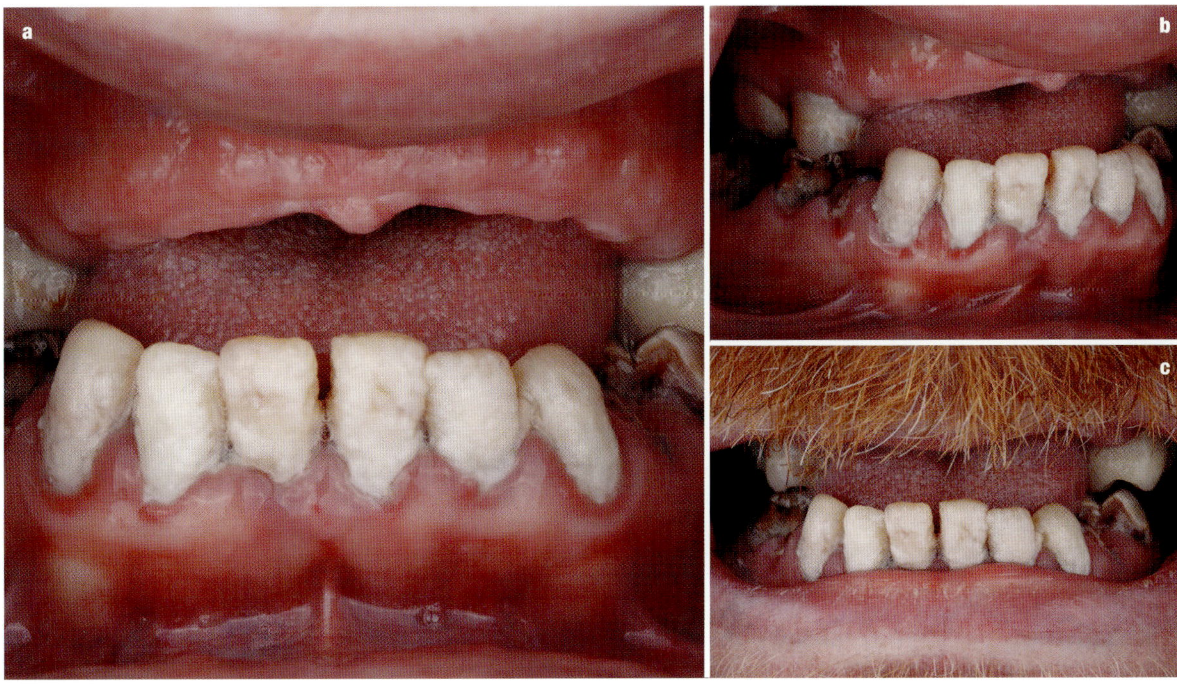

Figure 2.7 (a-c) Dental caries, periodontal disease, and tooth mobility in a patient diagnosed with terminal dentition.

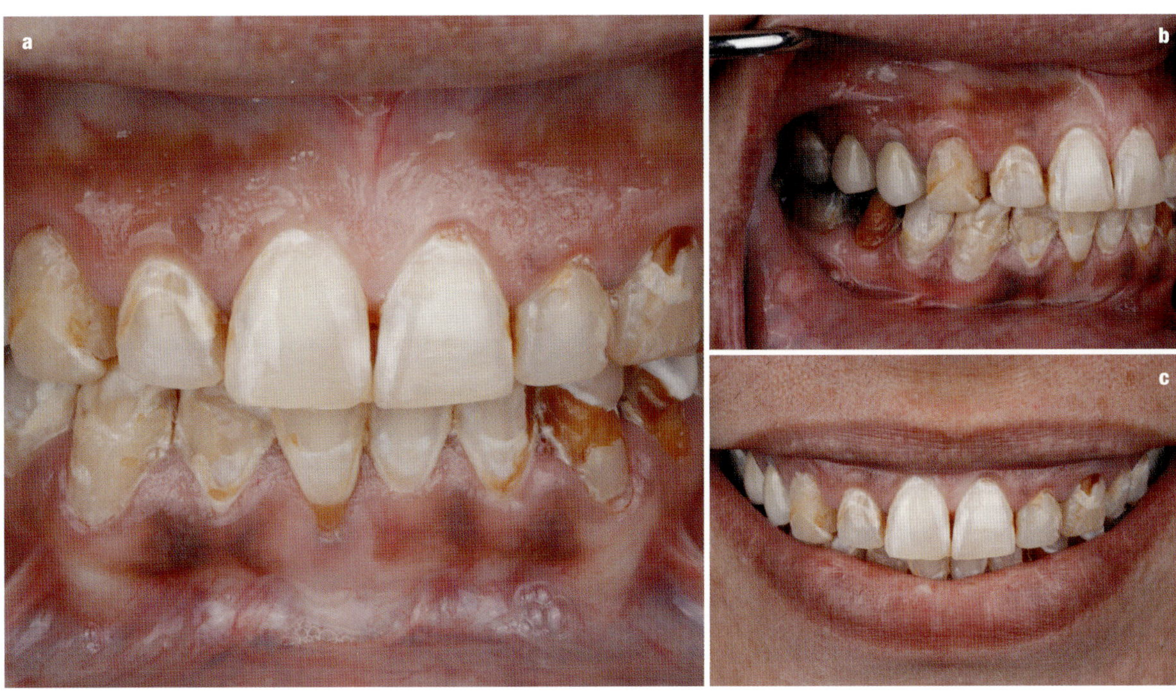

Figure 2.8 (a-c) Severe erosion and dental caries as well as gross recurrent decay under current restorations in a patient diagnosed with terminal dentition.

Data collection

Before considering a patient's final candidacy for fixed full-arch implant dentistry, it is wise to appraise the landscape of your potential surgical sites, take into consideration the prosthodontic ramifications, and obtain certain baseline measurements. I developed a Data Collection Checklist (Fig. 2.9) for gathering the information I need before proceeding on to case engineering and planning in collaboration with my guided surgery treatment planner.

Some of the data collected at the consultation appointment are used to assess the patient's candidacy for fixed full-arch implant rehabilitation. The rest are obtained at the patient's second appointment, which is covered in Chapter 3. In your practice, you may choose to do this in one visit. The reasoning behind my workflow is that I first want to quickly establish whether the patient is a candidate for fixed full-arch implant dentistry as time-efficiently as possible and begin developing a relationship with him or her. I also want to provide this assessment free or at a very low cost to the patient. In other words, I want to avoid spending an inordinate amount of time only to find out that this procedure is not a good fit for them. In this way I am being respectful to them as well as my practice, my team, and myself.

DATA COLLECTION CHECKLIST

PART I SURGICAL AND PROSTHETIC CONSIDERATIONS

Medical History Review: ☐ Completed

Maximum Pt. opening (inter-arch space): ________ mm ☐ Adequate ☐ Inadequate

CBCT EVALUATION

Adequate Bone Volume: ☐ Yes ☐ No

Is additional bone augmentation necessary? ☐ Yes ☐ No

Consider: sinus lift ridge grafting

Adequate Bone Quality/Density: ☐ Yes ☐ No

Bone Type

Maxilla:	type I	type II	type III	type IV
Mandible:	type I	type II	type III	type IV

consider osseodensification: ☐ Yes ☐ No

Radiolucencies and/or pathology present? ☐ Yes ☐ No

Where? ______________________________

SOFT TISSUE RELATED CONSIDERATIONS

Oral Cancer Screening ☐ Negative ☐ Suspicion ______________________________

Attached Keratinized Tissue adequate? ☐ Yes ☐ No

Excessive gingival display ☐ Yes ☐ No

If yes: ☐ High smile line ☐ Hyperactive upper lip
☐ Short upper lip ☐ Vertical Maxillary Excess
☐ Altered passive eruption

Consider: Lip repositioning Botox Other ____________

Labial Position & Lip Support
☐ Lips supported properly
☐ Lip support inadequate
☐ Lip support exaggerated

Anatomical Midline & Facial Symmetry
☐ Midline is appropriate and good facial symmetry
☐ Midline discrepancy, move tooth midline Left/Right ________ mm

Figure 2.9 (a) Data Collection Checklist, Part I: Surgical and prosthetic considerations (developed by the author).

DATA COLLECTION CHECKLIST

TOOTH RELATED CONSIDERATIONS

Skeletal Classification ☐ I ☐ II ☐ III

Teeth Classification ☐ I ☐ II ☐ III

Malocclusion? ____________________

Tooth Mobility ☐ Yes __________ ☐ No

Incisal Edge Position ☐ Keep

☐ Move: Bucco-Labially Lingually

Horizontal Plane of Teeth ☐ Level

☐ Canted: Keep or Change

Anterior Tooth Display ☐ Adequate ☐ Inadequate ☐ Exaggerated

Upper __________ mm

Lower __________ mm

Tooth Size & Shape ☐ Adequate ☐ Needs modification

Diastemas? ☐ Yes Locations __________ Size __________ ☐ No

Phonetics ☐ Speech is acceptable ☐ Needs to be changed (video)

VDO Considerations ☐ Appropriate ☐ Collapsed ☐ Excessive

JR (jaw relation) try-in? ☐ Yes ☐ No

Smile Simulation ☐ Yes ☐ No

Terminal Dentition? ☐ Yes ☐ No

Thoughts? ____________________

____

____

Figure 2.9 (a) *(cont.)*

DATA COLLECTION CHECKLIST

ANESTHESIA OPTIONS AND CONSIDERATIONS:

Mallampati airway classification:

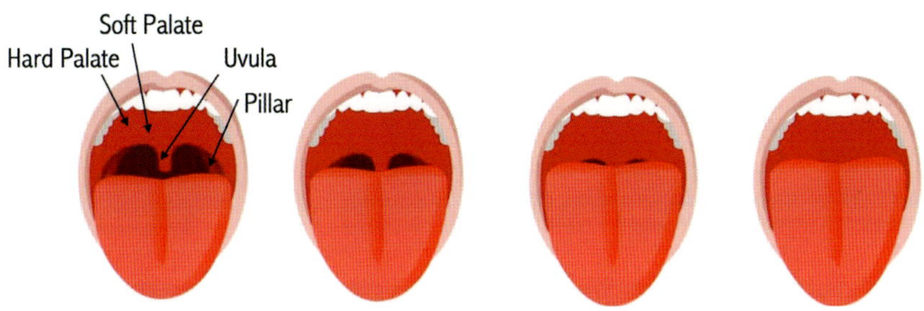

Class I ☐ Class II ☐ Class III ☐ Class IV ☐

Personal or family history of anesthesia complications? ☐ Yes ☐ No

Anesthesia considered for case: ☐ GA ☐ Conscious IV ☐ Local/N2O/Other

Patient Logistical and Fit Issues:

____

____

____

____

Patient Chief Concerns:

____

____

____

____

____

____

____

Figure 2.9 (a) *(cont.)*

DATA COLLECTION CHECKLIST

PART II RECORDS VISIT

Photo Set: ☐ Obtained

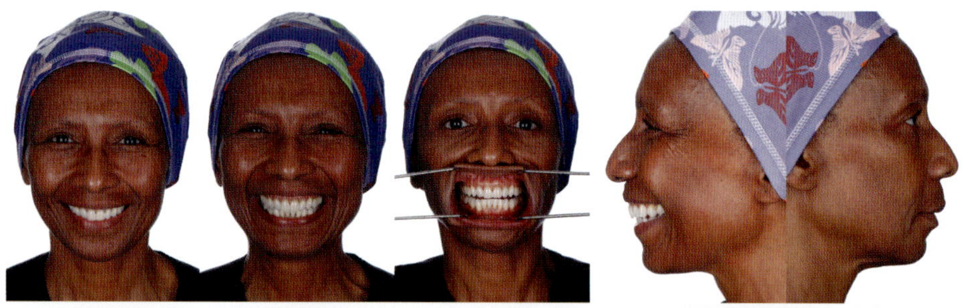

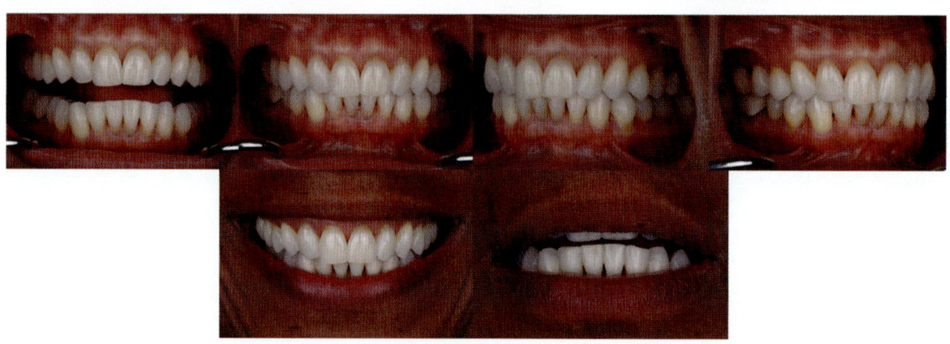

Digital Impressions: ☐ Obtained

Patient Medical Clearance: ☐ Obtained

Vitamin D Levels: __________ ng/ml

Patient Consent Forms: ☐ Obtained

Financial Arrangements: ☐ Completed

Prosthetic Design Considerations: ____

____

____

____

Shade: ______________________

Figure 2.9 (b) *(cont.)* Data Collection Checklist, Part II: Records visit (covered in Chapter 3).

Surgical and prosthetic considerations

Trismus/interarch space

One of the first parameters to assess is the patient's maximum vertical opening. My rule of thumb is that if I cannot get at least two vertically stacked fingers between the patient's teeth (assuming the teeth are in the appropriate position in a dentate or partially dentate patient), I question my ability to move forward. Causes for restriction of the range of motion of the jaws, or *trismus*, can vary and are sometimes reversible. However, a patient with a limited opening for whatever reason can be very difficult to work on. Remember that guided dental implant drills are longer and require more room for access than drills used in nonguided surgery. It is good to know this limitation on the front end and to have a game plan.

CBCT evaluation

Prior to discussing a patient's candidacy for fixed full-arch implant dentistry, I use the CBCT scan to assess bone volume and density, tooth positioning, pathology, and a host of other anatomical features that may be present in the jaws. Analyzing the CBCT can help me determine how I might engineer the case and whether I might need to consider bone augmentation or more specialized dental implant options such as those designed for use in the pterygoid and zygomatic regions.

Soft tissues

An intra- and extraoral cancer screening should be performed on all patients. In my career, I have referred a handful of patients to specialists for suspicious findings during an oral cancer screening. Four of my patients were diagnosed with operable cancer and returned to thank me for "saving their life." In every one of these cases, the patient was unaware of their condition.

Keratinized tissue is necessary to have around dental implant abutments for predictable longevity. I look at the keratinized tissues: Does the patient have an adequate or limited amount? Also, is it attached and nonmobile? Adequate non-mobile keratinized tissue is key to long-term survival of dental implants.

Gingival display is another important assessment to make when inspecting the soft tissues (Fig. 2.10). Excessive gingival display in the maxilla can be a red flag when it comes to fixed full-arch implant rehabilitation, so it is important to catch this on the front end and determine its cause. The fact that a patient has some gingival tissue showing does not necessarily mean he

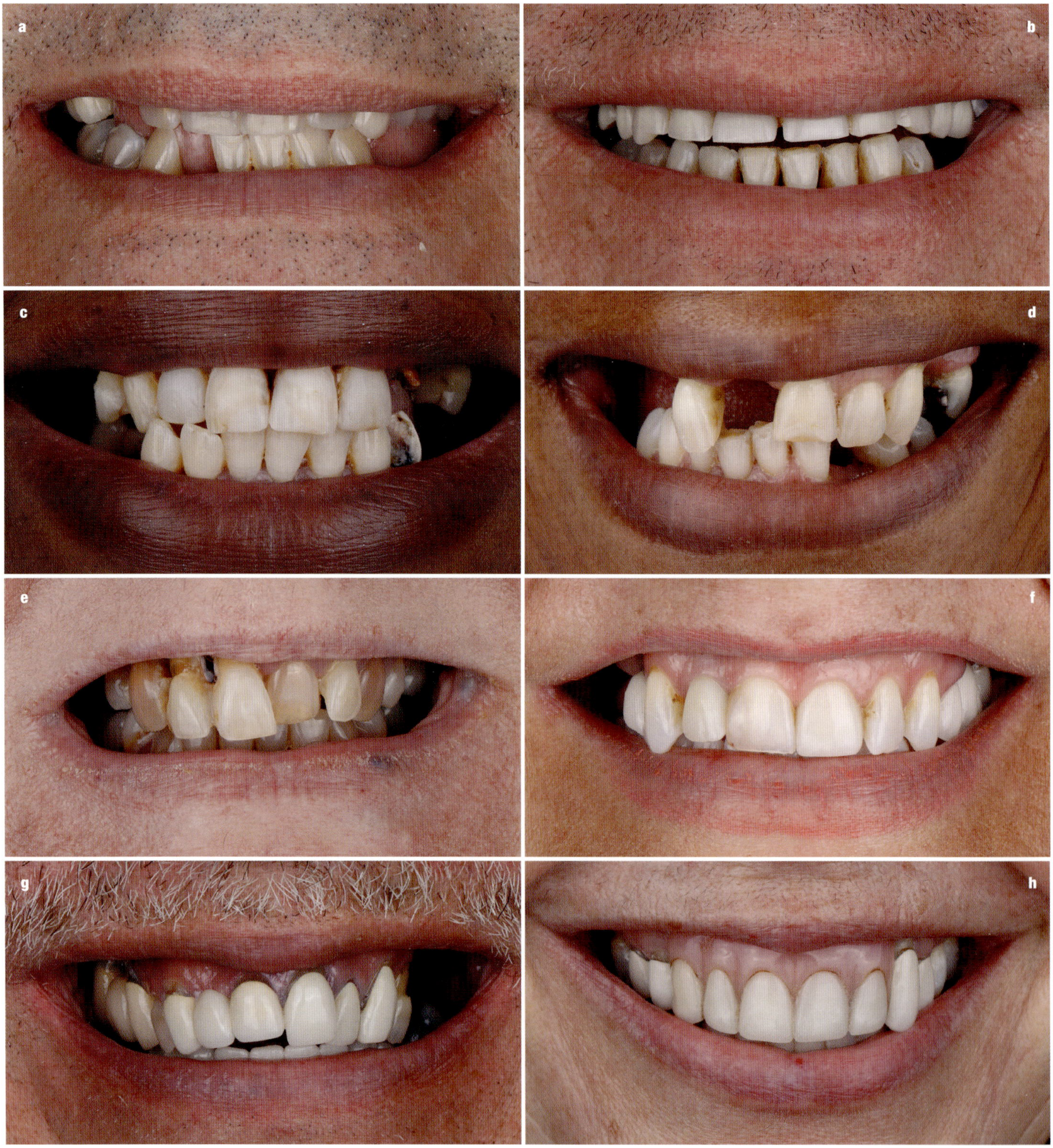

Figure 2.10 (a-h) Examples of patients with varying degrees of gingival display in the maxilla during full smile.

or she is not a candidate, but excessive gingival display may create limitations and require undue amounts of bone reduction, lip repositioning surgery, Botox, or other treatment modalities. Nothing is more off-putting cosmetically in these cases than a patient who exposes the transition line between their ridge and the prosthesis. When a patient has 3 to 4 mm of gingival tissue exposed in their exaggerated smile position, consider that a "gummy smile."

Labial position and lip support

The labial position of the lips in relation to the premaxilla may be the primary criterion for determining whether a fixed restoration is best for a patient. If appropriate labial positioning cannot be achieved with a fixed full-arch implant prosthesis because of a facially deficient edentulous arch, it may be advisable to consider a maxillary overdenture with a flange, or bone grafting/ridge augmentation. In *Fundamentals of Implant Dentistry* (2022), Beumer et al. identify the characteristics that make patients poor candidates for fixed maxillary arch implant prosthetics: insufficient lip support, a pseudo-Class III occlusion, excessive resorption of the premaxilla, and large defects in the premaxilla[8]. In such patients, it may be more appropriate to consider an implant-supported removable appliance such as an overdenture. I evaluate a patient's labial position by observing the patient profile or taking a portrait profile photograph.

A colleague of mine, Dr. Akil Alexander, taught me a technique for evaluating lip support in patients with the proper VDO. The first step is to visualize or draw two lines on a photo of the patient's profile (Fig. 2.11). The first line is the Frankfort horizontal; we can call this the true horizontal. Then draw or visualize a vertical line perpendicular to the true horizontal line; we will call this the true vertical. The true vertical line should intersect the subnasale point (SP). If the most anterior point of the upper lip is 1 to 2 mm anterior to the true vertical line, there should be appropriate upper lip support.

Another simple and widely accepted method to assess lip support uses a construct developed by Dr. Robert Ricketts known as the *esthetic plane*. The esthetic plane is a line drawn from the tip of the nose to the tip of the chin (Fig. 2.12). In a deficiency, the upper lip will be more than 4 mm behind the esthetic plane and the lower lip will be more than 2 mm behind the esthetic plane. The closer the lips are to this plane, the more dominant the teeth and lips will appear[9].

Assessing lip support and determining whether it is appropriate should ultimately involve the patient. Lip support and profile attributes can be something that varies between people of different races. Some patients may not be as concerned about the esthetic outcome of their

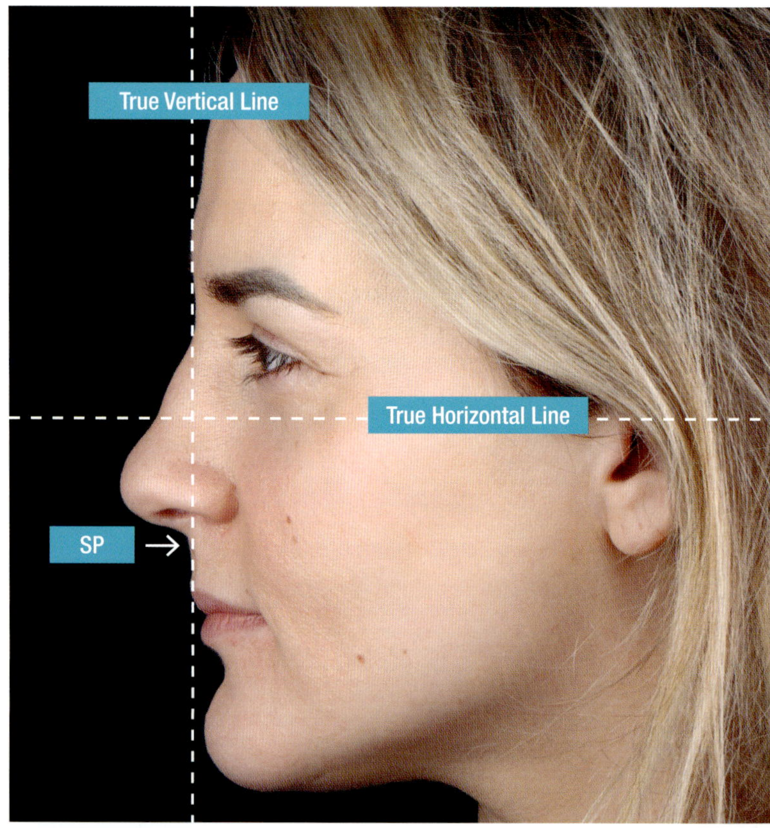

Figure 2.11 Technique for assessing lip support using vertical and horizontal planes and the subnasale point (SP).

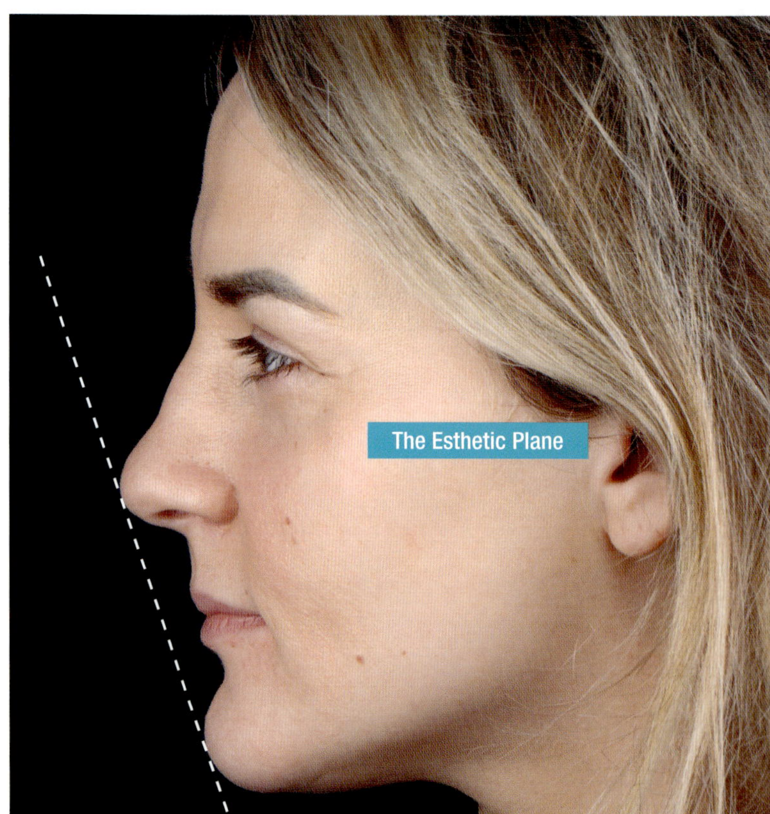

Figure 2.12 Technique for assessing lip support using the esthetic plane.

external features. An important point in recording lip support is to make sure the patient knows what your limitations are and has realistic expectations about what can be achieved.

Anatomical midline and facial symmetry

I evaluate and record the patient's midline as it relates to their anatomical features as well as their teeth. Most people have some discrepancies in this area and often do not consider the entire face when they evaluate the location of the midline of their teeth. There are several different techniques for measuring the patient's midline in relation to their features, but the one I have found most useful is to take a portrait photograph of the patient and draw a series of vertical and horizontal lines on it (Fig. 2.13). I generally use the eyes to establish the horizontal lines and then draw a vertical line through the center of the forehead, nose, and chin. Sharing this information with the patient helps them understand that there are certain factors that limit us based on their facial characteristics. Where their teeth midline is before treatment and where it will end

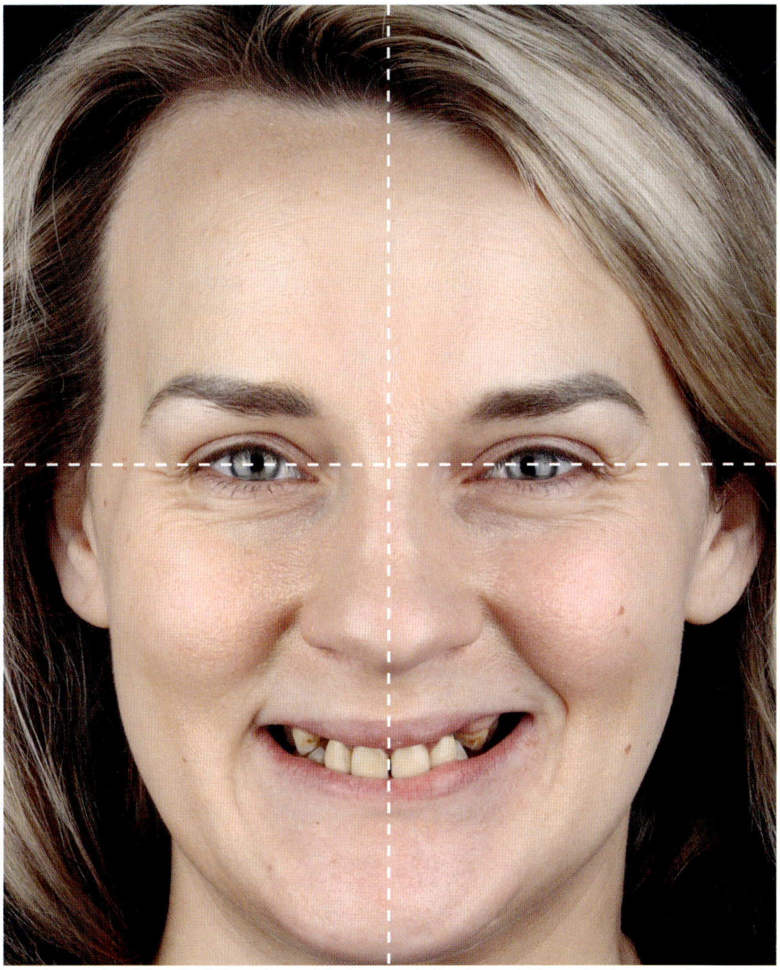

Figure 2.13 **Technique for determining the facial midline and assessing symmetry.**

up is somewhat flexible. The most important factor of midline evaluation is the vertical angle of the midline. During the data collection stage, you will be able to gain input from your laboratory, use your own judgment, and involve the patient in this process.

Tooth-related considerations

Next, I take a careful look at the teeth themselves: I measure tooth mobility, identify the horizontal plane of occlusion, note the incisal edge position, and record anterior tooth display while the patient is in repose. I also take into consideration the size and shape of the patient's teeth and any diastemata that may be present. More than once I have had a patient ask me to keep the diastema between certain teeth and replicate that in their interim and/or definitive prosthesis.

If the patient is struggling with their phonetics, I record it now. There are some phonetic issues that we can resolve, but sometimes patients have phonetic challenges that will persist even after rehabilitation.

Skeletal and teeth classification

Recording a patient's skeletal and teeth classifications is important. In my practice, I use the Angle Classification, which divides occlusion and malocclusion into four distinct classes (normal occlusion, Class I, II, and III) and is widely used by orthodontists. With some patients, I (or they) want to change the relationship of their teeth for esthetic and functional purposes. Although this can be done, in some cases there are limitations. It is helpful to record these attributes prior to moving forward with the case and to have discussions with the patient about what is possible and what is not.

Vertical dimension of occlusion

A few edentulous and partially edentulous patients will have lost some vertical dimension, and it is important to reestablish the appropriate VDO for them. Like occlusion, this is an area where several different schools of thought exist. Instead of getting into a long discussion about condylar positioning, muscle activity, and a host of other variables, I offer one simple way to help you decide whether the VDO might need to be changed (Figs. 2.14, 2.15):

1. With current dentures or other appliances in place, have the patient open their mouth and then close until the lips just touch: This is the physiologic rest position. Make one mark above the lip and another on the patient's chin and then measure the distance between them.

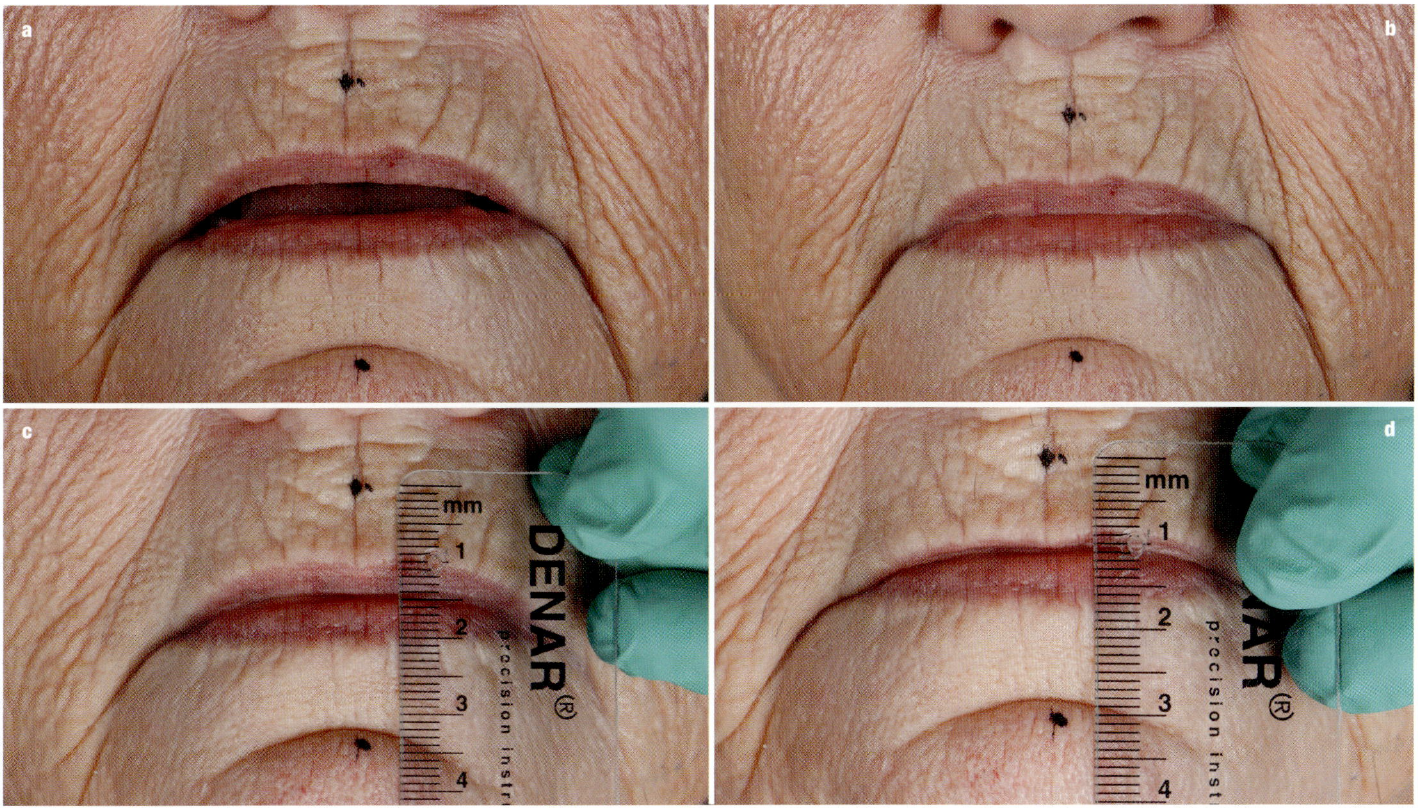

Figure 2.14 Technique for determining physiologic rest position and freeway space. In this patient, the distance between physiologic rest position and maximal intercuspal position (MIP) was approximately 5 mm, which represents her freeway space. (a) To begin, place a mark above the upper lip and on the chin and have the patient open their mouth. (b) The patient then closes until the lips just touch. (c) The distance between the two marks is measured. This is the physiologic rest position. (d) The patient now brings the teeth or ridges into MIP, and a second measurement is taken. The distance between the two measurements is the freeway space.

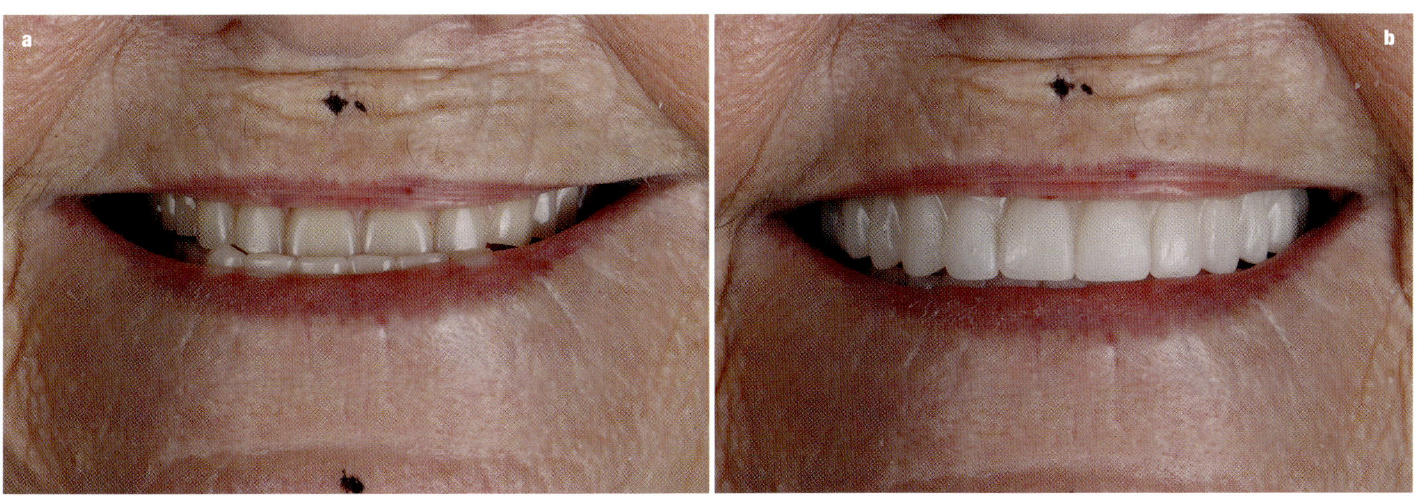

Figure 2.15 Patient shown in Fig. 2.14 (a) with current dentures and (b) with prototype mockup showing the change in her vertical dimension of occlusion (VDO) and considerably improved esthetics.

2. Have the patient close until their teeth or ridges touch in occlusion and measure the distance again: This is the maximal intercuspal position (MIP). The difference between the two measurements is your patient's interocclusal rest distance, or freeway space. I generally consider a difference of 2 to 4 mm to be acceptable.

If a patient's vertical dimension is collapsed and you plan to open the patient's occlusion (or if you are contemplating opening a patient's VDO to address a vertical overlap, or deep bite), you will want to consider an intermediate step, which would come after patient data collection and before case design, engineering, and planning. This step, using a jaw relation device, is covered in detail in Chapter 3.

Smile simulation

I like to do a smile simulation on almost every patient at their initial consultation (Fig. 2.16). A smile simulation is a wonderful tool that allows me to show my patients what I can accomplish with fixed full-arch dentistry, and it requires only one photo. (I take additional photographs of the patient at a future visit.) For the smile simulation, one of my auxiliary team members takes a full-face portrait photograph of the patient, smiling as big as they can. Taking a picture of the patient's face (and not just their teeth) captures emotion and creates ownership for the patient. Moreover, giving my patient a simulated before-and-after photo almost always helps to create confidence and trust as well as desire.

There are several smile simulation software programs available in the marketplace to choose from. I have used PreVu dental imaging software for many years. It is easy to train a dental team member to use it, and the entire process can be delegated. Generally, it only takes a few minutes for my dental assistant to snap a picture, upload it into the software, design the patient's smile, and print a hard copy for the patient to take home. Although it may not be an entirely accurate version of what their final teeth design will be, it gives patients an idea of what a full smile with straight teeth and a pretty color might look like. Recently, I started exploring other cosmetic imaging software options. Smilecloud® Biometrics has a promising platform for cosmetic imaging and planning. It is a robust program and allows users to export files into other software such as Exocad®. Although it is less user-friendly than PreVu for team users, dentists will appreciate the added features and ability to communicate more effectively with dental laboratories.

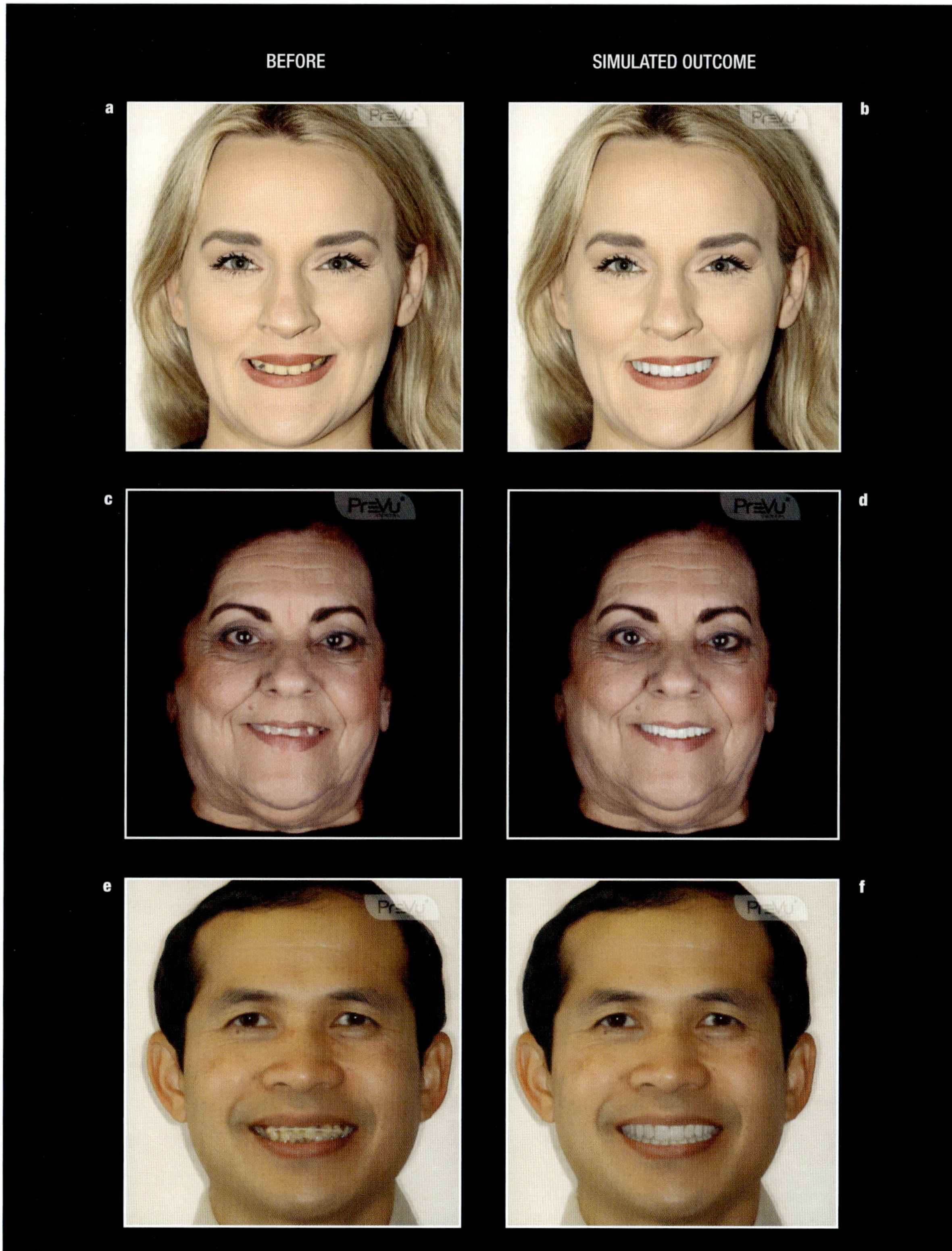

Figure 2.16 (a-f) Examples of smile simulations in PreVu®.

Anesthesia options and considerations

You and your patient may not be entirely settled on what types of anesthesia will be used at this early stage. Although it may not be definitively decided during the patient's initial visit, I like to discuss what the patient's expectations are for their potential surgery and make note of it.

There are a variety of choices for anesthesia. Obviously, every patient will have local anesthesia during surgery, but whether a sedation procedure is performed should be decided by you and your patient. Consider the comfort and safety of your patient, the efficiency with which you will be able to deliver care, the patient's personal and family history regarding anesthesia complications, the cost of having an anesthesiologist or certified registered nurse anesthetist (CRNA) present during surgery, and your country, state, and/or licensing board regulations regarding different types of anesthesia.

Most of the patients I perform fixed full-arch implant surgical procedures on prefer to be "asleep", which means that we will be discussing deep sedation or general anesthesia. I have developed a professional relationship with an anesthesia provider who sedates almost all my patients undergoing fixed full-arch implant dentistry. We built a surgical suite several years ago with enough room to accommodate an anesthesiologist or CRNA and the necessary equipment they utilize. For me, the best surgeries occur when I can stay entirely focused on the surgical procedure itself and not have to worry about monitoring my patient's anesthesia at the same time.

In every case, whether a sedative will be used during the procedure or not, you should always assess the upper airway of your patient based on the Mallampati classification (Fig. 2.17). It is helpful to have your patient's Mallampati score documented should you need to use an endotracheal tube for anesthesia or in an emergency because it helps you predict how difficult it might be to intubate your patient. The Mallampati classification is not the only predictor of whether a patient will be difficult to intubate, but it is widely used by anesthetists to assess whether the upper airway can be seen during tracheal intubation. The Mallampati classification assigns a score of I to IV to describe the size and shape of the patient's tongue and esophageal airway. The higher the Mallampati score, the greater the risk of having a difficult intubation. To conduct an upper airway assessment, have the patient seated and instruct them to open their mouth and stick out their tongue.

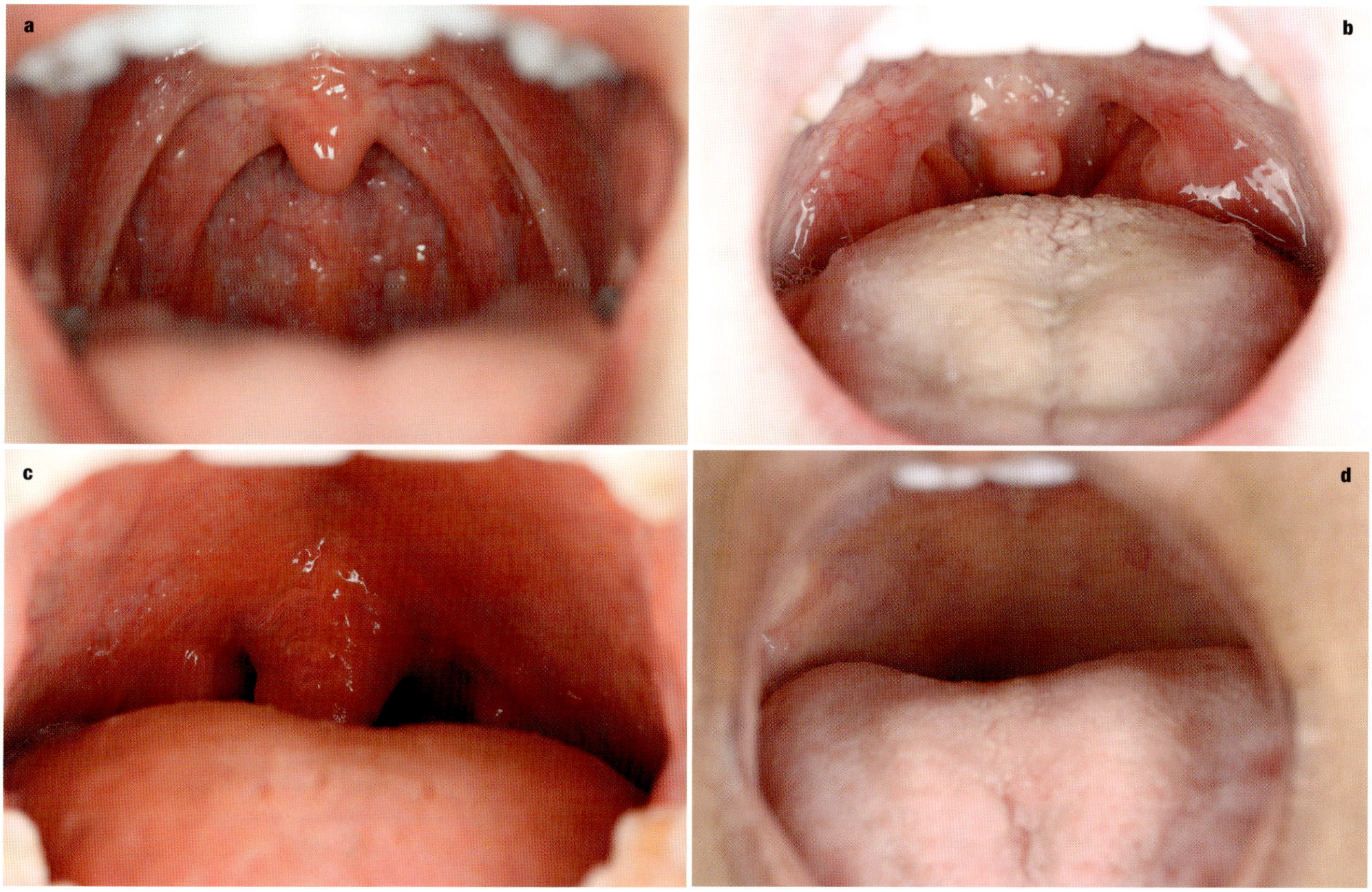

Figure 2.17 Examples of pharyngeal structures in the airways of four different patients representing Class I to IV in the Mallampati classification. (a) Class I; (b) Class II; (c) Class III; and (d) Class IV.

Logistical and "fit" issues

After a patient has been qualified as a candidate for fixed full-arch implant rehabilitation, one of my patient-care coordinators will take over and discuss "fit" issues with them. Fit issues usually involve finances, timing and scheduling, fear/pain/emotion, and overall readiness. There is a science and art to helping patients through their fit issues, and an entire textbook could be devoted to it.

We generally block 1 hour on our patient-care coordinator's schedule to go over the concerns a patient might have and discuss the financial obligations and logistical details of the process. If a patient does not make a definitive decision to move forward during their initial visit or consultation, we are okay with that. The key is to start to develop trust and a relationship and then follow up with them consistently. The best advice I can offer clinicians on helping patients proceed with care is to understand the importance of follow-up. It can frequently take three to seven follow-up calls or touchpoints with patients considering procedures before they accept treatment. Most offices my team and I speak to and consult with do not spend enough time working on the relationship and building trust. Having a dedicated patient-care coordinator or key member of your team for your patient to be able to follow up with is important. This individual, along with a lead clinical assistant, can help you manage the patient's case and all its moving parts.

Once a patient decides they are ready to make the commitment to move forward, it is time to schedule their next appointment.

References

1. American Society of Anesthesiologists [Internet]. Washington, DC: ASA; 2023. ASA Physical Status Classification System; 15 Oct 2014 [updated 13 Dec 2020; cited 15 June 2023]. Available from: https://www.asahq.org/standards-and-guidelines/statement-on-asa-physical-status-classification-system
2. US Food and Drug Administration [Internet]. Silver Springs, MD; 2023. Dental cone beam computed tomography: Information for patients and parents; updated 28 Sep 2020 [cited 15 June 2023]. Available from: https://www.fda.gov/radiation-emitting-products/medical-x-ray-imaging/dental-cone-beam-computed-tomography#patientsparents
3. Al-Rafee MA. The epidemiology of edentulism and the associated factors: A literature review. J Family Med Prim Care 2020;9:1841-1843.
4. Emami E, de Souza RF, Kabawat M, Feine JS. The impact of edentulism on oral and general health. Int J Dent 2013;2013:498305.
5. Chen J, Ren CJ, Wu L, et al. Tooth loss is associated with increased risk of dementia and with a dose-response relationship. Front Aging Neurosci 2018;10:415.
6. Tupac RG, Gillis RE Jr, Guichet GN, et al. Parameters of care for the specialty of prosthodontics. J Prosthodont [Internet]. 2005 Dec;14 (4 Suppl 1):14. Available from https://onlinelibrary.wiley.com/doi/10.1111/j.1532-849X.2005.046_2.x
7. Mitrani, R. Terminal dentition: Where do we draw the line? [Internet]. Scottsdale, AZ: Spear Education LLC; 11 June 2019 [cited 15 June 2023]. Available from: https://www.speareducation.com/spear-review/2019/06/terminal-dentition-where-do-we-draw-the-line
8. Beumer J, Faulkner RF, Shah KC, Wu BM. Fundamentals of Implant Dentistry, Vol 1: Prosthodontic Principles. 2nd ed. Chicago: Quintessence, 2022.
9. Spear F. Evaluating facial esthetics: The esthetic plane [Internet]. Scottsdale, AZ: Spear Education LLC; 9 Mar 2017 [cited 15 June 2023]. Available from: https://www.speareducation.com/spear-review/2013/08/evaluating-facial-esthetics-the-esthetic-plane

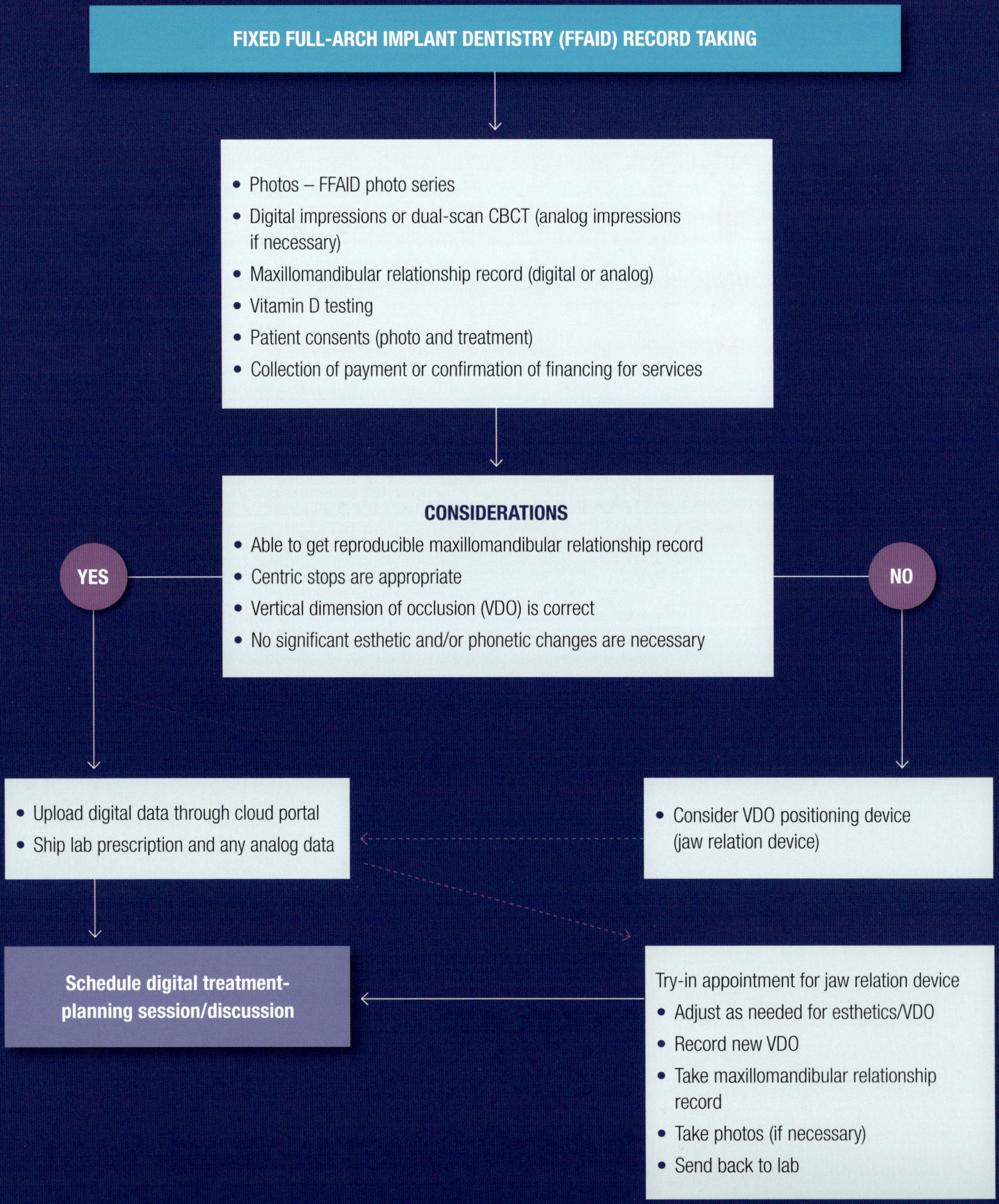
FIXED FULL-ARCH IMPLANT DENTISTRY (FFAID) RECORD TAKING
• Photos – FFAID photo series
• Digital impressions or dual-scan CBCT (analog impressions if necessary)
• Maxillomandibular relationship record (digital or analog)
• Vitamin D testing
• Patient consents (photo and treatment)
• Collection of payment or confirmation of financing for services
CONSIDERATIONS
• Able to get reproducible maxillomandibular relationship record
• Centric stops are appropriate
• Vertical dimension of occlusion (VDO) is correct
• No significant esthetic and/or phonetic changes are necessary
YES
NO
• Upload digital data through cloud portal
• Ship lab prescription and any analog data
• Consider VDO positioning device (jaw relation device)
Schedule digital treatment-planning session/discussion
Try-in appointment for jaw relation device
• Adjust as needed for esthetics/VDO
• Record new VDO
• Take maxillomandibular relationship record
• Take photos (if necessary)
• Send back to lab

DATA COLLECTION, PART 2. FINAL RECORDS

CHAPTER 3

Commitment: Be generous and avoid scarcity.
Generosity is a virtue recognized around the world,
and being generous helps one avoid falling into a scarcity mindset.
Giving is scientifically proven to increase happiness.

Once the financial arrangements have been reviewed and accepted by the patient, an appointment is scheduled for the remainder of the digital data collection. This appointment may take 1 hour or more depending on how much additional information needs to be obtained and if further clinical examination is necessary. Part II of the Data Collection Checklist (see Fig. 2.9b) can be used to document this visit.

Because the CBCT scan was taken at the patient's initial visit, no further radiographic data is needed unless something is unclear. Additional studies may be necessary though if you need to establish a different vertical dimension of occlusion (VDO) and the maxillomandibular relationship for the patient's interim prosthesis. These are discussed later in this chapter.

DIGITAL PHOTOGRAPHY

Digital dental photography has permanently changed the landscape of dentistry. Here is why I think it is critically important to use it in fixed full-arch implant rehabilitation.

- **Diagnosis and treatment planning.** Having patient photographs available to look at while developing a patient's diagnosis and treatment plan is essential. Too often in dentistry, the process of getting the actual diagnosis is overlooked, and we jump right into planning the treatment needed to fix a patient's problem. Our colleagues in medicine understand the importance of diagnosis, and the insurance companies require it as a condition of coverage. Diagnostic codes in medicine are the norm but are not commonly used as a prerequisite to treatment in dentistry. Nevertheless, having a diagnosis is important, and photographs can aid in this. In addition, planning cases when the patient is not sitting right in front of you can be much easier if you have the appropriate series of photographs to work from.

- **Documentation and medicolegal protection.** Full-arch implant dentistry is much more complex than placing a class 2 composite restoration, performing a root canal, or even placing a single implant. Unlike general restorative dentistry, where problems or mistakes can often be "fixed" easily and cost effectively, fixed full-arch implant dentistry can be disastrous for a patient if things go wrong, or for you if a malpractice lawsuit is brought against you. Having good photographs can protect you as well as defend other colleagues if you end up in a legal situation.
- **Patient communication and education.** When presenting options to a patient, you can use photographs to help them understand the different procedures they may be a candidate for. Many patients absorb information better when it is presented visually rather than verbally. I have been known to pull out my smartphone during an initial consultation with a patient to show them photographs of previous patients who have given their written consent and undergone similar procedures. When a patient can "see" someone with issues related to theirs, they will often have an "a-ha" moment and be more inclined to develop trust and believe that you can help them.
- **Laboratory communication.** We sometimes forget that the dental laboratory is our partner in fixed full-arch implant rehabilitation, and that it is helpful for them to see what we do. Photos and video can be vital in showing and explaining design, relationships of the mouth and lips to the teeth, shade, gingival characteristics, and so forth. When a lab technician can see a patient's face and the anatomy surrounding the teeth, it gives them insights as to how they can help us get the best results for our patient.
- **Marketing.** There is truth in the cliché "a picture is worth a thousand words." Just as they can be used to explain a procedure to a patient, photographs can also be used to create emotion in your marketing. We have used full-face before-and-after photographs of our patients in internal and external marketing for over 20 years, and they have been a powerful aid in helping potential patients not only see the quality of our work but generate desire and motivation to move forward with treatment. Patient photographs can also build credibility for you and your team. (The importance of obtaining written consent from your patients before using their likeness for marketing purposes is discussed later in this chapter.)

Cameras

With so many camera options to choose from, some dentists may find themselves in a "paralysis by analysis" situation. Keeping it simple (as is my mantra) may be the best course of action, so this discussion is limited to an overview of the main options. For those of you who want a deeper dive into dental photography, I recommend the recent book by Dr. Amanda Seay entitled *SEE: Art, Esthetics, Dental Photography* (Edra Publishing, 2022). This and other similar texts can be very helpful to those learning the basics as well as more advanced dental photography.

Smartphone cameras

One of the simplest ways to document these cases is to use the camera on your smartphone, because it is straightforward and requires little more than a steady hand and basic light attachment. PhotoMed makes a very good light attachment called the SDL® (Smartphone Dental Light) (Figs. 3.1, 3.2). I have used this setup in my practice for several years, and it has served me very well. Many smartphones can easily shoot photos and videos that can be uploaded to the laboratory more quickly than any other method allows. However, be aware of regulations under HIPAA (Health Information Portability and Privacy Act) in the U.S. and GDPR (General Data Protection Regulation) in the E.U. that protect sensitive information, including how you save the photos

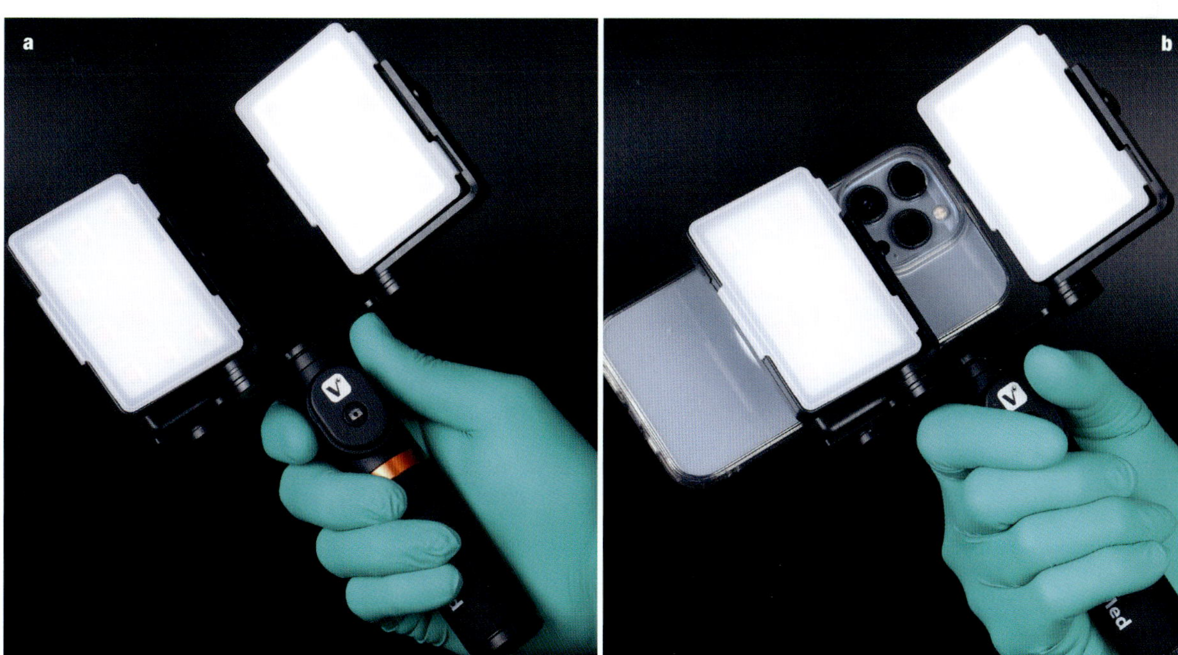

Figure 3.1 PhotoMed SDL® - Smartphone Dental Light (a) without and (b) with a smartphone camera attached.

and/or transfer them to a patient's digital chart. It is important to stay in compliance with these regulations (or whatever patient privacy regulatory agencies exist in your country) before sending photos and videos from your smartphone to your laboratory. Patient privacy and confidentiality are important and worth investigating. (See further discussion of this topic later in this chapter.)

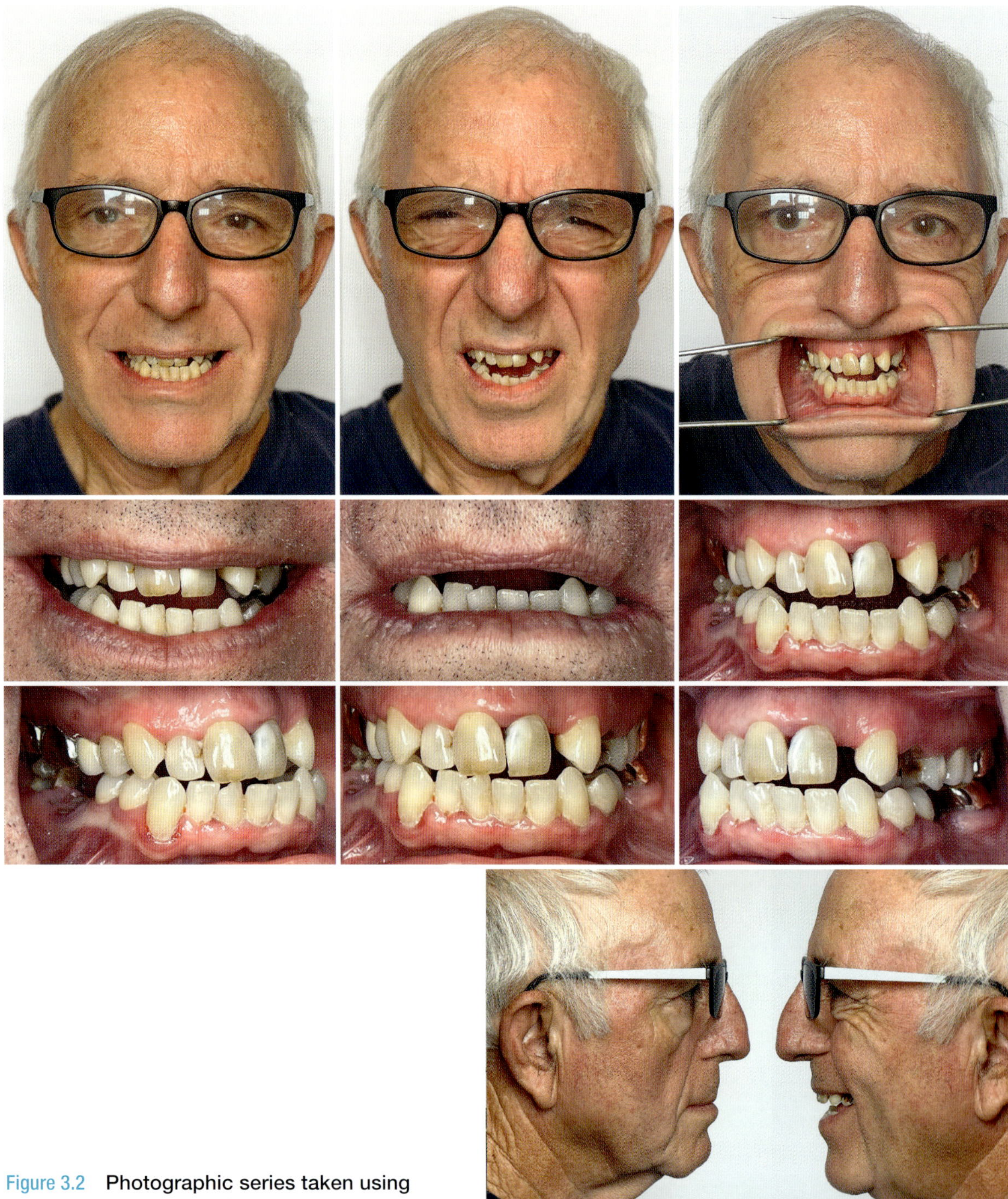

Figure 3.2 **Photographic series taken using a smartphone with the SDL by PhotoMed.**

Digital single-lens reflex (DSLR) cameras

There are a multitude of digital SLR options to choose from. If you decide to use a digital SLR camera, you can either purchase a camera "system" or setup from an online dental photography retailer or order individual pieces of camera equipment separately and create your own system. PhotoMed has several packages that can get you started. They have been very helpful to me and have provided great advice over the years. You may spend a little more money than if you purchased pieces separately, but their customer support has been outstanding, and you only have one call to make if you run into any issues with your setup (Fig. 3.3).

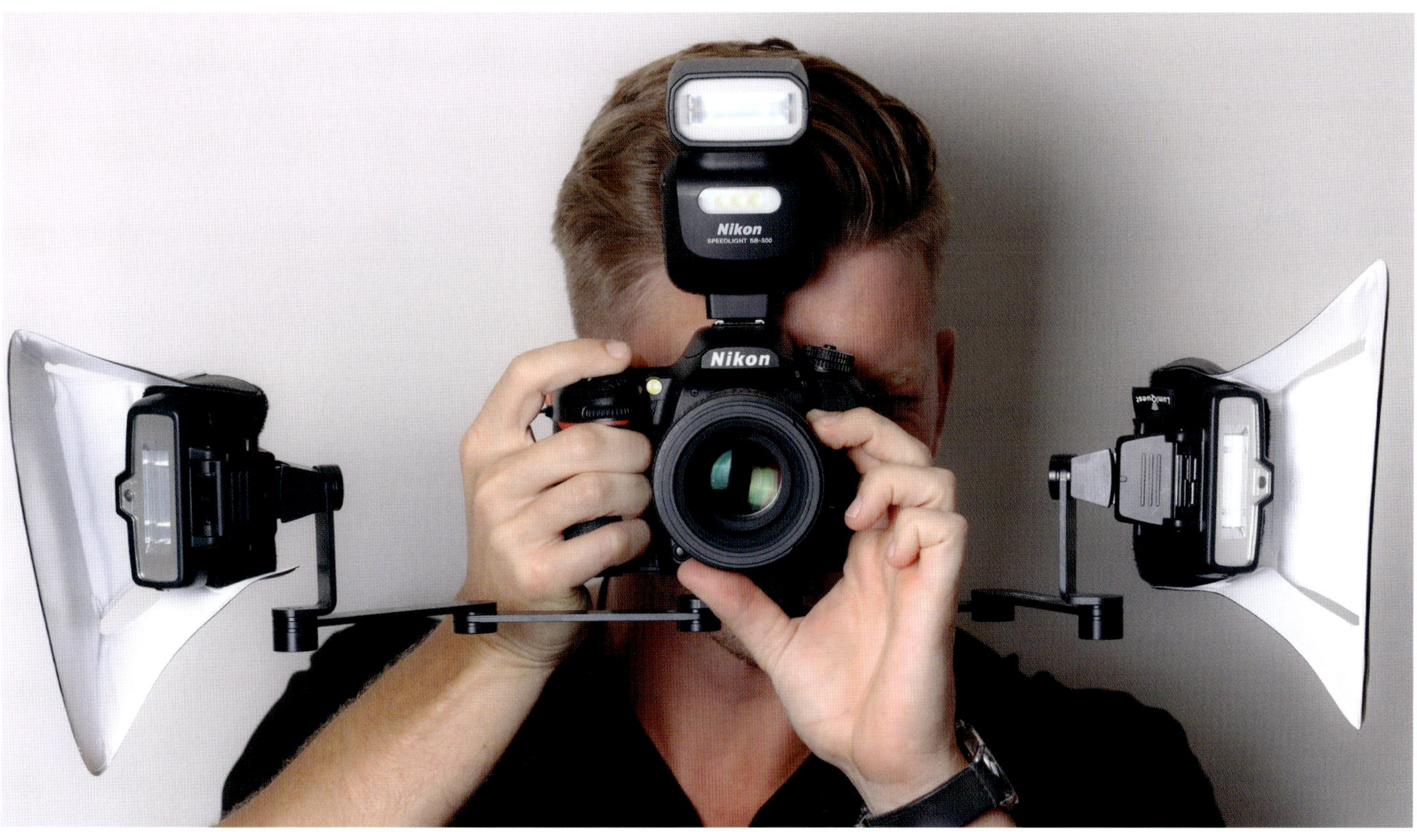

Figure 3.3 Digital single-lens reflex (SLR) camera system. This setup features the SLR camera body, a macro lens, a dual-point flash bracket, a shoe-mounted speedlight, and twin flash attachments.

While writing this book, I found that I needed to "up my game," so to speak, when it came to dental photography. I started using a simple DSLR setup with a ring flash and graduated over time to more advanced setups and higher-quality lenses and lighting systems. Figures 3.4 to 3.6 show a portable photo studio setup that we frequently use. However, there are several different ways to take the photos you need for fixed full-arch implant dentistry using a variety of camera and lighting setups. The general idea is to get high-quality photos, and the lighting and camera system you use depends on what is right for you. As you make the move into dental photography, you should be able to find a setup that meets your needs if you understand the rationale for your pictures and know what you want to use them for.

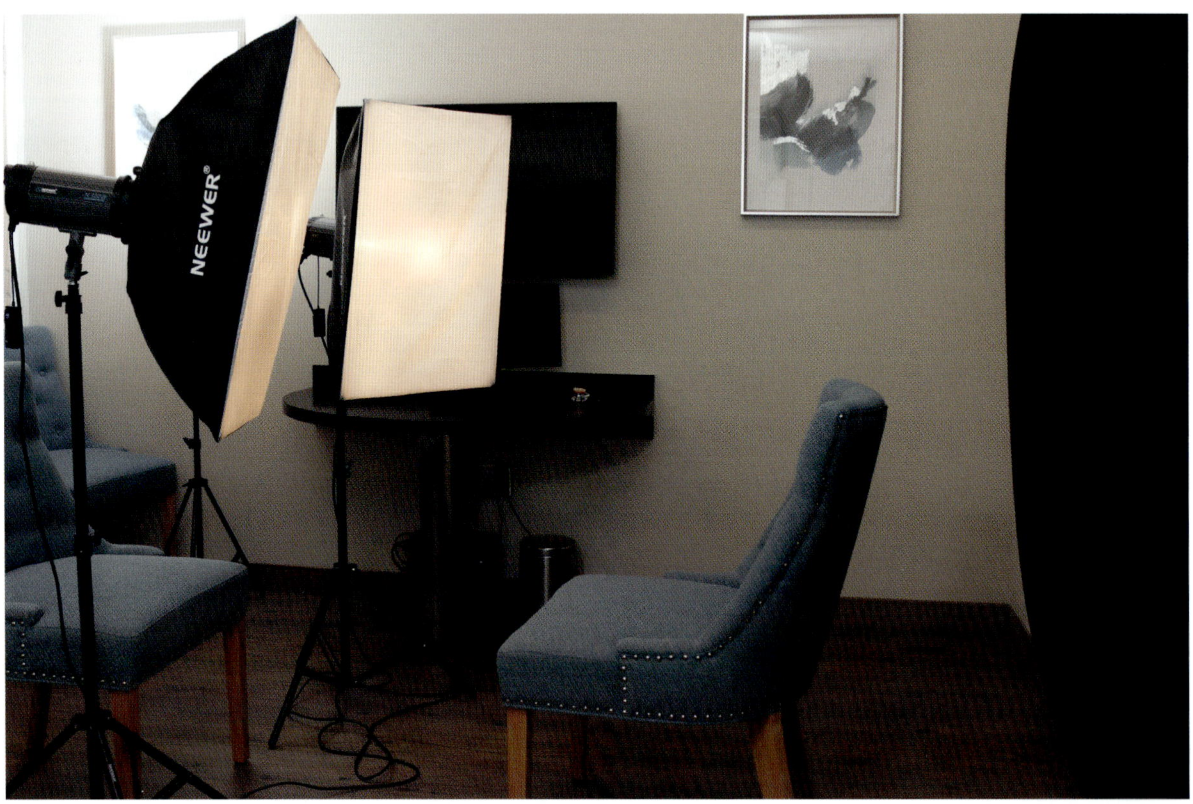

Figure 3.4 **Photo studio with strobe flashes and patient seating.**

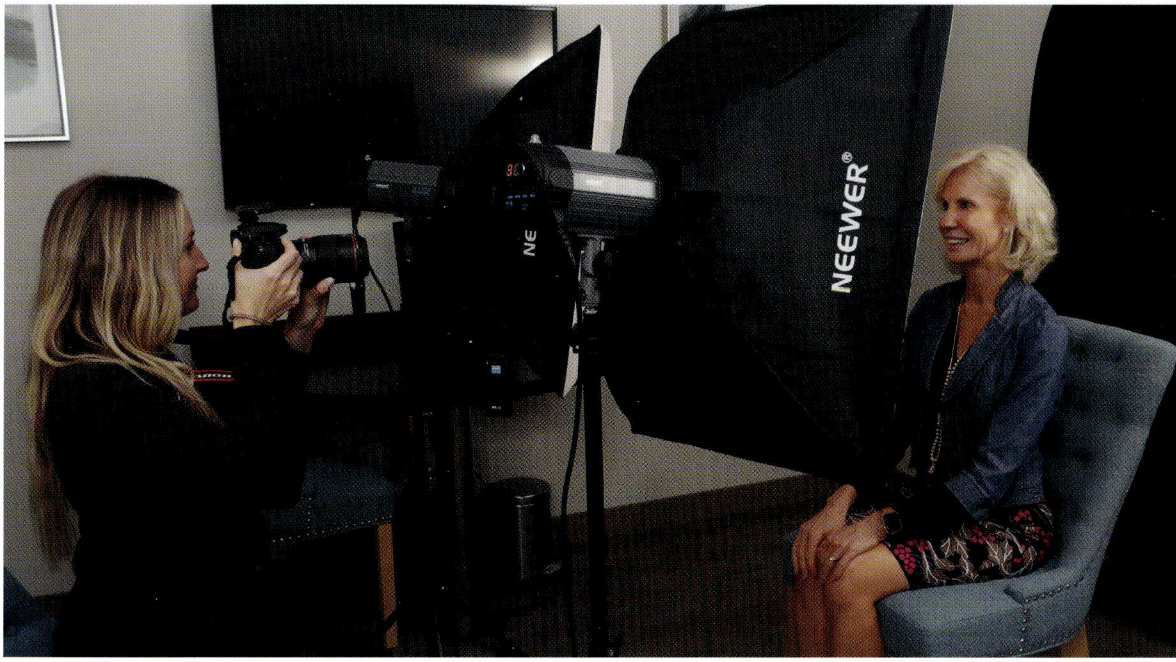

Figure 3.5 Team member shooting photos in the photo studio.

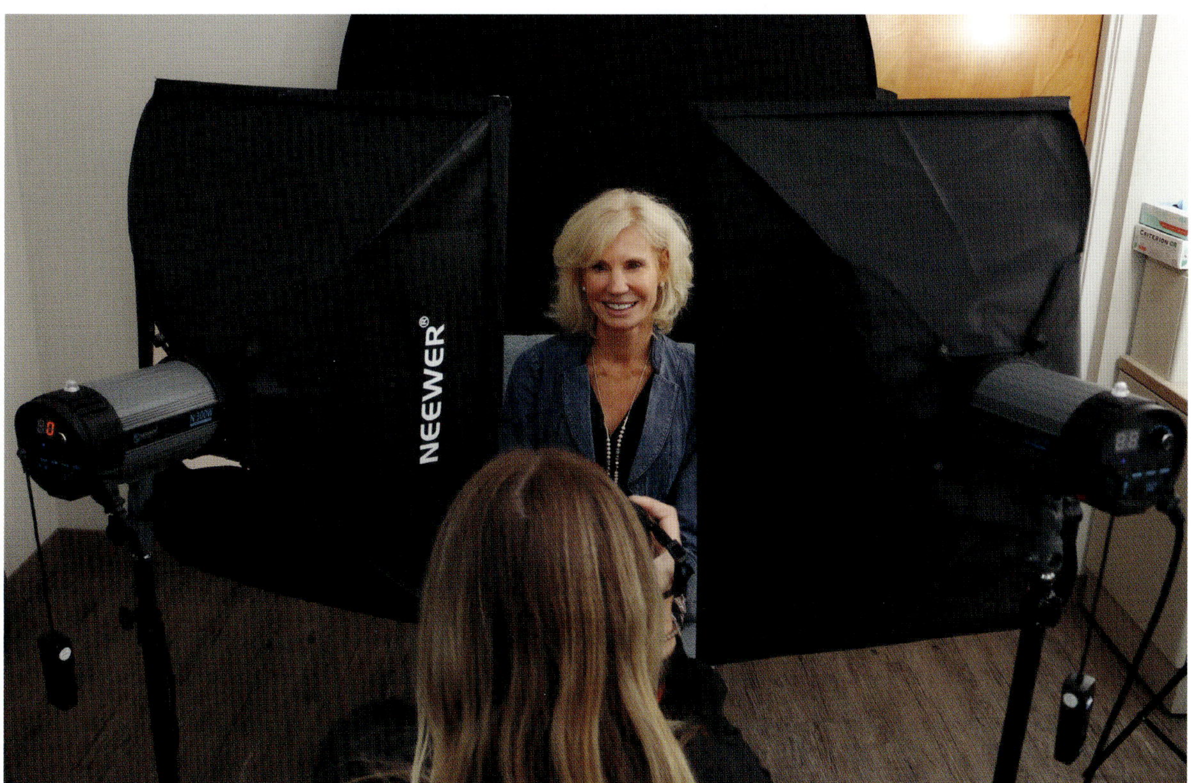

Figure 3.6 Photo studio with strobe flashes and solid background.

Software

Different types of software can be used to catalog and edit your photographs. The simplest and most practical way to store your photos is to import them into your patient chart software, which works okay for many clinicians but has significant limitations when it comes to editing and using your pictures in your marketing. I have found that keeping copies of patient photographs in their charts is only step one. After my team uploads photos to our patient chart software, I have the photos transferred into a program called Adobe Lightroom® (Fig. 3.7). This cloud-based software allows me to access, view, and edit photos on all my work and home devices (computers as well as smartphones) and on different operating systems. Because photographs are stored in the cloud, they do not take up space on my devices. Other software programs provide similar functionality along with more robust organizational and editing tools, such as Adobe Bridge® with Adobe Photoshop®. Using a cataloging and editing software product instead of simply storing your photos in your patient charts gives you more flexibility and allows you to have more customized options. From simple to complex, there are plenty of software options available.

Video

Although dentists have been using photography for many years, video documentation in dentistry has only recently started to be more common. In the years before digital video, storing and then reviewing analog video was cumbersome, and it was also very difficult to catalog efficiently. Today, thanks to cloud software and less-expensive hard drives, video can be cataloged, stored, and viewed much easier. Although we do not regularly use video for documentation in my practice, I often take small clips for communicating with laboratories, patient education, lectures, and webinar content, as well as marketing. One of the most powerful methods of marketing to patients considering fixed full-arch dentistry is through video testimonials and educational clips. Patients who are actively looking for a clinician that provides advanced and more expensive procedures appreciate the chance to observe their provider in video. Websites like YouTube, Vimeo, Dailymotion, and other social media platforms work well. Video testimonials of patients who have gone through the process of fixed full-arch implant rehabilitation in your practice can carry a particularly powerful endorsement. Videos can also be used as educational tools for new team members who are hired into your practice. As technology advances, I think video will become more and more common and useful.

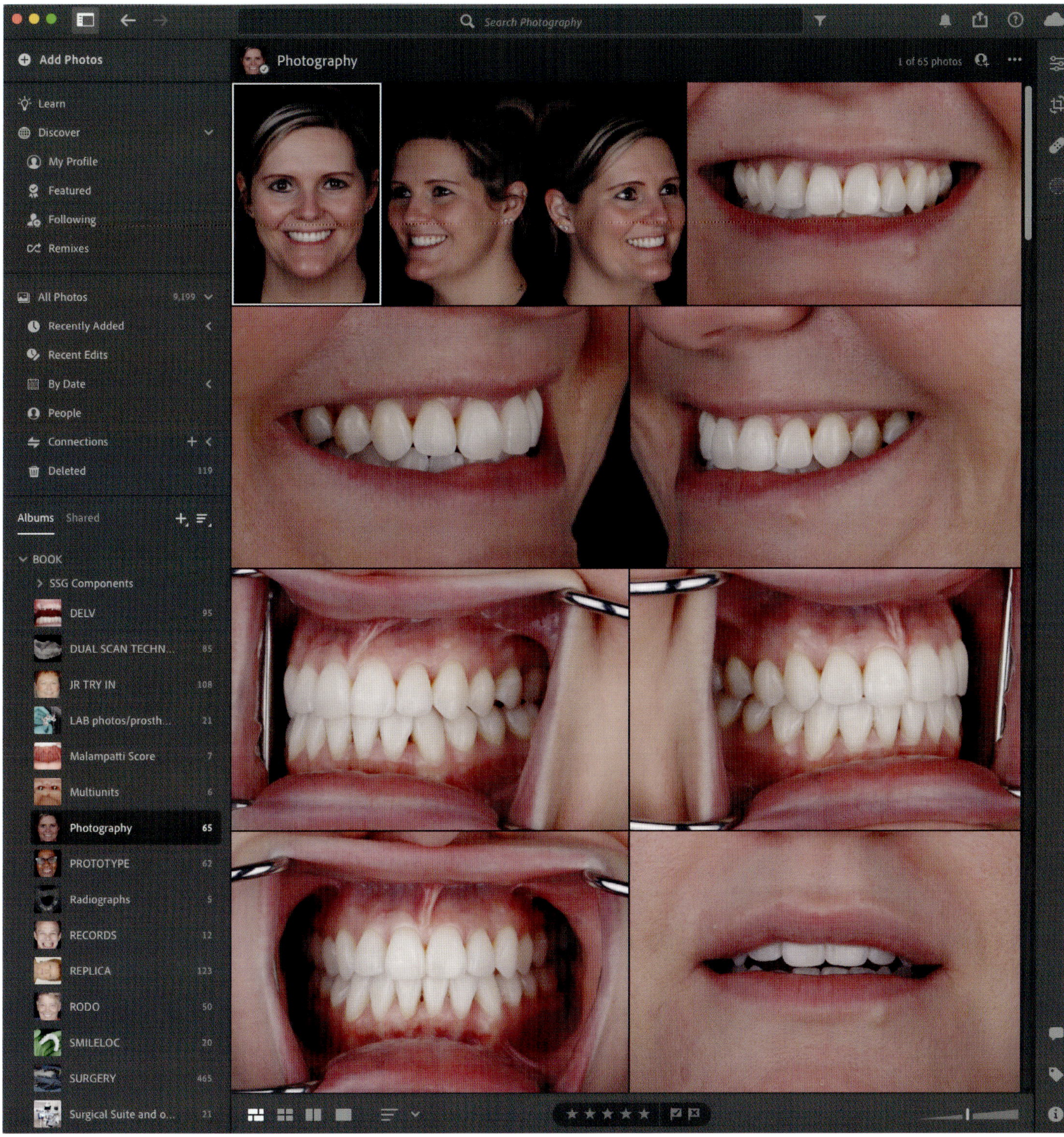

Figure 3.7 Adobe Lightroom® software designed for cataloging and editing photographs.

FIXED FULL-ARCH PHOTO SERIES

Being organized generally saves time and increases efficiency, and the same is true when it comes to photography. Most dental educators and associations recommend following a consistent method when documenting patient cases with photos. Many of the series are similar, but there can be variations in the number of photos and perspective. Based on long-term experience and discussions with multiple laboratory partners, I have found that taking a series of 11 photographs allows us to diagnose, treatment plan, and document our cases (Fig. 3.8). Remember that the photographs are not just for your own documentation but also for communicating important data to members of your team.

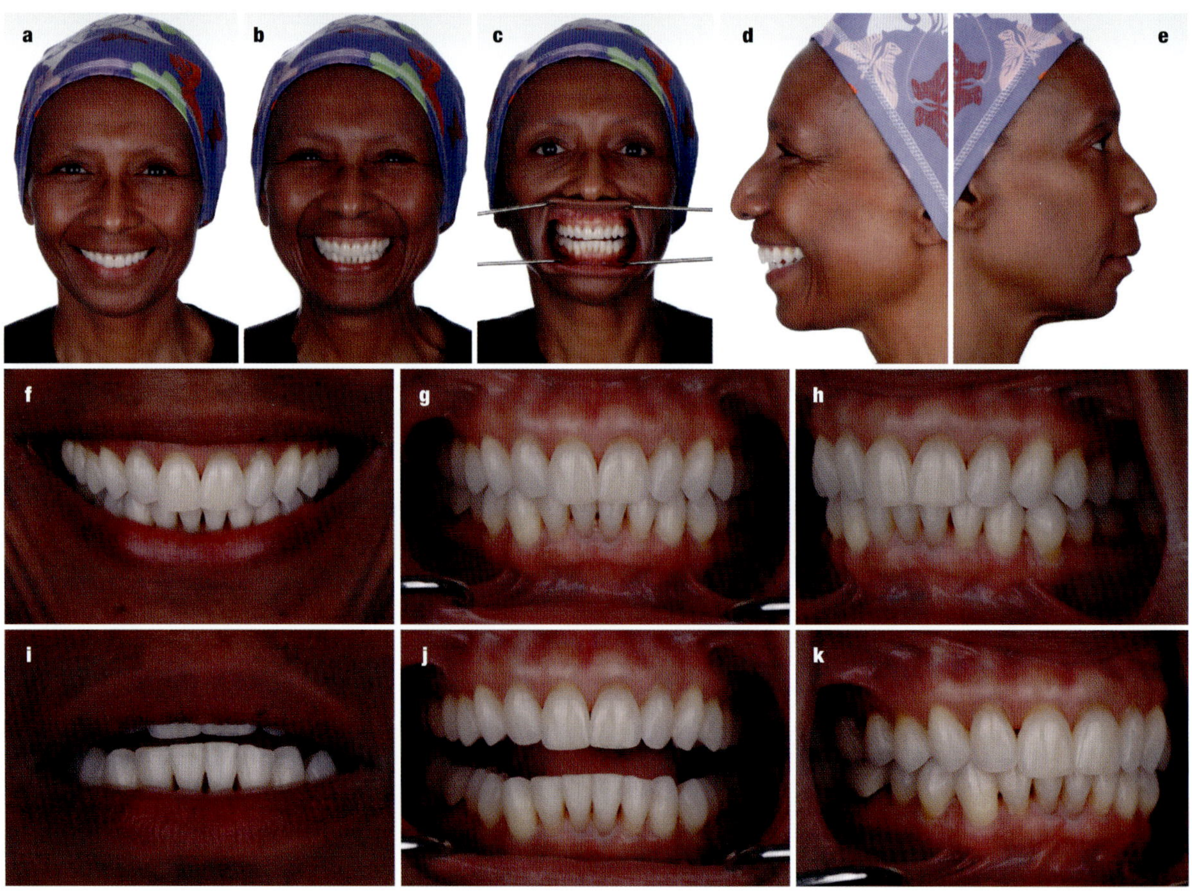

Figure 3.8 The fixed full-arch photo series for initial data collection featuring Marcia, the author's wonderful hygienist of 15 years. (a) Portrait view of natural smile; (b) Portrait view of exaggerated smile; (c) Retracted portrait view; (d, e) Profile views; (f) Close-up frontal view of smile; (g) Retracted close-up frontal view in maximal intercuspal position (MIP); (h) Retracted close-up lateral view of left side in MIP; (i) Close-up frontal view in repose; (j) Retracted close-up frontal view in open position; (k) Retracted close-up lateral view of right side in MIP.

In some circumstances I will take different or additional photographs and even video throughout the course of treatment, especially if I am planning to use the case for marketing or advertising. However, the photos described on the following pages are the core shots that I take of my patients before and during the process.

Portrait photos

Five portrait photos are taken as the first part of the series of photographs. These pictures will allow you and your lab partner to visualize not only the teeth but the whole face and how the patient's mouth and smile relate to their other features. To take these photos, the patient should be seated or standing comfortably in an upright and relaxed position. The photographs should be taken straight on in a horizontal plane as if you were lining the camera up with the patient's eyes. Your camera should be set up for portraits, with the F-stop and lighting adjusted accordingly.

Photo 1

The natural smile (Fig. 3.9)

Patients with deteriorated or terminal dentitions often have a hard time smiling. For years they have been trying to hide their smile, and their smile muscles consequently "forgot" how to work. Ask the patient to smile and show their teeth. For patients having difficulty, you may have to take a few minutes to teach them how to smile again. Coaching a patient by using a team member as a model and having the patient mimic their gestures has proven helpful in our practice.

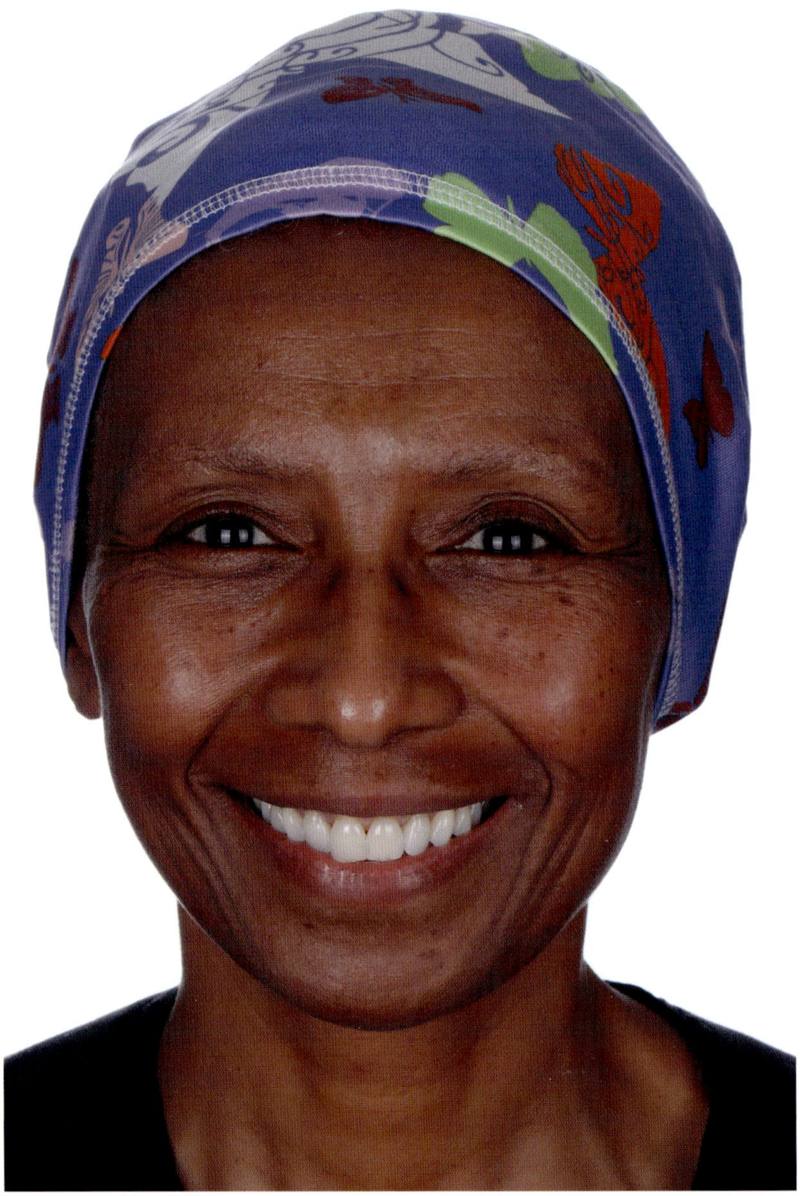

Figure 3.9 **Natural smile portrait photograph.**

The exaggerated smile (Fig. 3.10)

This photo is important in fixed full-arch implant dentistry cases because we need to be able to see how active a patient's upper lip can get. Patients with high smile lines—those who lift their upper lip considerably during smiling, laughing, or speaking—could present concerns in a fixed full-arch type of implant prosthesis (particularly with FP2 and FP3 designs). They may potentially show the transition line where the prosthesis and their natural gingival tissue meet. This can be esthetically unappealing. It is essential in case planning that you and your lab partner know where this transition line is. For patients in whom the exaggerated smile is significant, it can be helpful to use a clear ruler and measure the distance from the apex of the anterior teeth or edentulous ridge to the bottom of the upper lip. You can then use this information to determine what limitations exist in developing certain types of fixed full-arch prosthesis designs for that particular patient. Getting a patient to show you an exaggerated smile may also take some coaching. Showing them photos of others or having them observe someone doing it is useful. I have asked patients on occasion to "snarl", which is a good way to observe the mobility of the upper lip.

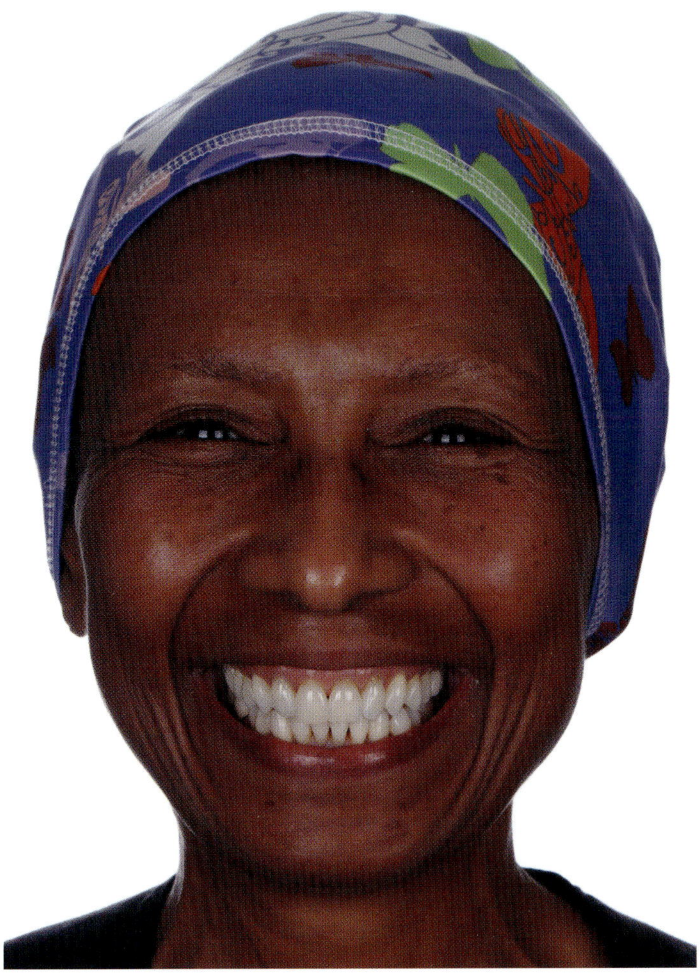

Figure 3.10 **Exaggerated smile portrait photograph.**

The profile—Smile and no smile (Fig. 3.11)

When a patient is turned to the side, you can evaluate their profile and gain a better understanding of how the lower third of their face fits into the big picture. Skeletal classification, lip support, chin position, and other data can be gathered from these photos. Have the patient smile normally for one photo and then take another of them not smiling.

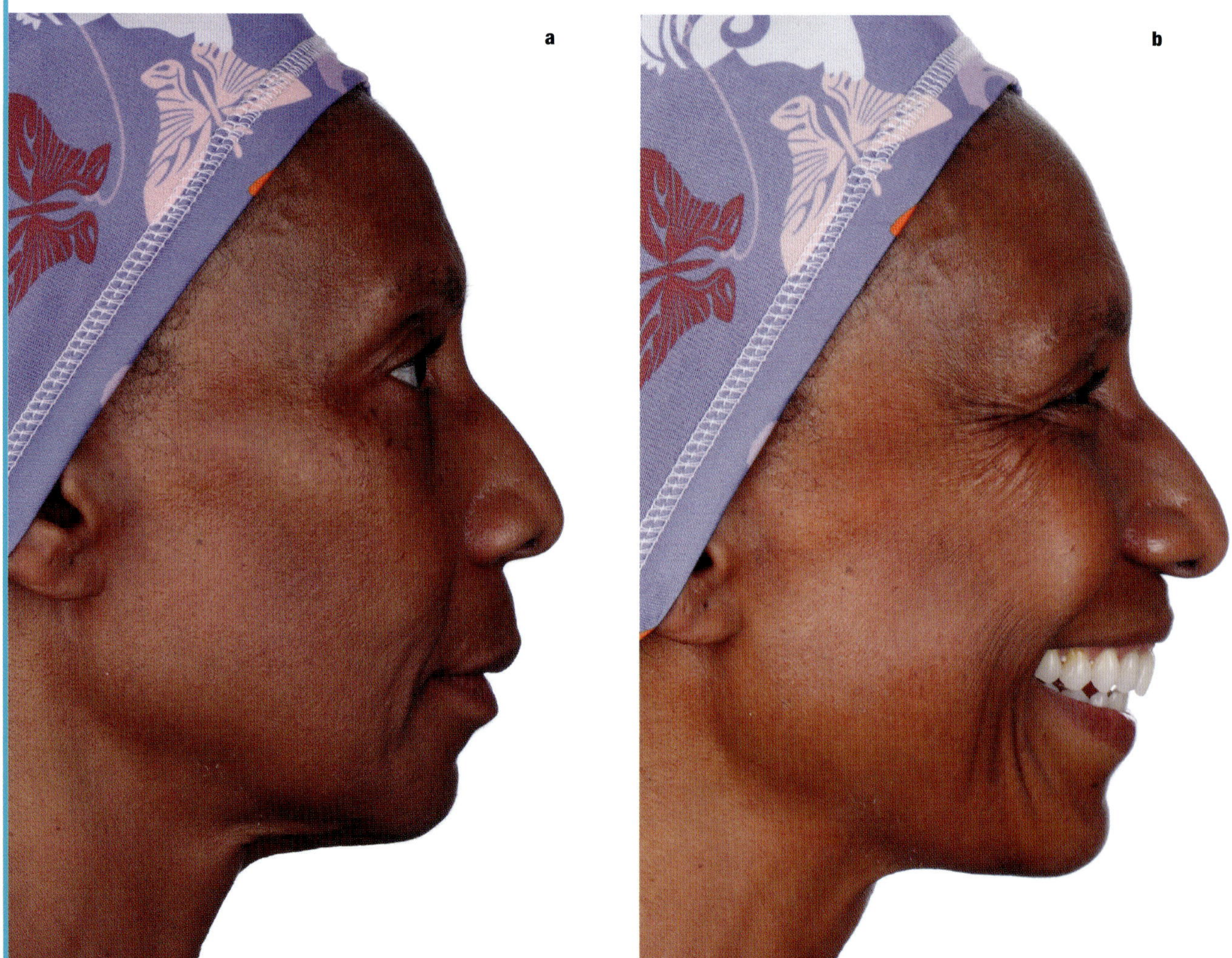

Figure 3.11 Profile portrait (a) no smile and (b) smile photographs.

The retracted portrait (Fig. 3.12)

The retracted photos are usually the most challenging. It may require a little patience and some assistance from a team member, but have the patient hold the cheek retractors in a position that allows you to capture a photograph of their entire mouth. I prefer to use stainless steel retractors, but you can use whatever gets you the best results. Have the patient relax their lips and pull the retractors to the side and forward just slightly to allow light to come in and expose most of the teeth and oral cavity.

This photograph is very helpful for observing a patient's horizontal occlusal plane. It can also provide additional information about the midline and other landmarks. Have the patient hold the retractors in place and open slightly so it is easier to define where the incisal edges are.

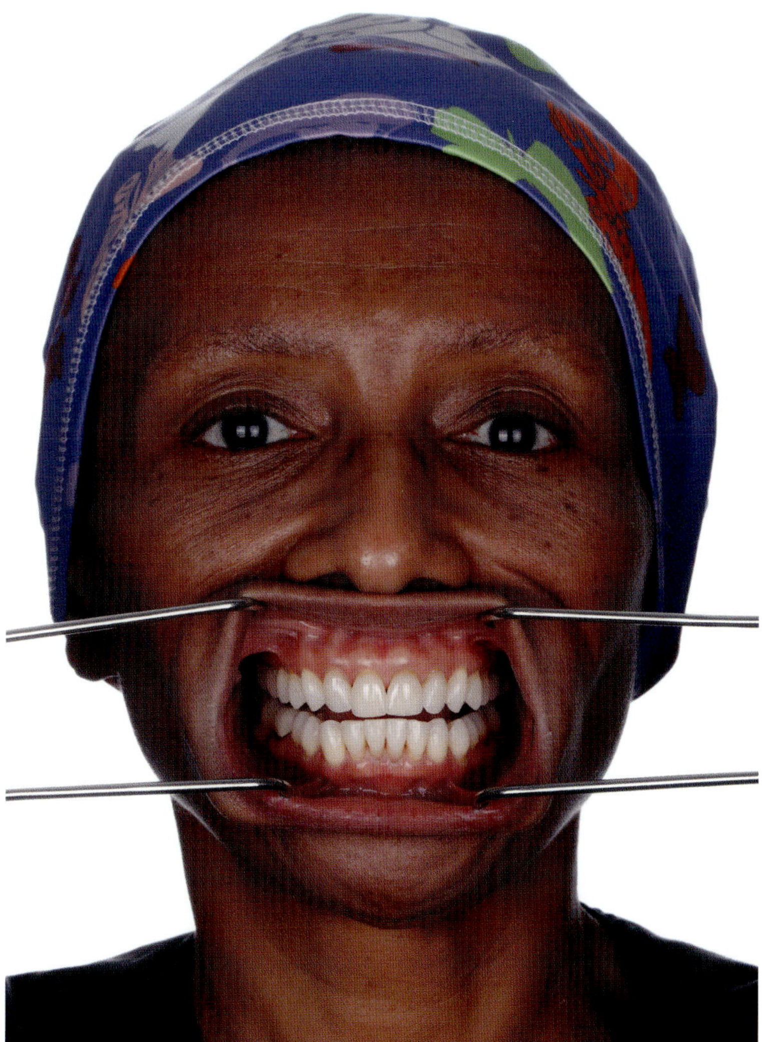

Figure 3.12 **Retracted portrait photograph.**

Close-up photos

The next series of photographs can also be taken with the patient in the same seated or standing position. As you move closer, the F-stop should increase, and less light will be needed. For efficiency, have the patient continue using the retractors and simply change the settings on your camera from portrait to close-up. You can then move in and take the following six photographs.

Photo 6

Retracted—Open (Fig. 3.13)

For this picture, have the patient open slightly to expose the occlusal and incisal edges of their dentition.

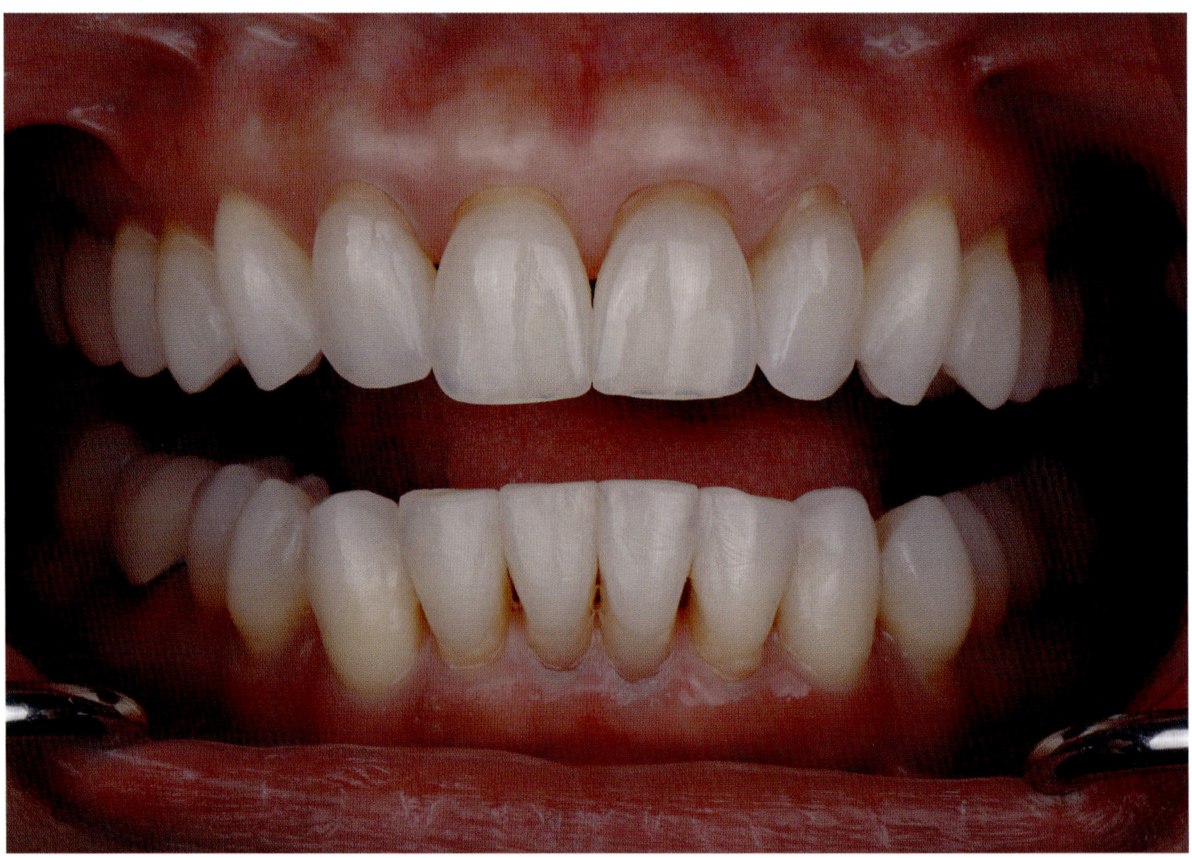

Figure 3.13 **Close-up retracted open photograph.**

Photo 7

Retracted—MIP (Fig. 3.14)

Have the patient go from slightly open to biting down into maximal intercuspal position (MIP) for this picture.

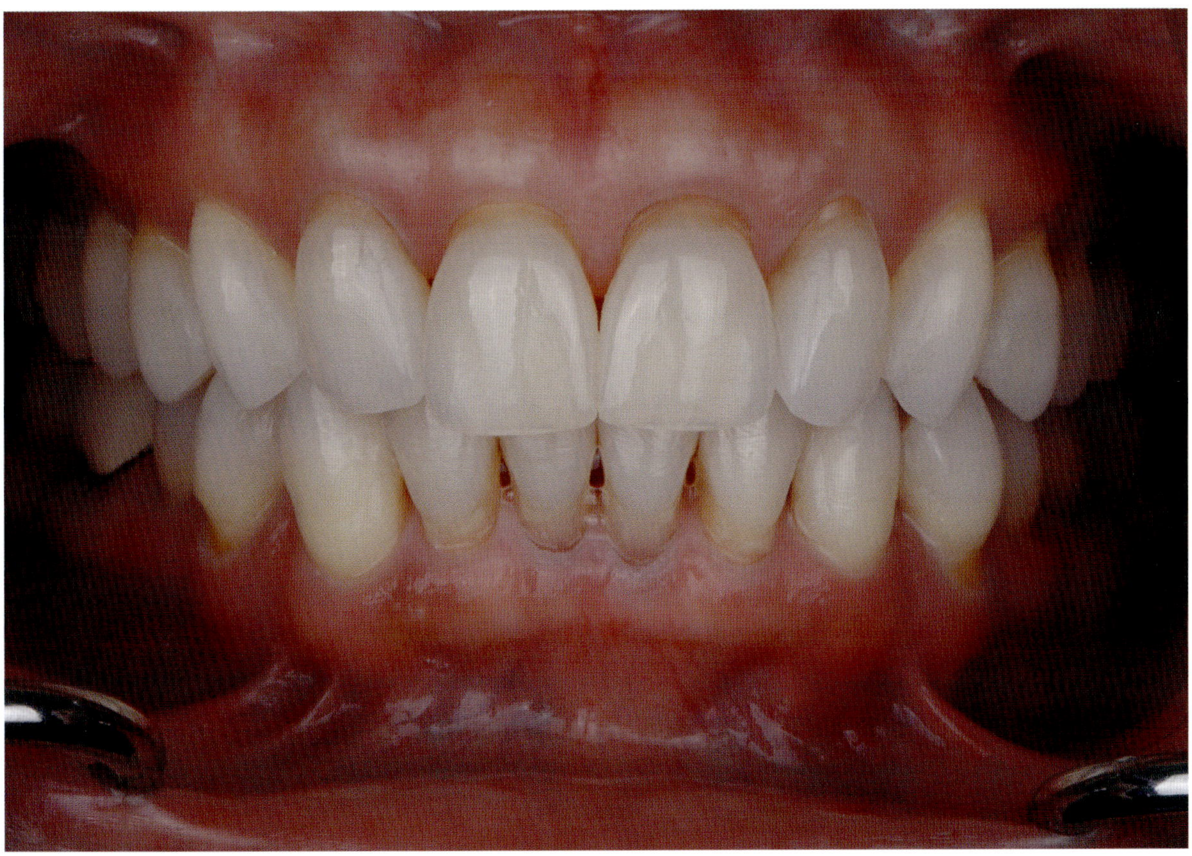

Figure 3.14 Close-up retracted in MIP photograph.

Retracted right and retracted left—MIP (Fig. 3.15)

With the patient closed in MIP, ask them to turn their head right and then left to get these shots. Patients may need to pull a bit more on the retractor on the side you are shooting; this is easier when they allow the retractor on the opposing side to release a bit. Try to get the mesial line angle of the maxillary canine on the opposite side in these shots.

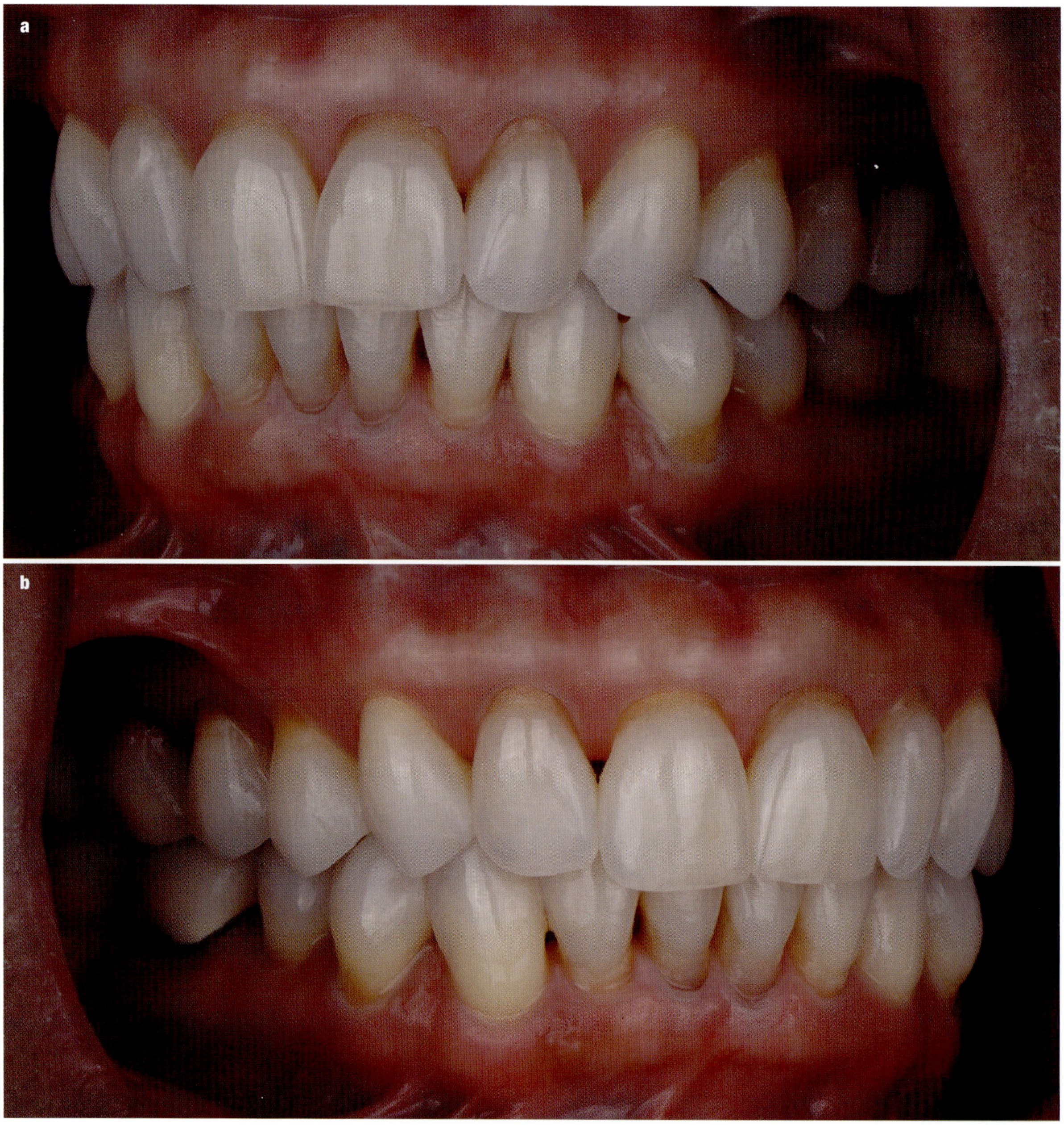

Figure 3.15 Close-up retracted (a) left and (b) right in MIP photographs.

Photo 10

The smile (Fig. 3.16)

The retractors can be removed for the last two photos, but you should stay in the same close-up position and have the patient give you a natural smile, just as they did in the first portrait photograph. This picture can capture more details of the patient's smile.

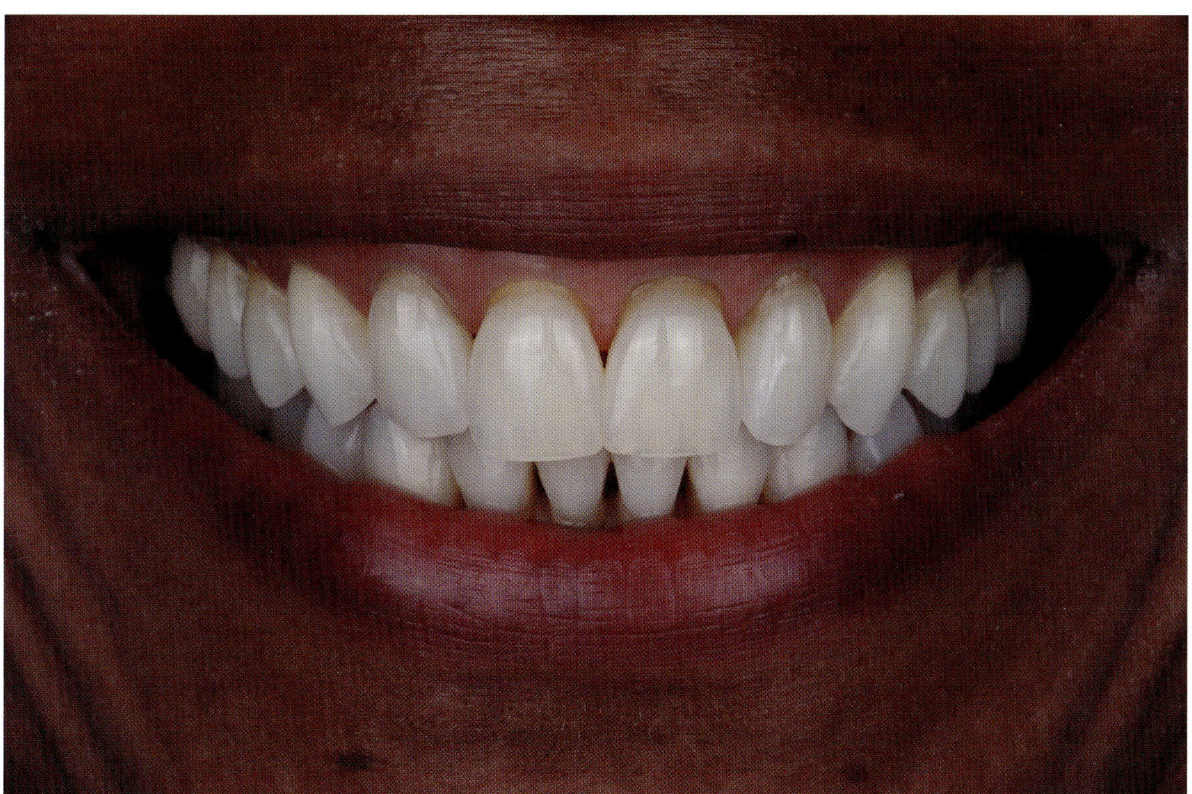

Figure 3.16 **Close-up smile photograph.**

Photo 11

Repose (Fig. 3.17)

This photo will allow you and your lab partner to better understand how the length of the teeth relate to the patient's lips at rest; it is sometimes referred to as the "Emma" picture. To get this shot, have the patient fully relax their face and say "Emma" and then hold their mouth completely still after the "a."

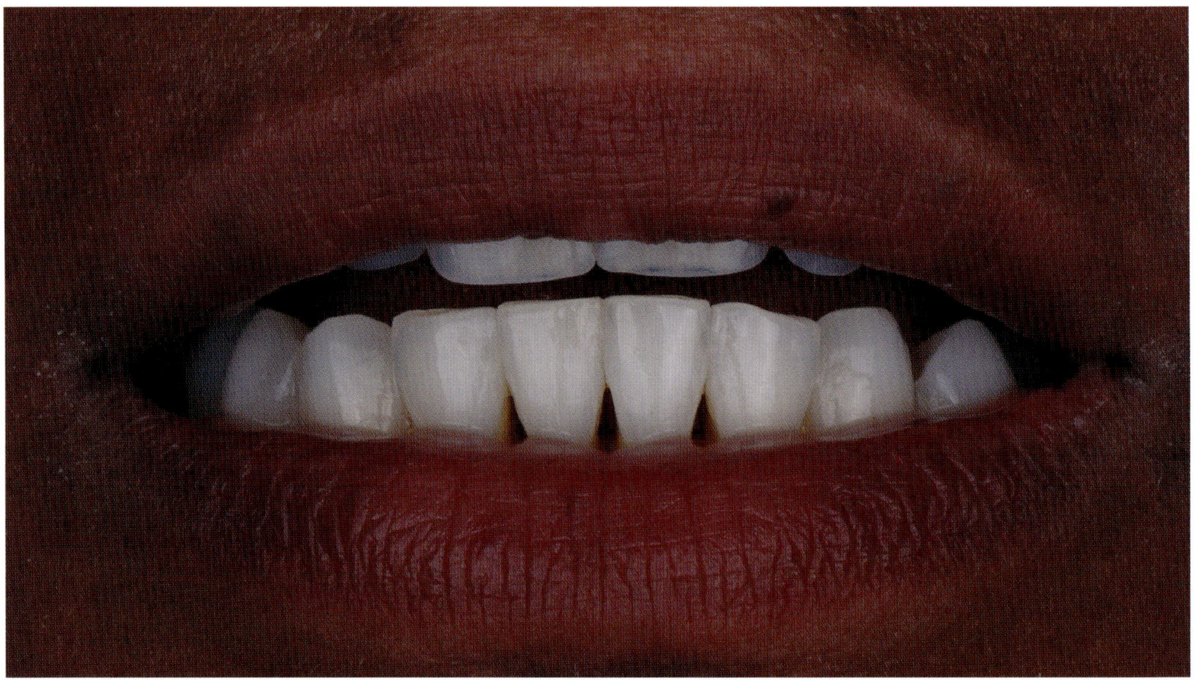

Figure 3.17 **Close-up in repose photograph showing the incisal edge positions of the teeth.**

PHOTO PRO TIP. A final word on photographs

Most of your fixed full-arch implant patients will not have an entire set of teeth, unlike the model shown in the examples for this photo series. If a patient is edentulous or partially edentulous but has dentures or partial dentures, you may want to take additional photos of them with their prosthetics in place. If a patient does not have a sufficient dentition, getting good photos will be challenging. You may need to retake the photo series once the patient has had a VDO orthotic positioning or jaw relation device fabricated. These are discussed later in this chapter.

DIGITAL IMPRESSIONS

For efficiency, you can and should delegate the task of taking digital impressions to one of your auxiliaries. Make sure the person you designate is highly trained to take accurate digital full-arch scans. This can be done using one of the many intraoral scanners on the market today. The key is to be able to obtain a downloadable .stl file to use in your practice or upload to your dental laboratory. STL is an abbreviation for stereolithography, a file format commonly used for 3D printing and computer-aided design (CAD).

Digital intraoral scanners

There are several systems available for dentists, and the cost of owning an intraoral scanner has declined considerably over the last several years. Some dental laboratories will give you an intraoral scanning system to use if you agree to work with them. In my practice, we use several types of intraoral scanners, and each has its strengths and weaknesses. This is a piece of technology you should purchase only after determining how it will integrate into your practice and what you will be using it for. In addition, consider the following.

- **Accuracy and efficiency.** Does the accuracy of the scans allow you to achieve a level of accuracy acceptable to you, and does the amount of time necessary to complete a scan meet your expectations?
- **Cost.** A scanning system can cost as little as a few thousand dollars and up to tens of thousands of dollars. Generally, the more you spend on an intraoral scanner, the more features it will have and the more you will be able to accomplish with it.
- **Comfort.** Is the scanner comfortable in your hands and, maybe more importantly, can your team members and auxiliaries use it easily? The larger scanner handles and cameras make scanning less comfortable for the patient and harder for some females and small-handed individuals to use.
- **Versatility.** Does the scanner allow you to use it for multiple purposes? There are some systems that allow you to capture digital impressions as well as design and predict tooth movement. To utilize your scanner in the fixed full-arch workflow presented in this text, you will need it to be proficient at intraoral scanning and scanning extraoral objects in 3D, such as dentures, appliances, and other prostheses.

- **Proprietary status.** Software that is used in digital intraoral scanners can be open source or closed source. An open system means you can use the files generated from the scanner with other technologies from other manufacturers. A closed system may mean that you are required to use specific technologies developed by the same company that makes the scanner, be it software or something else. Open-system scanner technology is my preference.
- **Customer support, contract, warranty.** These are considerations that can make or break your happiness with your intraoral scanner. Find out from other users how happy they are with these details.
- **Obsolescence.** It is a fact of modern life that technology, especially software, becomes obsolete much more quickly than it used to. Knowing the upgradability of your intraoral scanner components and software is important.

Digital impression-taking

Dentate and partially dentate at correct VDO

If your patient has teeth and has the appropriate VDO, you can scan the maxillary and mandibular arches using the same method as for digital diagnostic casts. Have the patient take out any removable appliances that are in the arch or arches that will undergo surgery. If the patient has any removable appliances in the opposing arch that you will be leaving unrestored, leave them in place for the digital impressions.

There are several important landmarks to obtain in your digital impressions. Be sure to capture the full palate of the maxillary arch, the teeth, the buccal and lingual vestibules, the maxillary tuberosities, and the mandibular retromolar pad areas (Figs. 3.18, 3.19). It is a good idea to have a backup immediate denture in case you find that you are unable to load your implants on the day of surgery. If you do not capture the aforementioned landmarks, your laboratory will have difficulty making an acceptable denture for your patient to wear.

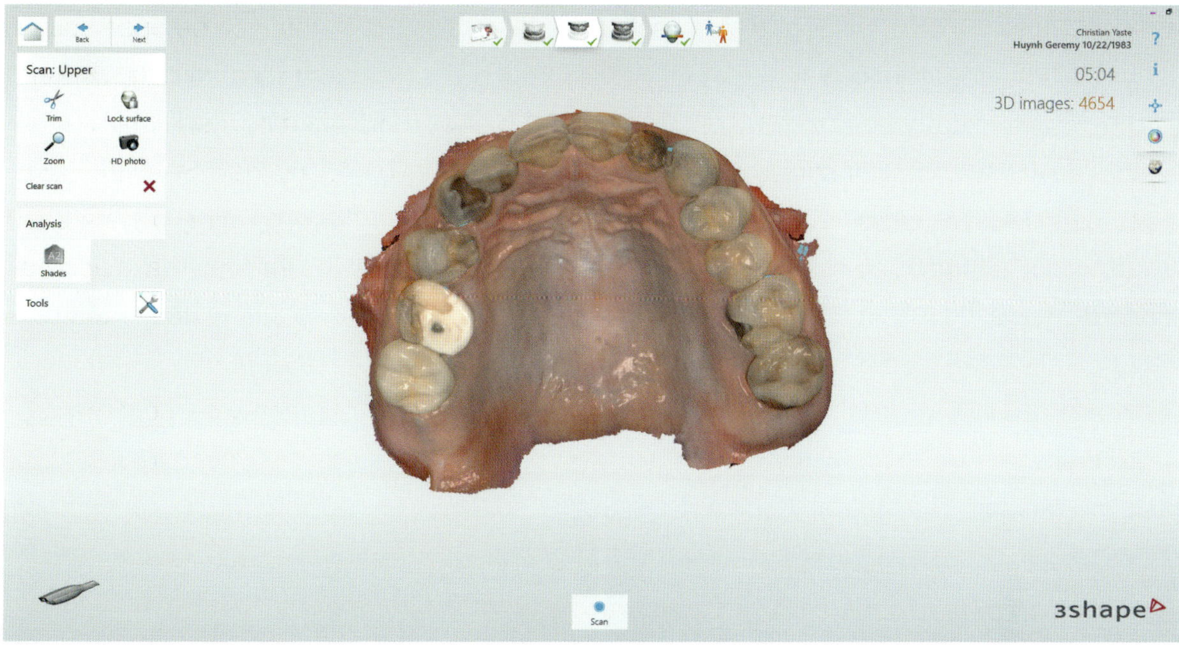

Figure 3.18 Digital scan of maxillary arch capturing the entire palate and maxillary tuberosities as well as the teeth.

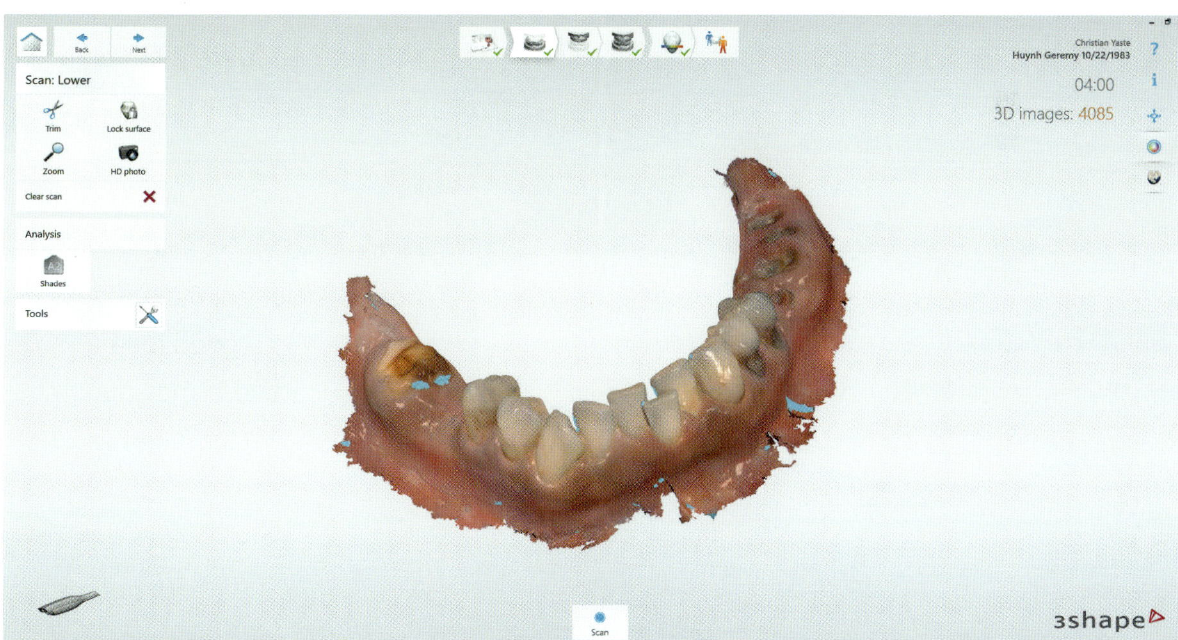

Figure 3.19 Digital scan of mandibular arch capturing teeth, ridges, retromolar pads, and vestibule.

Edentulous at correct VDO

If your patient is edentulous and has an appropriate VDO, and you have already taken a dual-scan CBCT at the prior visit, you may only need to take a digital impression if the opposing arch is dentate. As outlined in Chapter 2, the laboratory will use the patient's current denture with the fiducial markers to merge into the software as a record of where the patient's teeth are currently located in the arch. The lab will also be able to identify the morphology of the soft tissues covering the edentulous arch on the CBCT. After taking the scan of the patient with the denture and fiducial markers in place, be sure to also scan the denture separately, as shown in Figures 3.20 and 3.21.

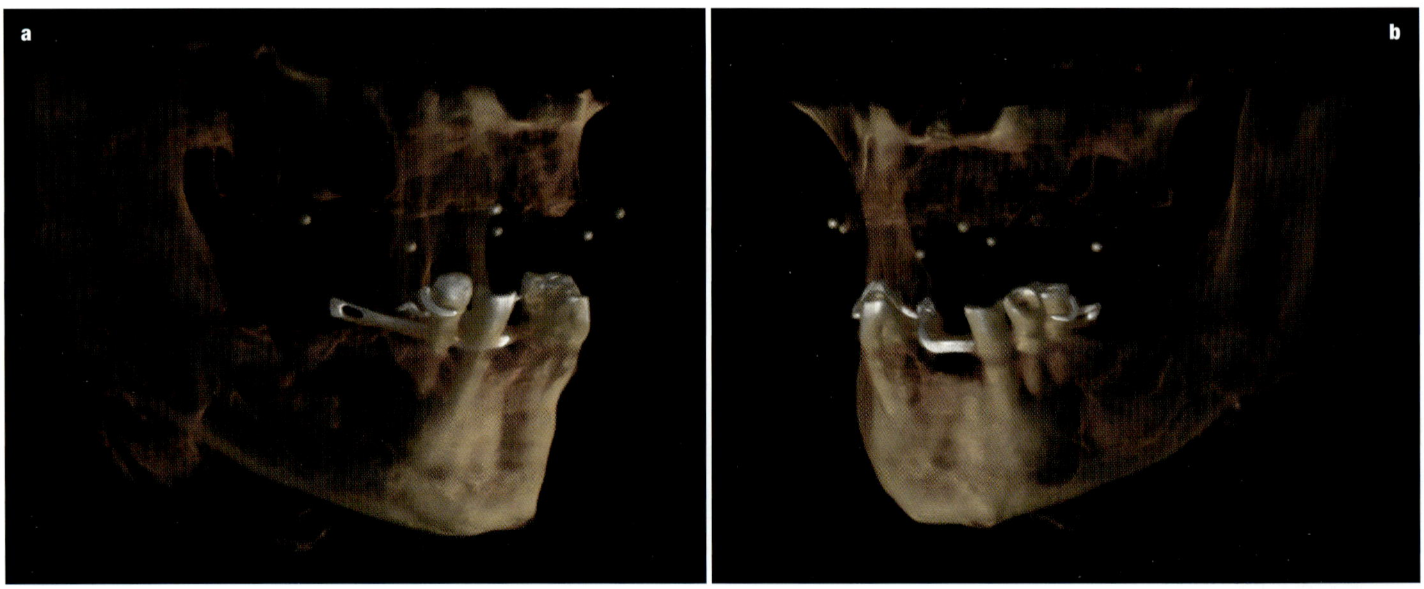

Figure 3.20 (a, b) CBCT scans of an edentulous maxillary arch with a complete denture and fiducial markers in place, taken with the dual-scan technique.

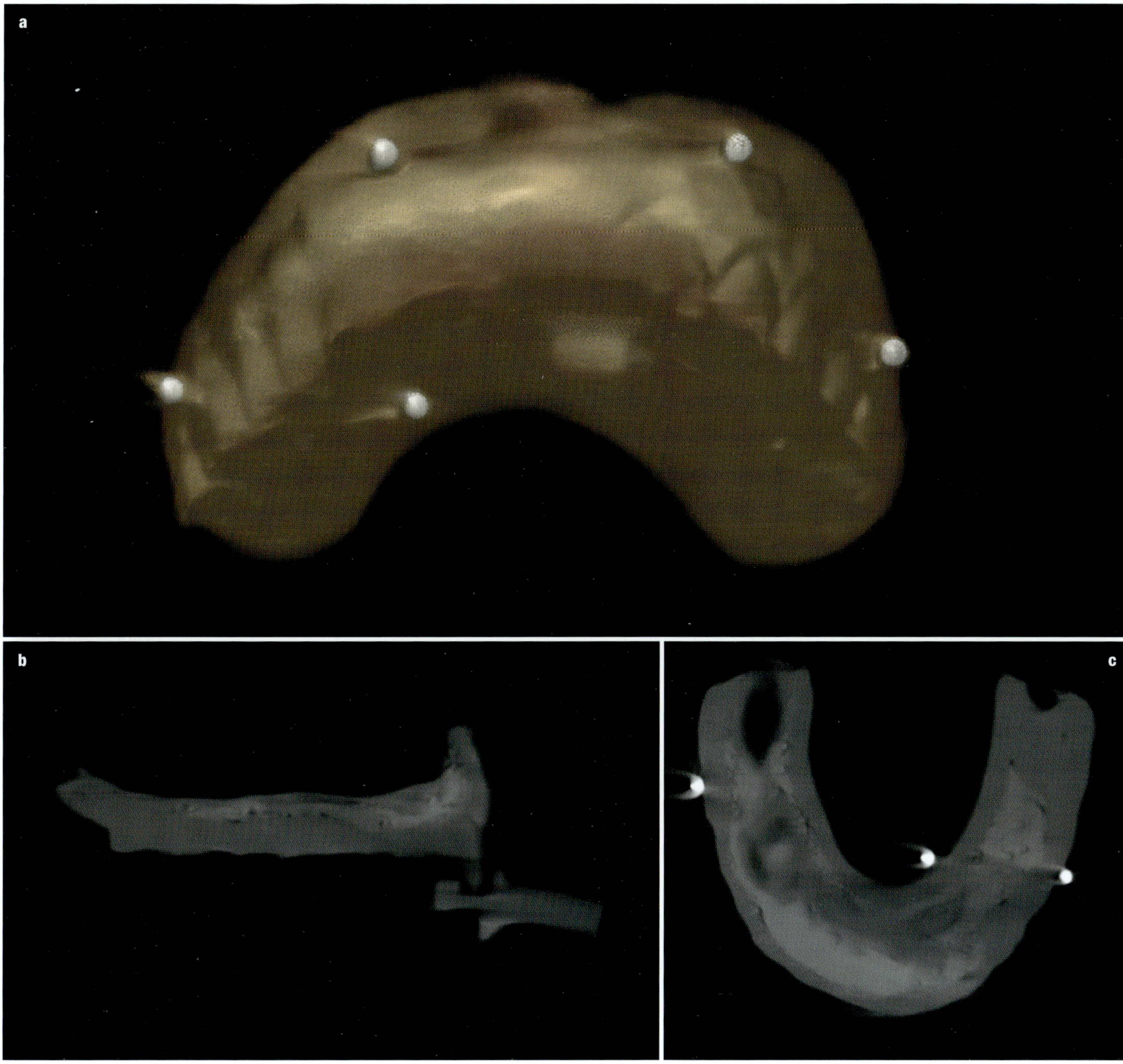

Figure 3.21 CBCT scans of a maxillary denture with fiducial markers representing the views obtained in the second scan of the dual-scan technique. (a) 3D view; (b) Cross-sectional view; (c) Axial view.

Maxillomandibular relationship record

Dentate and partially dentate at correct VDO

The next step is to obtain the patient's maxillomandibular relationship record, which is easy to do in patients who are dentate and at an acceptable VDO. Generally, I have the patient close into MIP and see if this is reproducible and comfortable. However, I have found it worthwhile also to determine if the patient can place the mandible in a more retruded position, or what is known as *centric relation* (CR). If the patient has a shift between these two positions, I record the maxillomandibular relationship in the patient's most retruded position, or CR. However, recording the maxillomandibular relationship in this position does not mean that the definitive restorations will function in the same position. After a patient has become fully edentulated, the masticatory system may change, and considerations will need to be made before restoring the patient into their final occlusion.

The patient's maxillomandibular relationship can be recorded with the same intraoral scanner used to obtain the digital impressions (Figs. 3.22, 3.23). I recommend that the dentist always be the one to record and evaluate the maxillomandibular relationship. If an accurate maxillomandibular relationship cannot be recorded in the software, you can veer off the digital highway, so to speak, and use analog occlusal registration material. In some cases where the patient is missing a significant number of teeth or has little or no posterior occlusion, I will often use polyvinyl siloxane (PVS) putty to record the positions of the jaws and teeth.

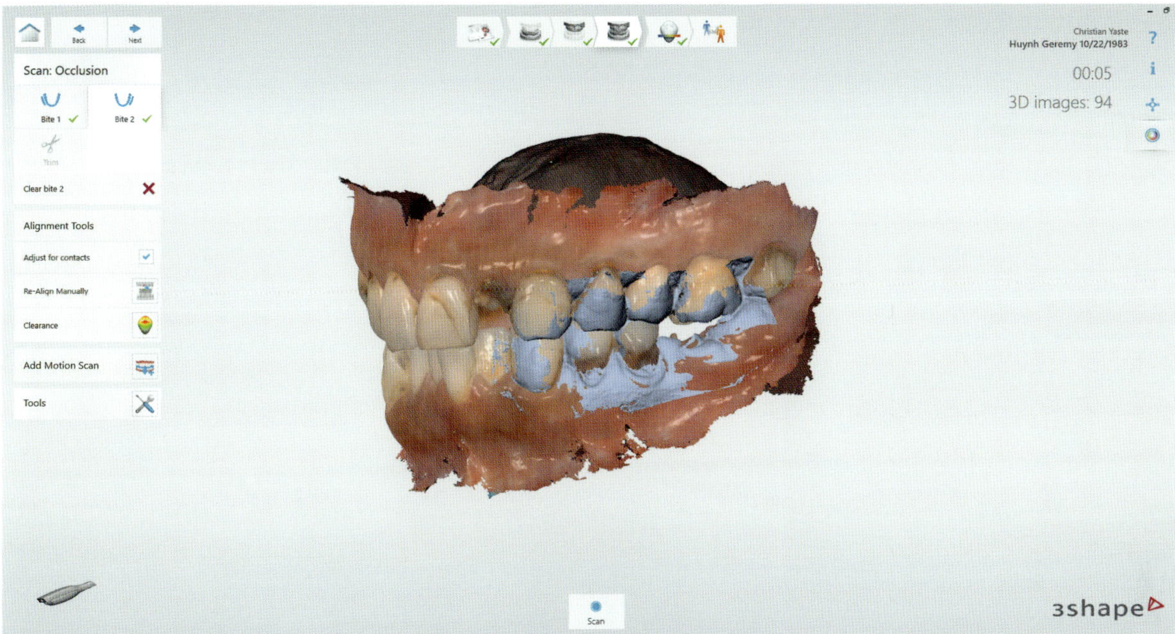

Figure 3.22 Digital scan of maxillomandibular relationship, left side.

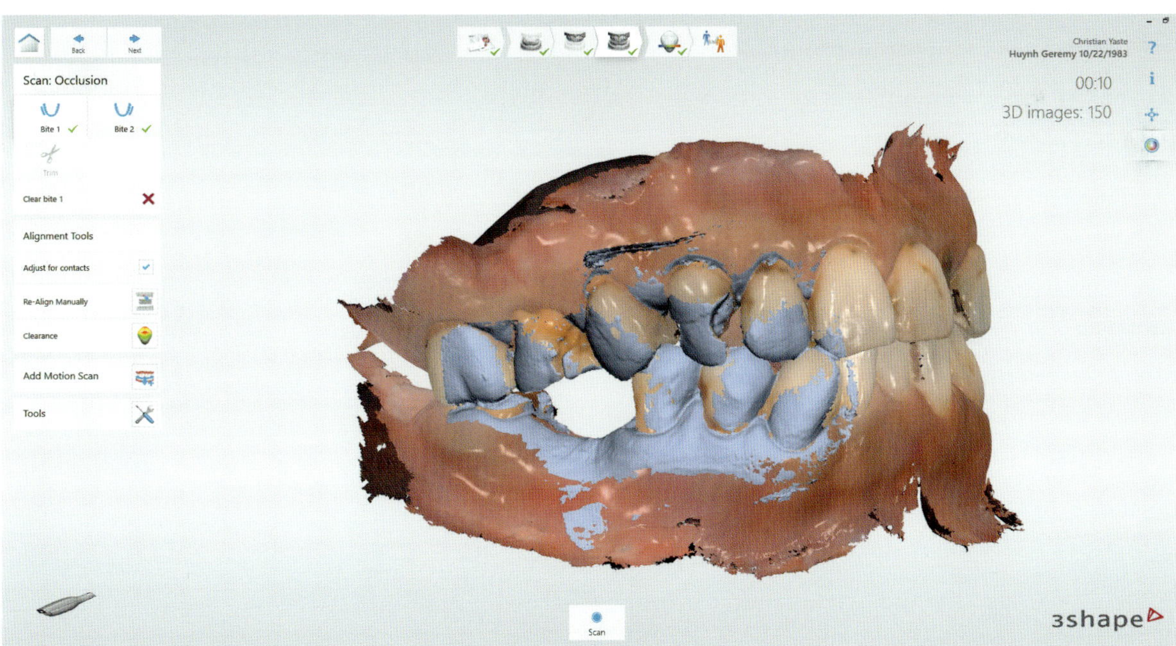

Figure 3.23 Digital scan of maxillomandibular relationship, right side.

Edentulous at correct VDO

As with digital scans or impressions, it is not necessary to take a maxillomandibular relationship record when a patient is fully edentulous and wearing a denture. Again, this is assuming that you took the initial CBCT using fiducial markers with the patient in MIP, and the maxillomandibular relationship was already recorded for the dental laboratory that will be creating the interim prostheses (Figs. 3.24, 3.25).

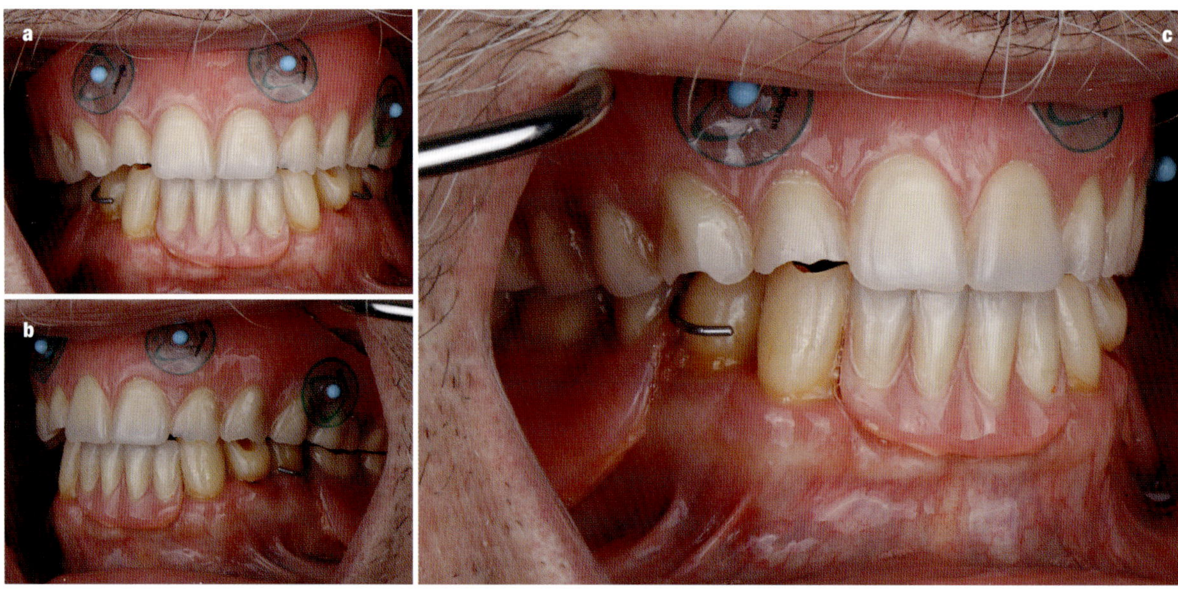

Figure 3.24 (a-c) Fiducial markers on maxillary complete denture with patient in MIP.

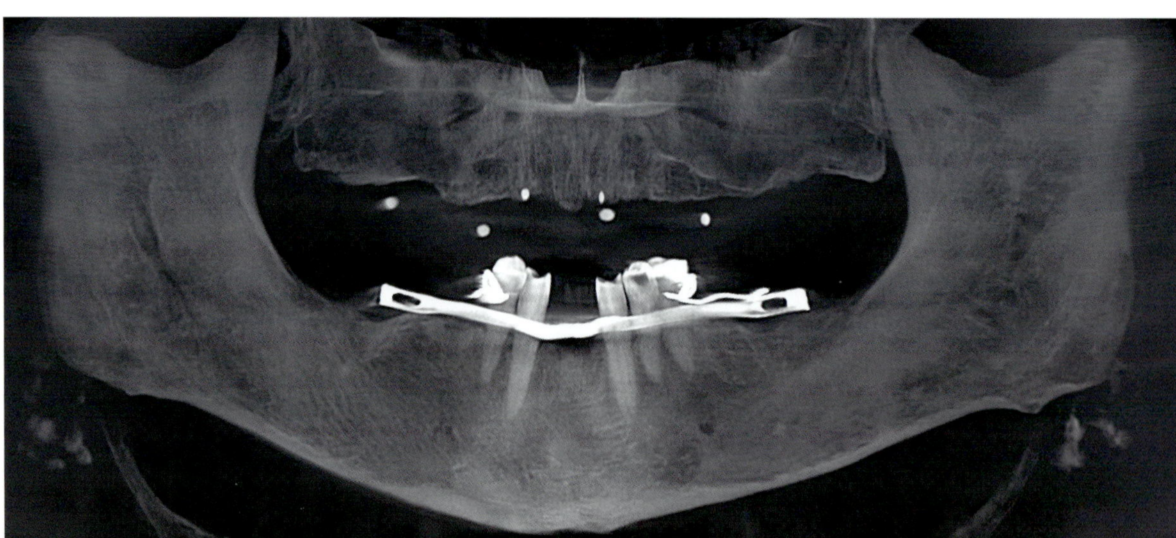

Figure 3.25 CBCT showing fiducial markers on a maxillary complete denture.

VDO ORTHOTIC POSITIONING DEVICE, OR JAW RELATION DEVICE

Engineering a patient's interim prosthesis with appropriate esthetics and function may be more challenging if certain conditions exist. Under any of the following circumstances, consider the jaw relation device (Figs. 3.26, 3.27):

- Patient is edentulous and does not have a current denture
- A predictable, reproducible maxillomandibular relationship record cannot be obtained
- There are no centric stops
- Patient (dentate or edentulous) is not at an acceptable VDO and needs to be opened or closed more than 3 mm (collapsed bite)
- Significant esthetic and phonetic changes are needed

I take this additional step with my laboratory and create an appliance or appliances that will help establish the VDO and the patient's occlusion in the interim prostheses. This is the VDO orthotic positioning device, or what I refer to as a *jaw relation device*.

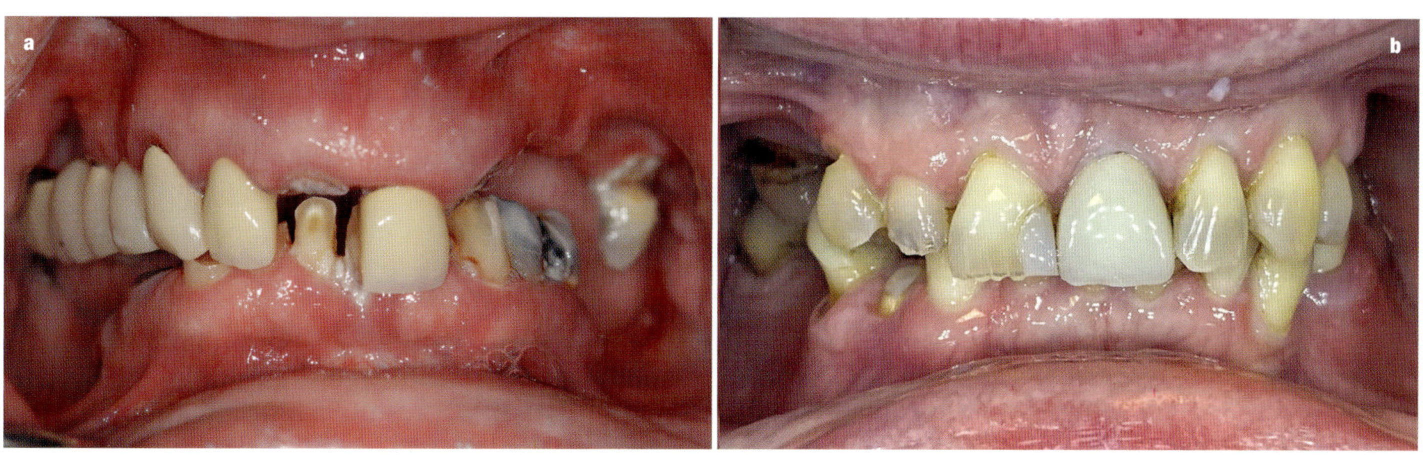

Figure 3.26 (a-b) Close-up retracted views of patients with terminal dentitions where vertical dimension has been lost and the occlusion has collapsed.

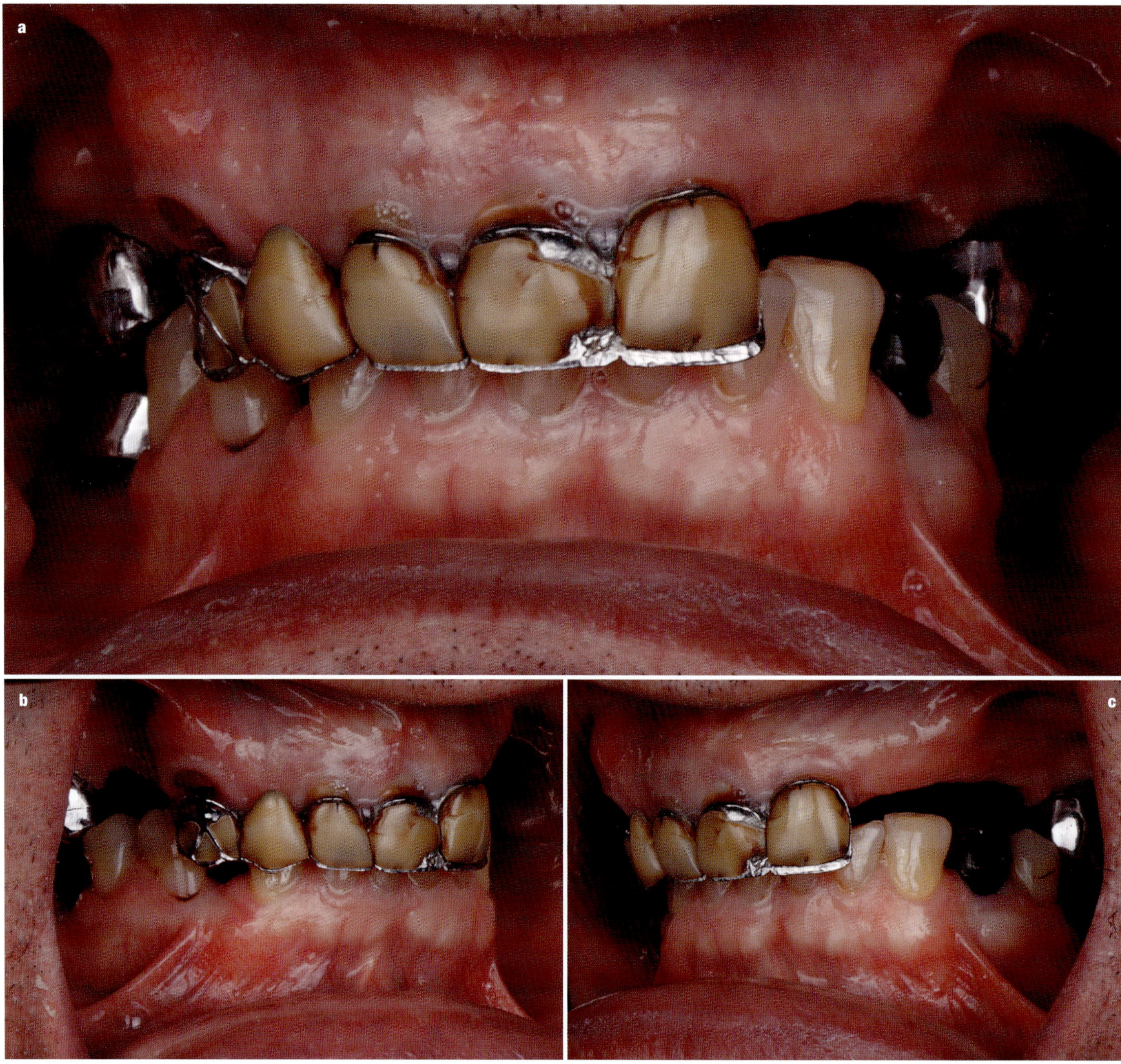

Figure 3.27 Close-up retracted (a) frontal and (b, c) lateral views of patient with a collapsed VDO.

A jaw relation device is a full or partial mock-up used to create a new vertical dimension and occlusion for the patient. This device is used to create a proposed design for the patient's interim prosthesis. In addition, it can be used to evaluate the esthetics and the patient's phonetics at this new position.

A jaw relation device can be made from printed clear or colored resin materials. Once the device (or devices) has been fabricated, you may decide to have the patient wear it at home and during functioning. Very similar to a denture or partial denture, this allows you and the patient to evaluate and test the new occlusion and vertical dimension.

To fabricate a jaw relation device, your dental laboratory will need all the current records (digital impressions or master casts, current maxillomandibular relationship, photographs, and CBCT) you have obtained of the patient. Once the lab has received the records, you should discuss the best design with them and have them fabricate a full denture, partial denture, or occlusal overlay to correct the patient's vertical dimension and establish the new occlusion. Ask your lab to place fiducial markers if you are having a prototype denture fabricated.

To use the jaw relation device (or devices), follow these steps:

1. Completely seat the jaw relation device(s) in the arch(es) (Fig. 3.28).
2. Adjust or equilibrate to an ideal maxillomandibular relationship and VDO.
3. Take new photographs of the patient with jaw relation device(s) in place (Figs. 3.29-3.31).
4. Record the new maxillomandibular relationship using an analog occlusal registration material. Alternatively, if a prototype denture with fiducial markers is part of the case, take a dual-scan CBCT with the appliance(s) in place (Fig. 3.32).
5. Verify the change in the vertical dimension by measuring it without and with the jaw relation device seated (Fig. 3.33).

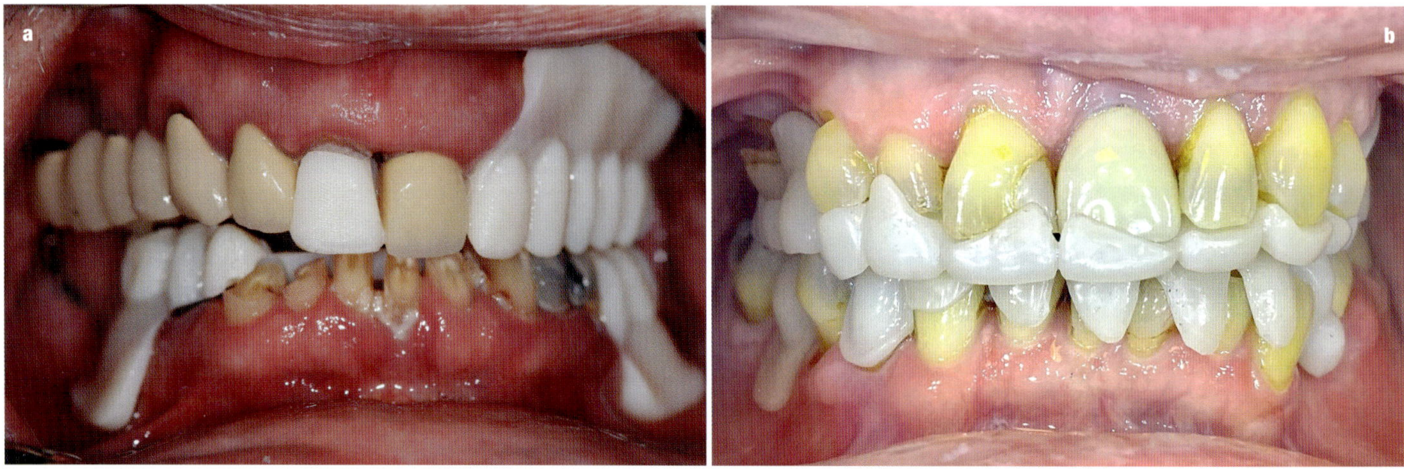

Figure 3.28 (a, b) Close-up retracted views of jaw relation devices seated in both maxillary and mandibular arches.

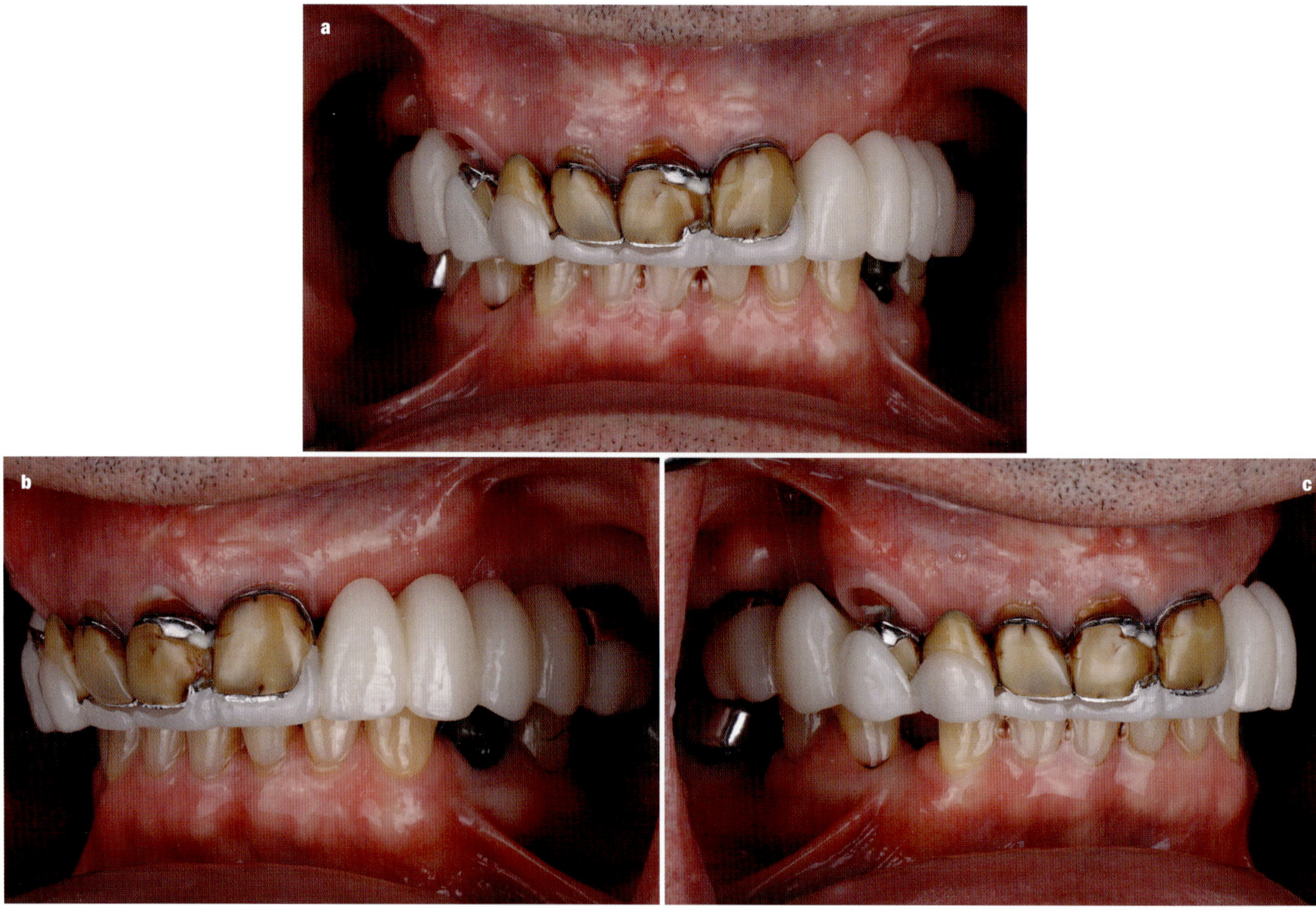

Figure 3.29 Close-up retracted (a) frontal and (b, c) lateral views of maxillary jaw relation device after adjustment of the occlusion.

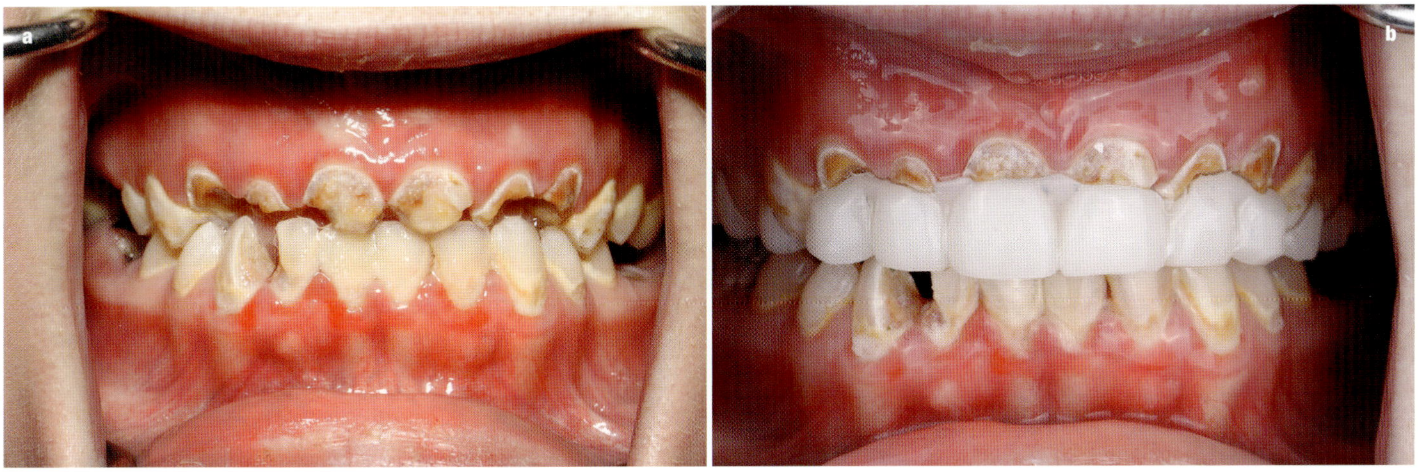

Figure 3.30 Close-up retracted frontal views (a) without and (b) with maxillary jaw relation device in place.

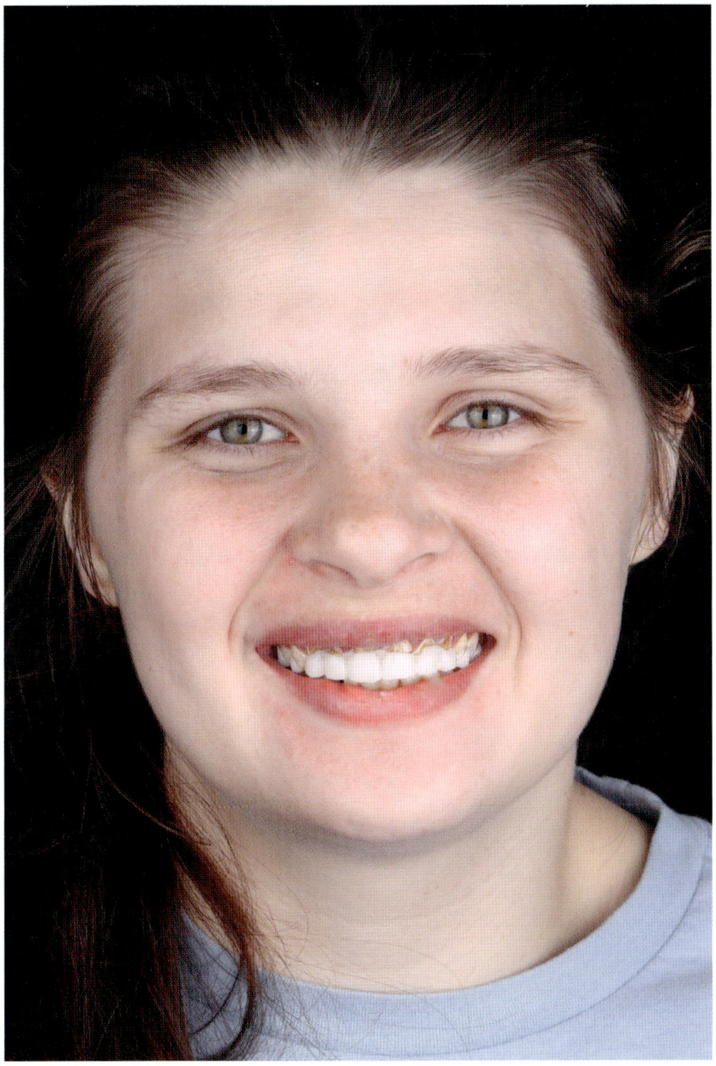

Figure 3.31 Smiling portrait view of patient with maxillary jaw relation device in place.

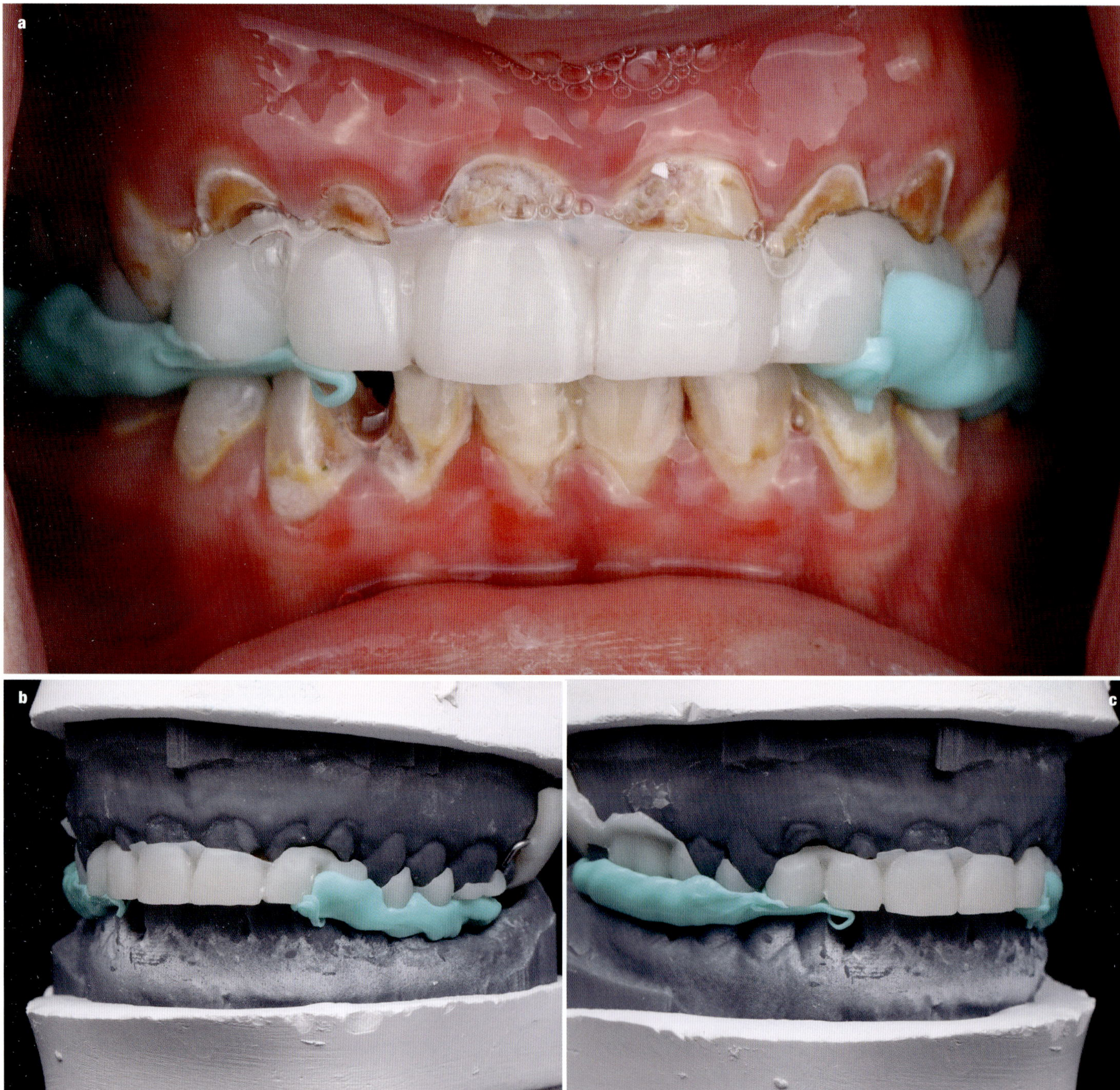

Figure 3.32 Maxillary jaw relation device with occlusal registration (a) recorded intraorally and (b, c) shown on the master cast.

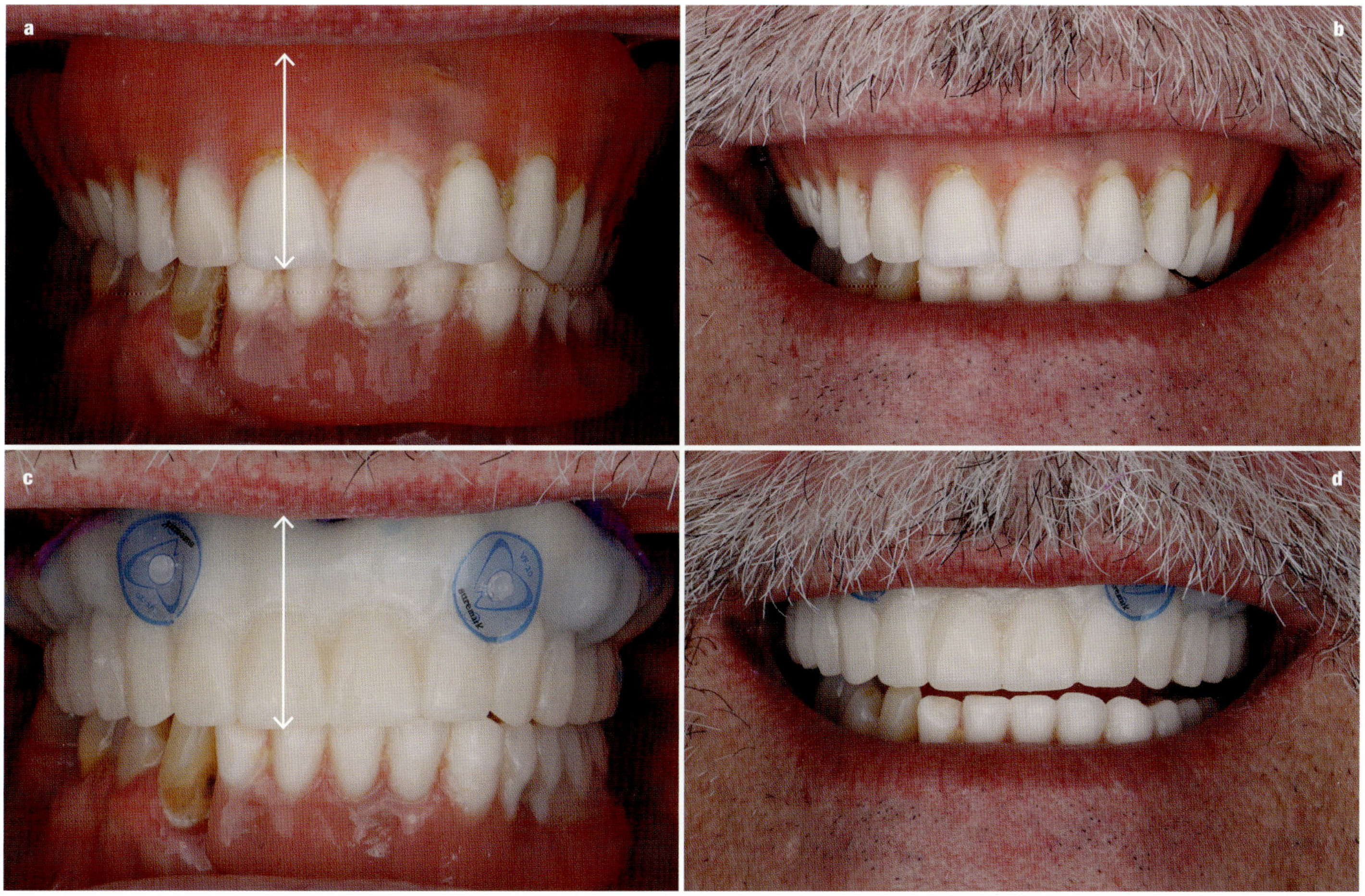

Figure 3.33 Close-up retracted and smile views (a, b) with the patient's current maxillary denture and (c, d) with the jaw relation device with fiducial markers in place. Note the change in the patient's VDO (arrows) as well as the esthetic improvement achieved with the new design in the jaw relation device. The occlusal plane on the left posterior quadrant was also corrected. An analog maxillomandibular relationship record or dual-scan technique can be used to record the occlusion.

A mandibular jaw relation device featuring just the missing teeth and a maxillary denture-style jaw relation device are shown in Figures 3.34 and 3.35, respectively. The patient they were made for, who presented with combination syndrome, had been wearing a maxillary denture for many years and had lost a significant number of mandibular posterior teeth. The anterior maxilla had resorbed considerably, and the posterior maxilla was collapsing. She had also experienced a considerable change in her VDO and developed a reverse smile. A set of jaw relation devices was used to correct the occlusal plane as well as open the vertical dimension (Figs. 3.36, 3.37). The patient's maxillomandibular relationship can be confirmed either digitally or with occlusal registration material, as shown in Figure 3.38, and the difference in the height of the VDO can be measured (Fig. 3.39).

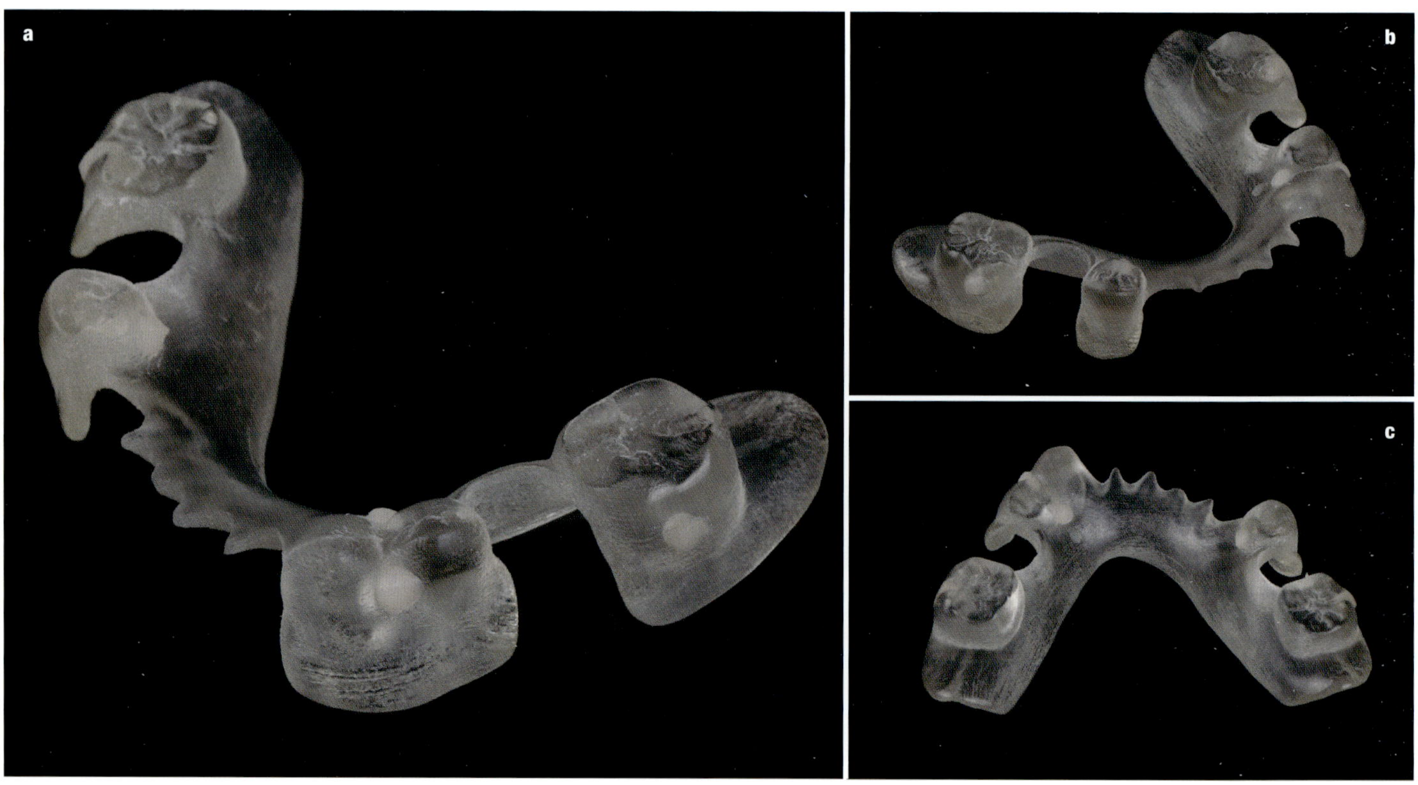

Figure 3.34 (a-c) Mandibular jaw relation device with radiographic markers.

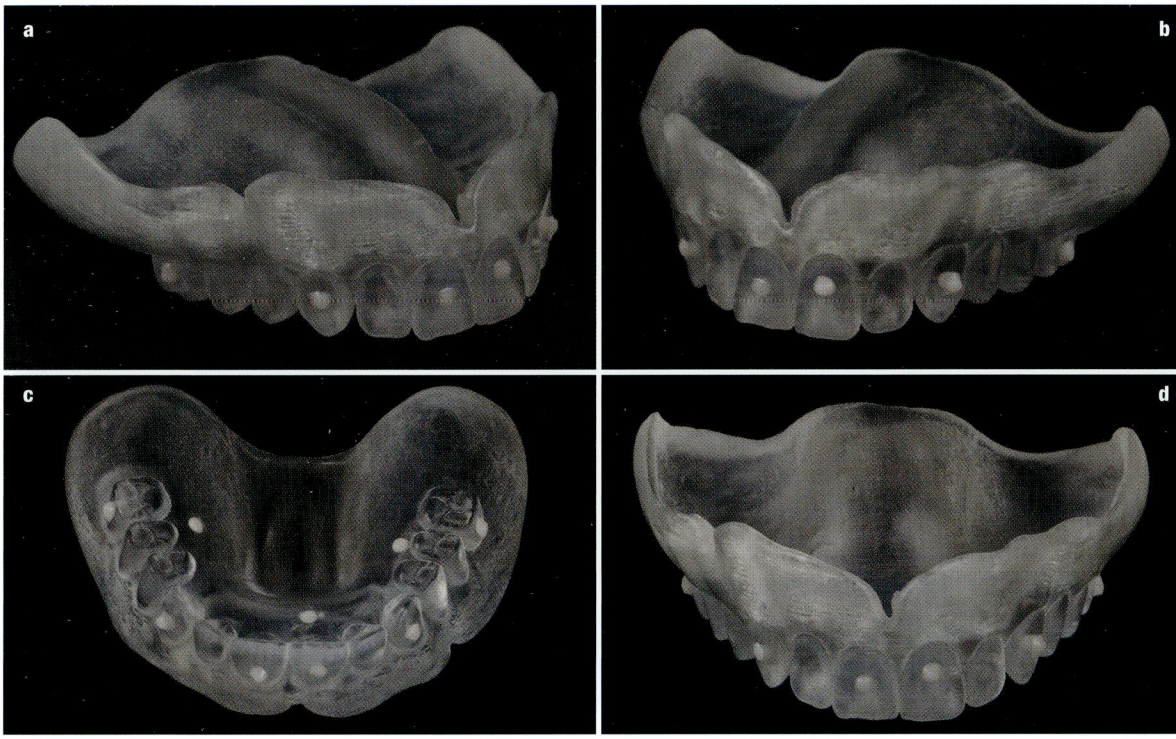

Figure 3.35 (a-d) Maxillary-denture style jaw relation device with radiographic markers.

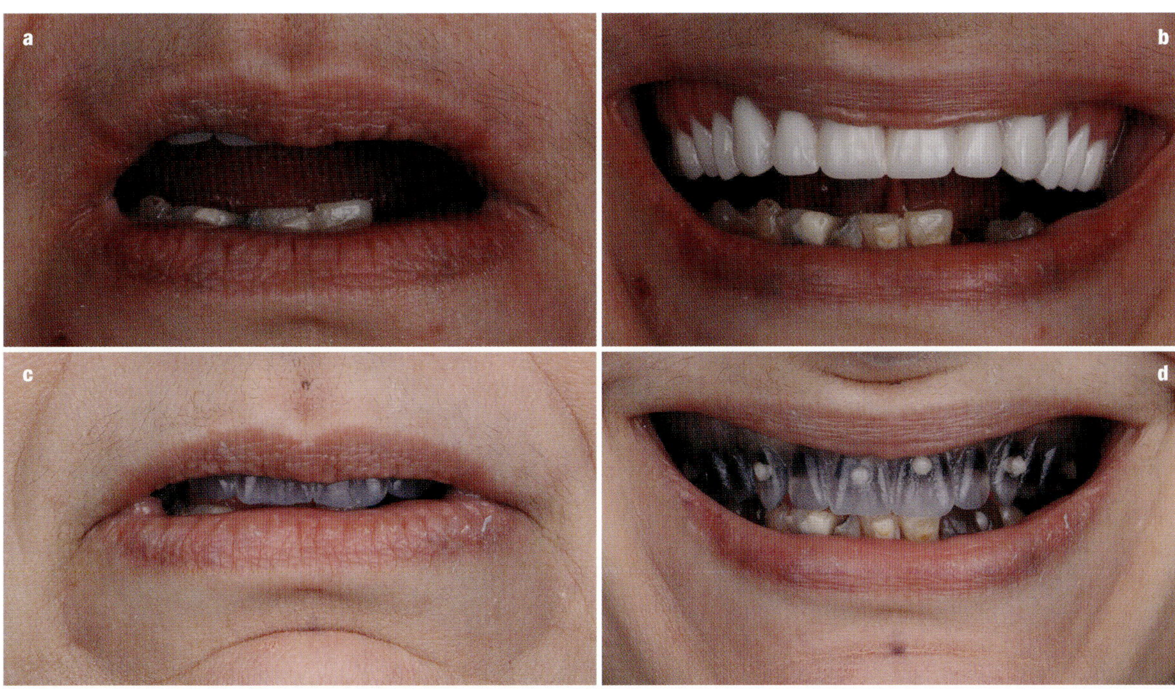

Figure 3.36 Correction of the reverse smile, incisal edge display, and occlusal plane with a jaw relation device. (a) Patient with current denture in repose with inadequate incisal edge display; (b) Patient with current denture displaying reverse smile; (c) Patient wearing jaw relation device displaying corrected incisal edge position; (d) Patient wearing jaw relation device displaying corrected tooth position in occlusal plane.

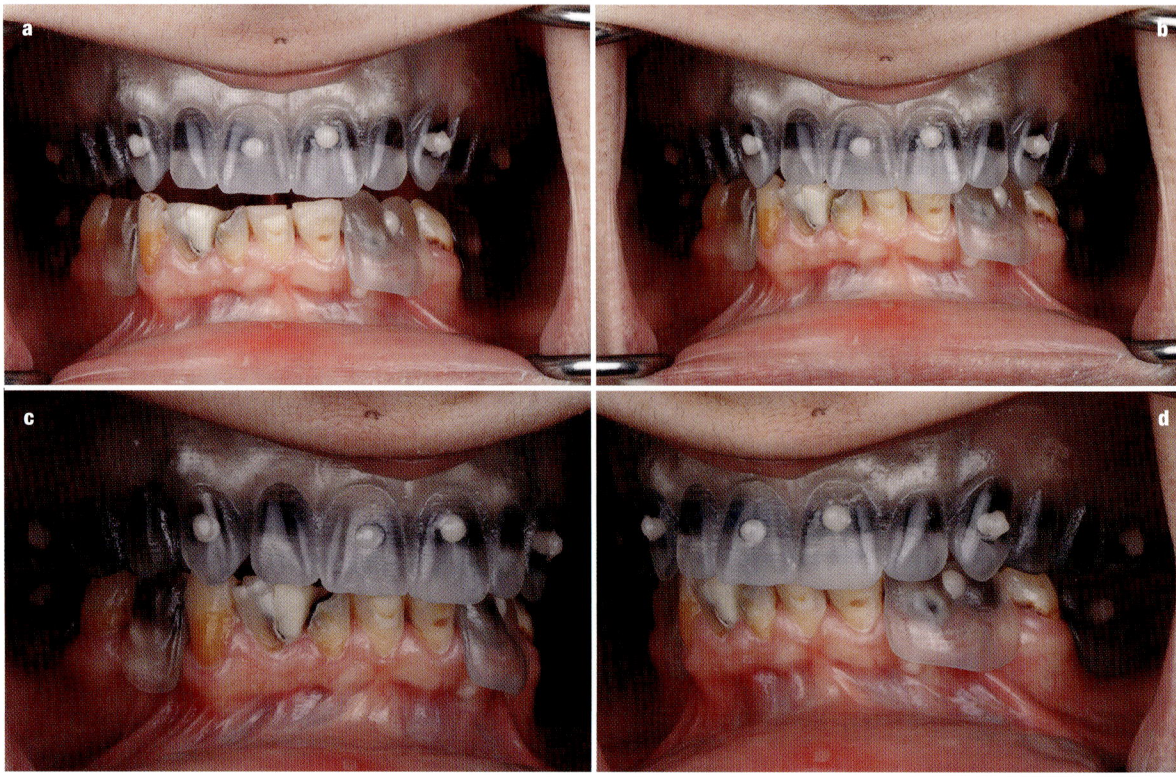

Figure 3.37 Retracted views of patient with jaw relation devices seated in maxilla and mandible. (a) Open; (b-d) In MIP.

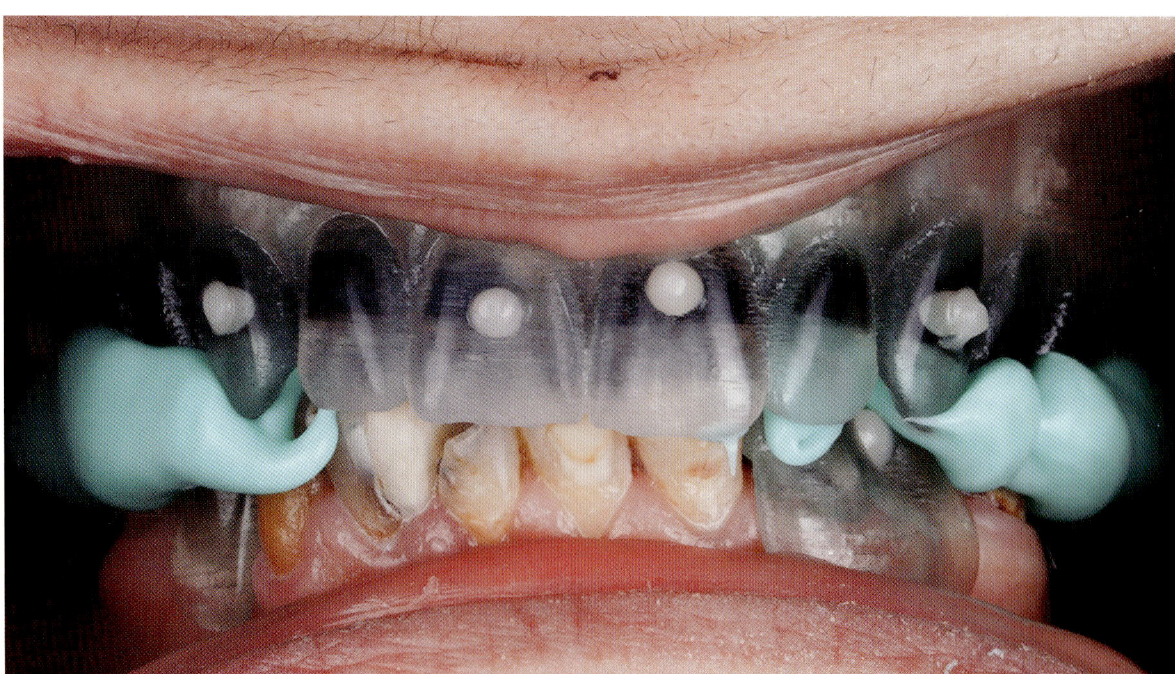

Figure 3.38 Analog occlusal registration material used to confirm patient's maximal intercuspal position.

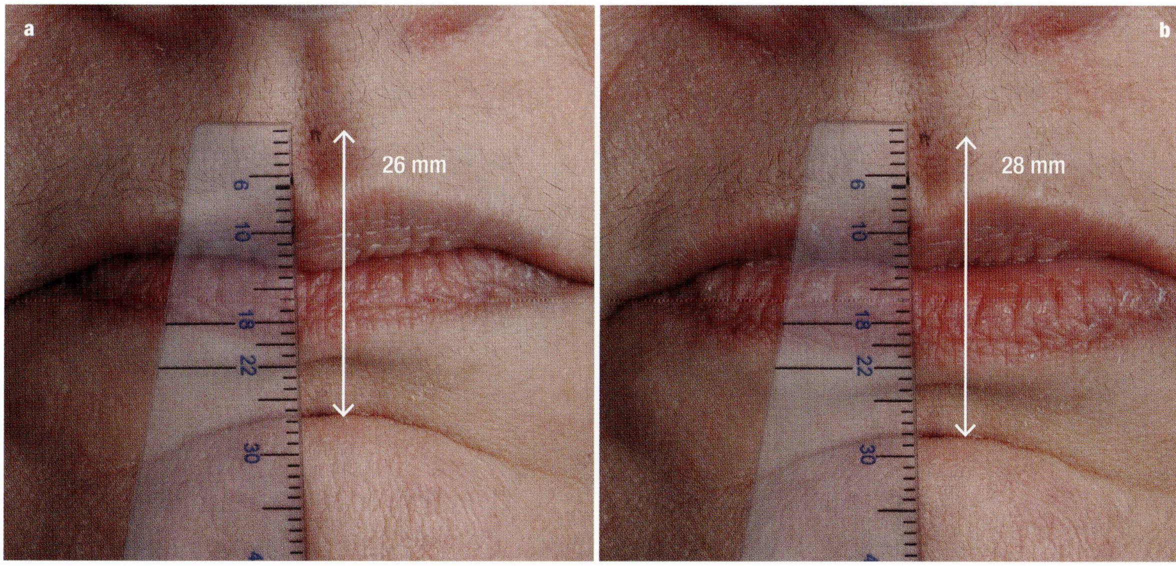

Figure 3.39 **Measurement of patient's VDO (a) with current maxillary complete denture and (b) with jaw relation devices in place.**

PROSTHETIC DESIGN CONSIDERATIONS

There are several matters to consider when sending patient data to the laboratory. Tooth color is important to most patients. The material I am currently using for interim prostheses is Flexcera™ (Desktop Health), a nanoceramic resin that comes in six shades (Bleach, A1, A2, A3, A3.5, and B1) **(Fig. 3.40)**. Most patients I see are displeased with the current shade of their teeth and prefer them to be whiter. To keep things simple, and also meet expectations, we let our patients see the shades and make the decision for themselves. For the gingiva, I almost always recommend medium pink because it looks appropriate on most people with most skin types.

When designing how a patient's teeth might look in their interim prosthesis, I usually start with the smile simulation that we create at the first visit. Sometimes patients will provide us with photographs of themselves from years earlier when they liked their smile, or with pictures from magazines. Smile design software and services are widely available and quite easy to use. Your dental laboratory can also be most helpful in assisting with this task. However you choose to design the interim prosthesis, be sure you involve the patient in the process to some degree. Most patients appreciate having a voice in the matter and will be happier during the time they are wearing a transitional interim prosthesis if they were able to participate in its design.

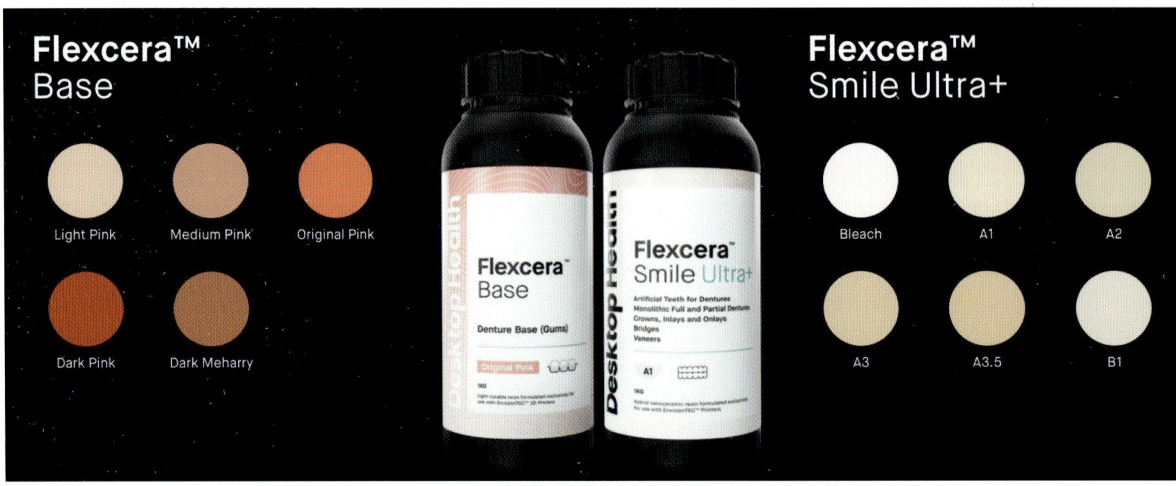

Figure 3.40 Flexcera™ (Desktop Health) printable nanoceramic resin showing currently available gingival and tooth shades.

PATIENT CONSENT AND PHOTOGRAPHIC CONSENT

Obtaining consent from a patient before delivering treatment is required in the U.S. Most state laws require patients to sign a written document as proof of consent; those that do not, require verbal consent. The number and type of consent forms and what they contain can be debated. I prefer to err on the side of caution by overdoing it. My personal experience is that obtaining patient consent before treatment helps avoid miscommunication and allows patients to make informed decisions.

Treatment consent forms

There are several treatment consent forms that we use in our practice before proceeding with fixed full-arch implant dentistry. Patient consent rules and laws differ from country to country; depending on where you practice, there may be different standards that need to be met and should be taken into consideration. In the U.S., according to the American Dental Association, there are three types of treatment consent a patient may give you[1]. The first is *implied consent* and it is reasonable for you to assume that you have this before you proceed with an examination and patient conversation because the patient traveled to your practice. The next is *general consent*, and this is usually obtained during a medical history and review of systems. General consent is when the patient gives you permission to proceed with treatment and releases you from the possibility of being charged with battery. It gives you permission to perform minor restorative procedures as well as give local anesthesia. The third type of consent is *informed consent*. Specific informed consent is necessary before providing most procedures that will be discussed in this text. It should be more than just a bunch of papers that a patient signs and instead be a process and discussion that helps you educate the patient about your treatment plan. The conversation you have with your patient should include discussion of:

- Dental health problems that you observed during your examination
- The nature and process of fixed full-arch implant rehabilitation
- Benefits and risks associated with fixed full-arch implant rehabilitation
- Potential alternatives to fixed full-arch implant rehabilitation
- The risks and benefits of alternative treatments as well as no treatment

Photo and video consent forms

Obtaining photographs of a patient is not the same as treatment, but as noted earlier, one of the reasons to take photographs is for record-keeping and medicolegal purposes. If you plan to use the patient's photo in any marketing, advertising, presentations, lectures, social media, etc., you should have a photography consent form. It could be argued that even sharing photographs with other dental professionals, such as referral sources, could be observed by some as a privacy issue. So, to protect yourself and to be completely transparent with your patient ask for their permission before taking their picture. In the process of writing this book, I changed my current consent form to be more explicit about how I might use my patients' pictures. I have provided the form I use as an example (Fig. 3.41). *Please be advised that this is not a legal document, and you should consult with your own legal professional before using this document in your practice.*

PHOTOGRAPHY AND VIDEO AGREEMENT & RELEASE

We kindly ask your consent to potentially use any photos taken of you in our office.
Dr. ______________________________ has been given the distinction of being retained by an international publisher to write a comprehensive textbook on dentistry.
He requests your assistance by granting him permission to use your case materials and your image (without your name or identification, in all cases) for his education endeavors. Photos may be used with the book, lectures, and articles under his authorship and that of the other dentists at Ballantyne Dentistry.

Photographs may also be used for marketing and promotional purposes.
Thank you!

Dr. Yaste and Team at Ballantyne Dentistry

Yes ☐ No ☐ I consent to the use of my photos for educational purposes.

Yes ☐ No ☐ I consent to the use of my photos for marketing and promotional purposes.

Yes ☐ No ☐ I do not consent to the use of my photos for the above mentioned.

Signed: ______________________________ Dated: ____________________

Figure 3.41 **Author's photo consent form.**

VITAMIN D TESTING

There is growing evidence in the current literature of a possible link between vitamin D deficiency and early dental implant failure[2]. Several leading dental implant clinicians have suggested patients should be tested for low vitamin D, and those with serum 25(OH)D values of less than 30 ng/mL be advised to take vitamin D supplements.

Research in this area is limited and it may be too early to prove definitively that low vitamin D levels cause early implant failure. However, I have implemented vitamin D testing in my practice. Considering that testing for vitamin D deficiency is relatively easy and cost effective, it makes sense for our practice to eliminate this potential risk factor. Testing and supplementation have been widely accepted by our patients, and many appreciate our taking the time to do it. Although this is only empirical evidence, we have not had any early implant failures among the patients we have provided vitamin D supplementation through the DentaMedica dental recovery support program www.stellalife.com/products/stellalifedentamedica-supplements. For information about this program, visit the StellaLife website (stellalife.com).

PATIENT MEDICAL CLEARANCE

Even if a patient seems healthy and without significant medical problems, it is important to gain clearance from a patient's physician to avoid the risks that come with fixed full-arch implant rehabilitation. Clearance from a patient's physician, especially if conscious intravenous sedation or general anesthesia will be used, should be obtained during the time frame between digital data collection and the surgical visit. My patient-care coordinators and I work with our patients and their physicians to obtain the appropriate forms and documentation before definitively scheduling their surgical visit.

References

1. American Dental Association [Internet]. Chicago: ADA; 2023. Guidelines for practice success | Managing professional risks | The consent process: Types of consent; 2023 [cited 14 Sep 2023]; [about 3 screens]. Available from: https://www.ada.org/en/resources/practice-management/types-of-consent
2. Miron RJ, Pikos MA, Bishara M. Vitamin D deficiency and early implant failure: What every clinician should know. Dent Today [Internet]. 2020 Apr 1;39(4):72-79. Available from: https://www.dentistrytoday.com/vitamin-d-deficiency-and-early-implant-failure-what-every-clinician-should-know/

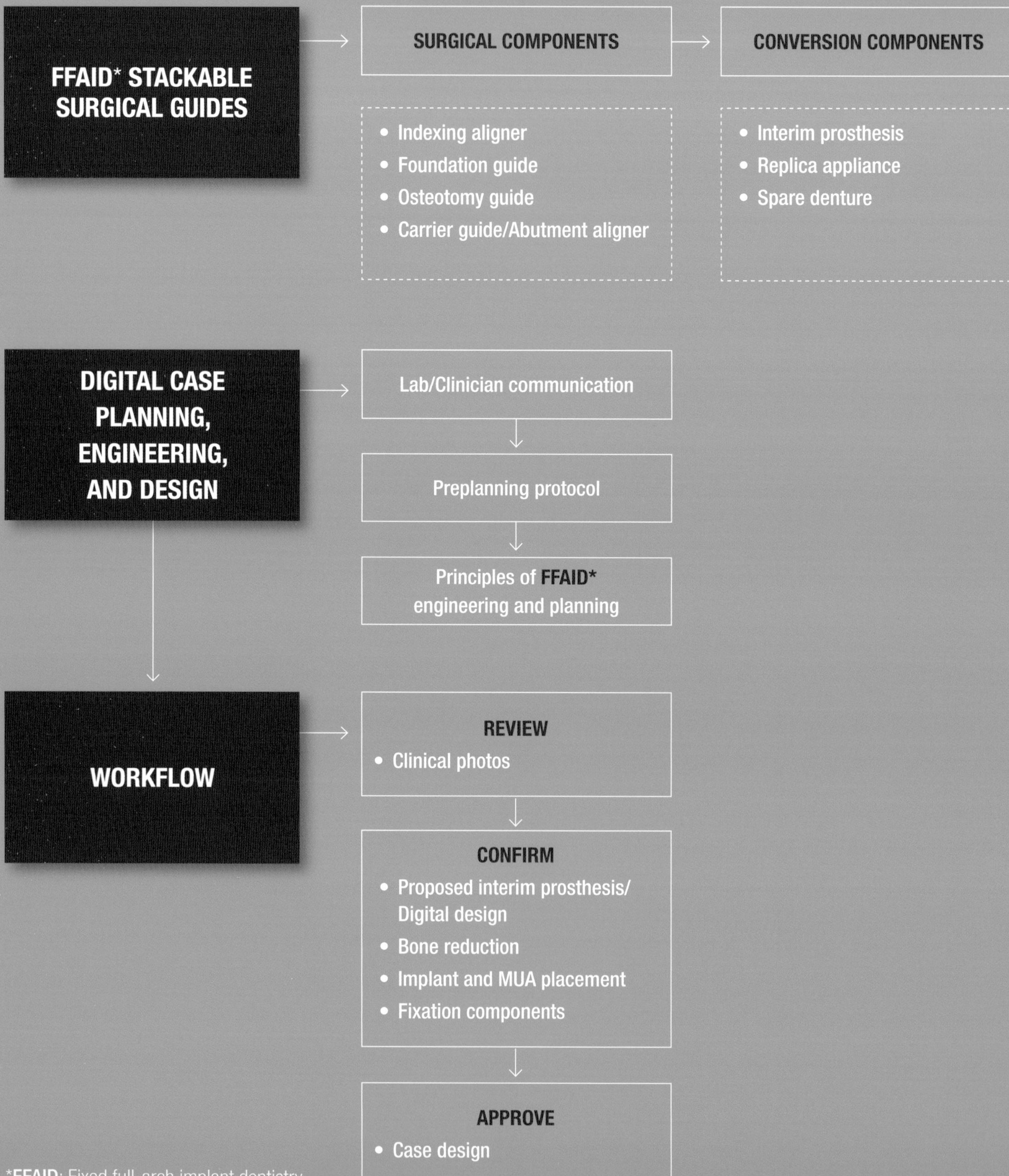

*FFAID: Fixed full-arch implant dentistry

PROSTHETICALLY DRIVEN TREATMENT PLANNING

SECTION III

FFAID STACKABLE SURGICAL GUIDES

SURGICAL COMPONENTS	CONVERSION COMPONENTS
• Indexing aligner • Foundation guide • Osteotomy guide • Carrier guide/Abutment aligner	• Interim prosthesis • Replica appliance • Spare denture

STACKABLE SURGICAL GUIDE SYSTEM

CHAPTER **4**

Commitment: Read, relax, meditate, pray, and reduce distractions.
On my best days, I have usually taken time to do these things.

The stackable surgical guide system is the method I employ for fixed full-arch dental implant rehabilitation in my practice **(Fig. 4.1)**. Understanding my method for providing fixed full-arch dentistry, digital case planning, engineering, and design requires detailed knowledge of each component and working part of this system. Stackable surgical guide systems have evolved dramatically over the past few years. Dental laboratories have developed numerous versions of full-arch stackable surgical guides that are printed and/or milled from various types of materials. I have used a variety of different stackable surgical guide systems for fixed full-arch implant dentistry, but they all work in the same general way, and the task they complete is essentially the same. This chapter provides an overview of how these guide parts are designed to function.

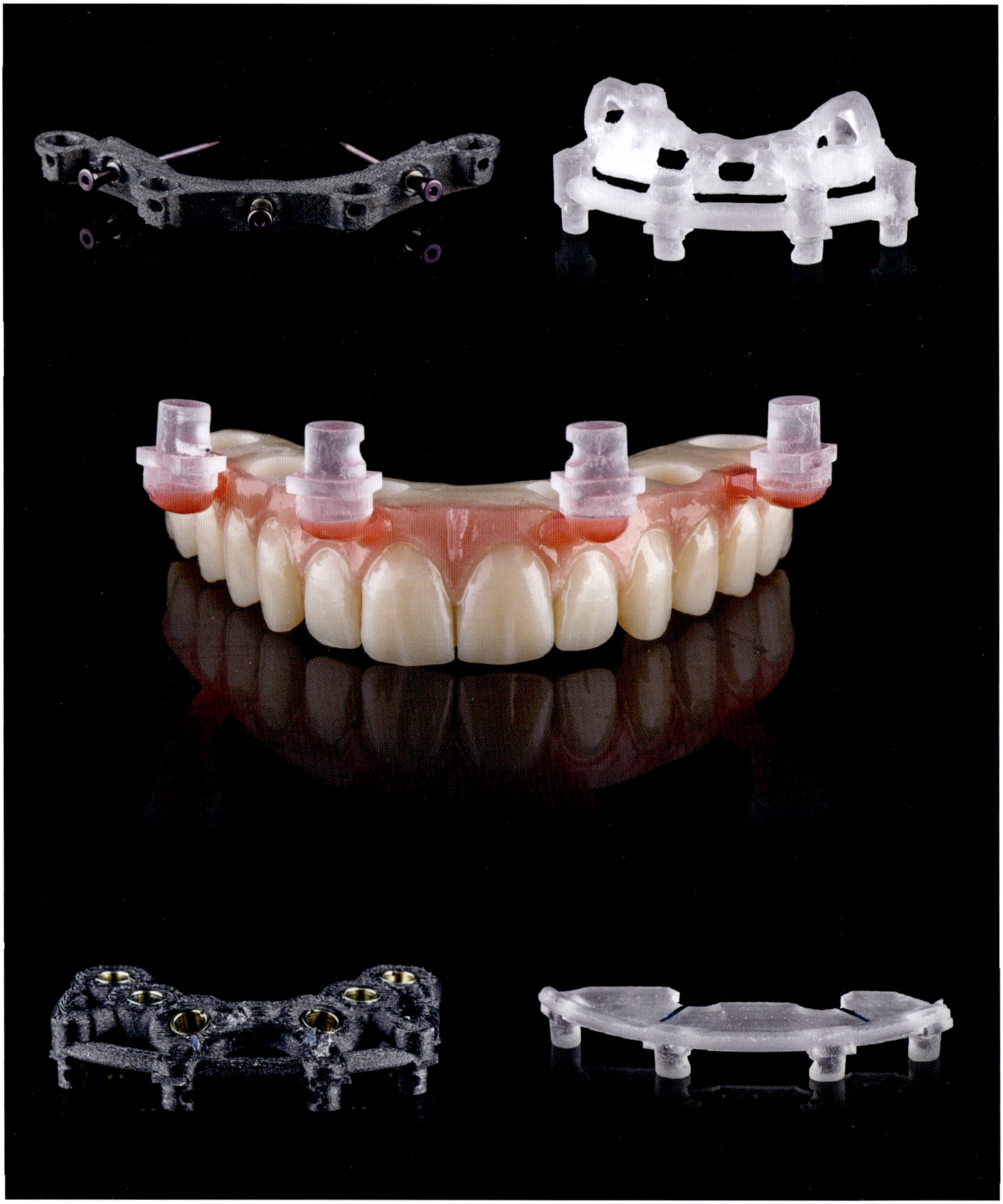

Figure 4.1 Components of a NavaGation® full-arch stackable surgical guide system for fixed full-arch implant placement, fabricated by Absolute Dental Services.

SURGICAL COMPONENTS

Indexing aligner

The indexing aligner, or *pin guide* as it is sometimes called, has one major purpose: to position and/or stabilize the foundation guide, which is the second component of the stackable guide system. The indexing aligner is generally made of printed plastic or acrylic resin. It is fabricated by the dental lab from either a digital scan (my preference) or an analog impression and can be designed to be tooth-, mucosa-, and/or bone-borne. The indexing aligner should be about 5 mm thick and, when made for a dentate arch, horseshoe-shaped to cover a minimal amount of tissue. The indexing aligner made for an edentulous ridge can be affixed to soft tissue or bone, depending on the design and preferences of the clinician (Figs. 4.2-4.5).

Figure 4.2 **Intaglio surface of a toothborne indexing aligner.**

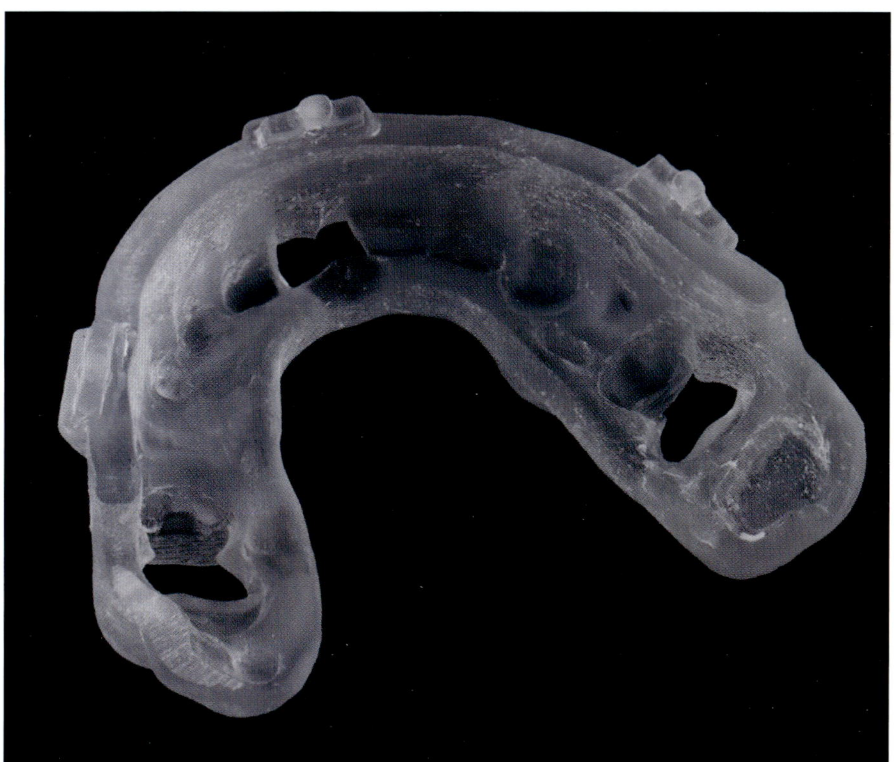

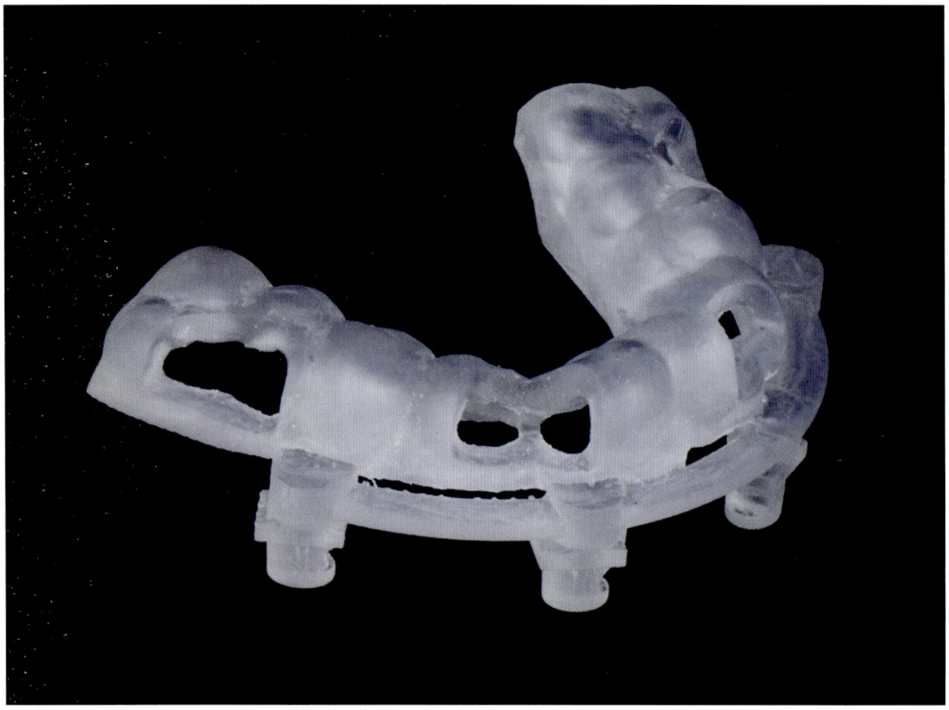

Figure 4.3 Occlusal surface of a toothborne indexing aligner.

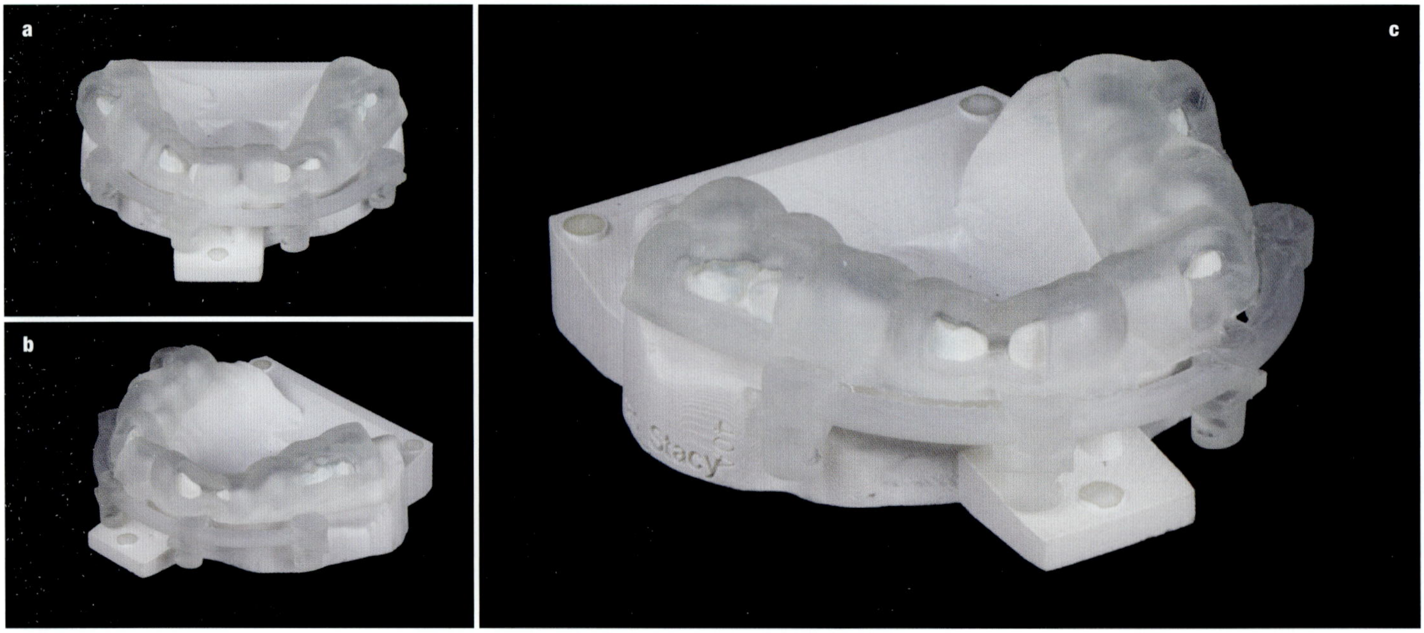

Figure 4.4 (a-c) Indexing aligner resting on a cast.

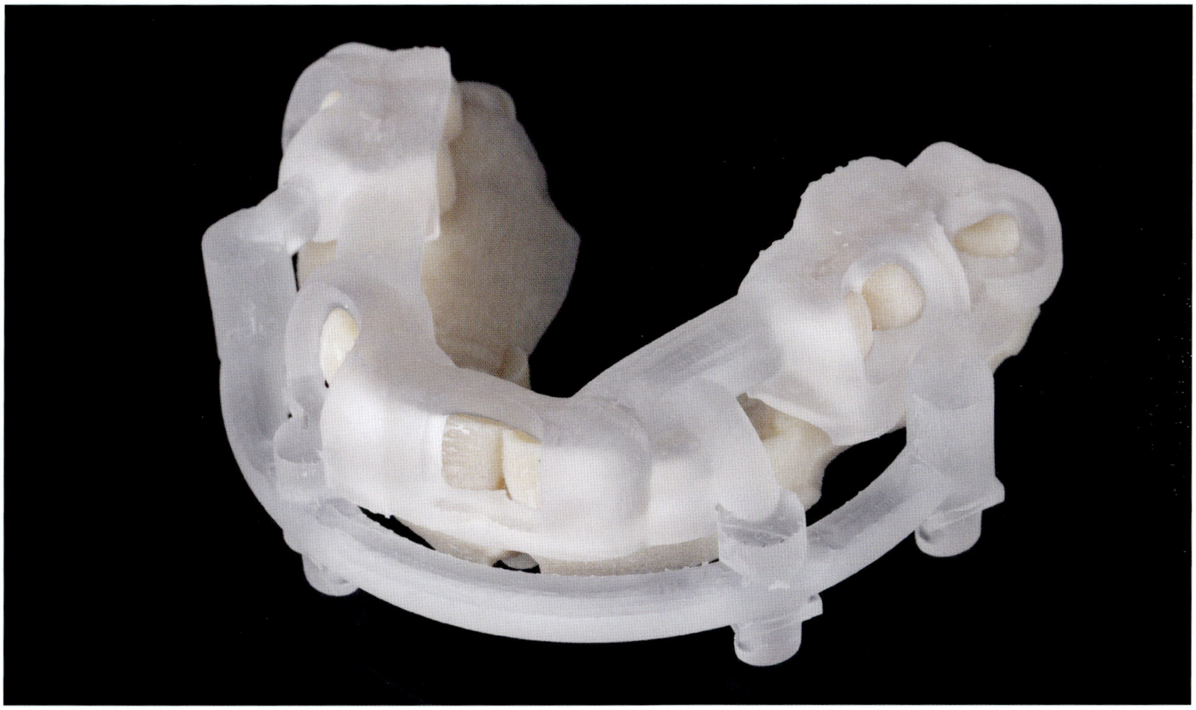

Figure 4.5 **Toothborne indexing aligner resting on a printed cast.**

In a system where the indexing aligner and the foundation guide are designed to work together, the aligner should fit intimately with the foundation guide (Figs. 4.6-4.8). Securing the foundation guide to the bone is a highly critical step that, if performed improperly, can put the entire surgery in jeopardy. Hence, it is very important that the indexing aligner and the foundation guide sync up properly.

In some guide systems, the aligner is not directly attached to the foundation guide but merely creates the osteotomies for the fixation pins of the foundation guide (Figs. 4.9, 4.10). In my opinion, this is a less desirable way to deliver and secure the foundation guide, but it can work nevertheless. I usually place the indexing aligner over the printed casts as well as in the patient's mouth several times to check for any undercuts or anomalies that may be present. Most indexing aligners feature small occlusal or edentulous cut-outs or windows for visualizing and verifying complete seating (Fig. 4.11). These windows should reveal no space between the guide and the teeth or edentulous ridge/bone. Make sure that no part of it is being hung up by the frenum, tongue, buccal vestibule, or any other soft tissue. The indexing aligner can attach to the foundation base with three or four plastic or metal pins, or locks (Fig. 4.12).

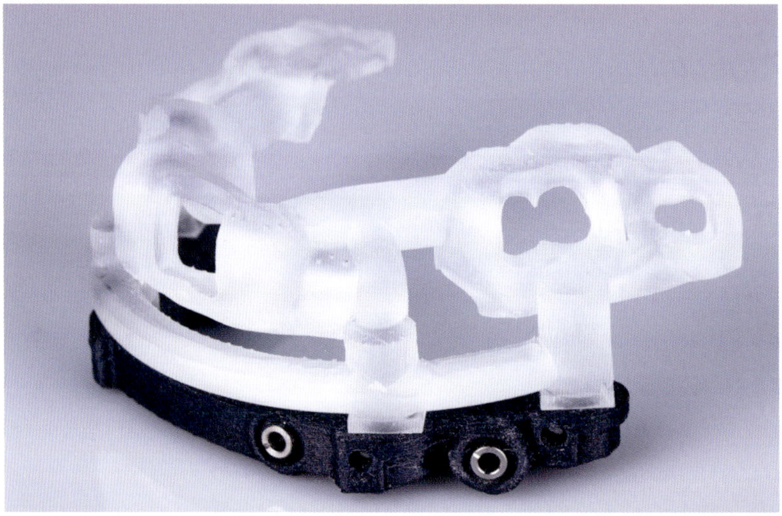

Figure 4.6 Toothborne indexing aligner attached to a printed carbon-fiber reinforced foundation guide.

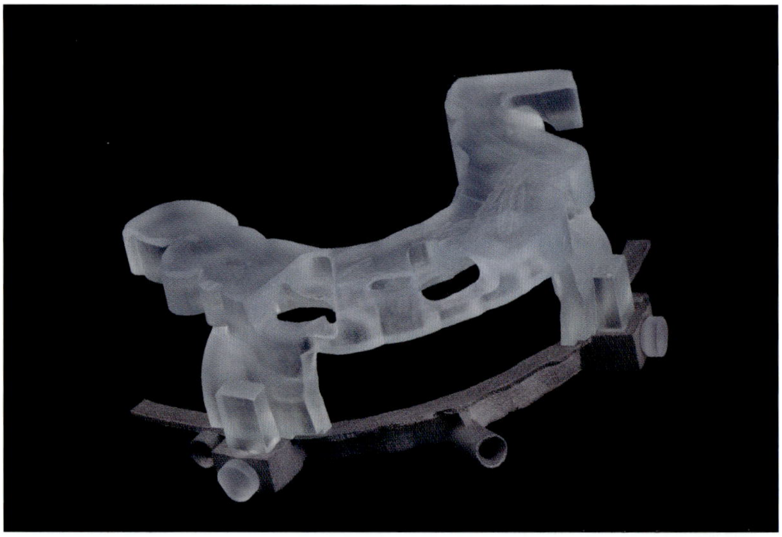

Figure 4.7 Toothborne indexing aligner affixed to an unfinished cobalt-chrome foundation guide.

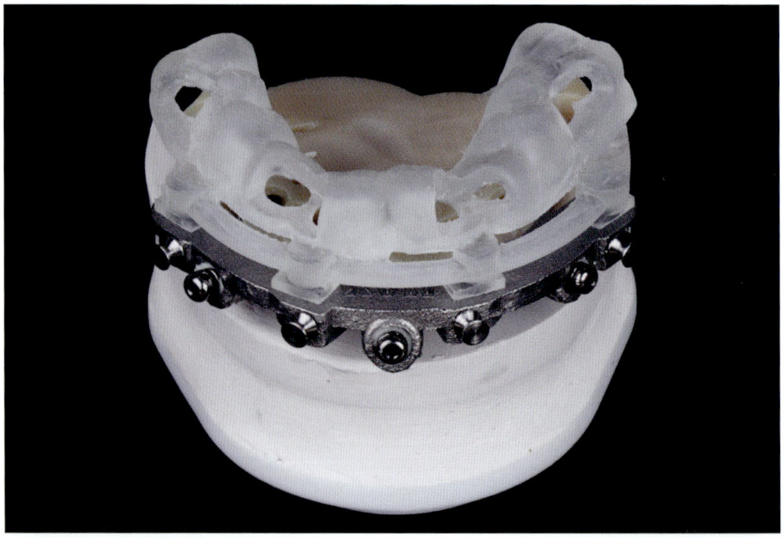

Figure 4.8 Toothborne indexing aligner affixed to a polished cobalt-chrome foundation guide.

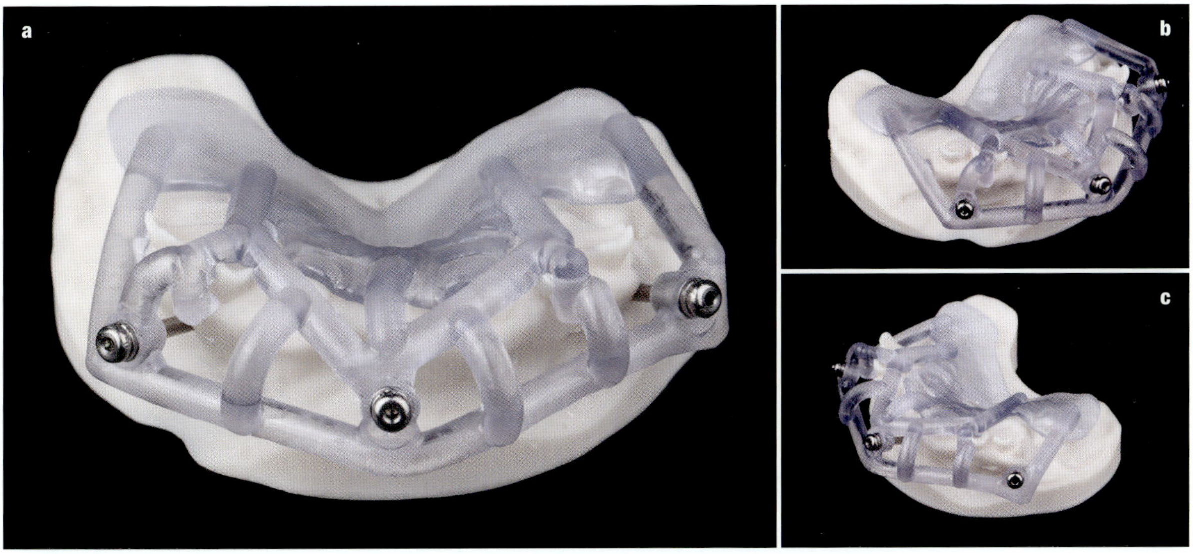

Figure 4.9 (a-c) Indexing aligner that does not affix to a foundation guide but is used to create positioning for it.

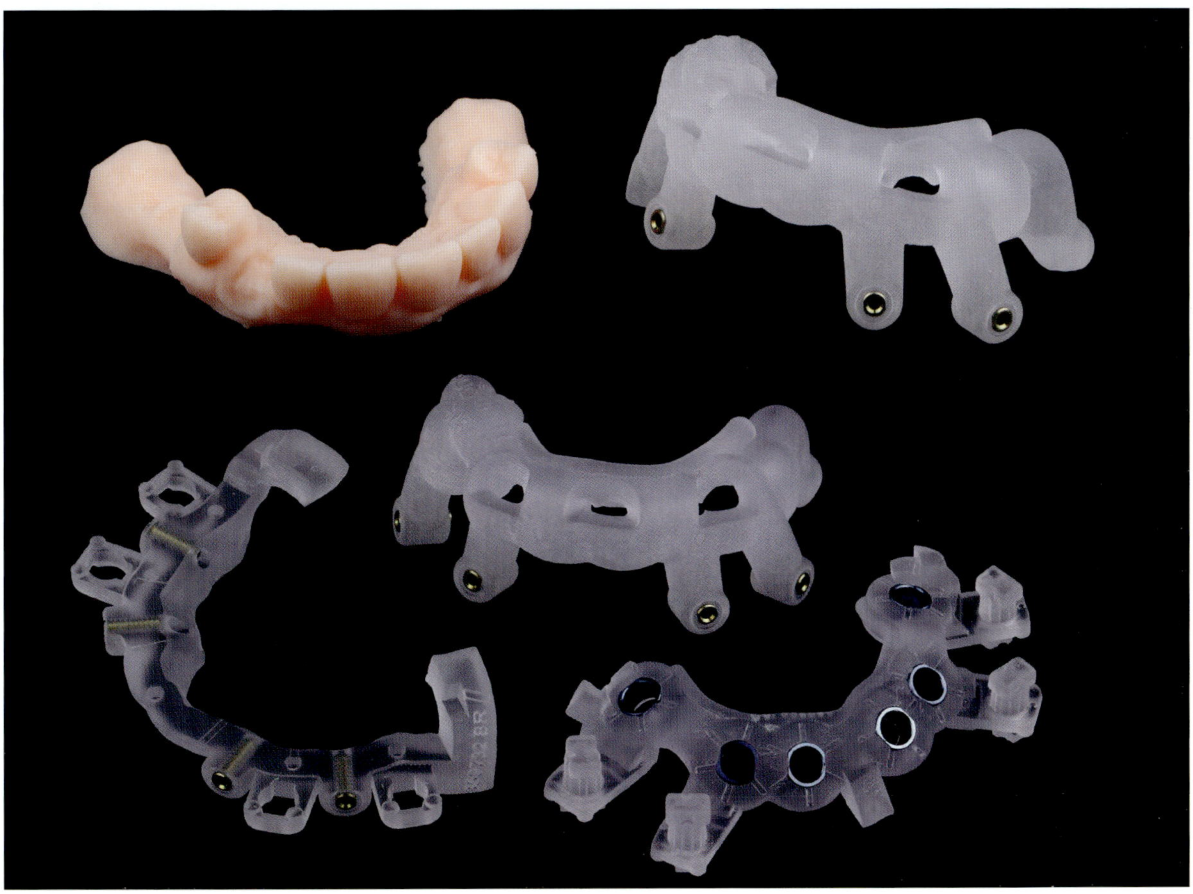

Figure 4.10 Stackable surgical guide system that creates pin fixation with an aligner guide but is not attached to the foundation guide. The lower left image is the foundation guide. The lower right image is the osteotomy guide that affixes to the foundation guide.

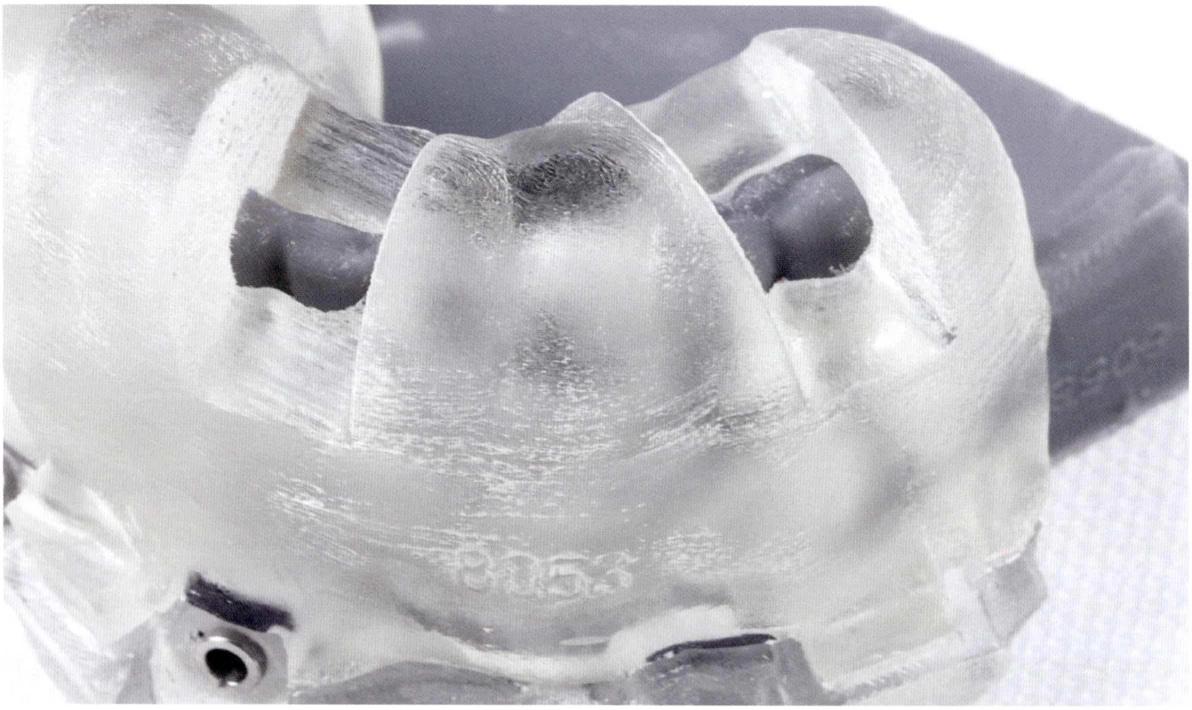

Figure 4.11 Occlusal window cutouts in indexing aligner to allow for seating confirmation.

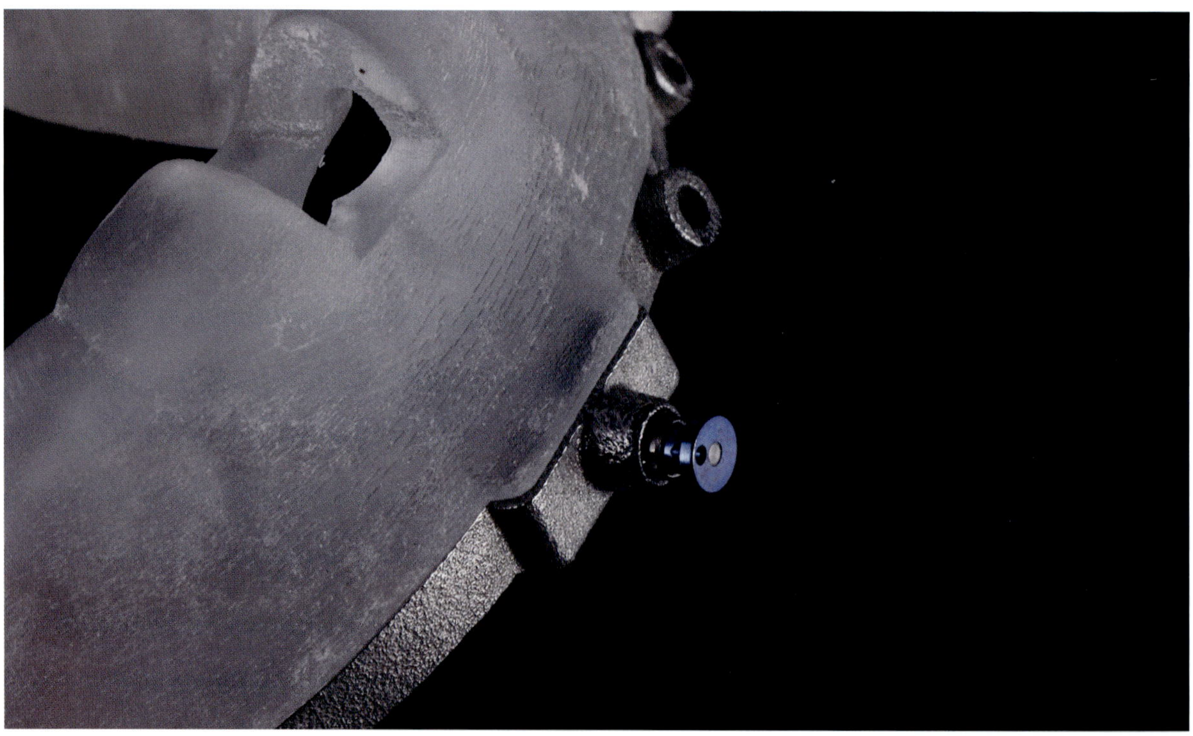

Figure 4.12 Indexing aligner attached to a cobalt-chrome foundation guide via a locking pin.

Foundation guide

The best way to describe the purpose of the next component of the stackable surgical guide system is as the foundation on which everything else follows. It is the "foundation" for the entire surgical process—hence the name *foundation guide* or *fixation base guide*. This is where the stack begins.

The foundation guide serves two functions:

1. **Bone reduction level indicator.** The vertical height at which the foundation guide is placed marks the level at which bone reduction will end. Following the general height of this guide ensures that enough space will be created for the interim and definitive prostheses.
2. **Support for the entire system**. The foundation guide provides a stable base for the guides that follow, including the implant osteotomy guide and the carrier and/or aligner guides used in some systems, as well as the interim prosthesis and the replica appliance (each of which is discussed on the following pages).

The foundation guide can be made of many types of material, including milled or printed polymethylmethacrylate (PMMA), laser-sintered cobalt-chrome, milled titanium, and more recently, carbon-fiber-reinforced materials (Figs. 4.13-4.17). At one time I considered laser-sintered cobalt-chrome guides to be superior because of their stability and rigidity, despite the fact that these guides require more work by the lab and are more expensive to manufacture. However, the recent introduction of printable carbon-fiber-reinforced materials and milled titanium, which are also very strong and lightweight yet avoid the limitations of cobalt-chrome, offers great promise. Carbon-fiber-reinforced materials can flex slightly without cracking or fracturing. Flexcera™ resin (Desktop Health) is another promising material that is printable and more fracture resistant than traditional printed resins. I predict that a number of other new materials will be introduced in the near future, giving dentists even more options to choose from.

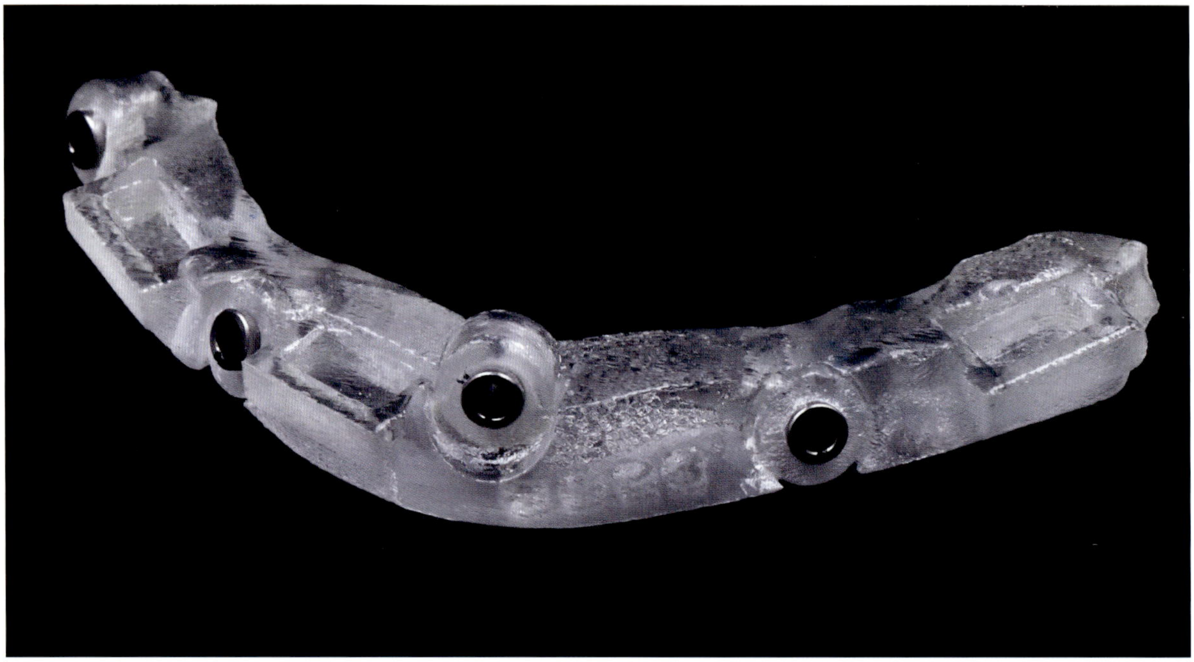

Figure 4.13 Printed resin foundation guide.

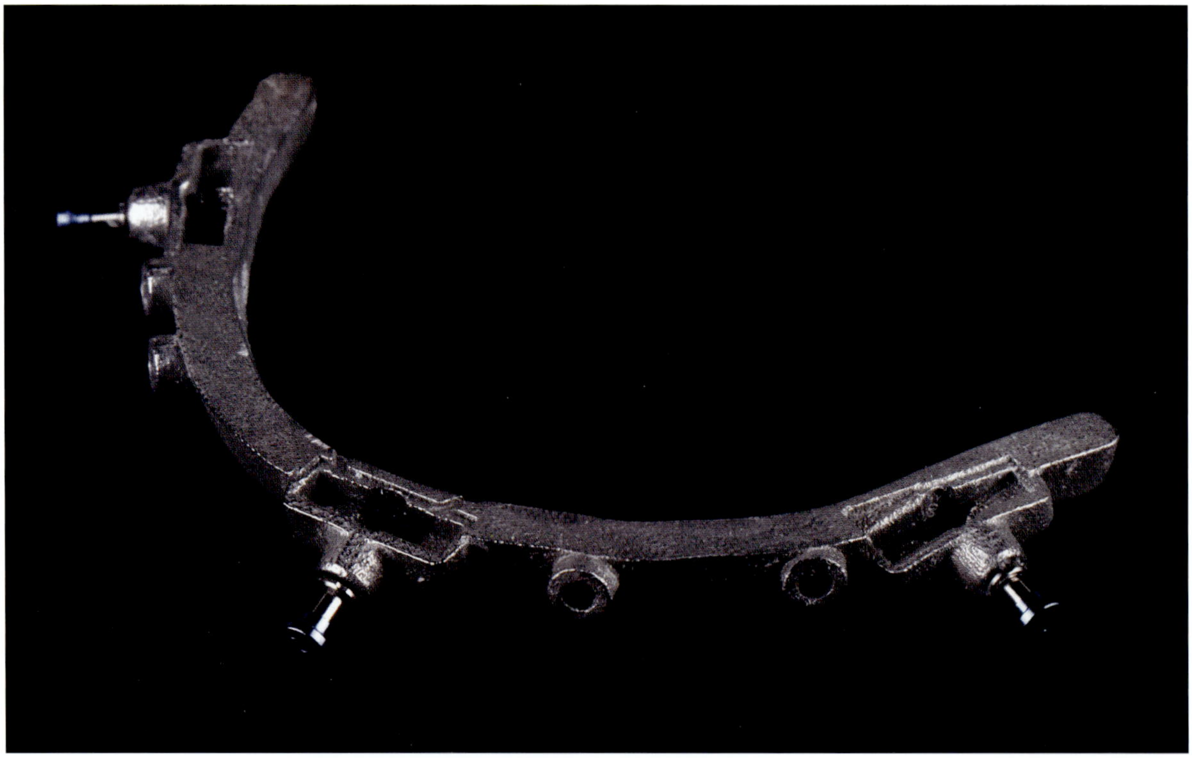

Figure 4.14 CHROME™ GuidedSmile fixation base made of cobalt-chrome.

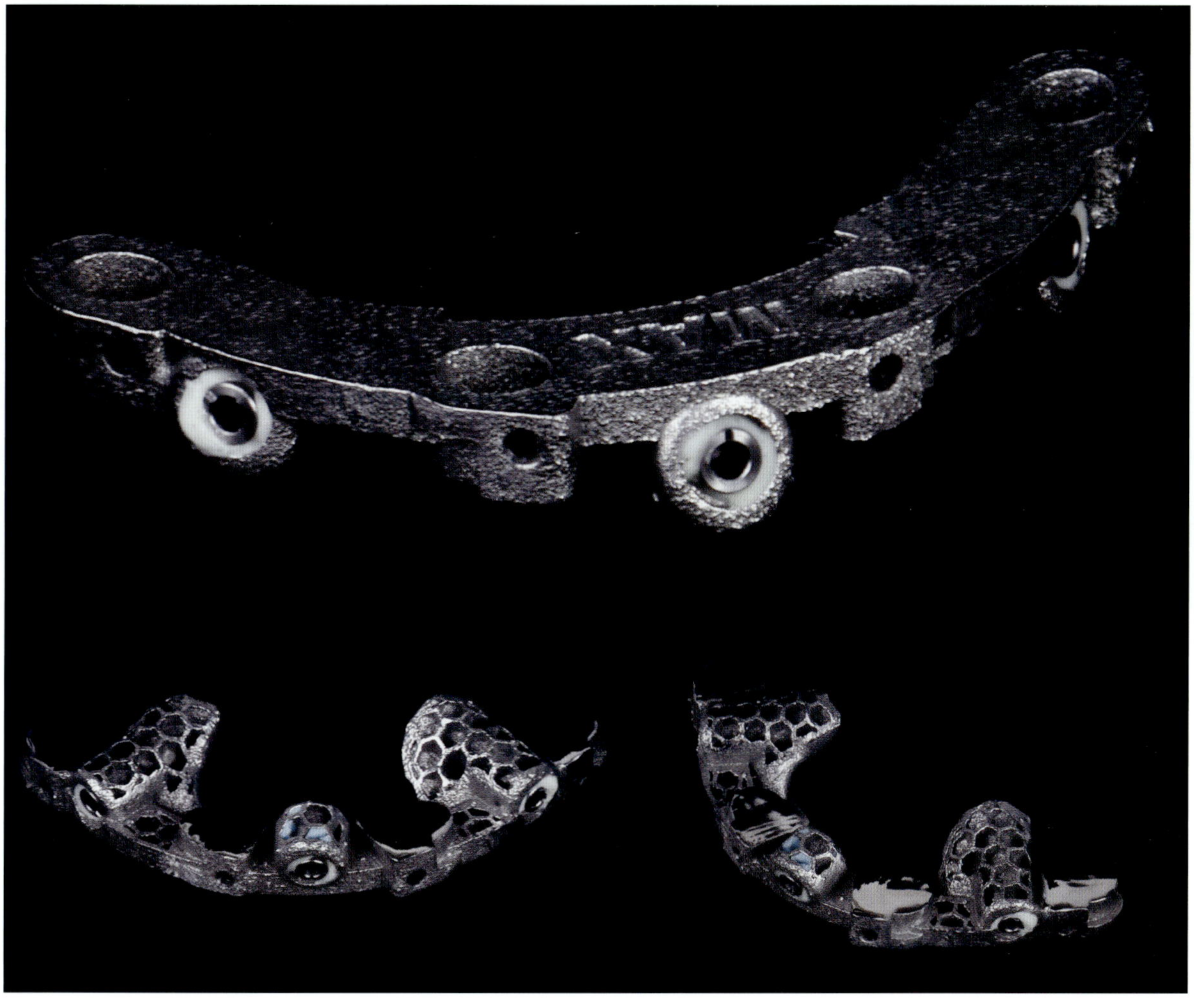

Figure 4.15 Synergy Plus foundation guide made from cobalt-chrome.

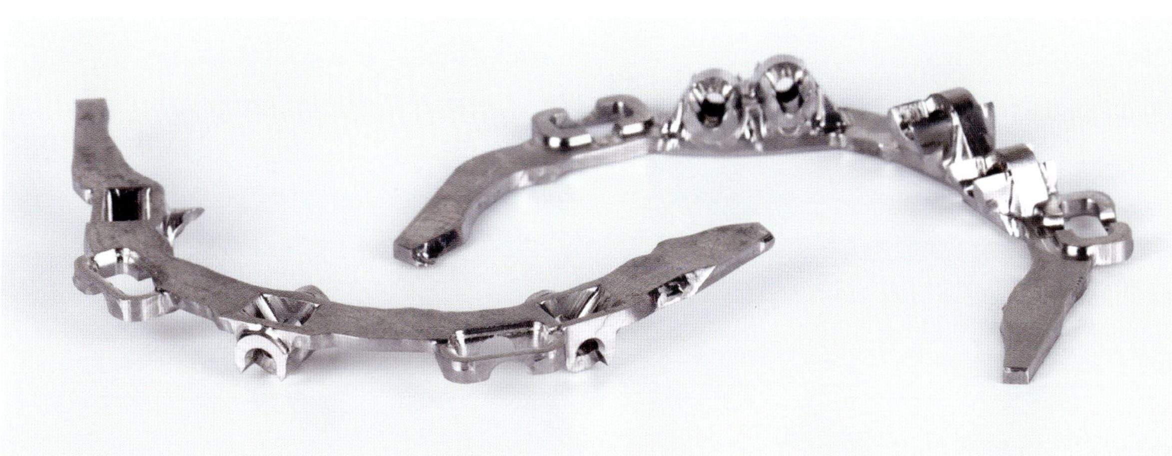

Figure 4.16 Milled titanium foundation guides from Renew Digital Design.

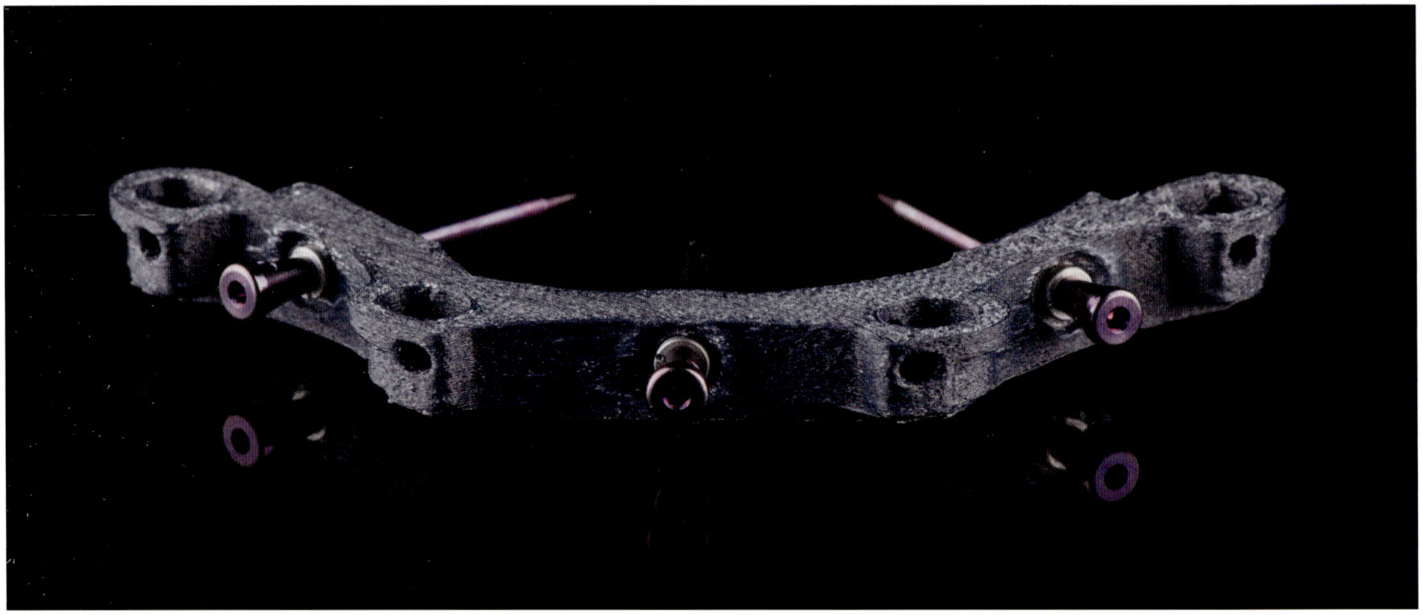

Figure 4.17 **Carbon-fiber reinforced foundation guide with fixation pins.** ***Source: Courtesy of Navagation Precision Guidance®.***

Foundation guides can be secured to the bone in one of three ways: anatomically, in a "floating" position, or in a hybrid combination of the two. Some systems use a floating guide that does not contact the buccal bone, but most require the foundation guide to touch the buccal plate or even sit against the bone in a 360-degree fashion. My preference is to use a hybrid foundation guide that combines the anatomical and floating styles. This hybrid design foundation guide fits intimately over a small portion of the buccal bone and creates more stability, but this cannot be achieved if the CBCT scan from which it was designed is not accurate. The floating portion or open area of the hybrid foundation guide is easier to work with, allows visibility, and eliminates the possibility of adding inaccuracy into the system. In the floating only foundation guide, it is necessary for bone fixation pins to be placed in a divergent pattern to support the foundation guide on and in the bone. Anatomical bone-supported and hybrid type foundation guide platforms can be secured to the bone with pins or screws inserted through channels created in the guide (Figs. 4.18-4.23).

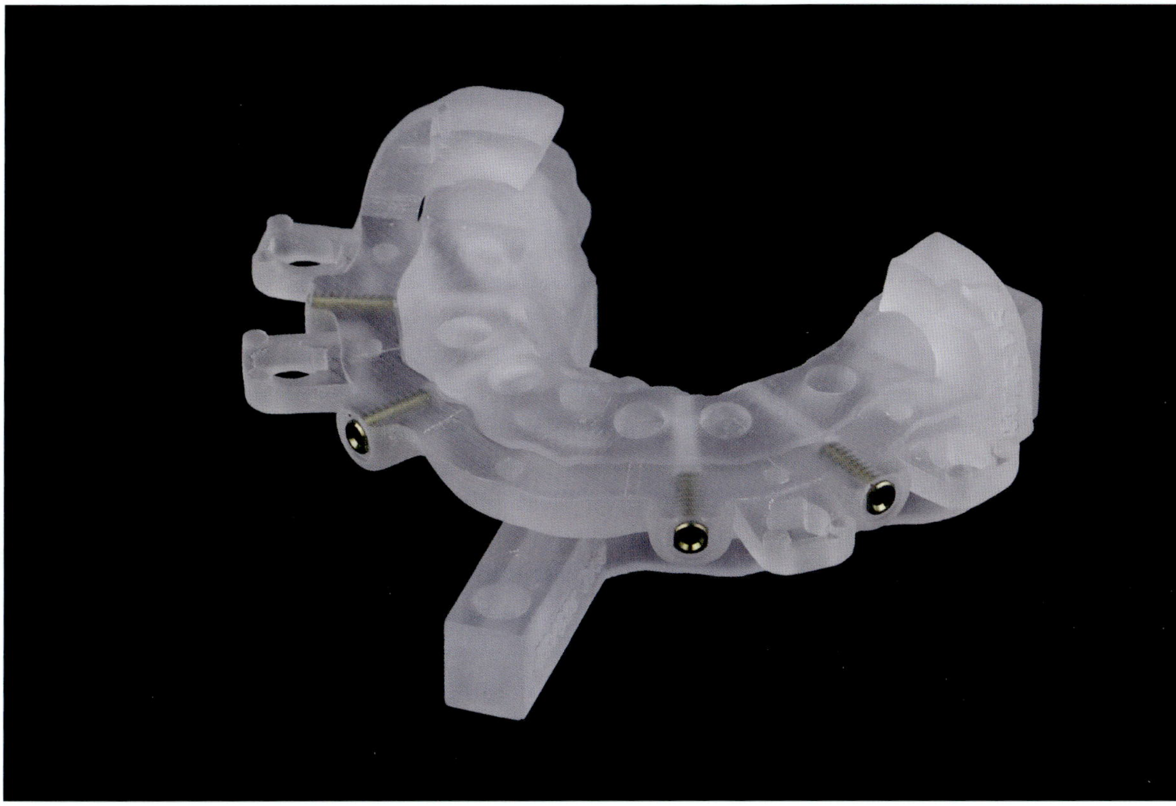

Figure 4.18 Anatomical-style resin foundation guide with distal bone support rests.

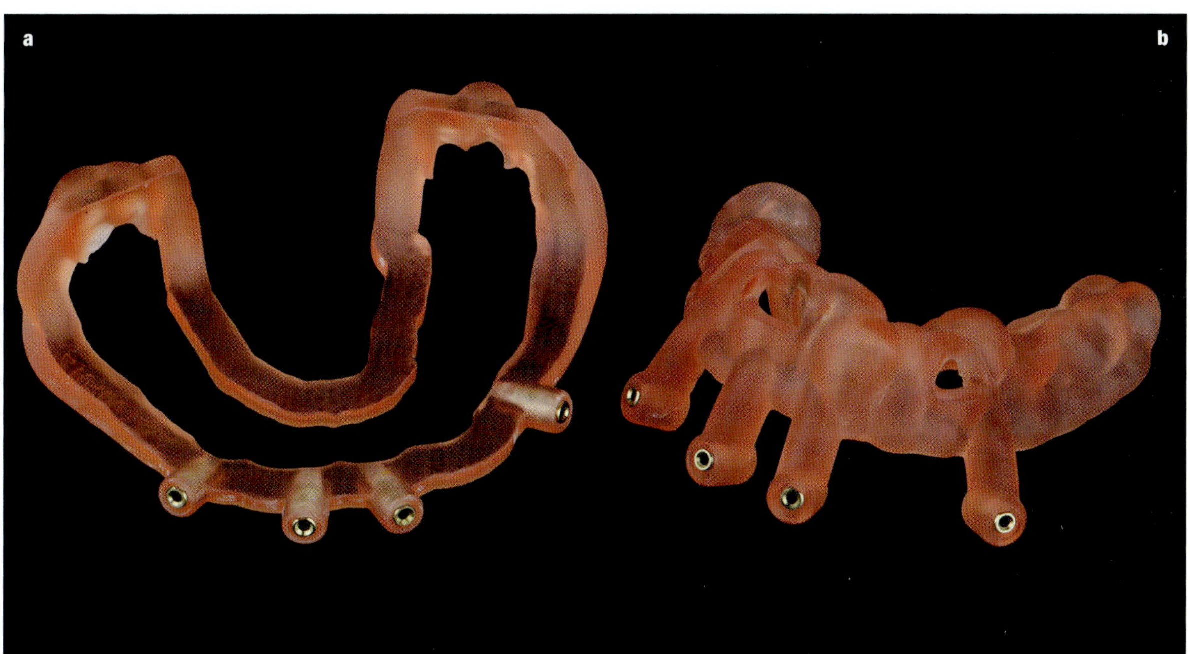

Figure 4.19 (a) Anatomical-style 360-degree resin foundation guide with (b) indexing aligner guide.

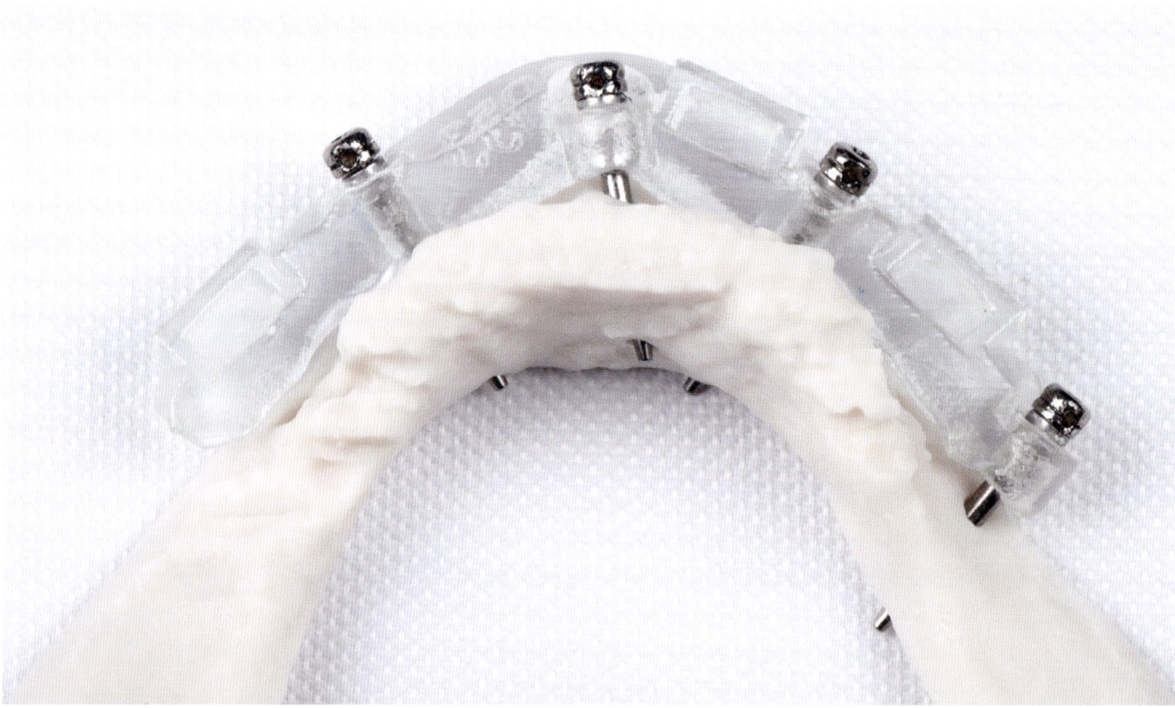

Figure 4.20 Floating-style buccal resin foundation guide.

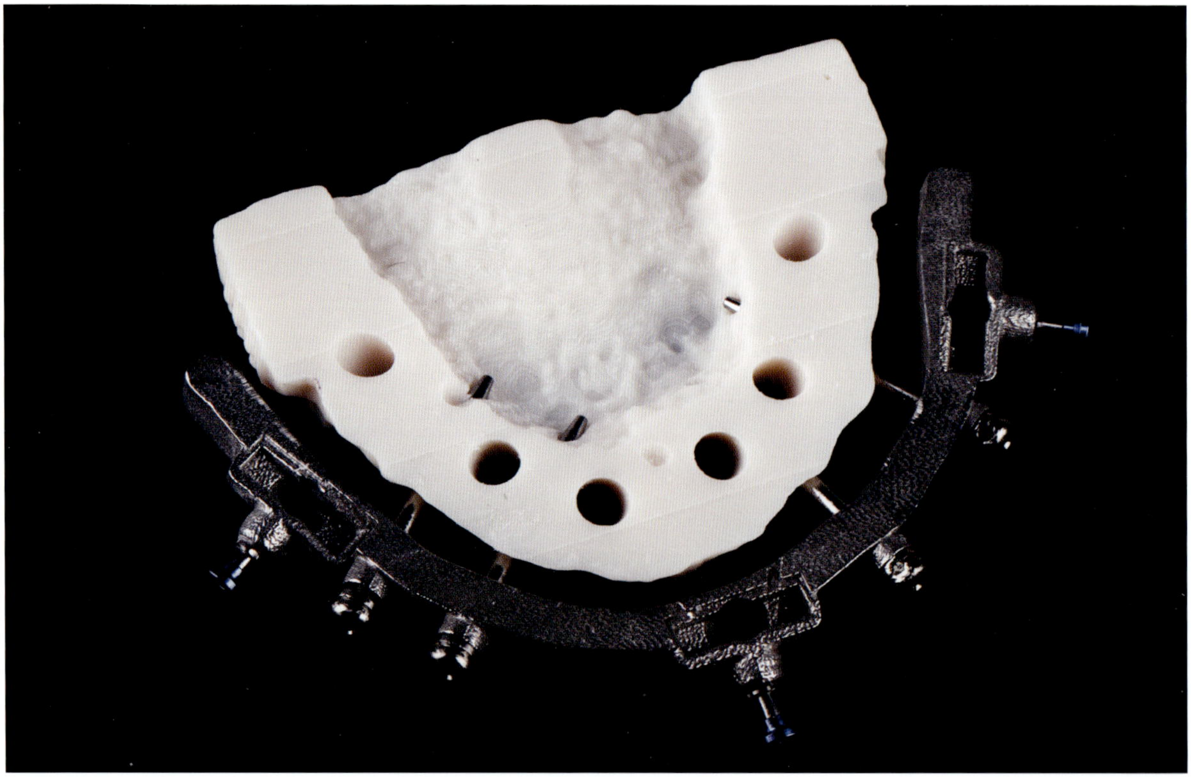

Figure 4.21 Floating-style cobalt-chrome foundation guide.

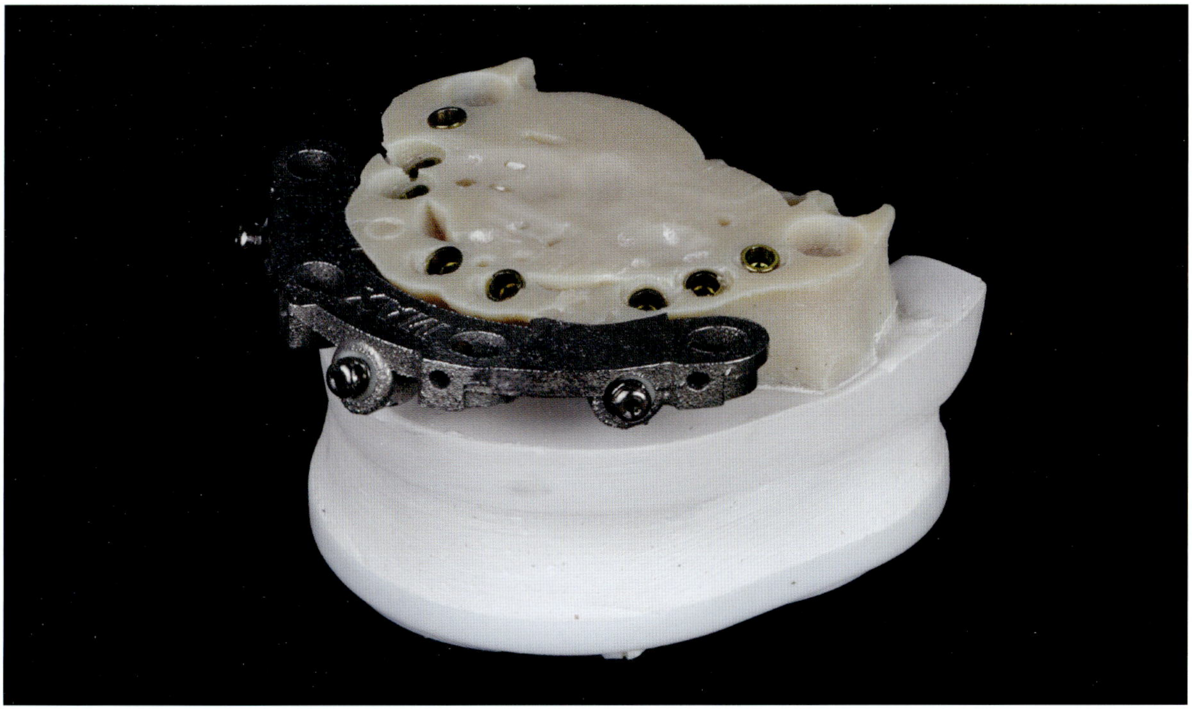

Figure 4.22 Hybrid floating- and anatomical-style cobalt-chrome foundation guide.

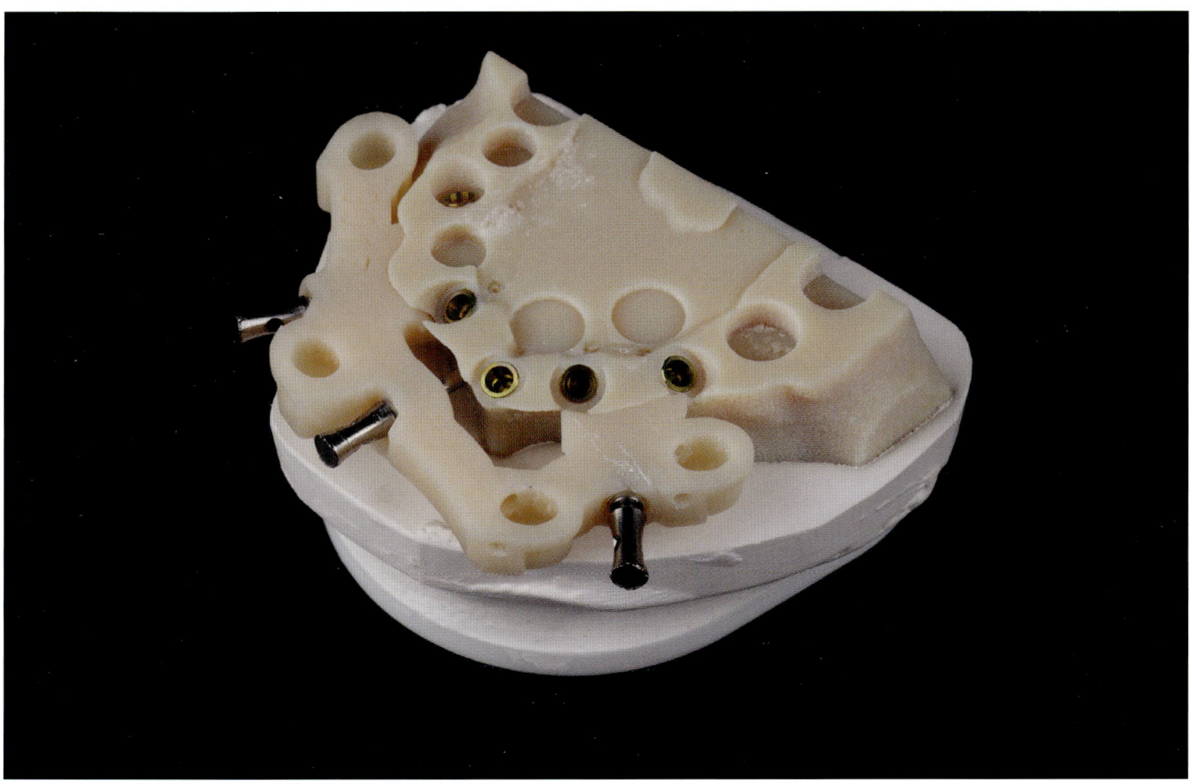

Figure 4.23 Hybrid floating- and anatomical-style foundation guide made of Flexcera™ resin (Desktop Health).

Three to five pins or screws are used to secure the foundation guide into the bone. Fewer than three points of bone fixation may allow movement and possibly destabilize the guide. Conversely, the external surface of the guide will not accommodate more than five pins or screws without potentially affecting the sequencing of the implant surgery.

Fixation pins and screws are available in varying lengths and diameters and require the use of a special drill to penetrate the bone and fasten the guide. The fixation drill should be made by the same manufacturer as the pins or screws, as mixing different-sized drills, pins, and/or screws can result in instability of the guide (Figs. 4.24-4.26). Also, the laboratory that is fabricating the foundation guide will need to know which brand will be used so that it can design the guide accordingly.

The foundation guide should only extend and be fixated distally as far as is necessary for stability and implant placement. The longer the distal extensions of this guide are, the harder it is to seat and access its pins and locks. The design of the foundation guide and the length of the distal extensions also must take into consideration the presence of the cheeks and allow for placement of the bone fixation pins in these areas without too much difficulty.

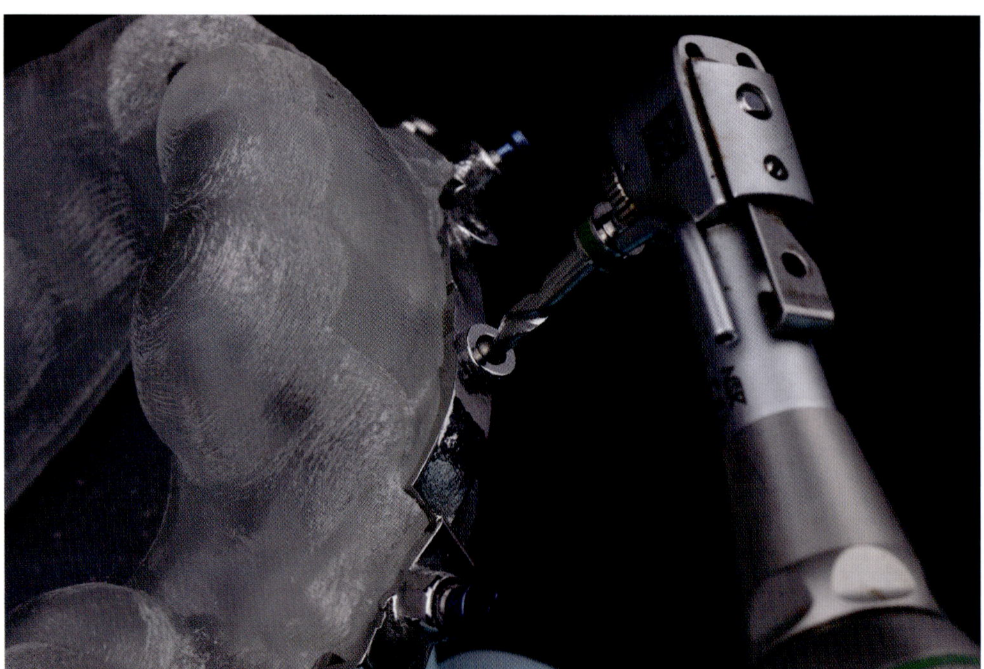

Figure 4.24 **Pin fixation drill inserted into foundation guide pin channel.**

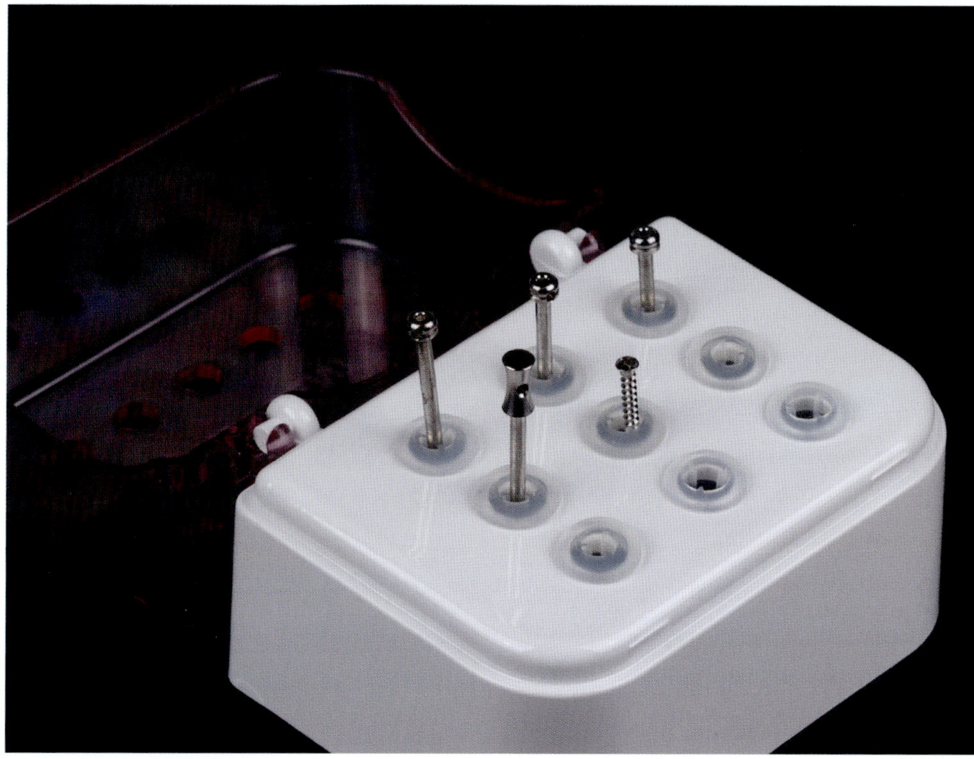

Figure 4.25 Foundation guide fixation pins and screws in a carrier.

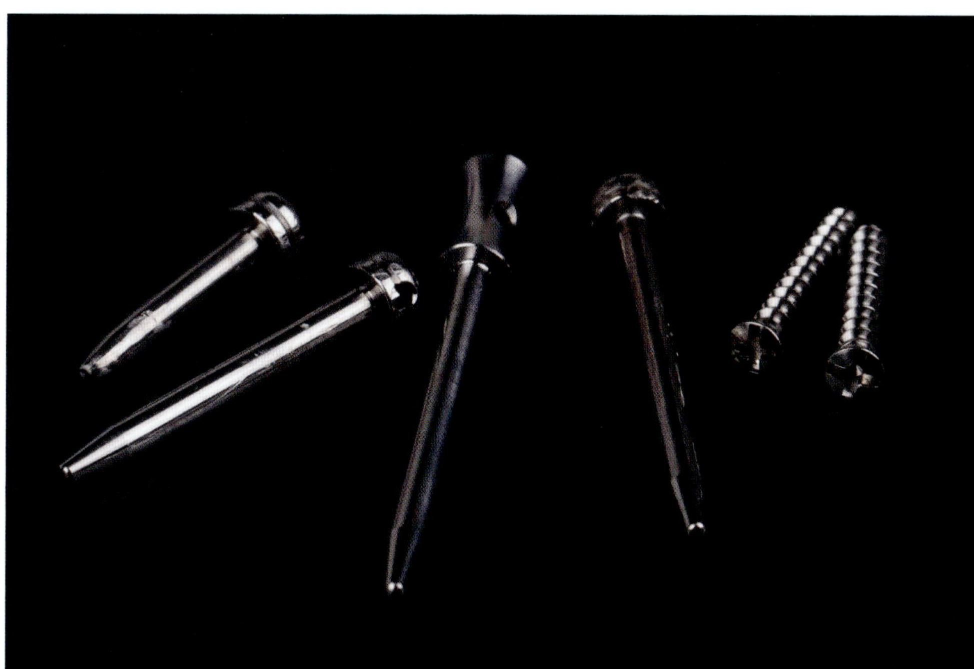

Figure 4.26 Foundation guide fixation pins and screws.

Osteotomy guide

The osteotomy guide, the third component of the stackable guided system, allows for accurate drilling and placement of the implants (Fig. 4.27). Like foundation guides, osteotomy guides can be made from various types of materials, although printed surgical resin is probably the most popular material being used today. Resin guides are less expensive and faster to manufacture than those made of other materials; the tradeoff is that they allow less visibility during drilling and placement of the implant than some other materials, and they can flex and break. Fracturing a guide during the process of drilling or implant placement can be stressful and potentially have a negative impact on the outcome of the surgery.

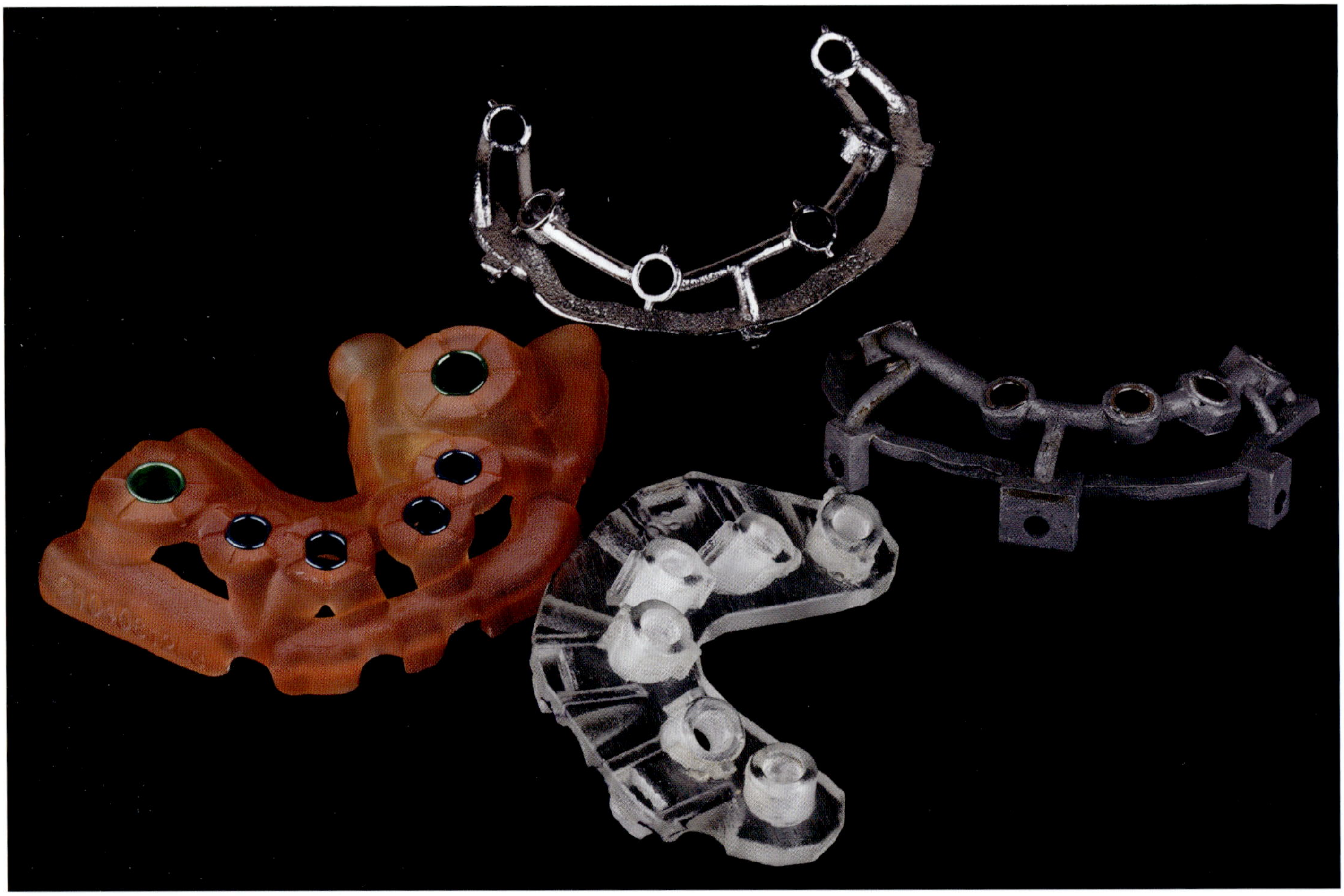

Figure 4.27 **Various osteotomy guides assembled from different stackable guide systems.**

My preferences are carbon-fiber-reinforced resin, laser-sintered cobalt-chrome, milled titanium, or Flexera resin material. An osteotomy guide made of cobalt-chrome is 3D printed by a process of direct metal laser sintering (DMLS), in which fine particles of the metal alloy powder are first melted down with a laser and then used to print the guide layer by layer. After the guide is completed, supports are removed, and the final design is finished by the laboratory (Fig. 4.28). Milling titanium for stackable full-arch surgical guides is a concept recently introduced to me by Dr. Nate Farley and Dr. Kent Howell of Renew Digital Design. The milling titanium process has had some limitations in the past, but I was very impressed with the system developed by Drs. Farley and Howell. The advantages of a metal guide are its strength and durability, which allow the guide's support arms to be very thin for maximum visibility and irrigation. Lack of flex in the metal also makes it very unlikely to break during use. One disadvantage of a metal guide is that it is more expensive and requires more time to manufacture.

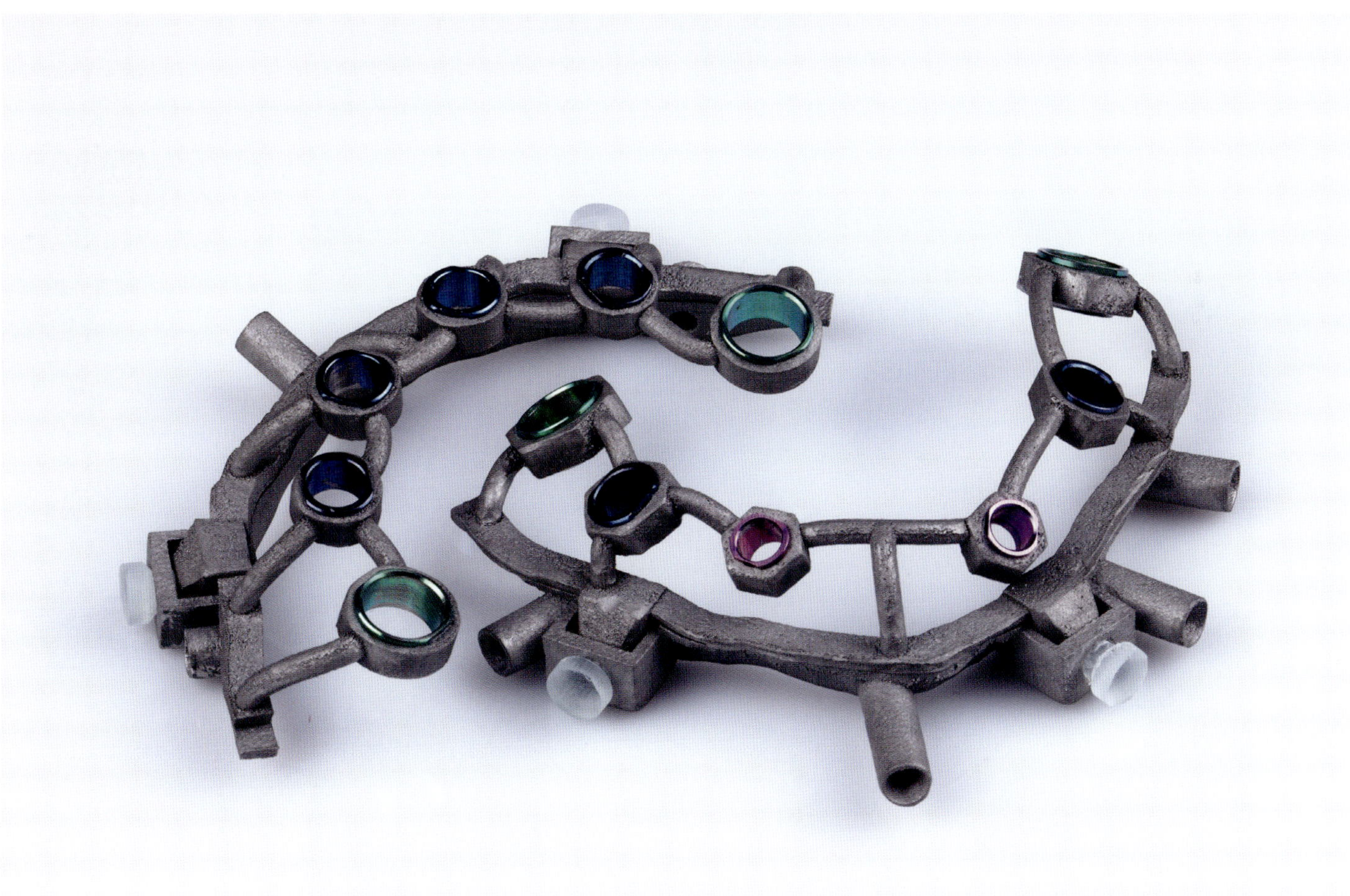

Figure 4.28 **Printed cobalt-chrome osteotomy guide with OEM guide sleeves fitted on a cobalt-chrome floating-style foundation guide.**

Printed carbon-fiber-reinforced material and Flexera resin currently have limited availability but are otherwise very good materials for the foundation and osteotomy guides. They offer all the benefits of metal but require less time and less expense to manufacture. The laboratories I partner with have the equipment to print these guides in their facility, which can reduce the amount of time needed for processing (Figs. 4.29-4.32).

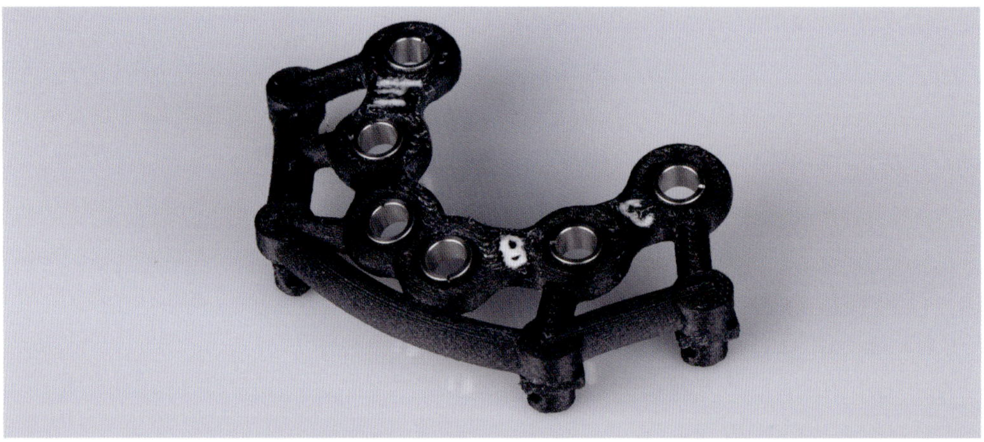

Figure 4.29 **Printed carbon-fiber reinforced osteotomy guide.**

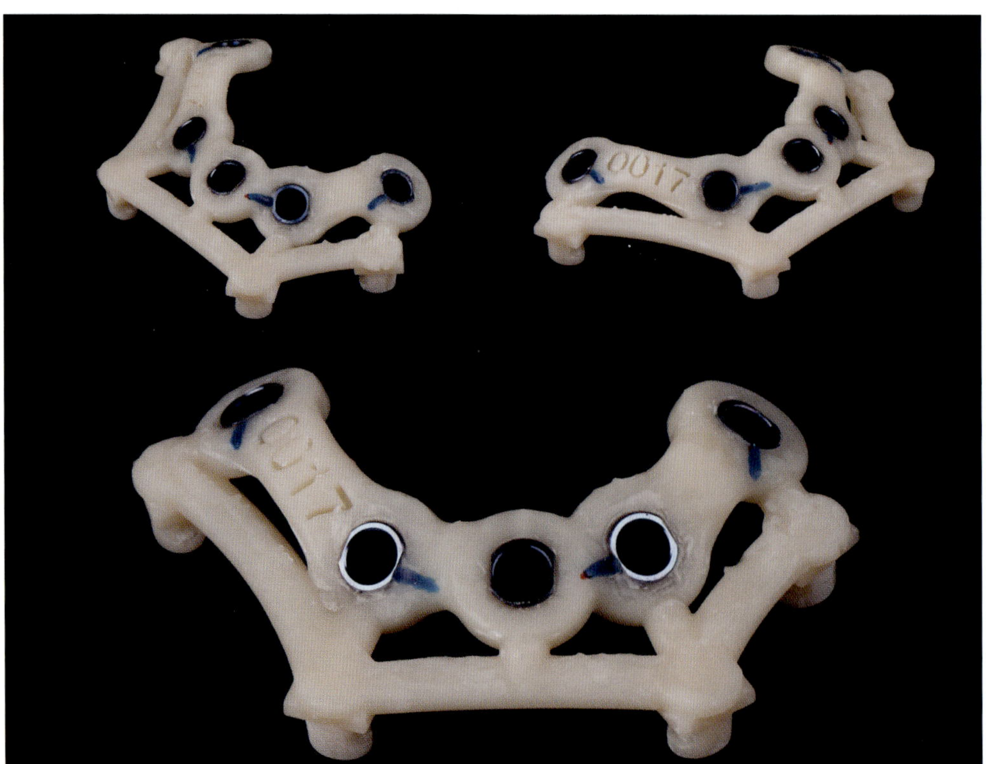

Figure 4.30 **Printed Flexcera™ resin osteotomy guide.**

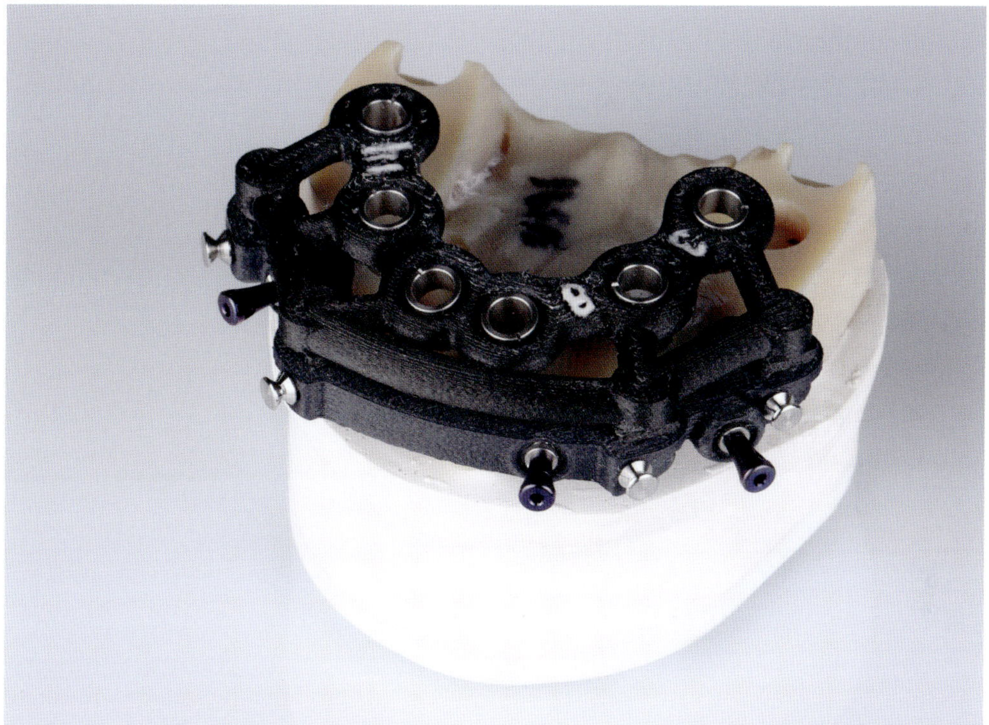

Figure 4.31 Carbon-fiber osteotomy guide affixed to a carbon-fiber reinforced foundation guide.

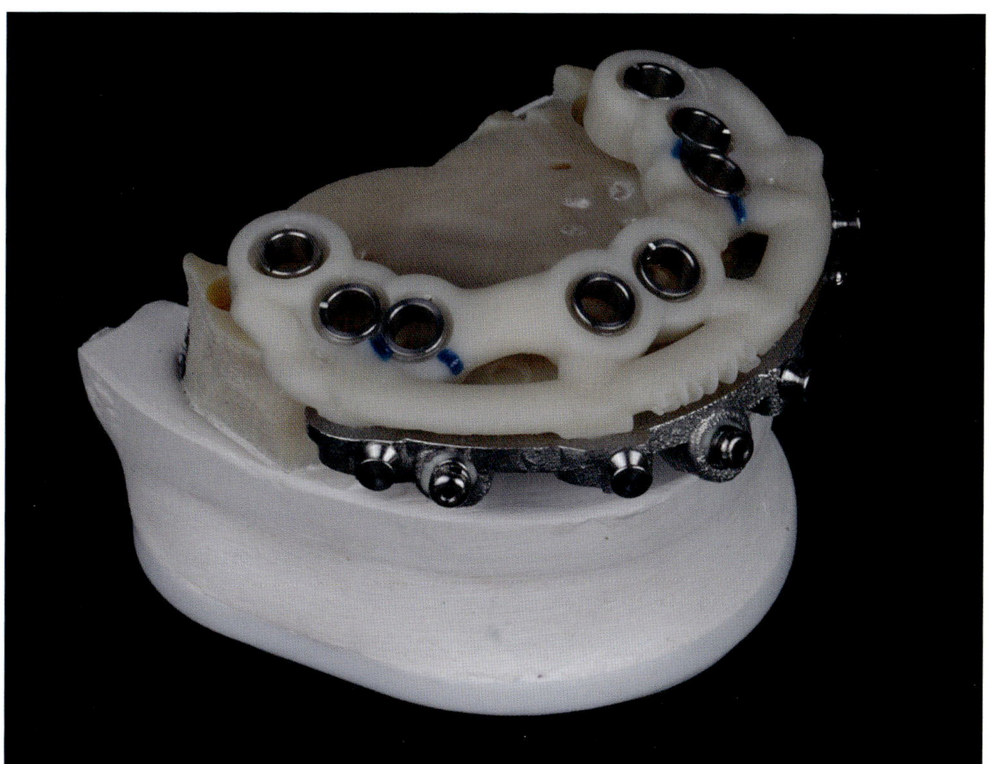

Figure 4.32 Flexcera™ resin osteotomy guide affixed to a cobalt-chrome foundation guide.

An osteotomy guide can be designed to function in one of three ways:

1. **As a pilot guide only.** In this design, the guide creates only the pilot osteotomy and path for the implant and should be used to drill to the final depth (Fig. 4.33).
2. **For partially guided implant placement.** This will allow the drilling of the pilot osteotomy and path and the subsequent drilling sequences to reach the final depth and width needed to accommodate the selected implant in the planned space. However, placement of the implant requires the guide to be removed and the implant to be placed in a manual "freehand" approach (Fig. 4.34).
3. **For fully guided implant placement.** With this design, which is my preference, the guide will support initial drilling for the pilot and full drill sequence as well as placement of the implant through the guide itself. This method of using a stackable guide system achieves the most accuracy (Fig. 4.35).

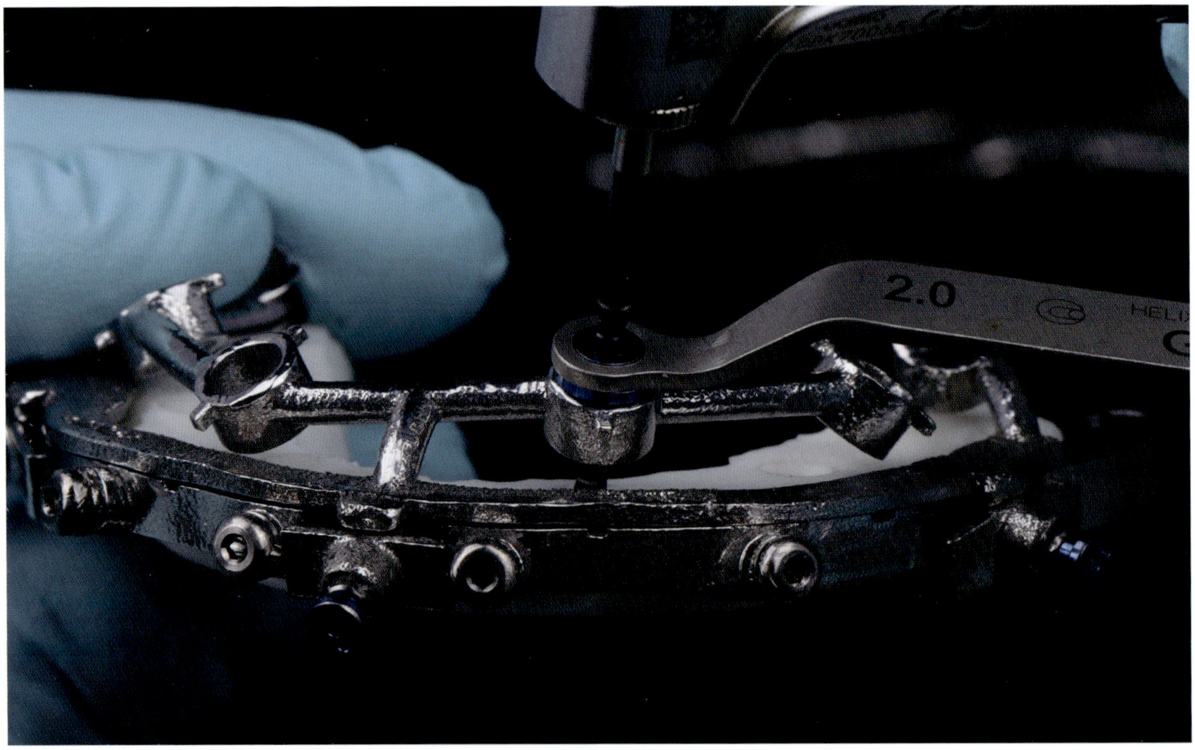

Figure 4.33 **Simulated use of a pilot drill through the osteotomy guide.**

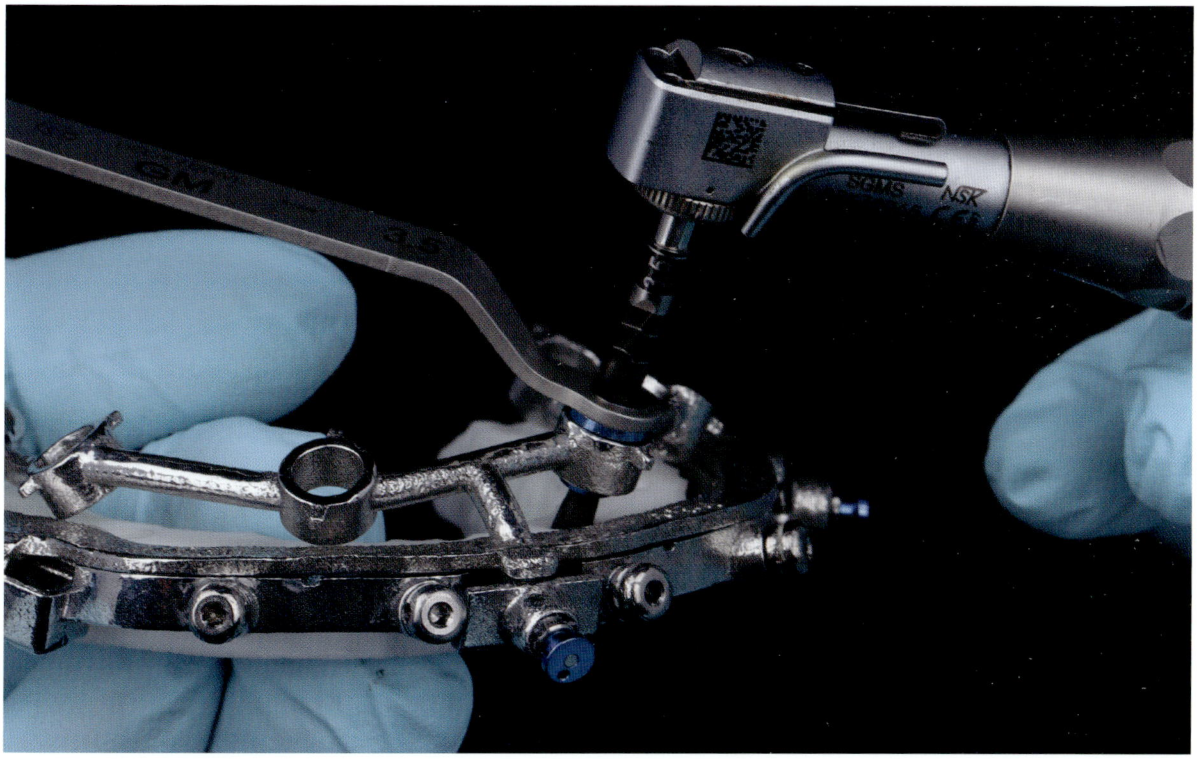

Figure 4.34 Simulation of drilling to final implant depth through osteotomy guide.

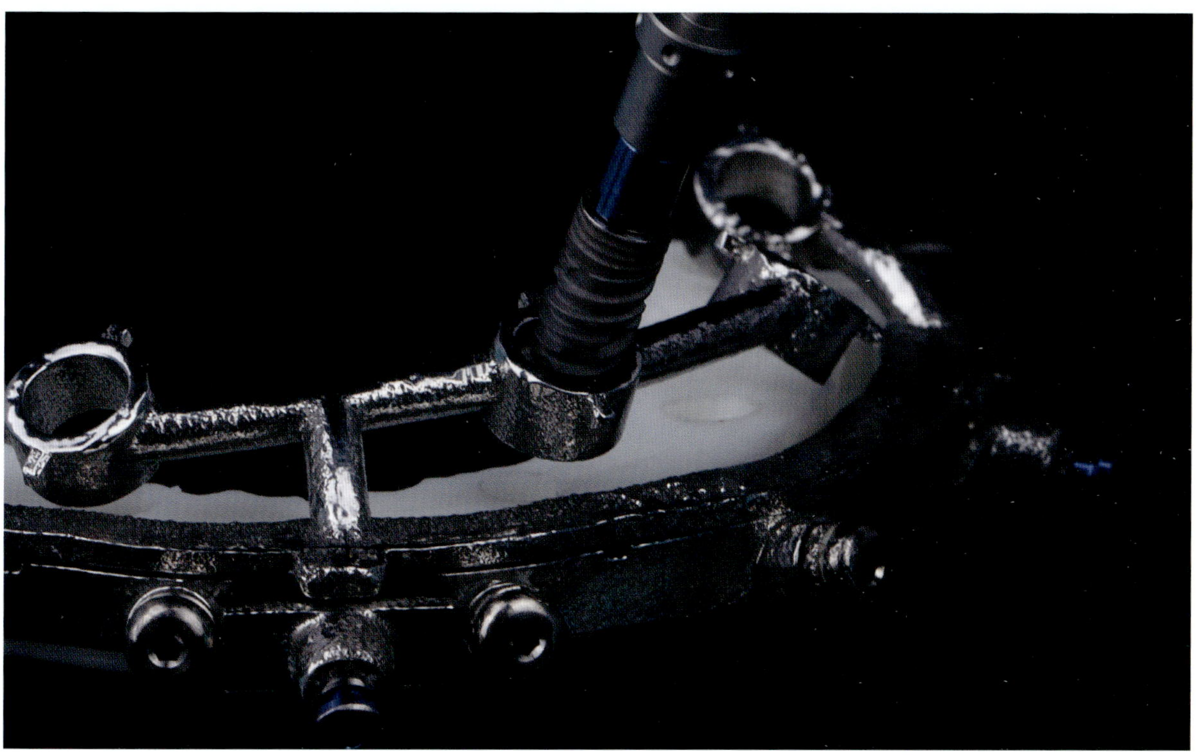

Figure 4.35 Simulation of implant placement through an osteotomy guide for fully guided surgery.

The osteotomy guide should be stable and adapt intimately with the foundation guide to which it is attached, via pins, locks, or friction fit (Figs. 4.36, 4.37). In some guides, the osteotomy sleeves are customized to fit the guide spoons or keys and possibly even the drills that come with some guided implant systems (Fig. 4.38). Guide spoons/keys control the position of the drill as well as the depth and trajectory of the osteotomy it creates. The osteotomy cylinders in the guide should have implant indexing marks that enable proper orientation of the implant for ideal placement of the multiunit abutment (MUA) in a fully guided surgery (Figs. 4.39, 4.40). Because MUAs are designed to be straight or angulated, the implant must be rotated into position based on the indexing marks on the sleeves or cylinders of the osteotomy guide in order for the interim prosthesis pick-up to be accurate.

The design of the osteotomy guide will depend in part on the brand of implant being used. Osteotomy guides can be designed to be implant-specific or generic to support multiple implant systems. It is important to inform the laboratory about the type of osteotomy guide that will be needed during the planning stage.

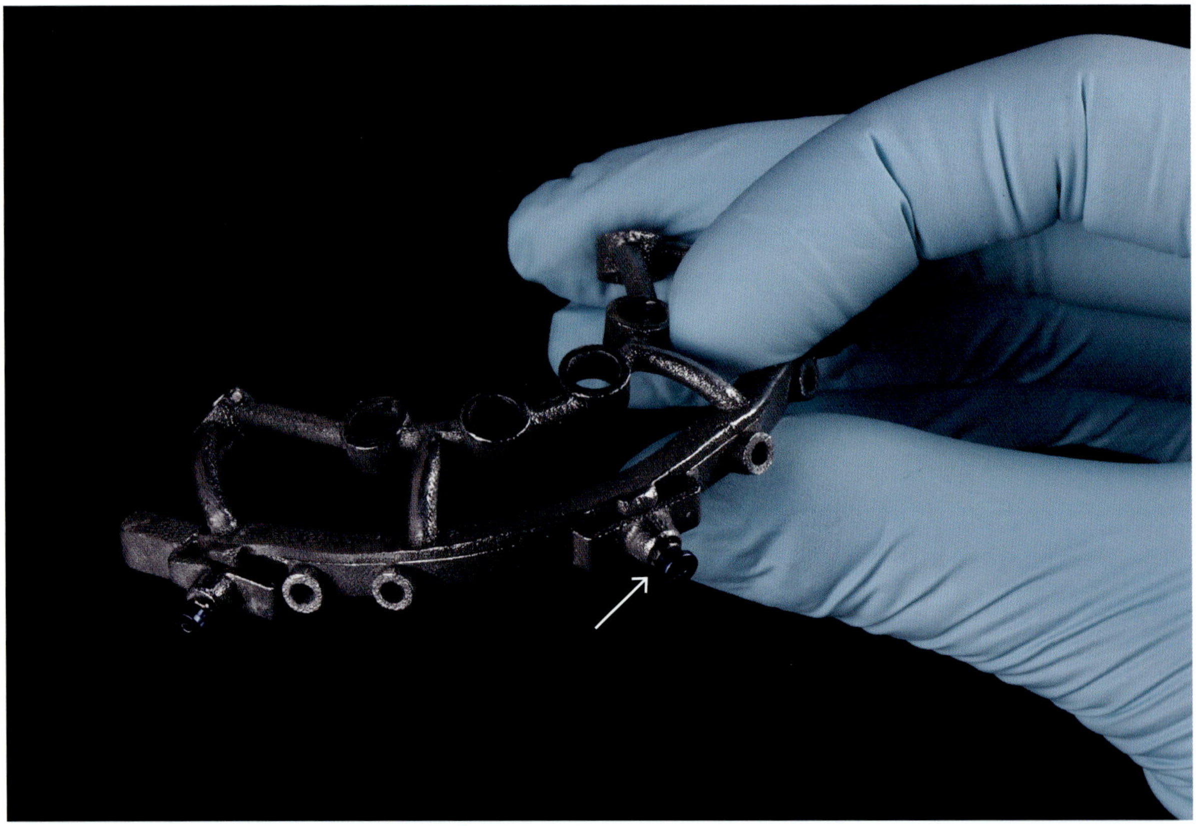

Figure 4.36 **Fixation of a cobalt-chrome osteotomy guide to a cobalt-chrome foundation guide via a locking pin (*arrow*).**

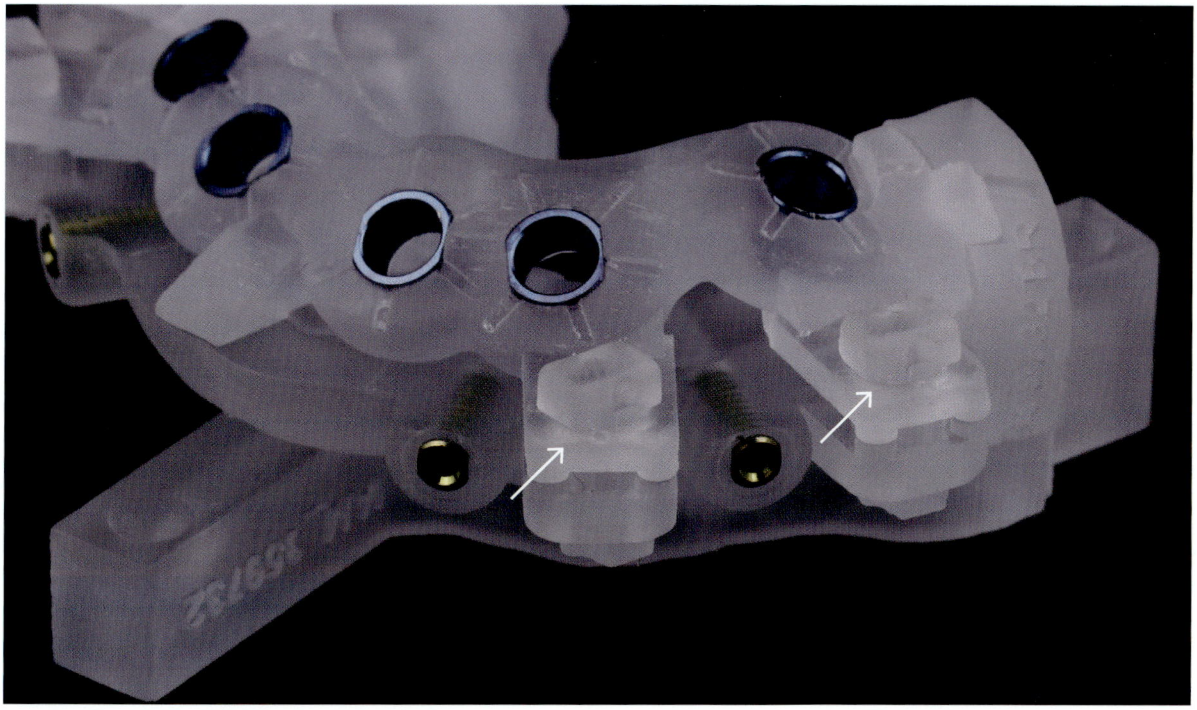

Figure 4.37 Resin locking pins (*arrows*) stabilize a resin osteotomy guide on a resin foundation guide.

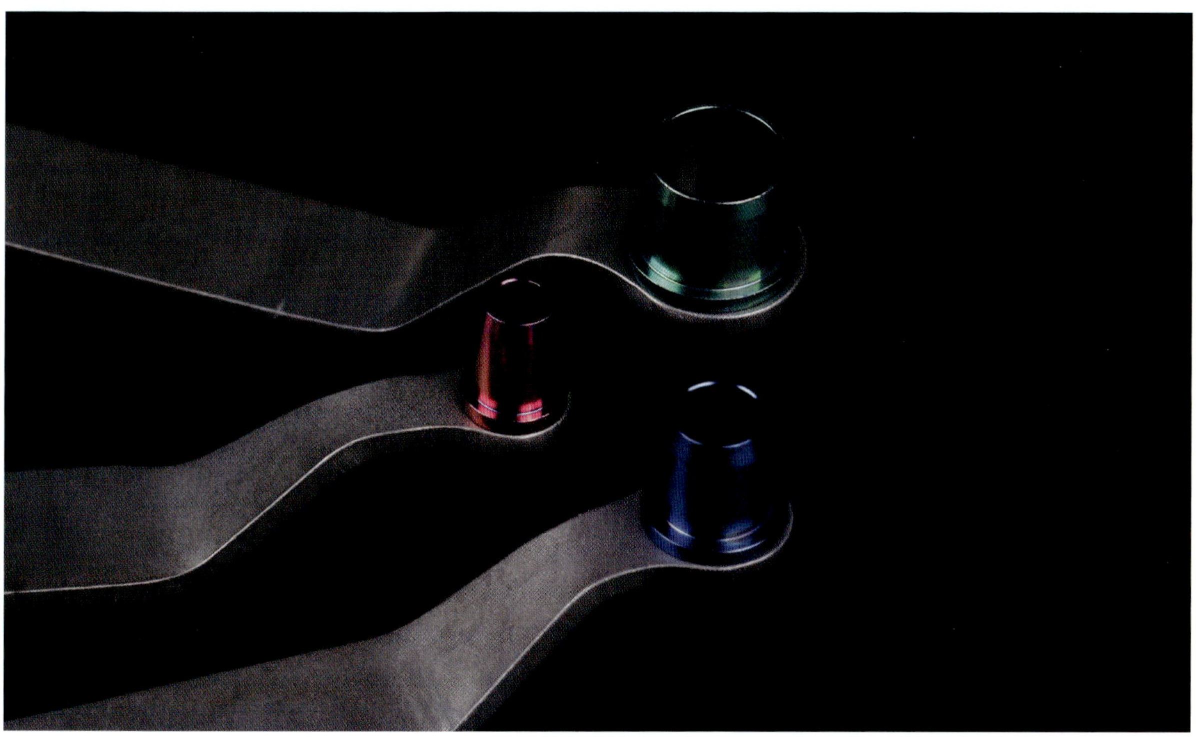

Figure 4.38 Guide spoons or keys designed to be placed in osteotomy guide sleeves.

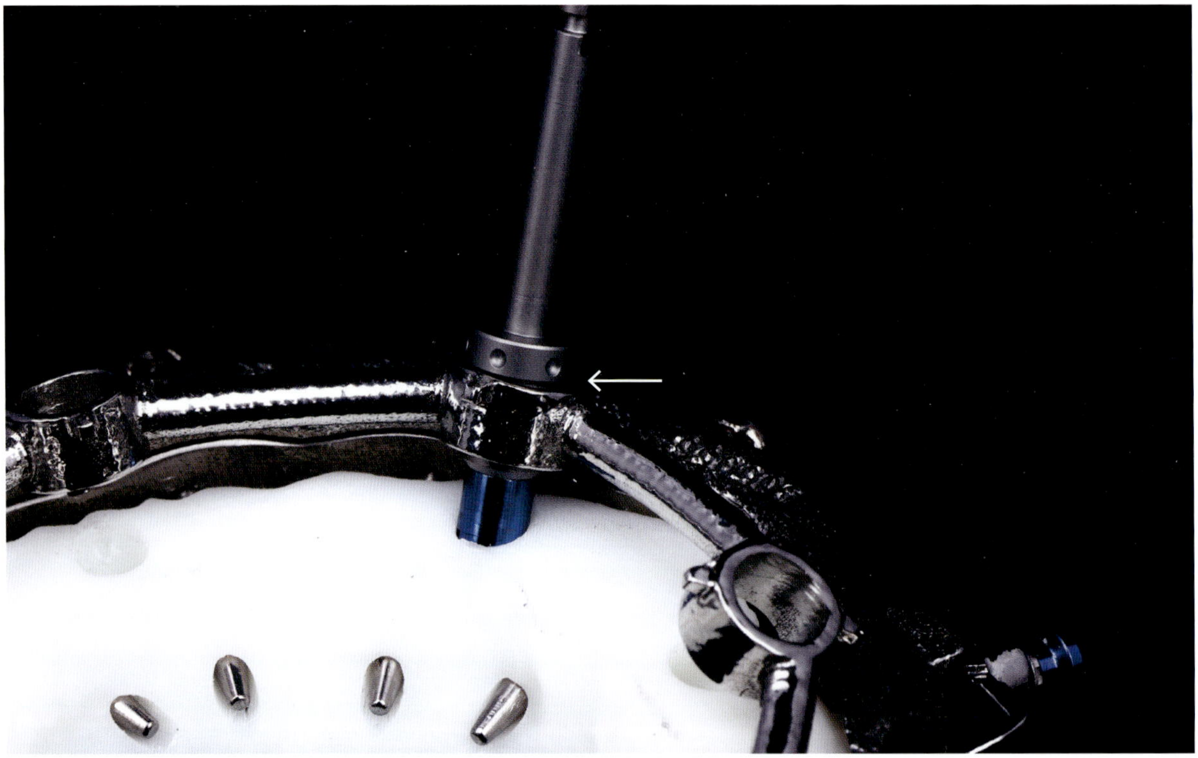

Figure 4.39 Points on the drill collar (*arrow*) serve as an index for proper implant orientation.

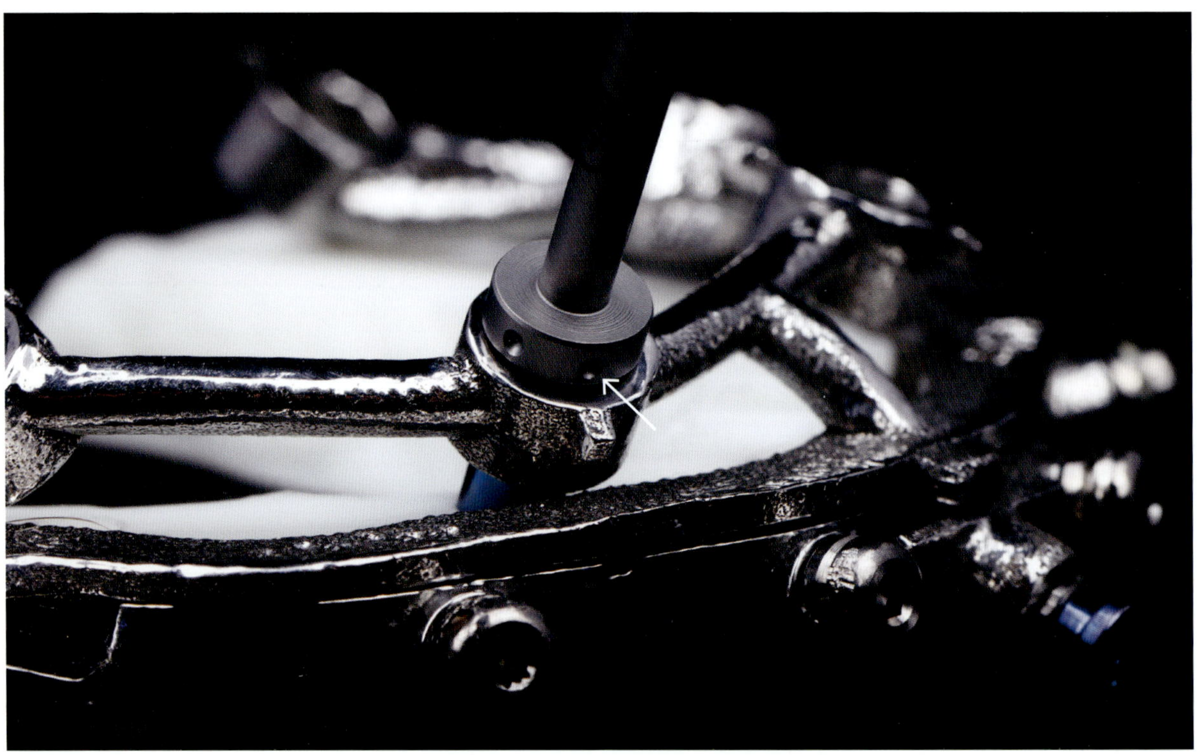

Figure 4.40 Alignment of a point on the drill collar with the indexing on the osteotomy guide (*arrow*).

Carrier guide and abutment aligner

A carrier guide and an abutment aligner are two optional components of some stackable surgical guide systems. Carrier guides and abutment aligners are thin pieces of printed or milled resin that fit on top of the foundation guide and are secured with the same pins, locks, or other retention mechanism used for the osteotomy guide. A carrier guide will remain positioned on the foundation guide during the prosthetic conversion to stabilize the prosthesis and should have indexing built into it. The abutment aligner will help orient the MUAs correctly (Figs. 4.41-4.44).

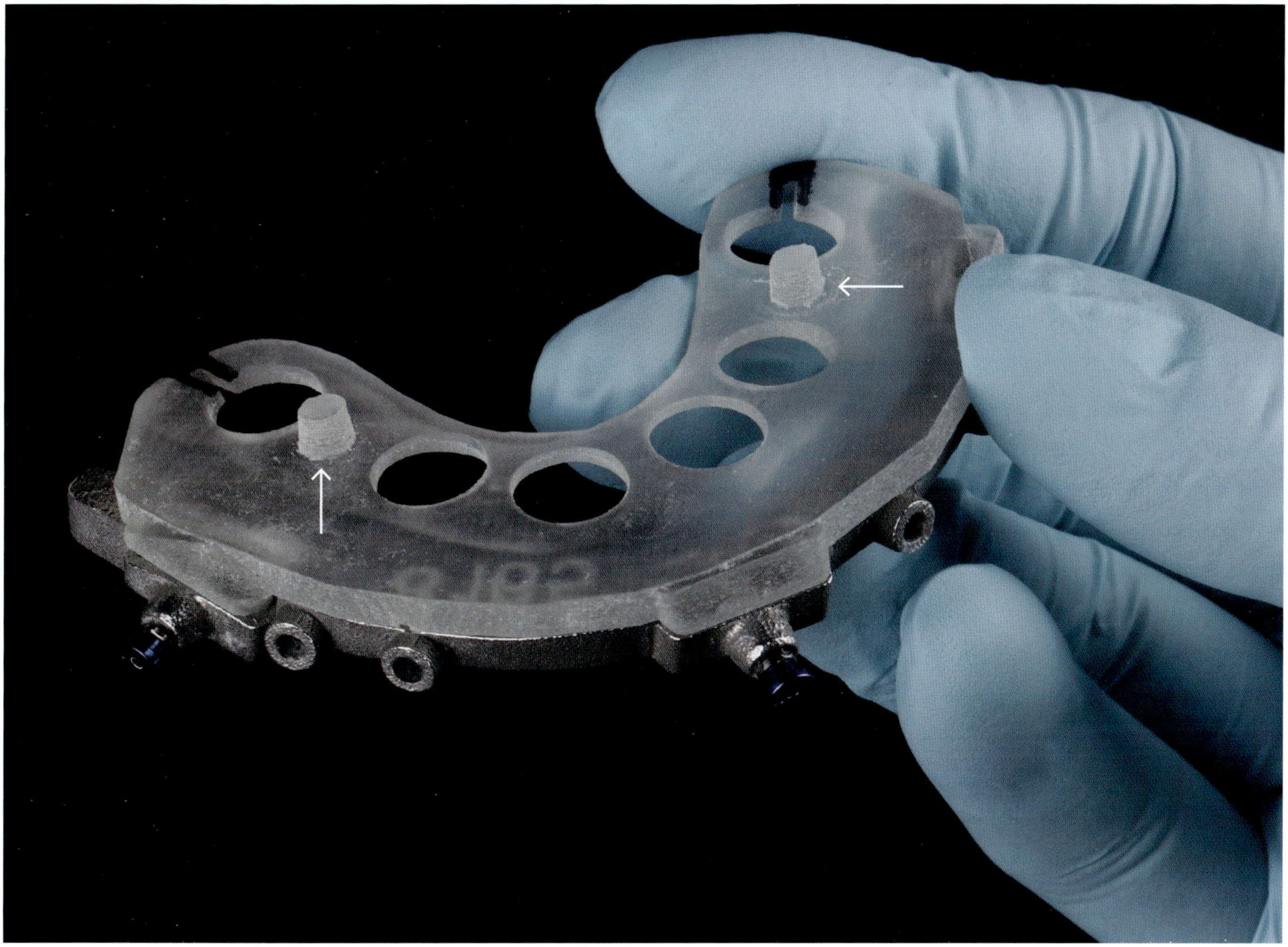

Figure 4.41 Carrier guide with projections (*arrows*) to index and stabilize an interim prosthesis.

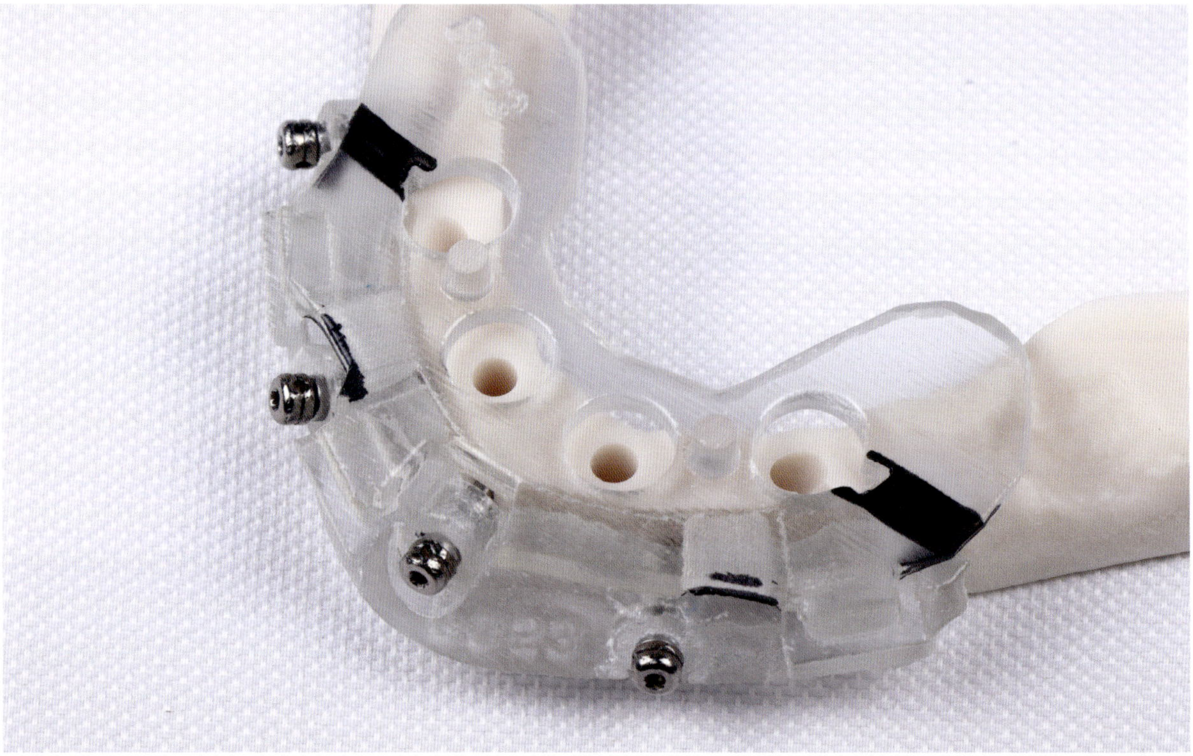

Figure 4.42 Carrier guide fixated to a resin foundation guide.

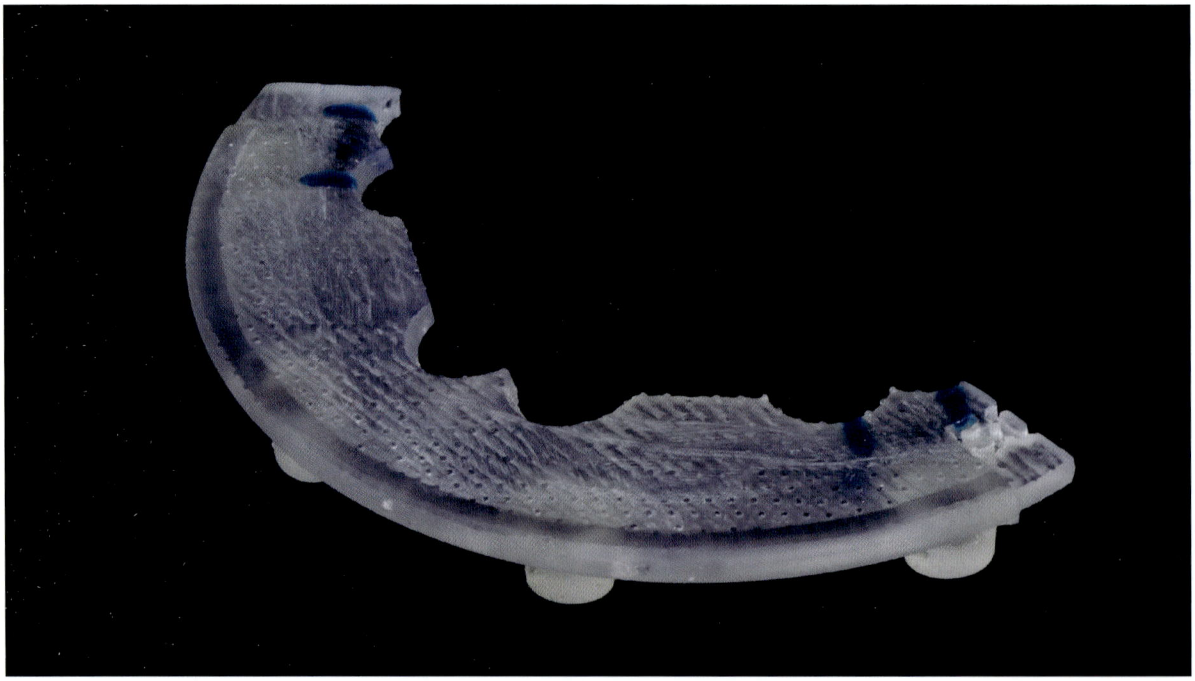

Figure 4.43 Printed abutment aligner.

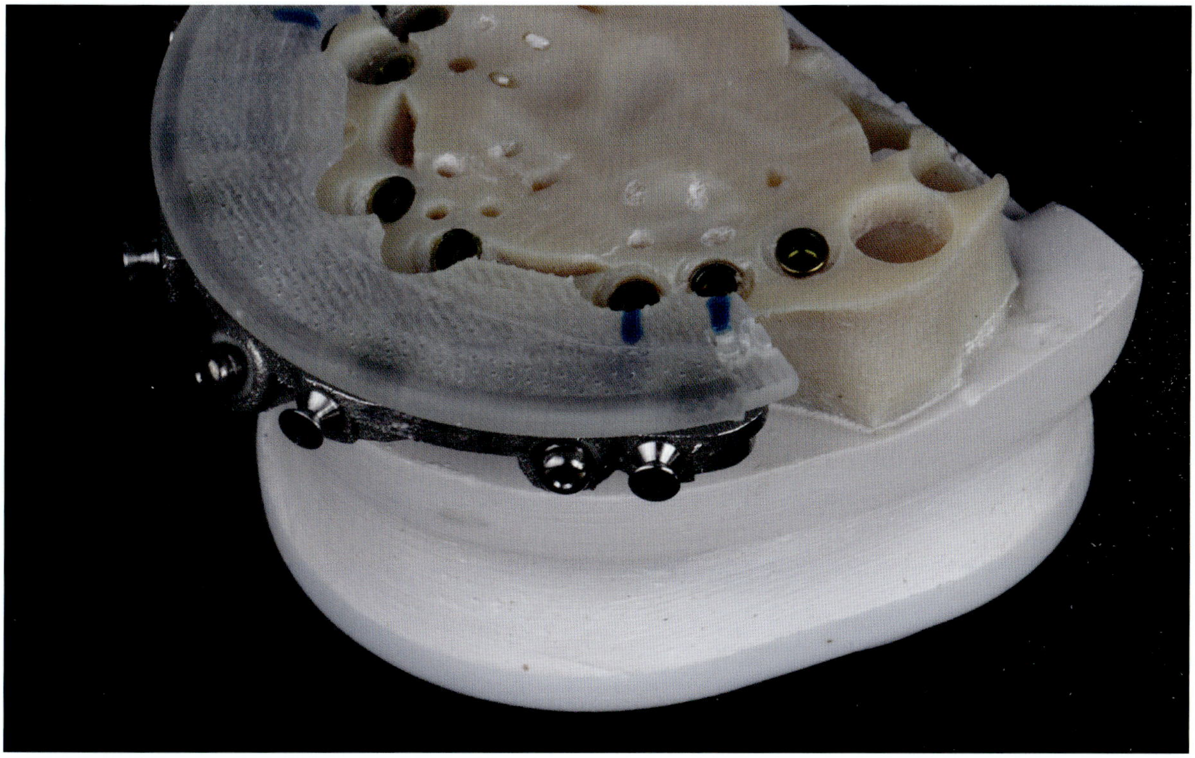

Figure 4.44 **Abutment aligner fixated to a cobalt-chrome foundation guide.**

The carrier guide and abutment aligner can serve the following purposes:

- **Bone reduction verification.** Positioned atop the foundation guide, the carrier guide shows how much bone reduction was planned and/or has been completed. It should fit passively and intimately with no gaps or space between it and the foundation guide. For this purpose the carrier guide is placed after bone reduction is completed and before the implants are placed.
- **Interim prosthesis and/or replica appliance indexing.** Once the carrier guide is in position, the interim prosthesis can be placed over it for added stability and security during the pick-up conversion of the interim prosthesis.
- **Tissue gap creation.** The carrier guide is a physical representation of the amount of space between the bone and the interim prosthesis occupied by the soft tissue. This gap will allow the tissue to heal and form properly around the MUAs without impingement. In some systems this component is unnecessary, and the space-for-tissue gap is accounted for during the digital planning workflow.

- **Direction and rotation indexing of MUAs.** The carrier guide and abutment aligner indicate the position of the implants and have indexing marks for the MUAs (Fig. 4.45). They should allow sufficient space for each implant to be seen and for each MUA to be placed. Straight MUAs are generally easiest and do not require much thought. Angled abutments will require alignment with the indexing on the guides, which show where screw access channels are located, thus allowing proper angulation.

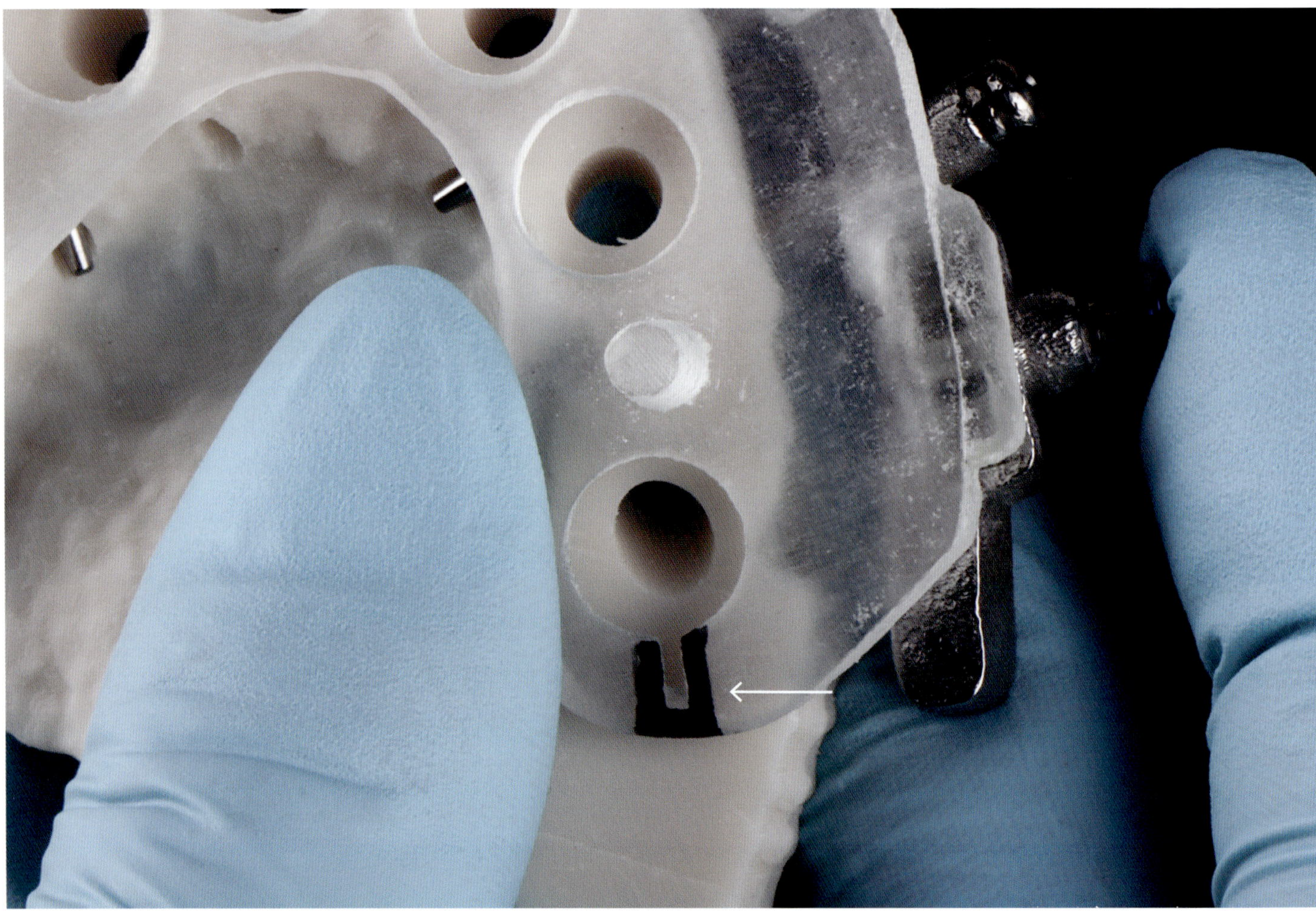

Figure 4.45 **Mark on a carrier guide denoting the position of a multiunit abutment (MUA) screw access channel (*arrow*).**

CONVERSION COMPONENTS

Interim prosthesis

For many years, the interim prosthesis that I used in my nonguided fixed full-arch implant rehabilitation was a denture that was then converted through a complicated technique utilizing self-curing acrylics, putty, or occlusal registration material and other paraphernalia. Most of the time, this workflow was carried out with a surgeon or another dentist and a laboratory technician. I soon learned that each clinician had their own way of doing it. Where exactly the teeth and access channels would end up, however, was something of a mystery to everyone. This lack of reproducibility and uncertainty made the process very difficult to teach. With the introduction of the full-arch stackable guide system, the surgical as well as the prosthetic phase of the process became systematic and more predictable.

The interim prosthesis is the first set of teeth that the patient wears during the implant-healing phase and immediately after the surgery is completed. The prosthesis should be esthetic and have good occlusion with the opposing arch, whether that is natural teeth, a denture, or another fixed full-arch implant-supported prosthesis. Because the case is worked up digitally and preplanned, the occlusion should not pose a problem. The exception to this is if changes are made during surgery, the plan is not worked up properly, or it is inaccurate.

Interim prostheses are generally made from milled or printed PMMA materials. Manufacturers offer several different PMMA materials, which have improved dramatically in esthetics as well as strength and durability over the past several years. The prosthesis may have holes or apertures for temporary copings or cylinders that are used during the conversion of the interim prosthesis. These holes should be wide enough to allow resin pick-up material to flow around each one. For esthetic purposes, all the channels or holes in the anterior portion of the prosthesis should be lingual to the teeth, whereas those in the posterior portion of the prosthesis should be through the occlusal surface or just lingual to it (Figs. 4.46-4.52).

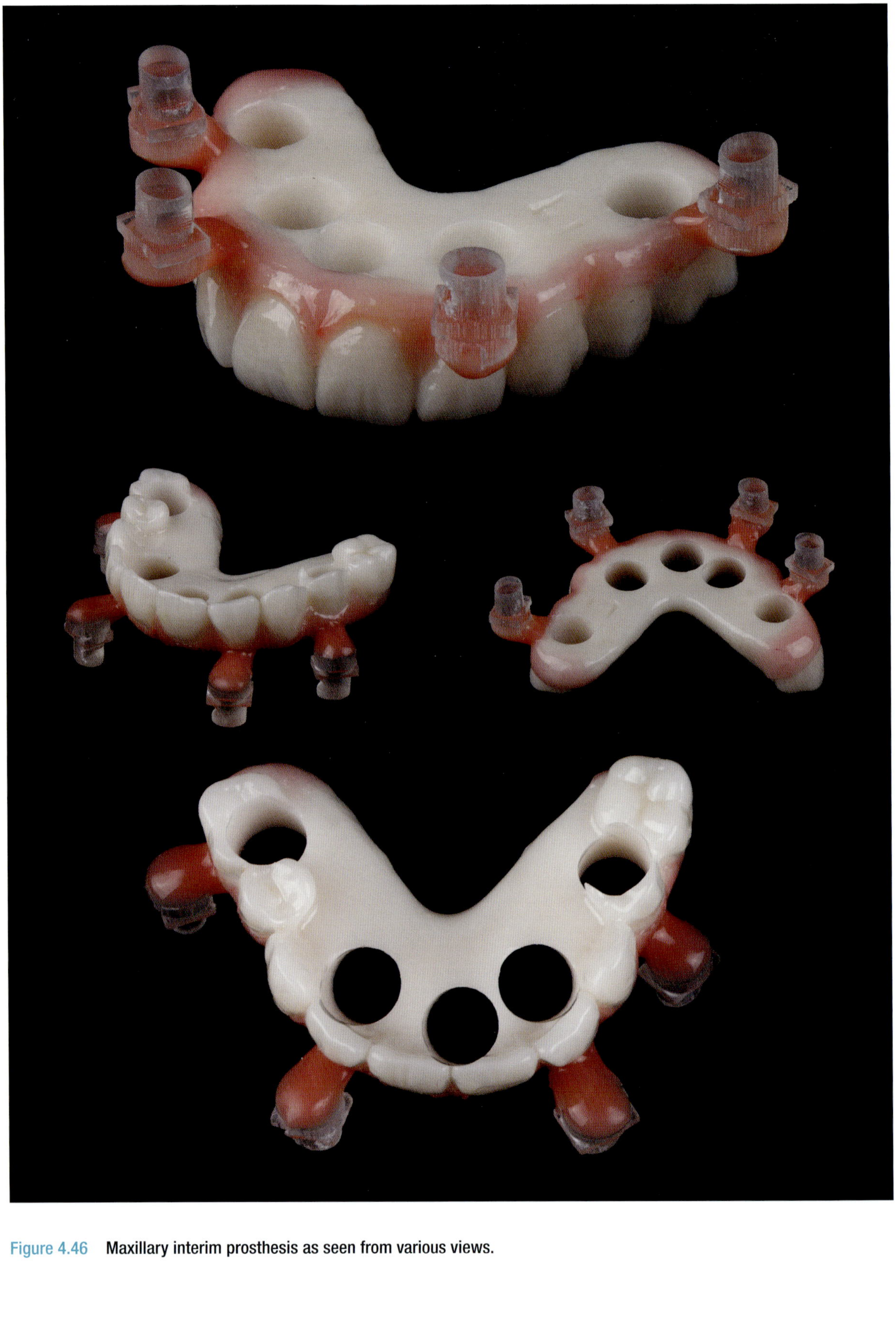

Figure 4.46 **Maxillary interim prosthesis as seen from various views.**

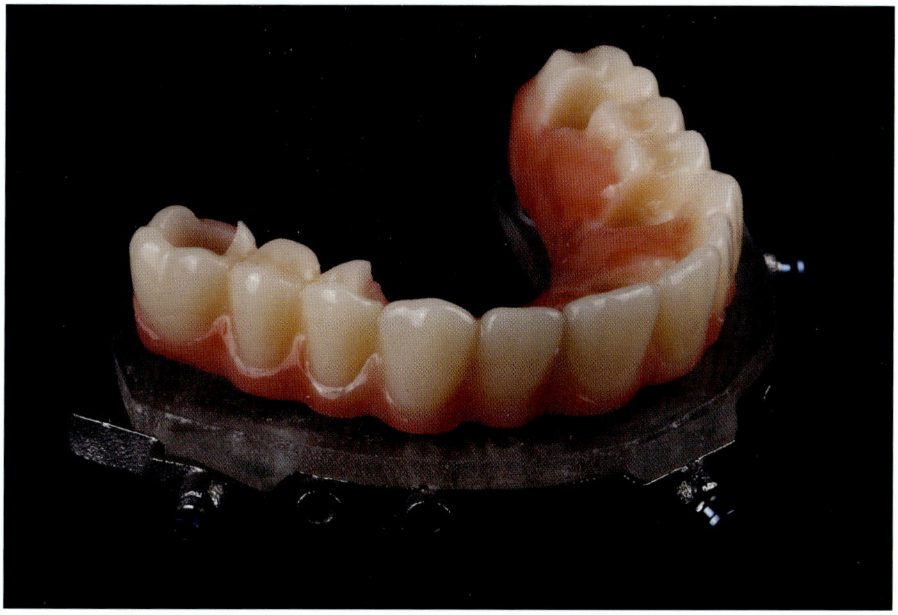

Figure 4.47 Maxillary interim prosthesis resting on a carrier guide attached to a foundation guide.

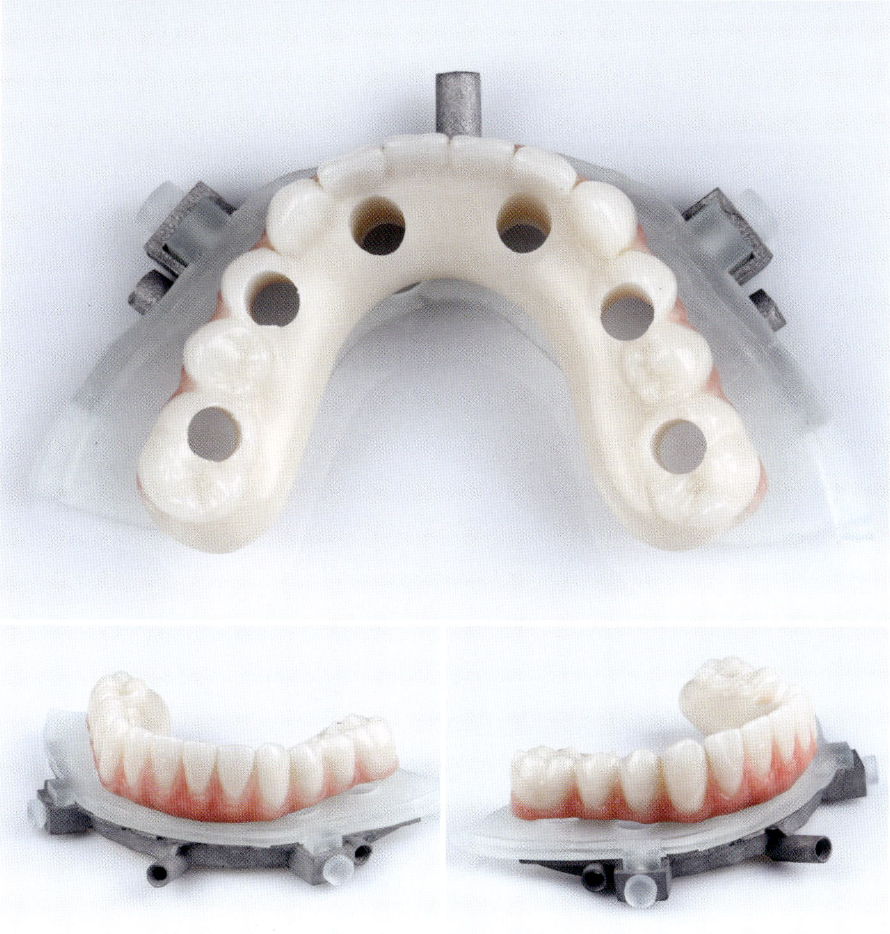

Figure 4.48 Mandibular interim prosthesis resting on a carrier guide viewed from different angles.

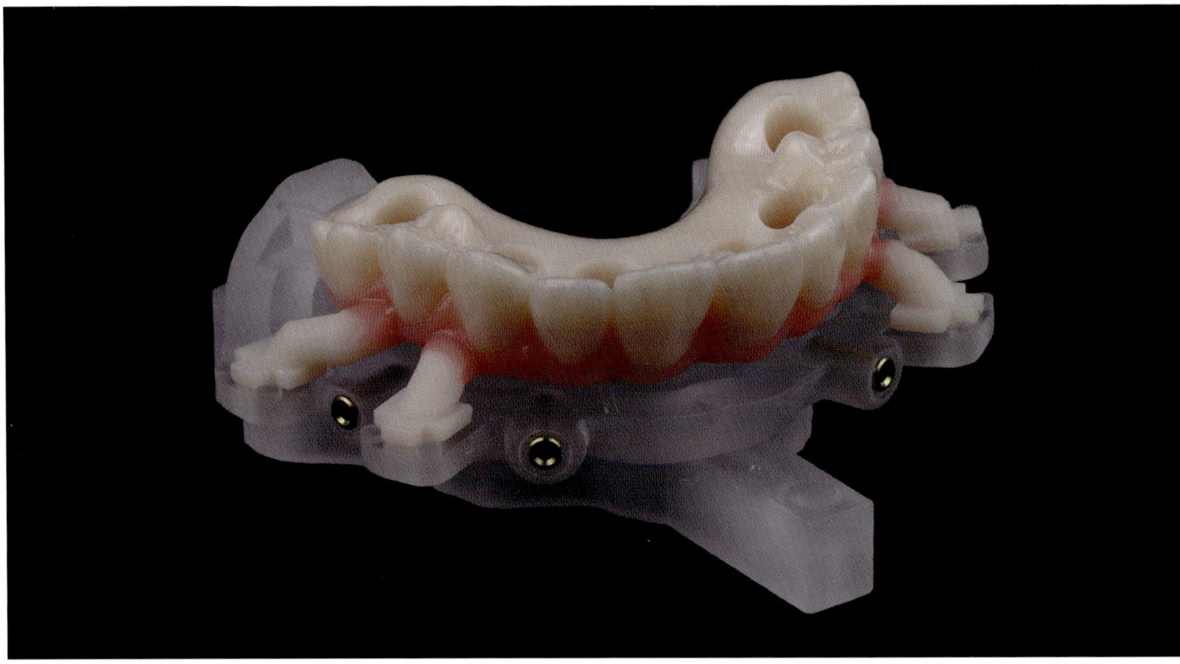

Figure 4.49 Maxillary interim prosthesis seated on a resin foundation guide without a carrier guide.

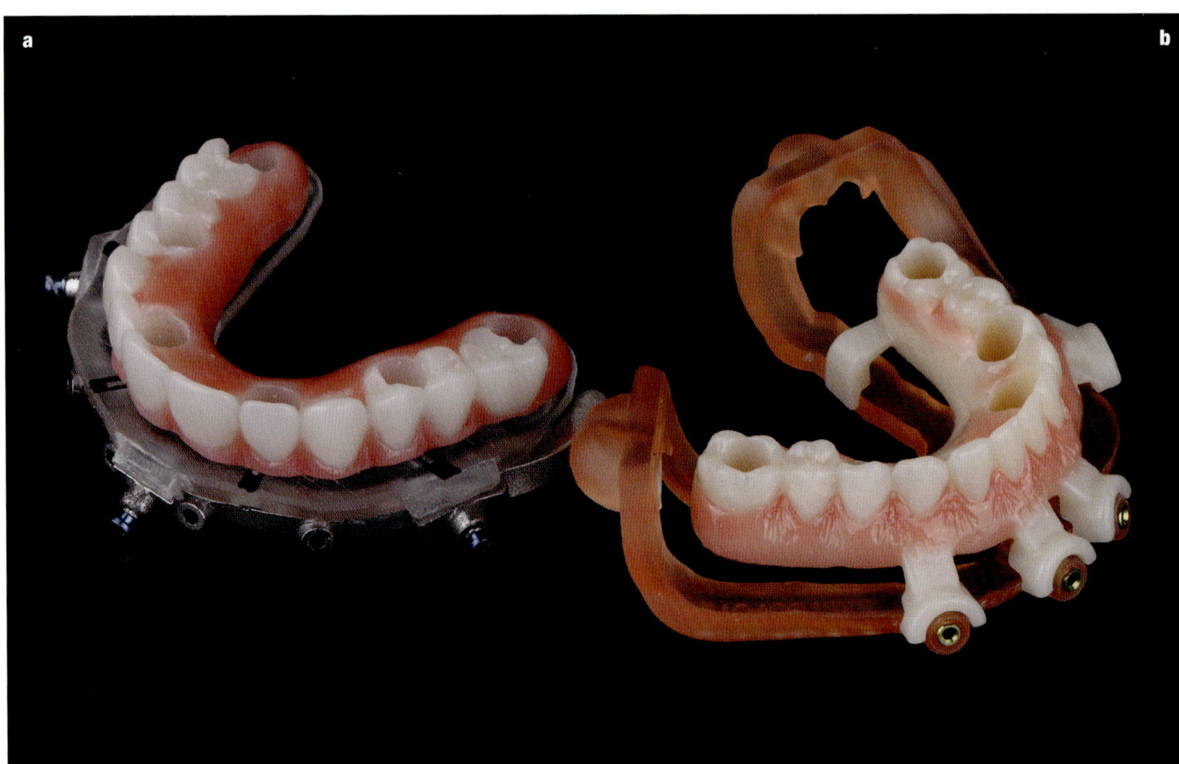

Figure 4.50 (a) Maxillary interim prosthesis seated on a cobalt-chrome foundation guide with a carrier guide; (b) Mandibular interim prosthesis seated on an anatomical-style 360-degree foundation guide without a carrier guide.

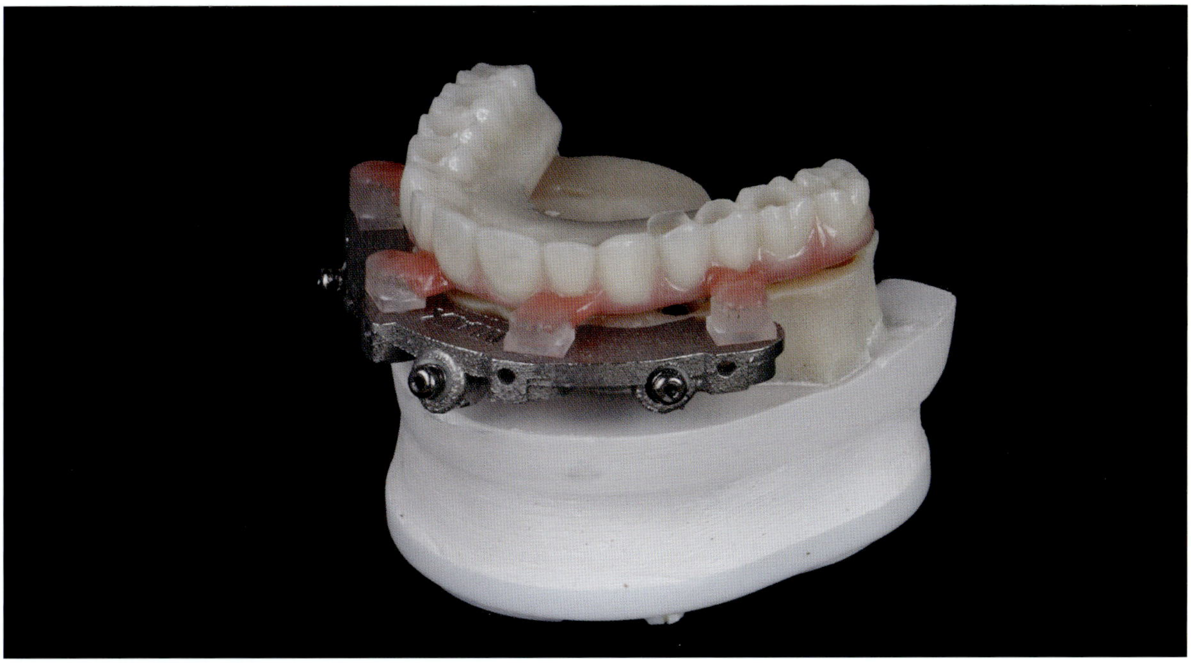

Figure 4.51 Maxillary interim prosthesis seated on a cobalt-chrome foundation guide.

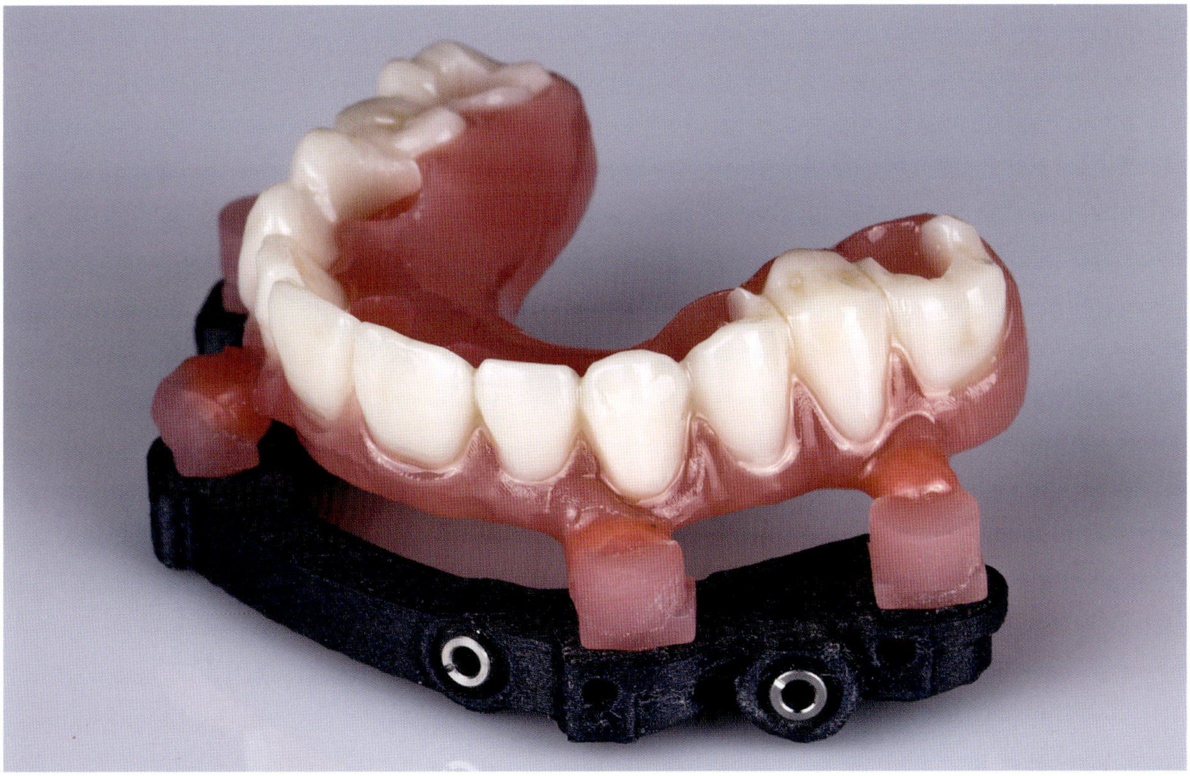

Figure 4.52 Maxillary interim prosthesis seated on a carbon-fiber reinforced foundation guide.

Replica appliance

In addition to the conversion of the interim prosthesis during surgical workflow, I will often do a pick-up of the replica appliance as well. This replica appliance can eliminate the need for some steps and appointments during the prosthetic workflow. In addition, it provides a secure record of the patient's implants, occlusion, current VDO, and tooth position during the implant healing phase (Figs. 4.53-4.55).

Replica appliances can be made of either milled or printed material. Milled PMMA has historically been stronger than printed PMMA, but it is more expensive. The printed materials being developed today actually rival their milled counterparts in strength and durability. I usually request a replica appliance that is made from an economical printed material to control costs unless I think the patient may need a stronger prosthesis as a potential backup (Figs. 4.56-4.59). In some higher risk cases I will ask the lab to just send two interim prostheses from the same material and same shades. That way, if something does happen to the patient's original interim prosthesis and it can no longer be used, I have a backup. I determine the risk based on whether the patient has any current parafunctional habits, how compliant they seem, the amount of wear and tear on their presurgical dentition, what the opposing arch is, and anything else that I think might make them more prone to fracturing their interim prosthesis.

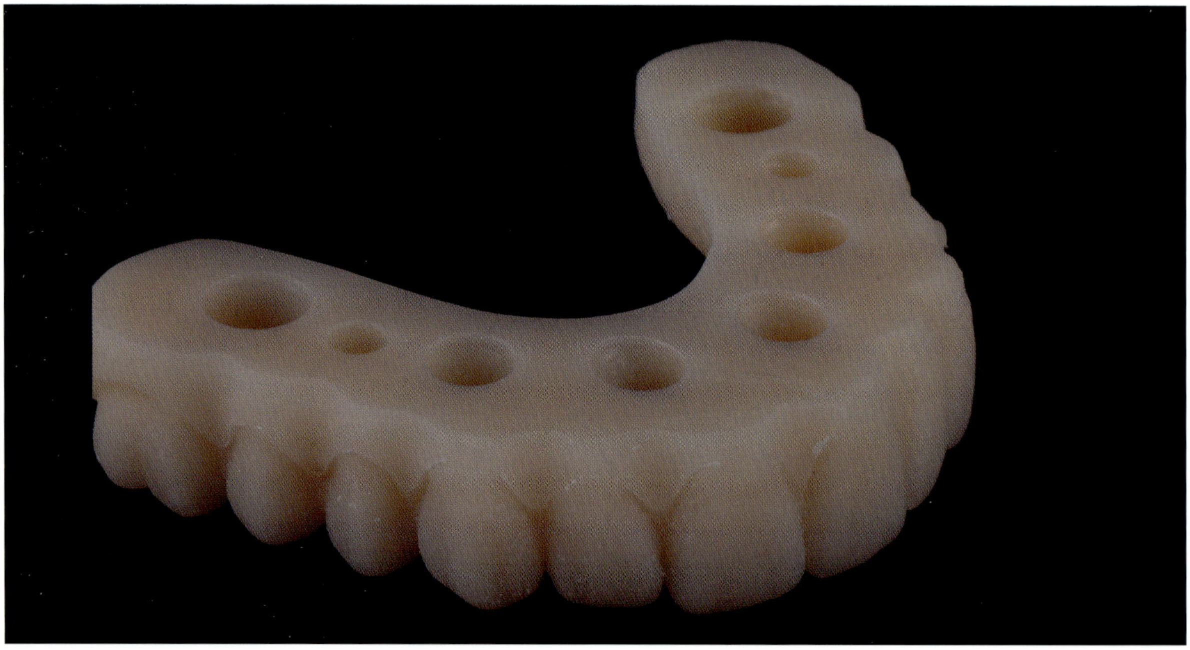

Figure 4.53 **Maxillary replica appliance with access holes and indexing divots for the carrier guide.**

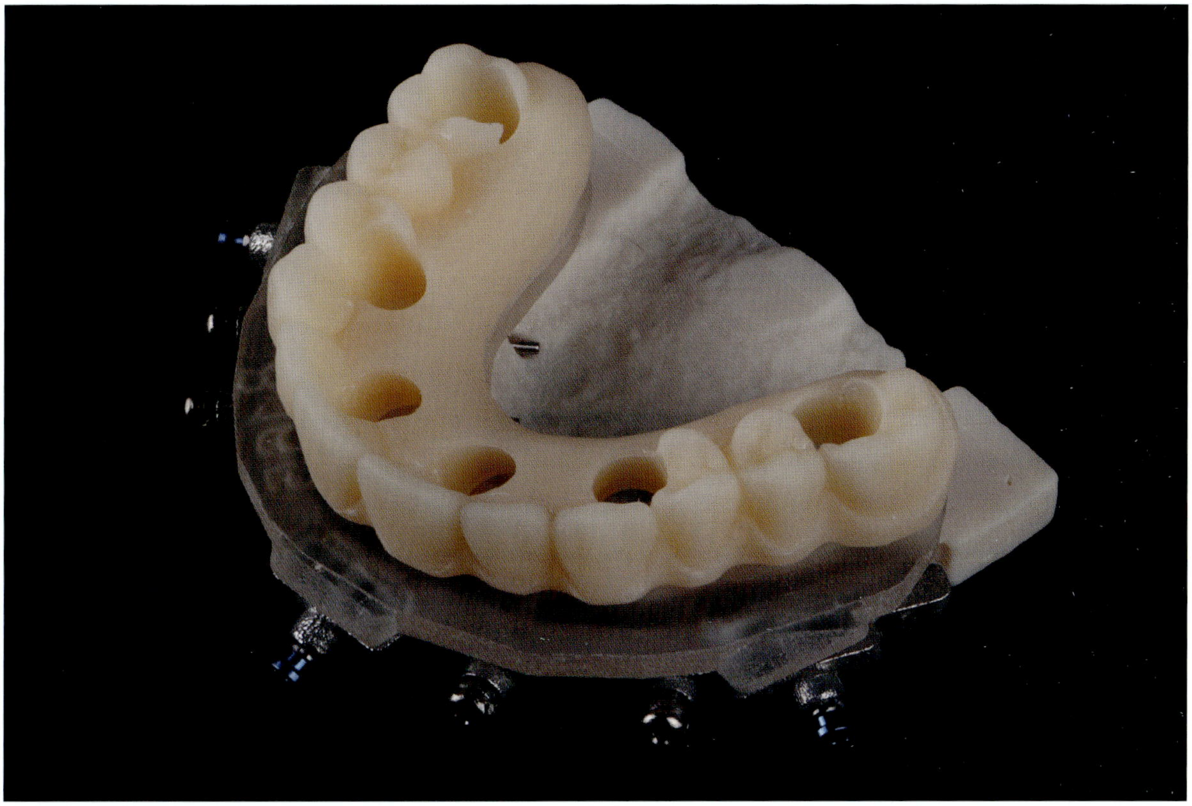

Figure 4.54 Maxillary replica appliance seated on a foundation guide with a carrier guide.

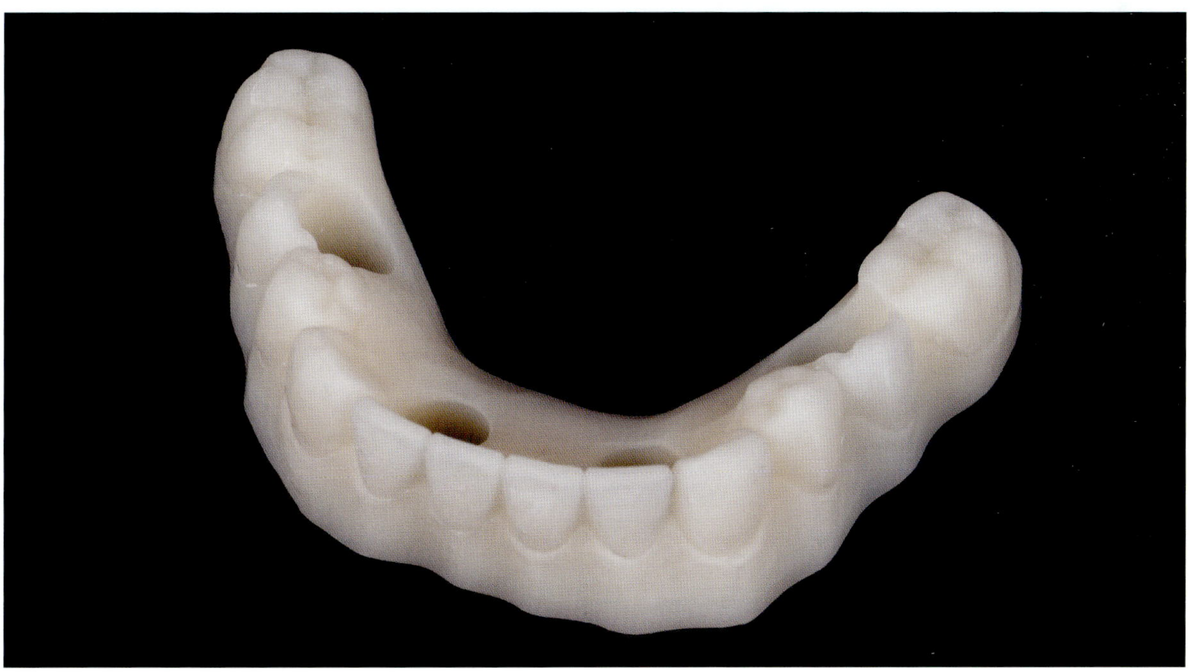

Figure 4.55 Occlusal surface of a mandibular replica appliance.

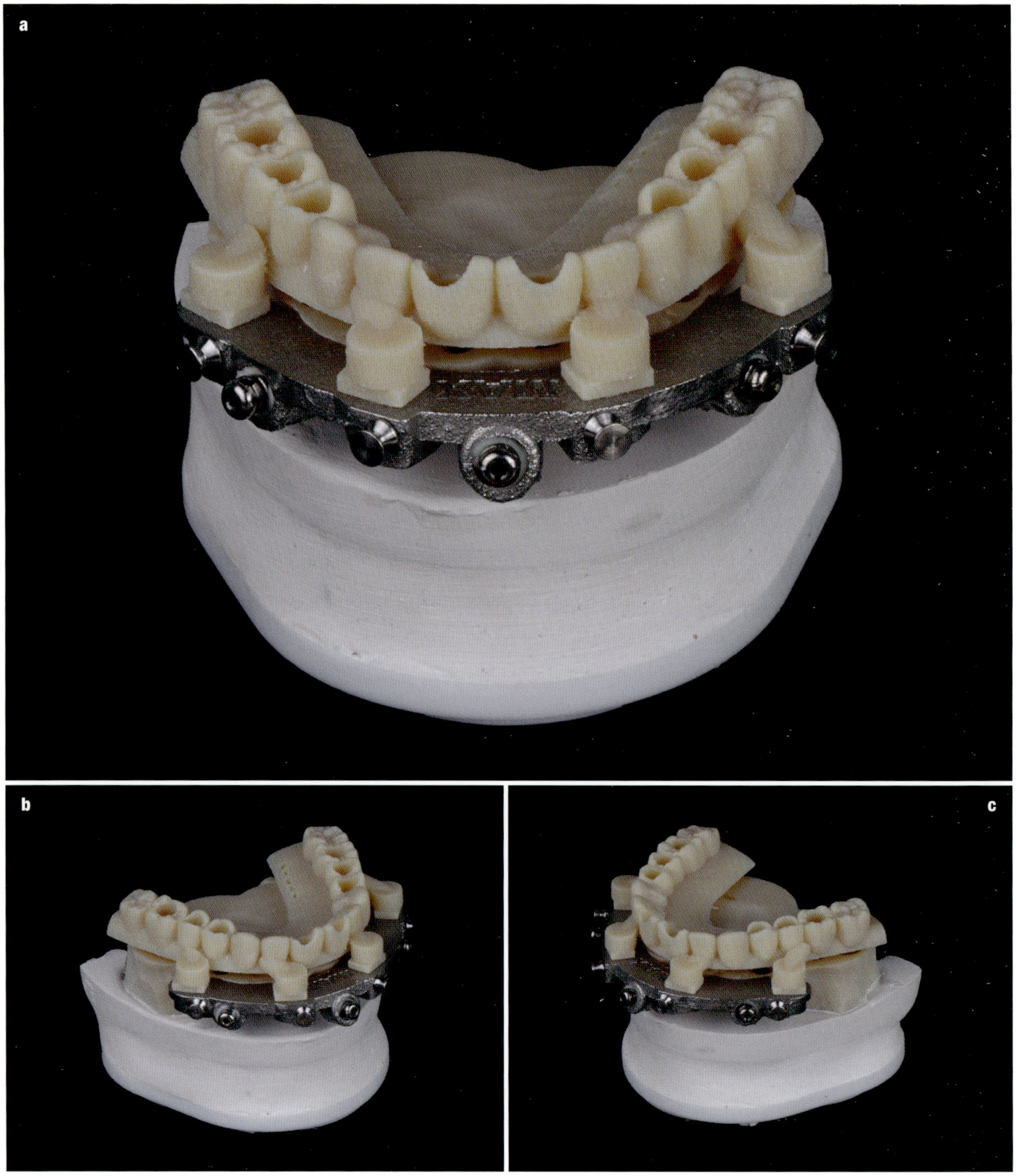

Figure 4.56 (a-c) Views of a maxillary replica appliance seated on a hybrid floating- and anatomical-style cobalt-chrome foundation guide.

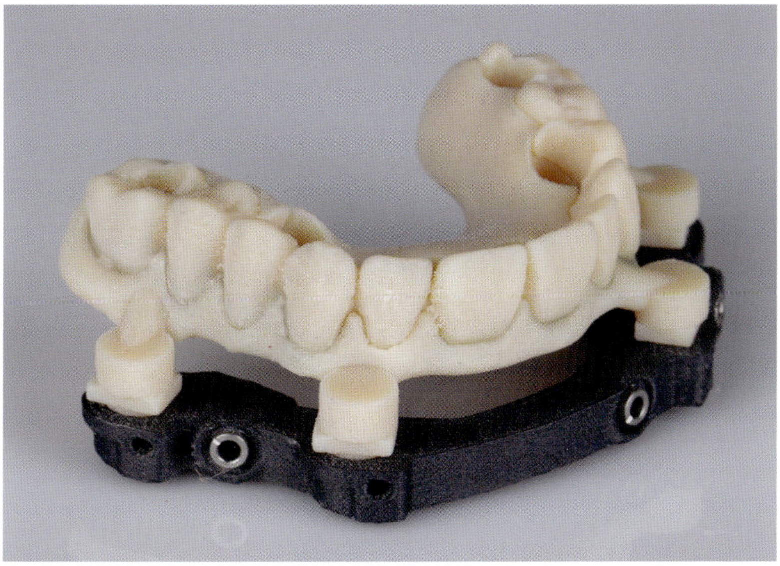

Figure 4.57 Maxillary replica appliance seated on a carbon-fiber reinforced foundation guide.

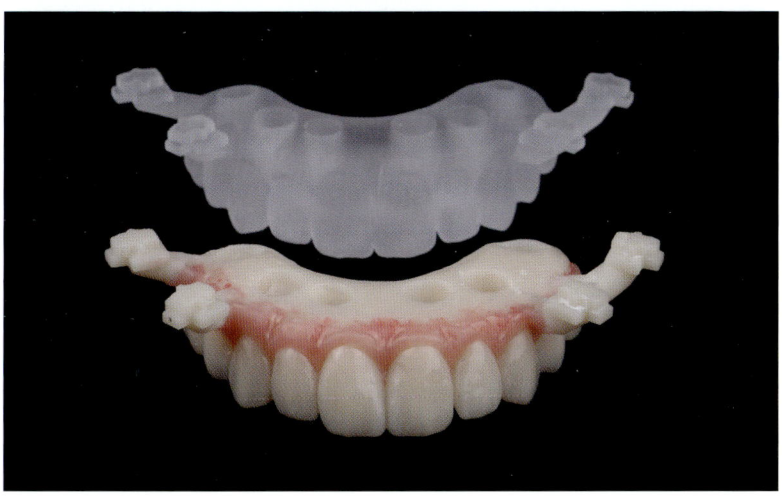

Figure 4.58 Clear resin duplicate (*top*) and interim prosthesis (*bottom*).

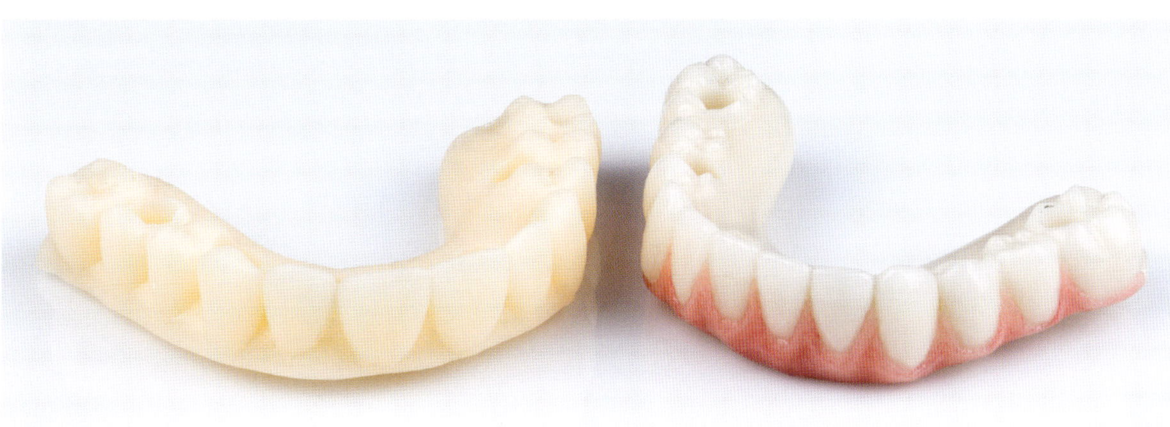

Figure 4.59 Maxillary replica appliance (*left*) and mandibular interim prosthesis (*right*).

The replica appliance can be used to accomplish three goals during the prosthetic phase of the workflow:

1. **Verification of the MUA-to-prosthesis relationship.** In this workflow, without a replica appliance, an implant indexing device or a verification jig would need to be created. The verification appliance (see Chapter 8) would have to be used to transfer this relationship to the laboratory. In earlier workflows, obtaining a record of this information would require one appointment to take an impression (whether digital or analog) and another appointment to verify the implant positions using a jig. Although this is an acceptable process, it lacks efficiency.
2. **Confirmation of VDO, tooth position, and maxillomandibular relationship.** In place of a traditional occlusion rim used in older analog workflows, the replica appliance captures a predetermined VDO (that can be modified). It also shows the general position of the teeth and the maxillomandibular relationship. This data offers a roadmap toward the definitive prosthesis and makes the process of developing a resin prototype for the patient much simpler and faster.
3. **Recording of soft tissues.** The laboratory can use the replica appliance to develop a soft tissue model from an impression of the intaglio surface of the appliance. Having an accurate intaglio surface for the definitive appliance is very important, and the replica appliance allows that anatomy to be captured quickly and easily.

Author note: *During the writing of this book, new features in ongoing planning software were under development that will eventually allow creation of very accurate soft tissue models via digital scanning of the patient's mucosa around the MUAs. We are evaluating specific MUA scan bodies for consistent accuracy and reliability. Success in this endeavor would mean that manual verification would be less important, and the entire prosthetic workflow can be done digitally. Until we have documented consistent success, the method outlined in this book continues to create excellent results that are duplicable and straightforward.*

Spare dentures

Clinicians performing fixed full-arch implant dentistry have found that the ability to obtain acceptable implant torque values and stability during surgery is unpredictable. In addition, unforeseen circumstances may prohibit immediate loading in these types of cases. For this reason, it is prudent to consider having the laboratory fabricate an inexpensive printed denture (Figs. 4.60, 4.61).

I order a printed denture to be at surgery for every maxillary case and for most mandibular cases I do. When the dental implants cannot be loaded immediately, the spare denture gives the patient a prosthesis to wear immediately after surgery so he or she does not have to go home toothless. In addition, there is always a small chance that one or more implants will fail during the healing phase, which could make an additional surgery necessary either to place more implants or do something else. Experiencing a failure like this, resulting in the loss of their prosthesis with nothing to replace it, can be emotionally traumatizing for a patient.

Having a spare denture has saved me from the distress of sending a patient home without teeth in these rare cases. A discussion about implant stability and the possibility of wearing a denture for a few months should always be part of the preoperative conversation with patients in order to establish appropriate expectations.

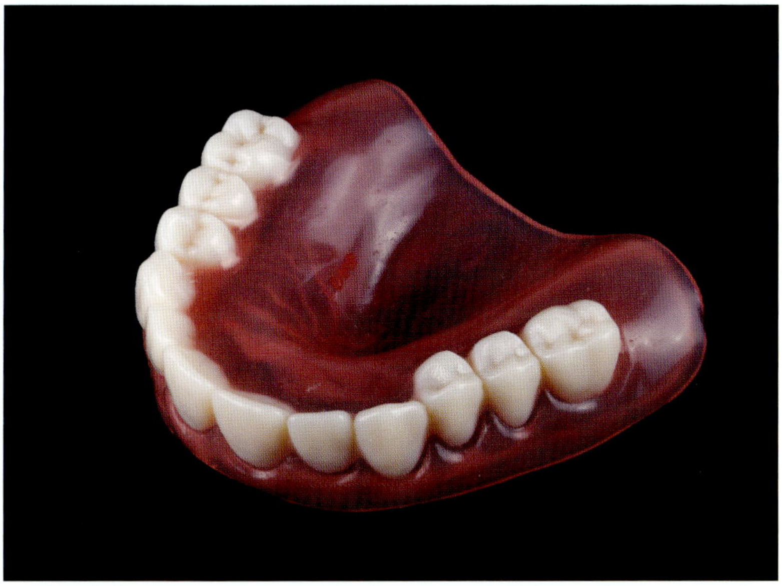

Figure 4.60 **Occlusal view of a printed maxillary complete denture.**

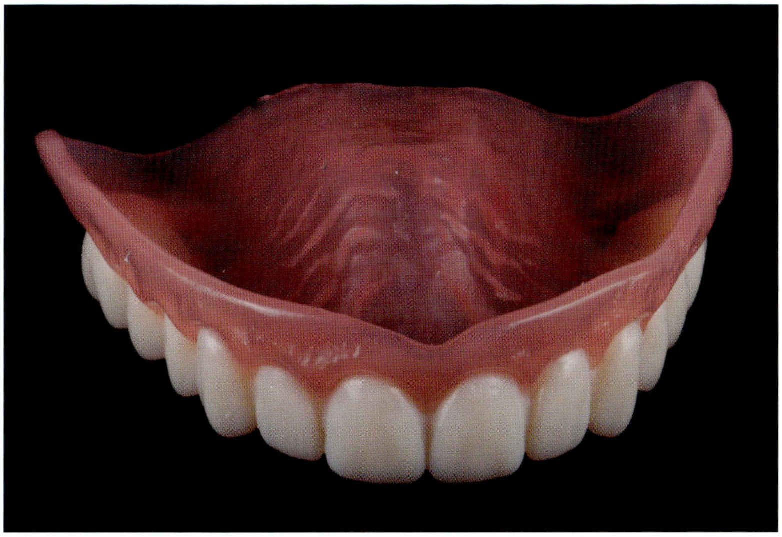

Figure 4.61 **Intaglio surface of a printed maxillary complete denture.**

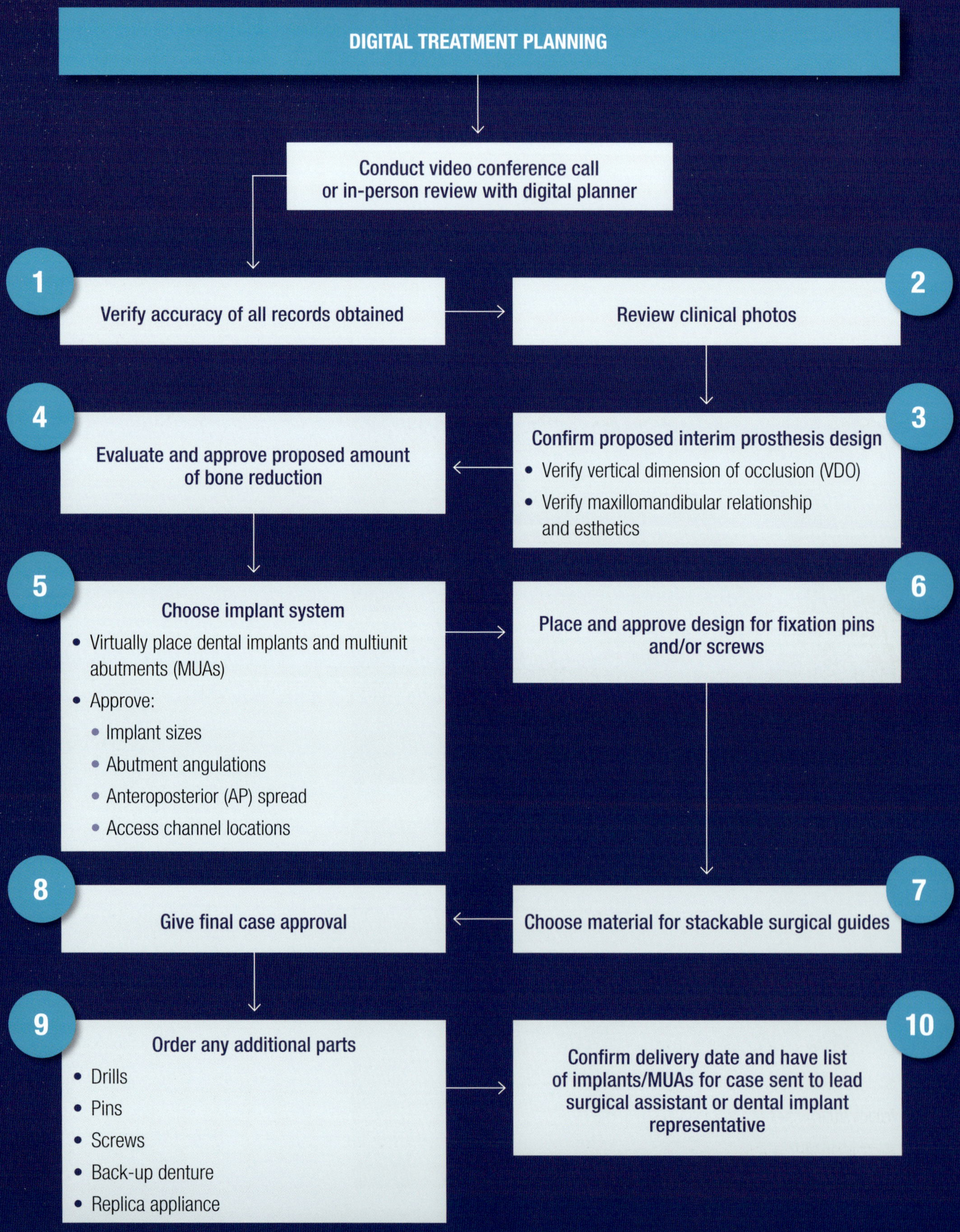
DIGITAL TREATMENT PLANNING
Conduct video conference call or in-person review with digital planner
1
Verify accuracy of all records obtained
2
Review clinical photos
3
Confirm proposed interim prosthesis design
• Verify vertical dimension of occlusion (VDO)
• Verify maxillomandibular relationship and esthetics
4
Evaluate and approve proposed amount of bone reduction
5
Choose implant system
• Virtually place dental implants and multiunit abutments (MUAs)
• Approve:
• Implant sizes
• Abutment angulations
• Anteroposterior (AP) spread
• Access channel locations
6
Place and approve design for fixation pins and/or screws
7
Choose material for stackable surgical guides
8
Give final case approval
9
Order any additional parts
• Drills
• Pins
• Screws
• Back-up denture
• Replica appliance
10
Confirm delivery date and have list of implants/MUAs for case sent to lead surgical assistant or dental implant representative

DIGITAL CASE PLANNING, ENGINEERING, AND DESIGN

CHAPTER 5

Commitment: Practice with integrity, strive for excellence.
This should be the mantra of every dentist.
We as a profession owe it to the patients that we serve.

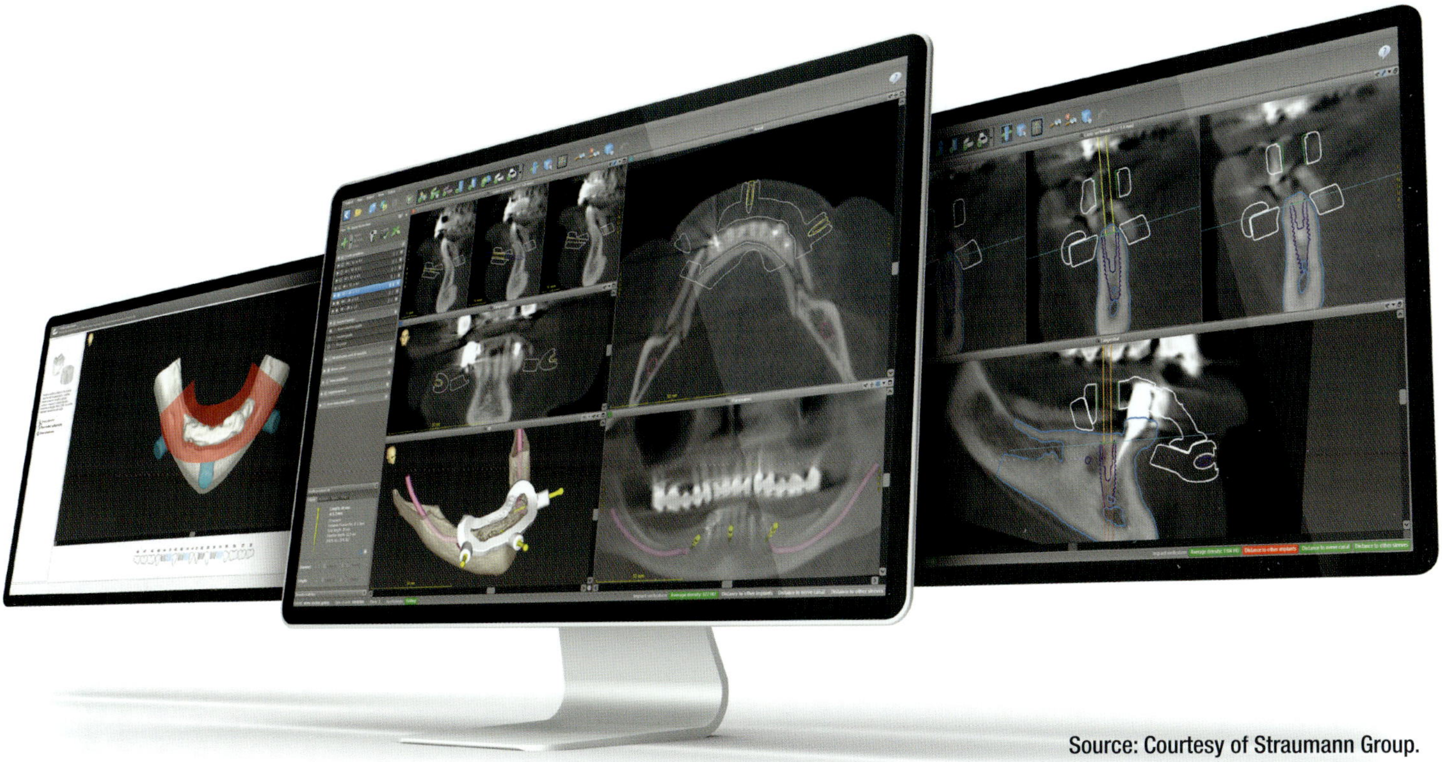

Source: Courtesy of Straumann Group.

After the patient data has been collected and logistics of the patient's case are finalized, the second stage—case planning, engineering, and design—can begin. This process is vitally important to a successful outcome for the patient. This stage involves communication with the dental laboratory, selection of the implants and multiunit abutments (MUAs), and confirmation of the surgical plan. You may also provide input and guidance on the design of the surgical stackable guides, interim prosthesis, and replica appliance.

CLINICIAN-LABORATORY COMMUNICATION

The first step in communicating with your lab is to upload all the digital data you have collected — namely, CBCT scan(s), digital impressions, and clinical photographs. Most labs that are familiar with the workflow outlined in this book provide an online portal that you can do this through. To maximize efficiency, this is a task I always delegate to my team after I have reviewed and approved everything. In addition to uploading data through a portal, you may need to fill out a digital or analog prescription, depending on your lab. I recommend filling out the final prescription yourself instead of having an auxiliary do it for you.

Once the lab receives the digital data, they will begin the process of organizing, segmentation, and merging it into software. I always request that the lab call my surgical coordinator once they have finished this process and schedule a time and date for the digital treatment planning of the case, which is then added into my calendar. In my practice, 30 minutes is scheduled for a single full-arch implant case and 45 minutes for a double-arch case.

DIGITAL CASE ENGINEERING AND PLANNING PRO TIP:
It is imperative that the lab receive accurate CBCT scans and digital impressions for your cases

Keep your CBCT and intraoral scanner calibrated and scrutinize your patient's records before sending them to the lab. One of the biggest frustrations for dental labs is getting flawed scans, impressions, and/or photos from the dentist. Although the lab's digital planners often can spot these problems before the guides and components are fabricated, they slow down the planning process and create frustration on both sides. Team training, attention to detail, and careful review of data are the best ways to avoid these problems. The saying "garbage in, garbage out" has never been more true.

Preplanning protocol

Before case planning begins, it is very helpful to have a basic understanding of your options related to dental implant planning software and dental implant systems as well as a working knowledge of important radiographic anatomical landmarks.

Planning software

Many different types of treatment-planning software are currently available, including Blue Sky Bio®, coDiagnostiX® (Dental Wings GmbH), Exocad® (Exocad GmbH), R2GATE® (MegaGen), and Simplant® (Dentsply Sirona), just to name a few. Your lab may use the one they find easiest to integrate into their workflow, or they may use more than one to plan, design, and fabricate the case. Generally, I let my lab decide which software to use based on what the technicians are most comfortable with and deem best. Dentists sometimes convince themselves that they should own the same software that the lab uses; this is unnecessary. As the dentist, you will not necessarily have to manipulate objects or make changes within the software. You will only have to review, provide guidance, and approve the plan that the technician creates during the planning and engineering video conference call. You should not have to invest in the cost of software or spend valuable time doing what they are best at. Remember that, as a dentist, you are spending your time most profitably and wisely doing dentistry. If you like to tinker and want to work directly in the software as a hobby, then do it. I am fascinated by what we can do in software and enjoy working with it. I realize, though, that I will not save time or money by doing the planning, designing, and fabrication of the stackable guide systems myself.

There is one important factor you and your lab will need to consider when choosing a planning software. The software must have an active and up-to-date catalog of the dental implants and (preferably) MUAs that you are planning to use available within the platform.

Dental implant system

Before case-planning begins, verify that the dental implant system you will be using for your full-arch dental implant cases has a guided solution. It needs to be compatible with the stackable surgical guide system your lab will be designing. Your laboratory and your dental implant representative should be able to clarify and/or resolve any potential issues you may encounter.

Some dental implant companies claim to having a dental implant specifically designed for full-arch dental implantology or promote their implants as having faster integration times, better initial stability, or superior design characteristics. I recommend choosing an implant based on these criteria but also taking into consideration the cost, simplicity, and ease of use of the surgical kit. Check the range of sizes offered, and the availability and versatility of the components. Having a range of implant diameters and lengths to choose from as well as MUAs that vary in height and angulation degree allows some flexibility in planning. MUAs with angulations of 0, 15, 17, and 30 degrees are standard, and although 45-degree angled abutments are also available, they are not as commonly used.

Radiographic landmarks

Most clinicians who have some dental implant experience have a basic grasp of the radiographic anatomical landmarks to be aware of when treatment planning for dental implants. In fixed full-arch implant dentistry, the same landmarks apply, but they may take on more importance than in single-tooth or partial-arch implant therapy. This is because of the greater amount of bone reduction and more aggressive flap designs that can be involved. Therefore, it is crucial to have a working knowledge of these structures and the consequences of impinging on them, and to recognize the advantages of working in the denser bone found near some of these areas. The landmarks listed below can be identified on a CBCT scan, and some are shown in Figures 5.1-5.6.

Maxillary landmarks

- Nasopalatine canal, incisive foramen, and neurovascular bundle
- Greater palatine foramen and neurovascular bundle
- Infraorbital foramen and neurovascular bundle
- Canalis sinuosus (a rare anatomical neurovascular variation from the infraorbital canal)
- Sphenopalatine artery
- Maxillary sinus
- Zygomatic buttress and pterygopalatine fossa

Mandibular landmarks

- Inferior alveolar canal and neurovascular bundle
- Mental foramen and neurovascular bundle
- Incisive canal and anterior loop
- Lingual foramen, lingual artery, and lateral canal

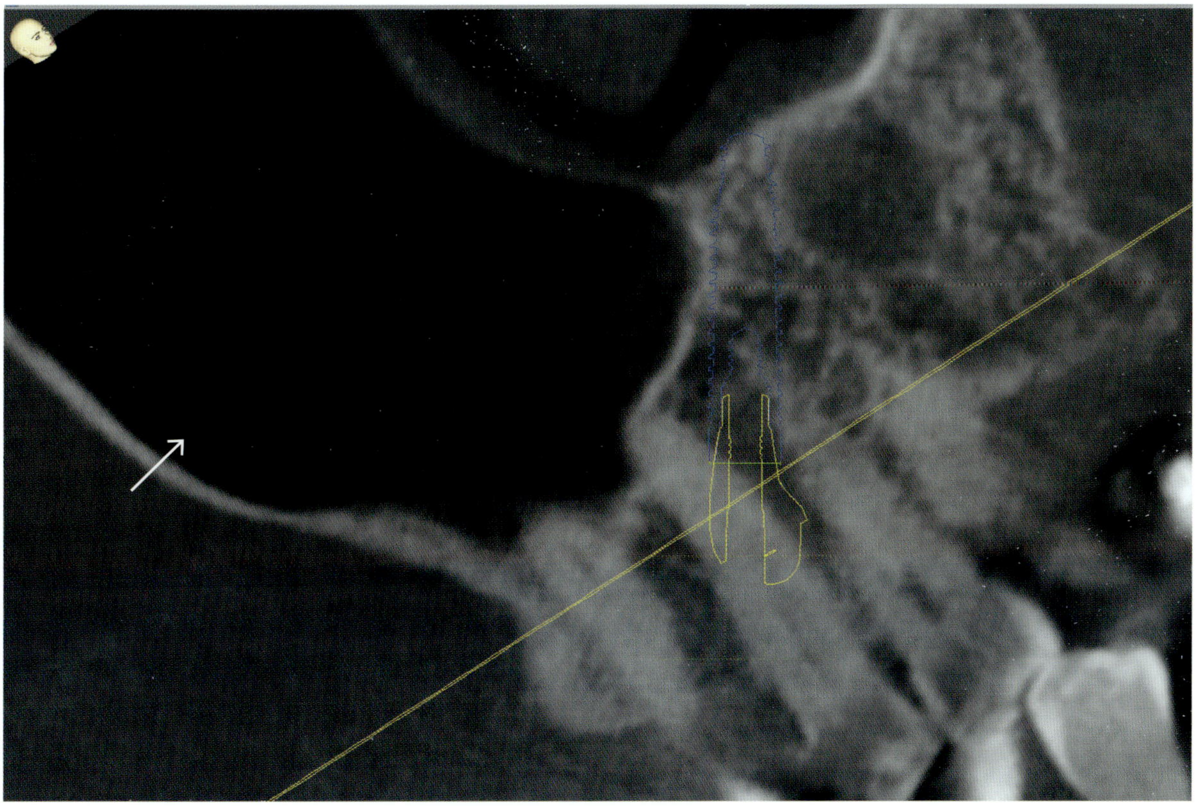

Figure 5.1 Detail showing the right maxillary sinus (*arrow*) from a panoramic CBCT.

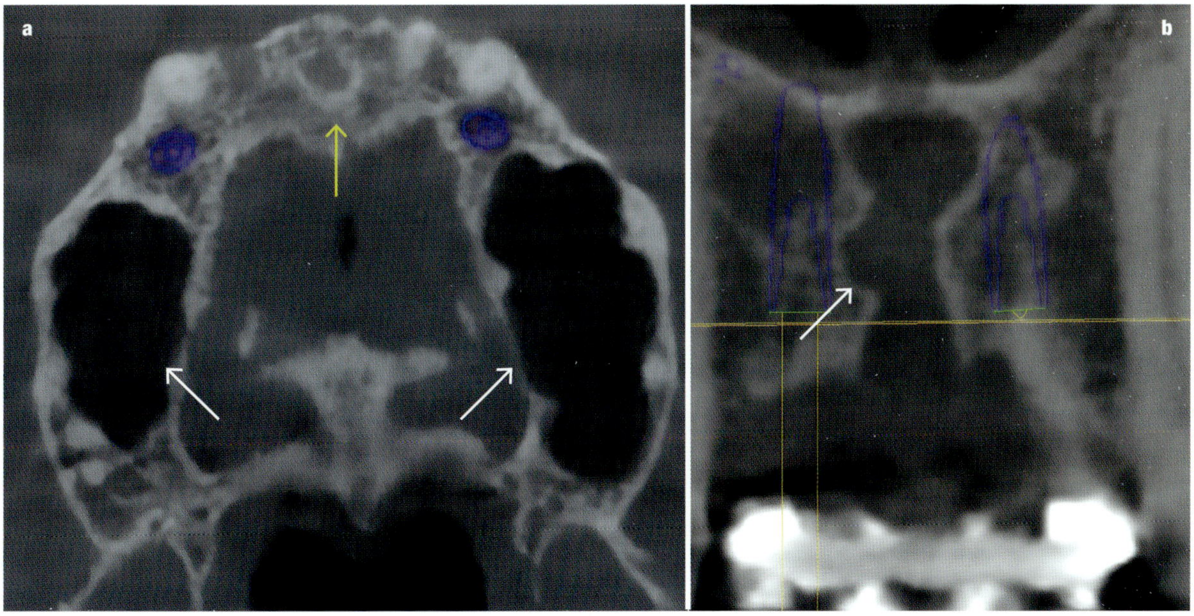

Figure 5.2 (a) CBCT showing an axial view of the maxillary sinuses (*white arrows*) and the nasopalatine canal/incisive foramen (*yellow arrow*); (b) Detail showing the nasopalatine canal/incisive foramen (*arrow*) from a panoramic CBCT.

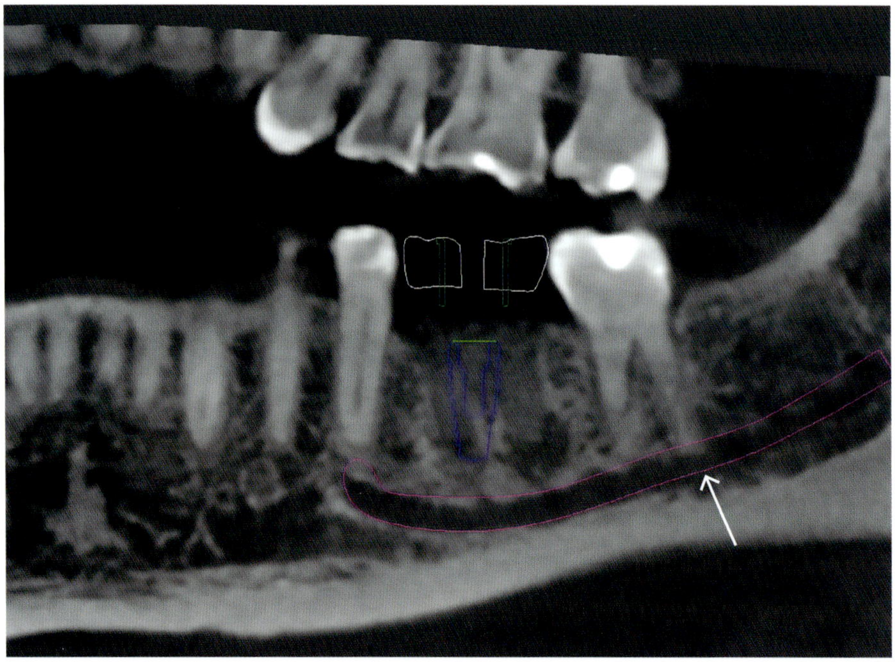

Figure 5.3 Detail showing the inferior alveolar canal and neurovascular bundle (*arrow*) from a panoramic CBCT.

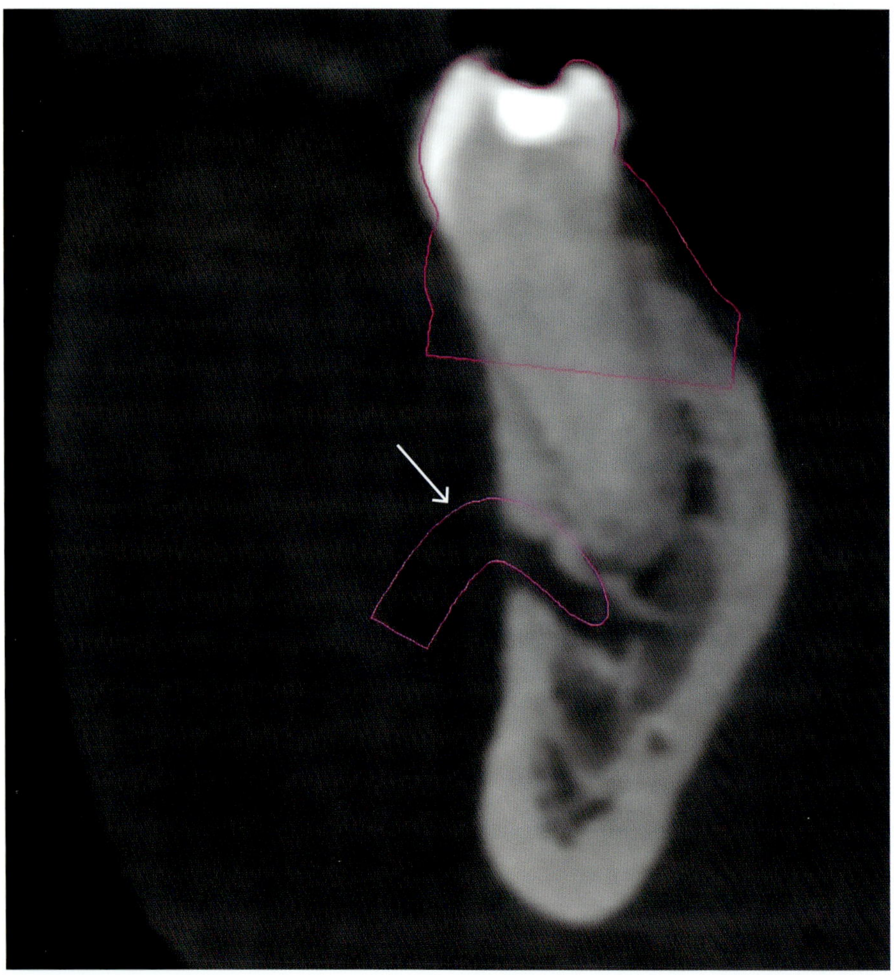

Figure 5.4 CBCT showing a sagittal view of the mental foramen and neurovascular bundle (*arrow*).

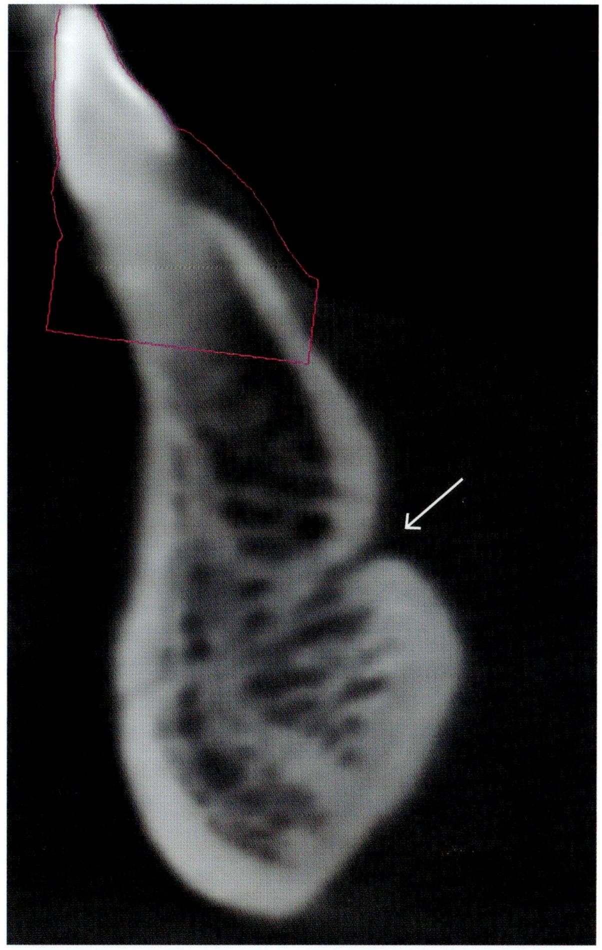

Figure 5.5 CBCT showing a sagittal view of the lingual vascular canal and foramen (*arrow*).

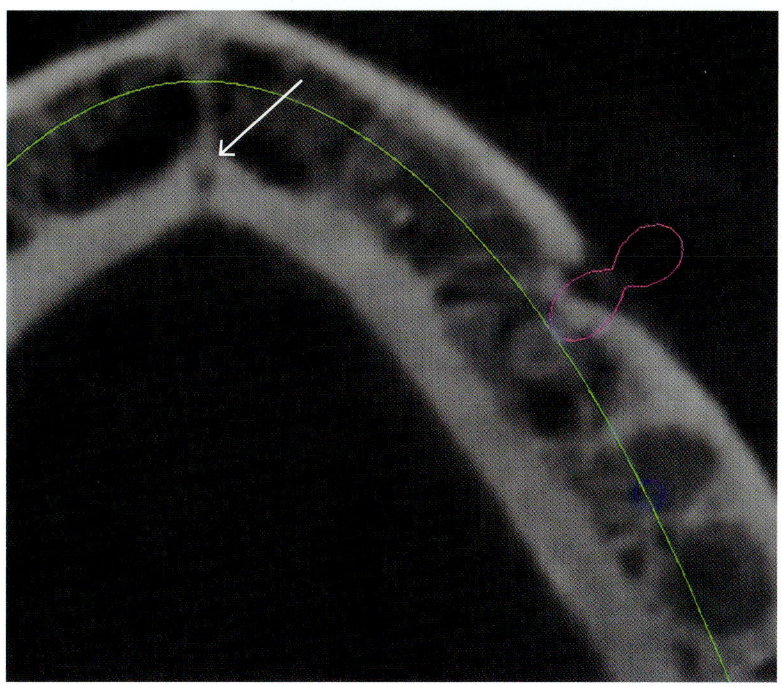

Figure 5.6 CBCT showing an axial view of the lingual vascular canal and foramen (*arrow*).

PRINCIPLES OF CASE PLANNING, ENGINEERING, AND DESIGN

When collaborating with a dental lab, some fundamental planning guidelines should be observed. Know the limiting factors in your case as well as what to look for and beware of. Your partner at the lab should also understand each of these factors. The principles I apply during my planning sessions are based on my understanding of the current literature, discussions with experts in the field, and personal experience.

Bone reduction principles

The amount of bone reduction to carry out should be guided by the need for adequate prosthetic space while taking into account the amount of bone available for the dental implants. A balanced approach is required to preserve as much bone as possible without compromising the prosthesis or creating a visible transition line when the patient speaks or smiles. You may also want to consider what design your final appliance may have and whether FP1, FP2, or FP3 may have limitations based on the amount of bone present. Bone reduction should be planned carefully, and arbitrary reduction should be avoided.

Implant-planning principles

Size

Consider using implants with a minimum length of 10 mm and a diameter ranging from 3.3 to 5.0 mm, which are widely accepted by most experienced clinicians.

Angulation

Implants can be angled or tilted to access denser, better quality, and more abundant bone; allow more implants to be placed; and increase the distance between implants. Angled implants can be corrected to be parallel with MUA abutments. Prosthetic screw access channels should be centered within the interim prosthesis.

Space between implants

At least 3 mm of space between implants is required coronally; less space is needed apically. Implants should not touch each other apically.

Anteroposterior (AP) spread

Allow as much distance as possible between the center of the most anteriorly placed implants and the center of the most posteriorly placed implants. The length of the prosthetic cantilever will depend on and be limited by this distance.

Intraoral access

Guided implant surgery requires the use of longer drills, so more intraoral space is needed than in unguided manual dental implant placement. Therefore, maximum mouth opening must be considered, especially for implant placement in the posterior regions.

Number of implants

A minimum of four and maximum of eight implants can be placed in each arch, depending on the case design and the patient.

MUA angulation and collar height

To establish a level restorative platform, implants require the use of MUAs, which are available in angulations of 0 to 45 degrees (although MUAs of more than 30 degrees can result in increased strain on the implant). Angulation correction is also needed to achieve parallelism and a more ideal path of draw for the future prosthesis. The height of an MUA collar ranges from 1.5 to 3.5 mm above the bone depending on the soft tissue height.

Bone density/quality

Dense bone (D1 and D2) is generally best for anchoring dental implants and achieving primary stability. D2 bone is best for osseointegration and stability. D1 bone has limited vascularity. Placing implants in lower-density bone (i.e., D3 and D4) may potentially limit torque values. In such cases, choose an implant with a more aggressive thread pattern and try to engage cortical bone when available. Also, consider using implant drills designed for osseodensification.

Bone volume

More bone is better. Minimal bone requirements for dental implants can be found in the literature and are affected by a variety of factors. As a rule, I plan to allow for at least 2 mm of bone circumferentially for predictable results. Otherwise, bone grafting or ridge augmentation procedures may be necessary.

Abscess or infection

Plan for areas of abscess or infection to be thoroughly enucleated and grafted. Such areas will not provide sufficient support for initial implant stability.

Anatomical landmarks

Implants should be placed at least 2 mm from the inferior alveolar nerve and at least 3 to 5 mm mesial to the mental foramen. Also, the anterior loop should be avoided as well as any small vascular branches, such as the lingual artery, whenever possible.

Stackable guide planning principles

Teeth/anatomy available for the indexing aligner

Know whether the aligner will be tooth-, mucosa-, or bone-borne and check to see if there is enough anatomy available to ensure its stability.

Mouth-opening space

Consider whether you will be limited by the amount of mouth-opening space available.

Size/position of the buccal vestibule, oral cavity, lips, tongue and muscle attachments

Consider where and how much flap elevation will be necessary and if there is enough space available to place the guides.

Number and positioning of pins or screws for stability of the foundation guide

Some teeth and/or existing implants may need to be removed before the foundation guide can be placed in order to accommodate the fixation pins or screws. Pins and screws should be placed as anteriorly as possible without compromising stability. Again, consider the mouth-opening space and the position of the cheeks and the lips and whether they will be in the way during screw or pin drilling.

Prosthesis-planning principles

Height/thickness of the prosthetic materials relative to the restorative space

Approximately 12-15 mm of height is required from the implant to the cingulum or occlusal surface in the FP3 design. The thickness of the interim prosthesis varies. When finalizing the design, check that the prosthetic screw access channels are centered within the prosthesis in the occlusal surfaces of the posterior teeth and just palatal/lingual to the anterior teeth, if possible.

Cantilevers

To be safe, cantilever length should not exceed the length of the AP spread, in most cases. With an ideal AP spread, 10- to 12-mm cantilevers can be planned in the mandible and 6- to 8-mm cantilevers in the maxilla, depending on the material used in the definitive prosthesis. When necessary, consider additional implants in the zygoma and/or pterygoid regions or performing sinus elevation and bone grafting. The choice of material to be used in the definitive prosthesis will influence the length of the cantilevers.

Positioning

Consider the vertical dimension of occlusion (VDO) and the position of the prosthesis over the arches in terms of their impact on function, phonetics, and esthetics.

Implant-protected occlusion

Consider whether the occlusal scheme is designed to provide long-term stability of the implants and the prosthesis.

DIGITAL TREATMENT-PLANNING STEPS

It is important to give your full attention during the appointment for digital treatment planning and case engineering, and to avoid interruptions. I generally get on a video conference in a quiet room of my office or home. Ask to have your video conference planning sessions recorded by your lab so that you have the ability to go back and review them if necessary. This can be especially helpful when you first begin this method of fixed full-arch implant dentistry.

The labs I have worked with pride themselves on having digital planners who put the case together prior to our meeting in order to save time. Thus, the next steps may only be a review and fine tuning of a proposed plan, depending on the digital planner and lab you are working with. Digital planners have knowledge and experience and can be a valuable resource as you learn this process. For those with little or no experience working with stackable surgical guides, I highly recommend taking a course with one of these planners or having a practice session to review what the expectations will be for both you and your planner.

Review, assess, and confirm the following at the time of case review:

Clinical photographs

Together with your planner, look at the photographs of your patient, including the preoperative photos you sent to the lab and any merged proposal(s) that you or the lab made by simulating where the patient's new teeth will be positioned. (These can appear in 2D or 3D, depending on the software being used and photographs taken in your office; either is sufficient.) Confirm that the proposal for the interim prosthesis design is placed properly and that the esthetics of the prosthesis are appropriate (Figs. 5.7-5.9).

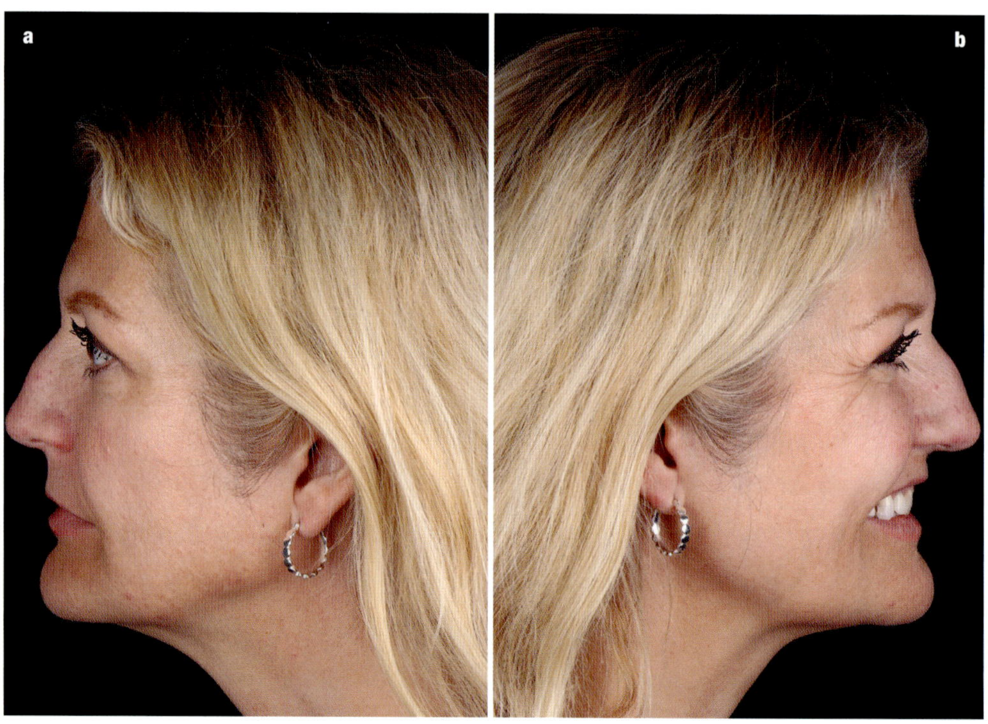

Figure 5.7 **Profile portrait views of patient (a) resting closed and (b) smiling.**

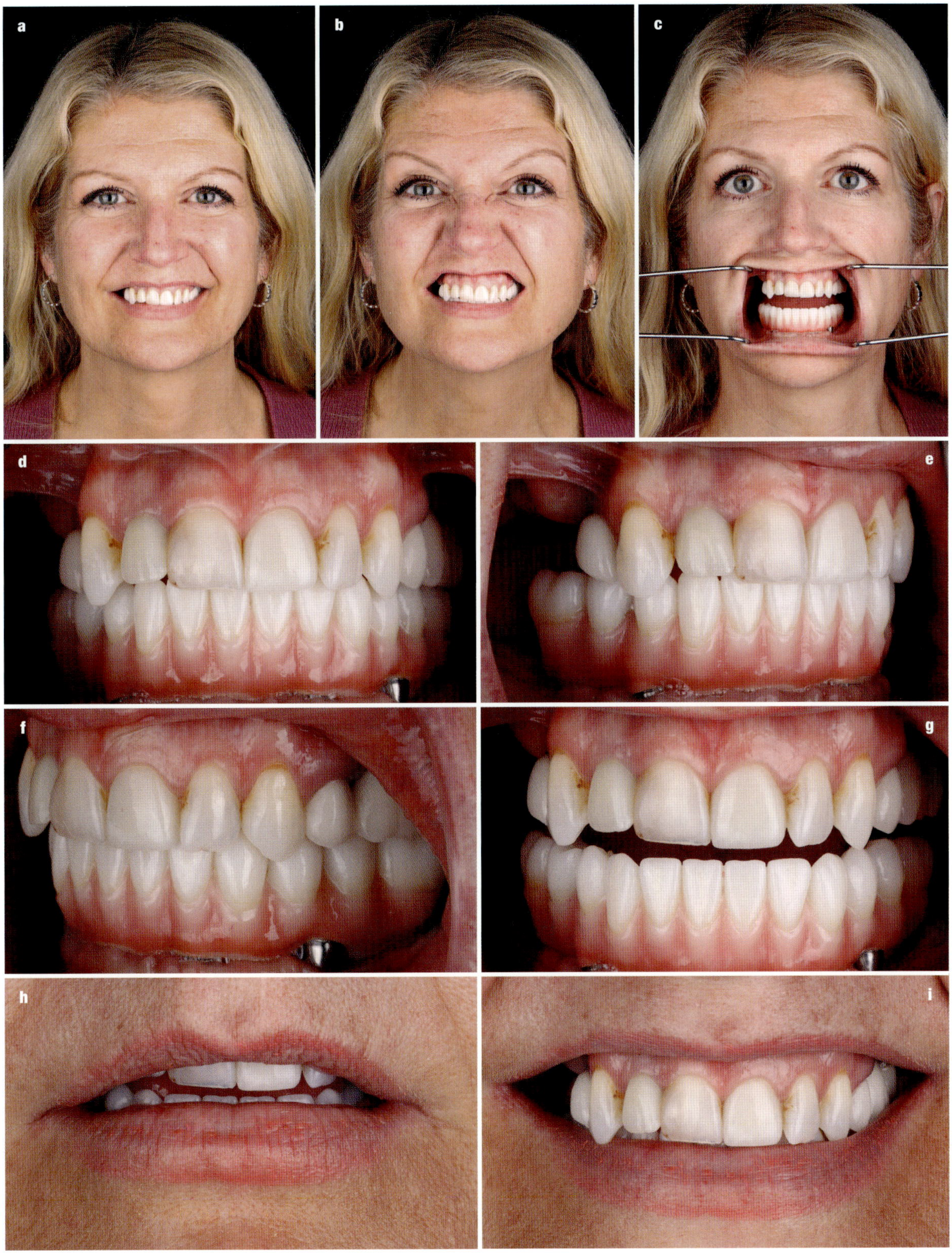

Figure 5.8 Patient photo series: (a) Portrait smile; (b) Portrait exaggerated smile; (c) Portrait retracted; (d, e) Frontal closed and right-lateral close-up retracted; (f, g) Left-lateral and frontal open close-up retracted; (h) Close-up repose; (i) Close-up smile.

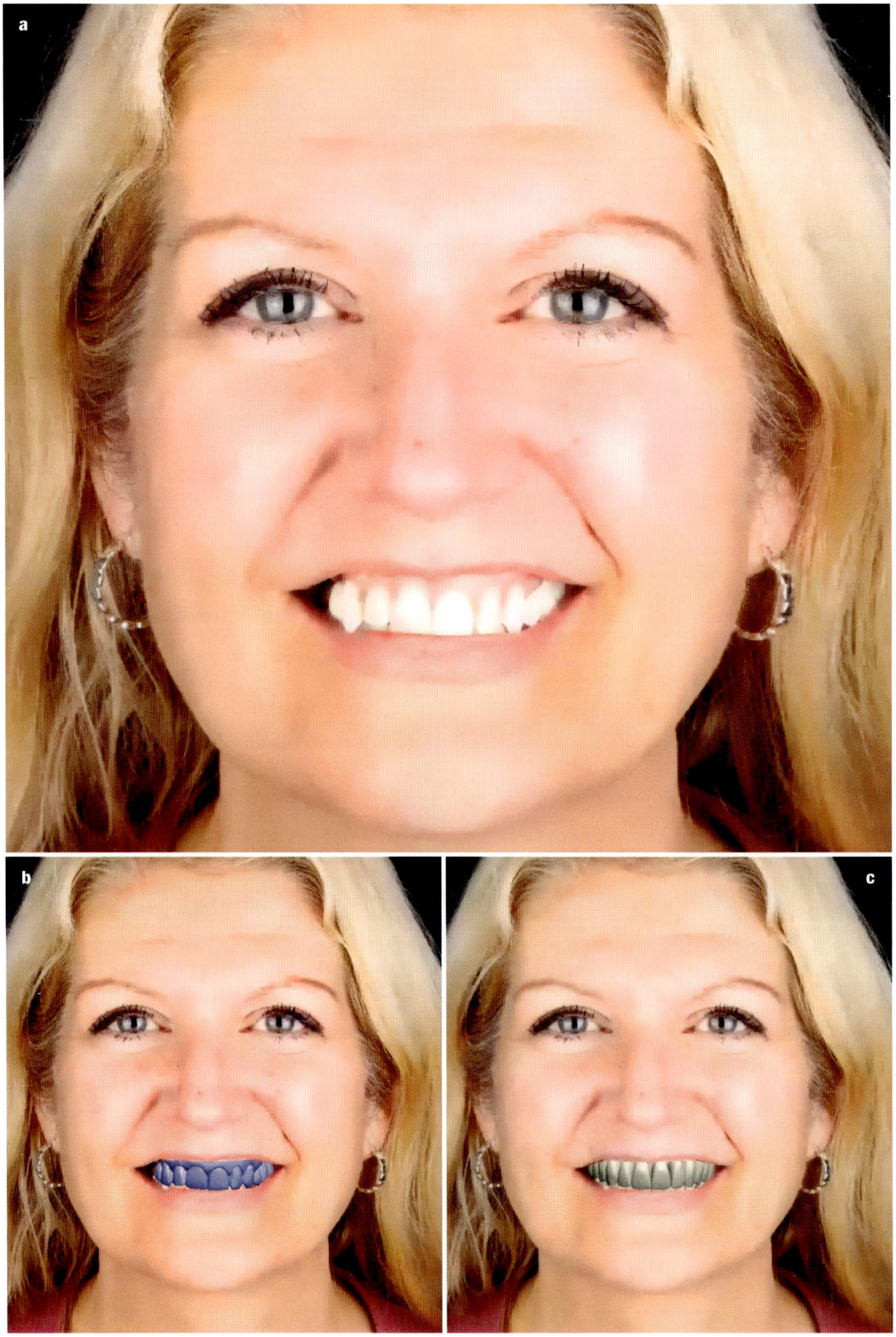

Figure 5.9 (a) Portrait smile photo used by the dental lab with (b) superimposed intraoral scan and (c) proposal of new teeth setup for interim prosthesis.

Proposed interim prosthesis/digital diagnostic design

As you carefully examine the prosthetic setup, remember that cases should be prosthetically driven, which means you want to see if you can put the teeth where they will eventually end up before deciding where you will place your implants. Compare the current and the planned maxillomandibular relationship and VDO. This planning session can often provide insights into potential challenges that might be encountered if they are not corrected with an orthotic positioning or jaw relation device. It is much better for you to make these corrections now and have the patient return for another appointment than to take unnecessary chances when significant changes are needed (Figs. 5.10, 5.11).

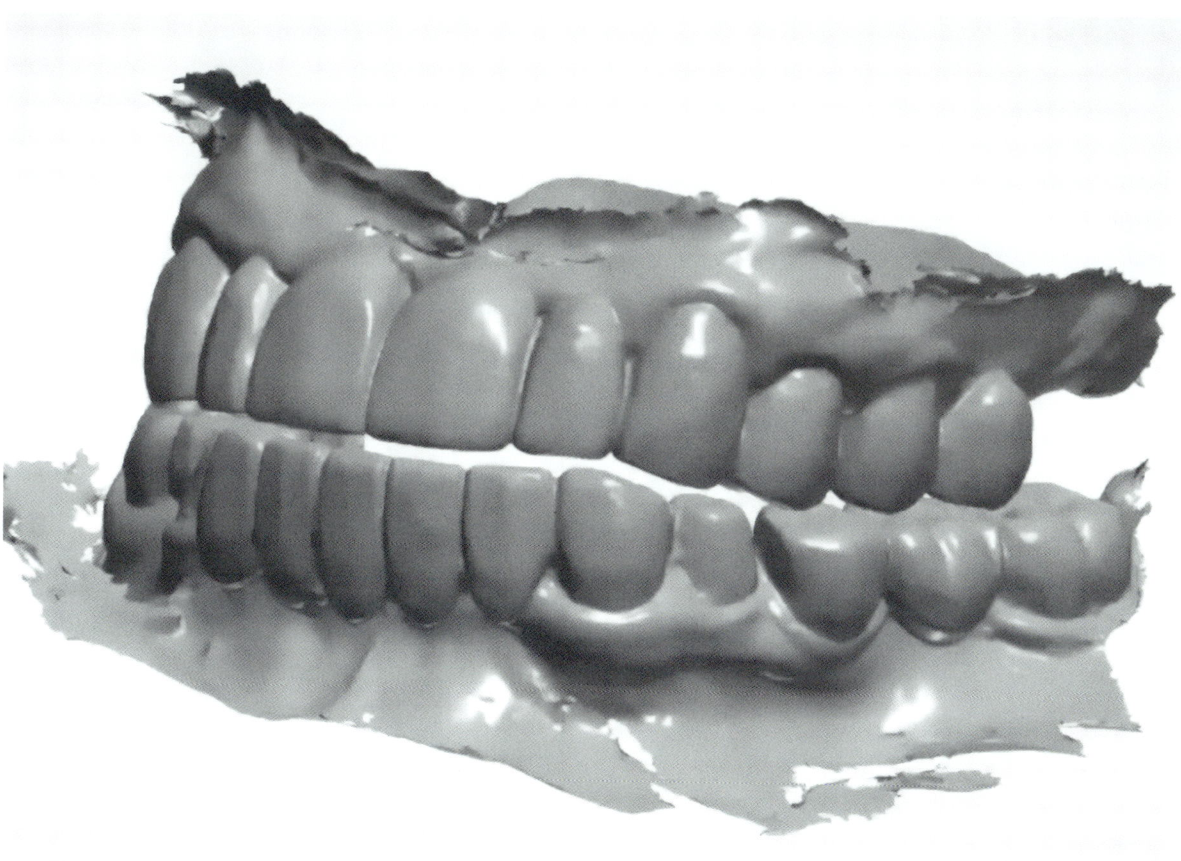

Figure 5.10 Intraoral scan of patient's teeth and occlusion. Note that the plan included opening the patient's vertical dimension of occlusion (VDO) by approximately 2 mm.

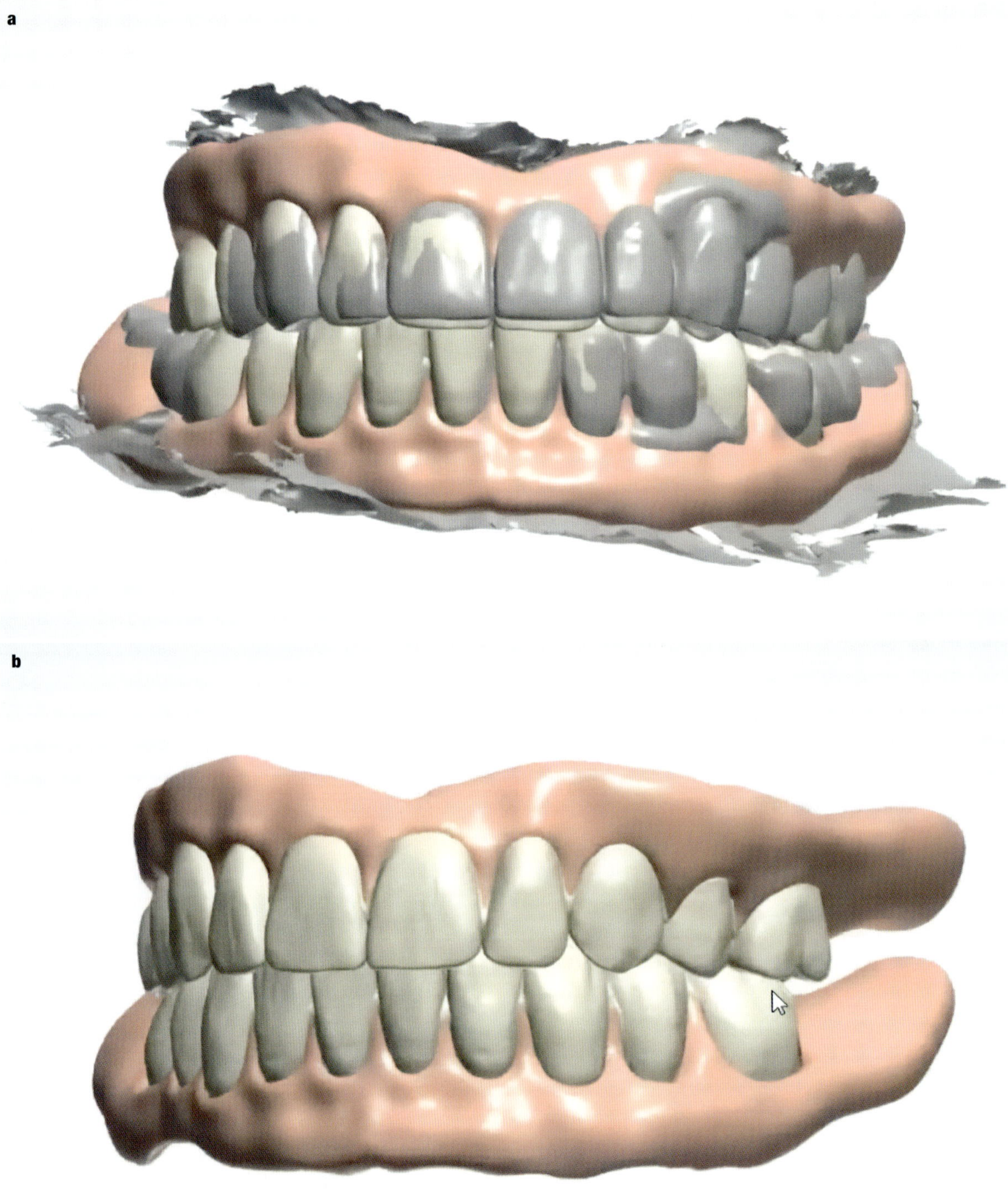

Figure 5.11 (a) Digital proposal, or digital design "wax-up," compared to and overlaid on preoperative scan; (b) Final proposal with the teeth in occlusion.

Bone reduction plane

Confirm that the appropriate amount of bone reduction is planned in the case before moving on to implant placement. My lab and I use a bone reduction plane that can be manipulated in the software to determine where the bone reduction will begin and end (Figs. 5.12, 5.13). The bone reduction plane allows for more predictable implant placement and provides assurance that the amount of restorative space will be adequate for both the interim and the definitive prosthesis.

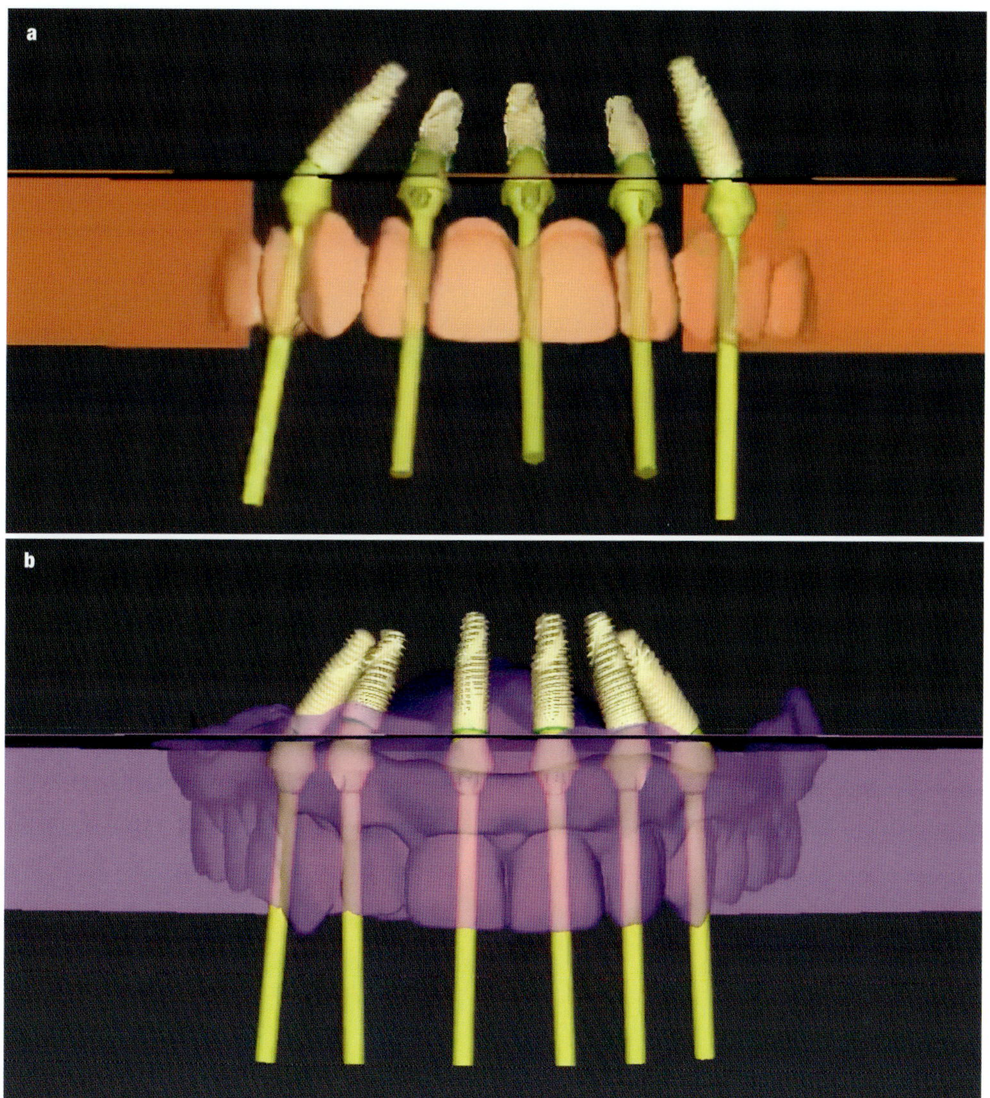

Figure 5.12 View of the digital bone reduction planes. (a) Proposed teeth position; (b) Current position of patient's teeth and tissues as captured by intraoral scan.

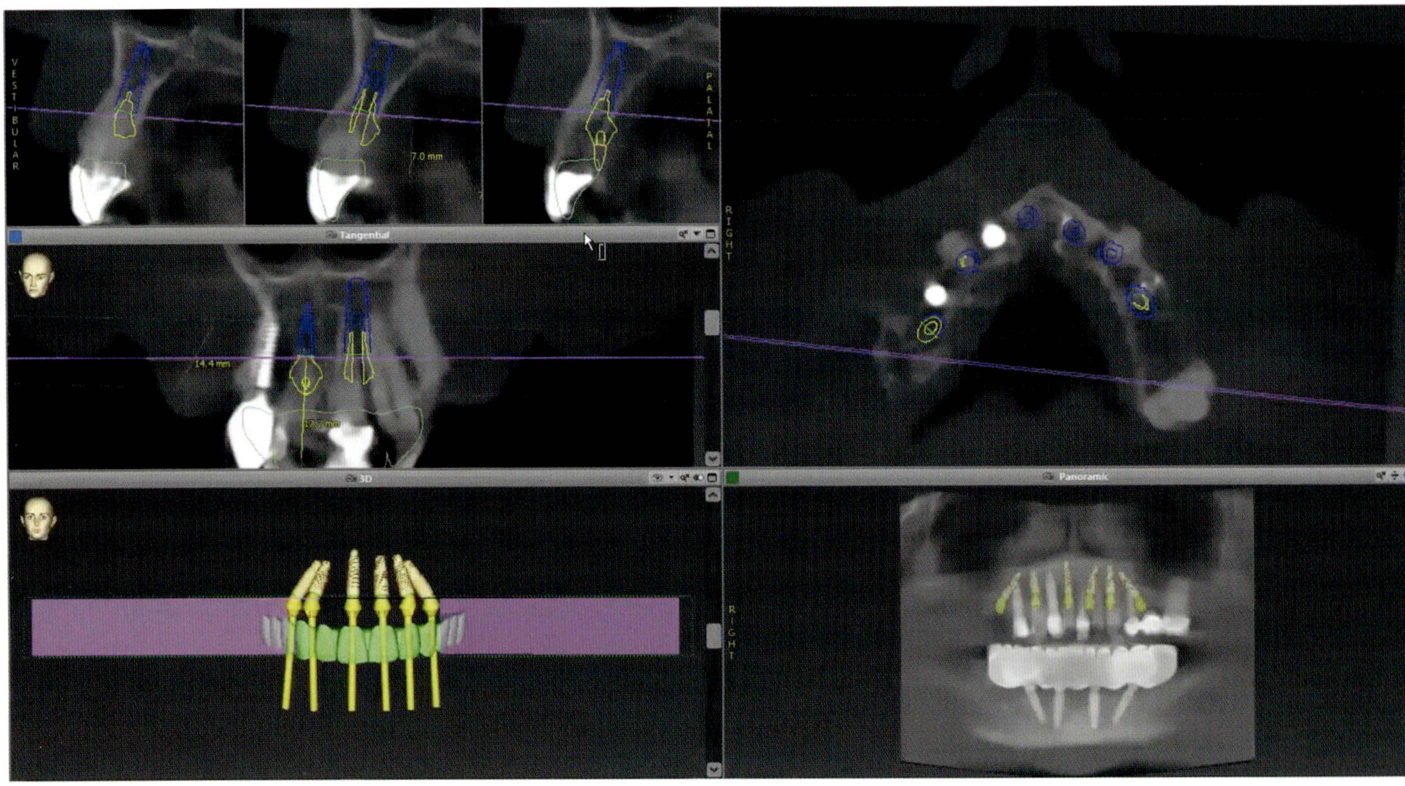

Figure 5.13 **Screen capture taken during the planning of a maxillary implant and multiunit abutment (MUA) positioning as well as interim fixed full-arch prosthesis, utilizing a bone reduction plane in coDiagnostiX® (Dental Wings GmbH) digital planning software.**

Implant and MUA placement

Once the bone reduction plane has been established, virtual placement of the dental implants throughout the arch can begin. The implants should be reviewed one at a time based on the implant placement principles discussed earlier. As you are virtually placing the implants, you will also want to consider positioning of the MUAs. The angulation of the implants and the MUAs will determine the path of draw for the interim and definitive prostheses. Achieving parallelism among the implants is important for ensuring the passive fit of your prosthesis (Figs. 5.14-5.19).

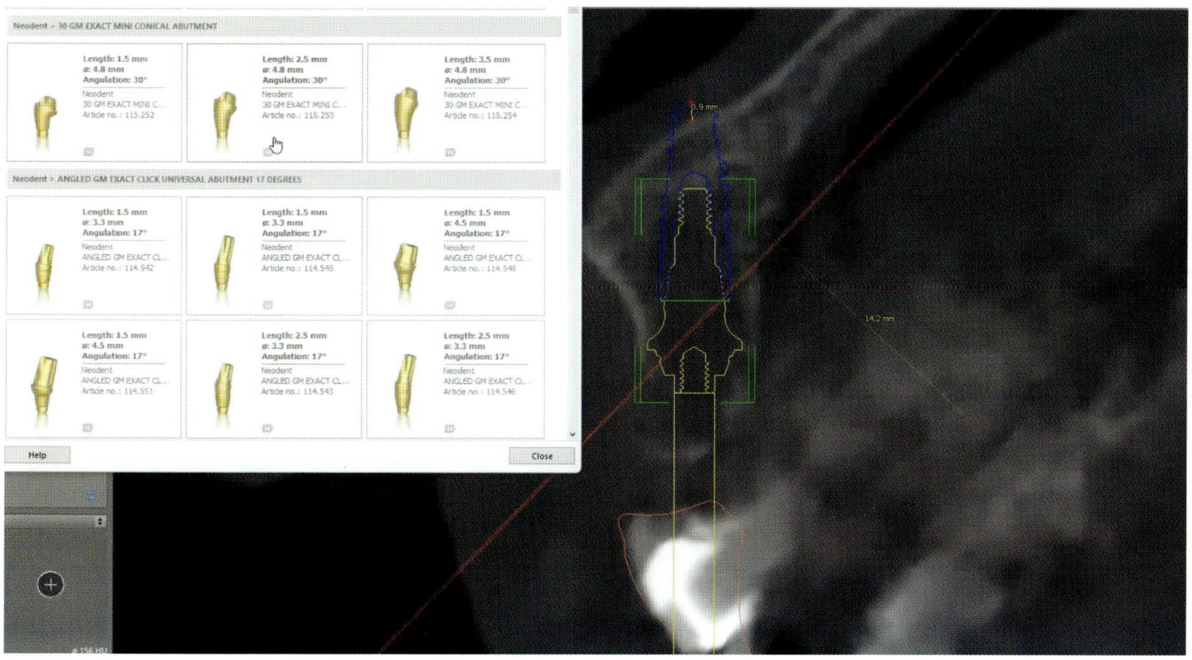

Figure 5.14 Screen capture taken during maxillary dental implant and MUA planning in coDiagnostiX software.

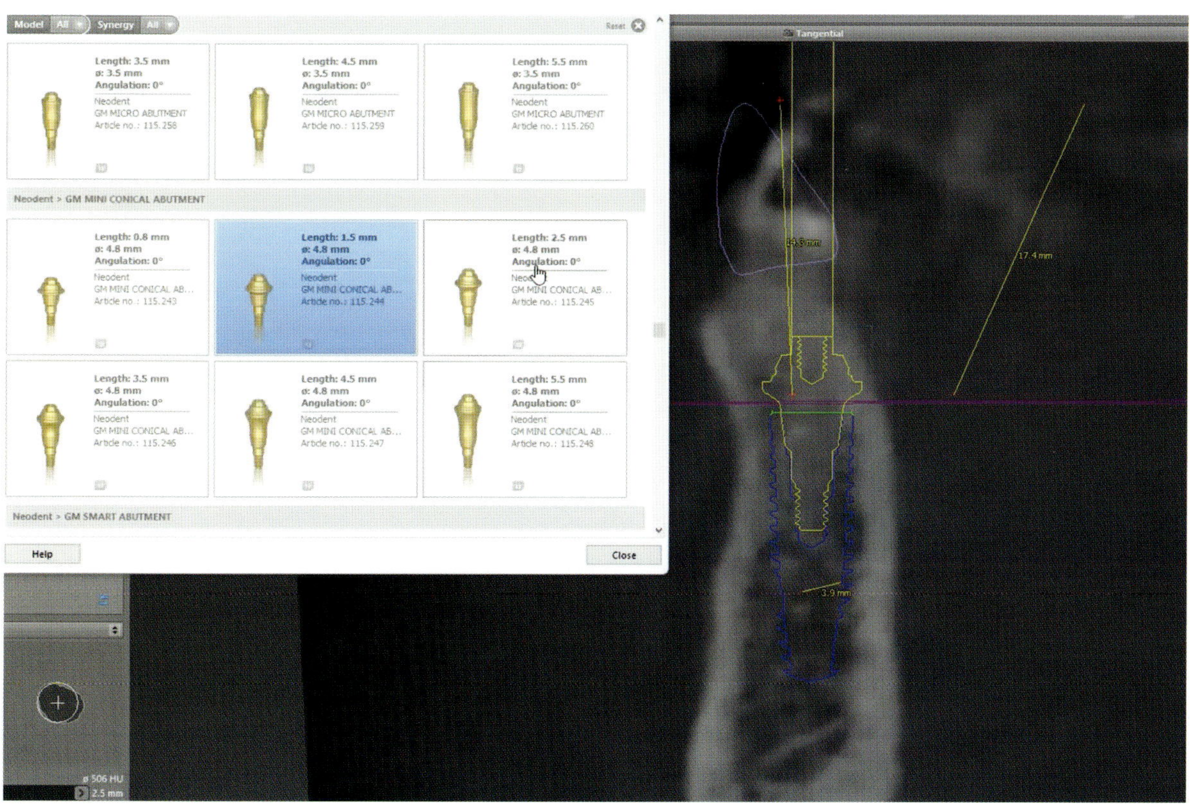

Figure 5.15 Screen capture taken during mandibular dental implant and MUA planning in coDiagnostiX software.

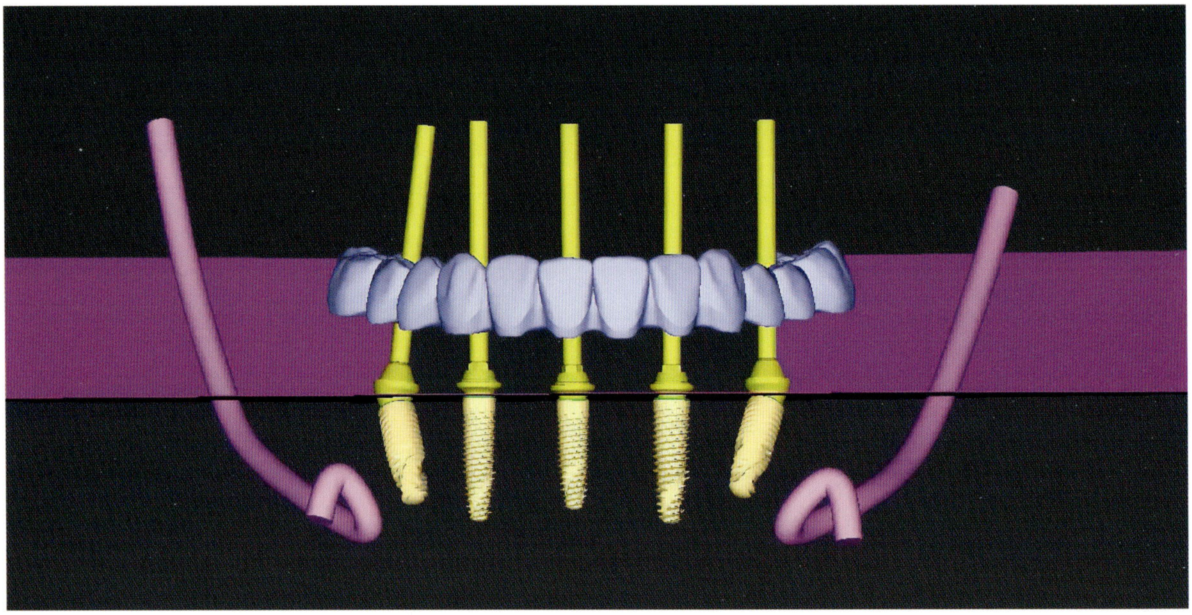

Figure 5.16 View of the digital mandibular bone reduction plane (*purple band*), proposed interim prosthesis teeth, dental implants with MUAs, and bilateral mandibular inferior alveolar nerves. Note the parallelism of the proposed access channels to achieve an ideal path of draw.

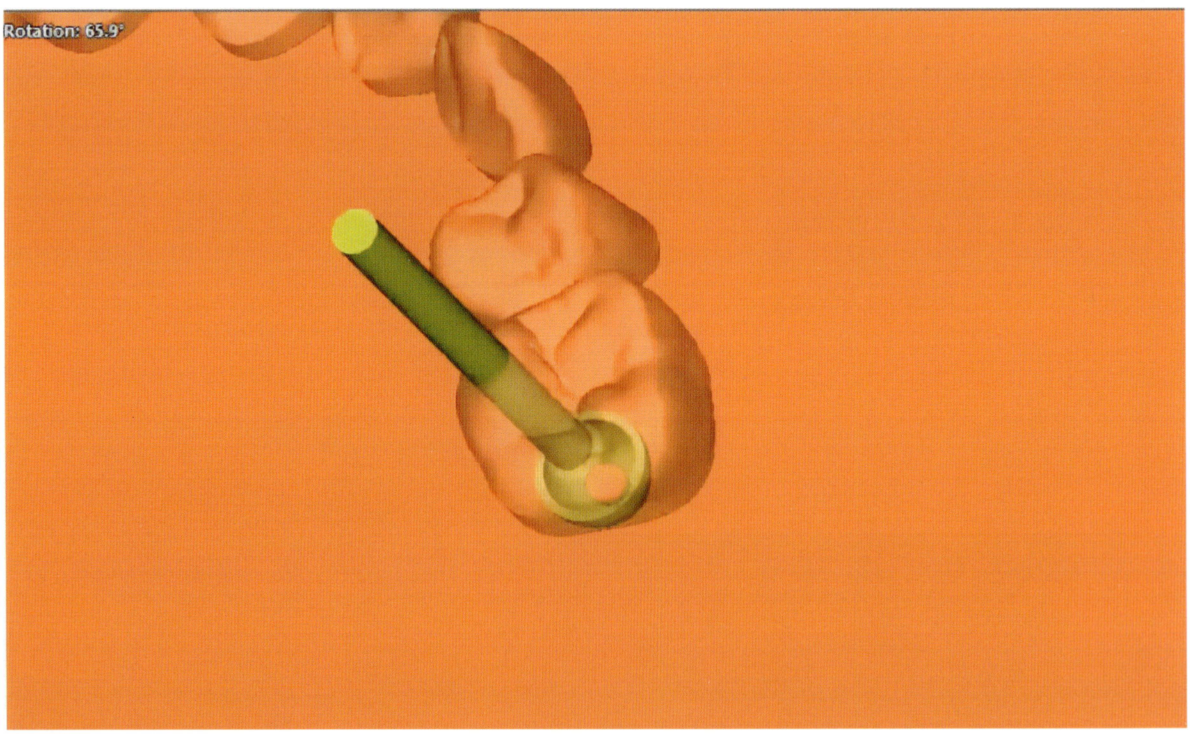

Figure 5.17 Digital screen capture demonstrating that the MUA can be rotated in the software to achieve proper angulation of the access channel through the surface of a proposed maxillary interim prosthesis.

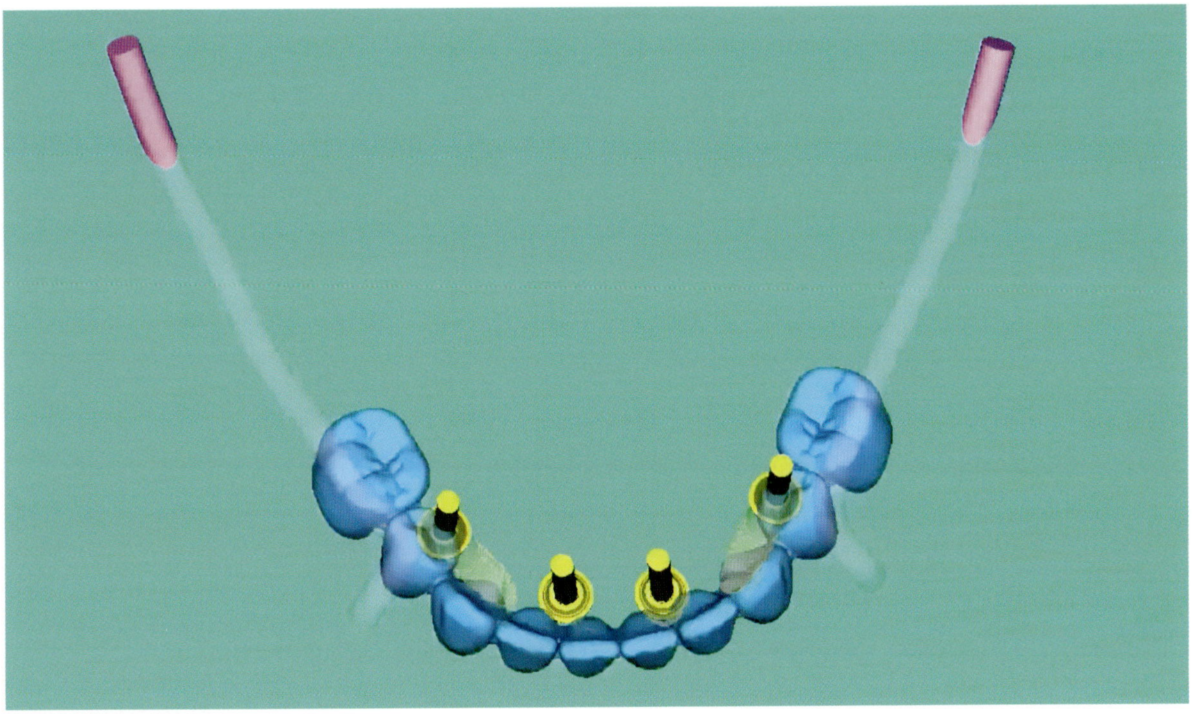

Figure 5.18 Digital occlusal view of the implants, the MUAs, and the screw access channels in a mandibular arch. Note the limitations of the AP spread.

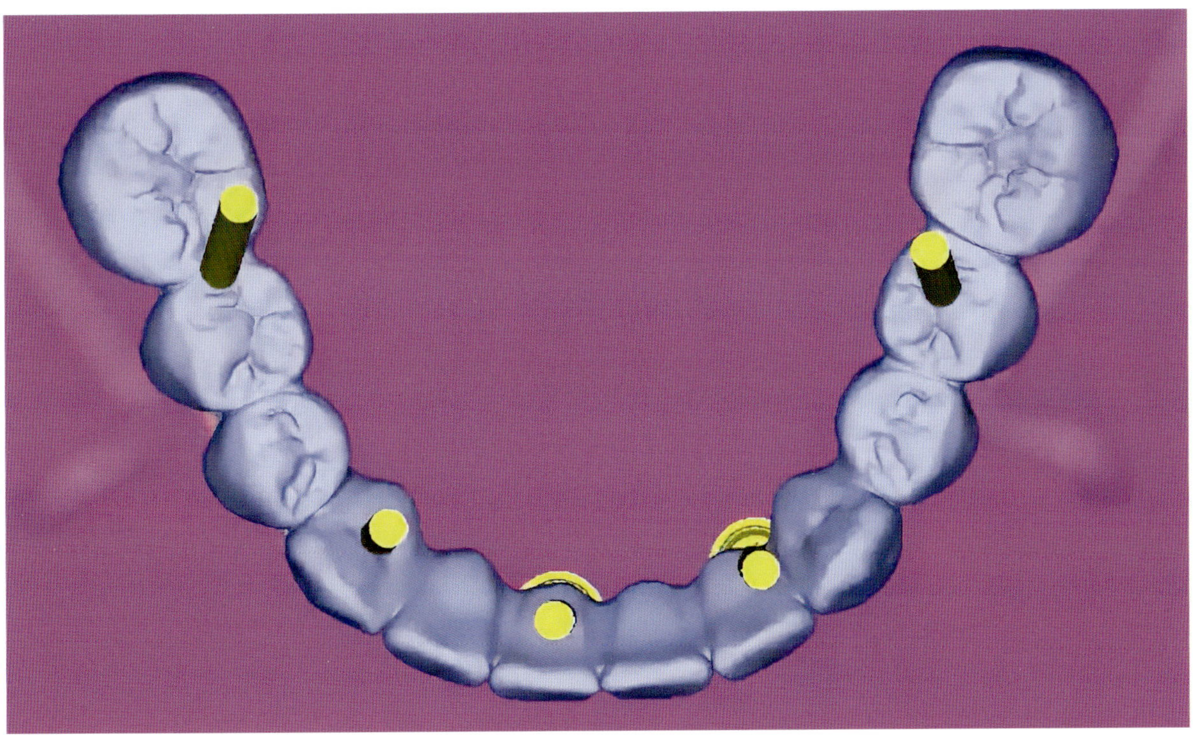

Figure 5.19 Digital occlusal view of the screw access channels and AP spread confirmation in the mandibular arch.

DIGITAL TREATMENT PLANNING PRO TIP:
Review each step before accepting the plan and giving approval for fabrication of the stackable surgical guide

During the implant engineering and guide design process, you will review each step in order. However, you can always go back and forth in the steps to confirm or change something. This is a fluid process, and the most important thing is to go through all the steps before validating the plan and approving it for the fabrication of your stackable surgical guide.

Fixation pin/screw design for the stackable surgical guide

Although the topic is not always addressed during the planning session, I recommend that the dentist participate in planning the design of the fixation pins or screws, or at least confirm where they will be placed with the digital treatment planner. The ability to visualize how the foundation guide will be fixated to the bone can be helpful, particularly when the patient has a small oral cavity or limited mouth opening (Figs. 5.20, 5.21).

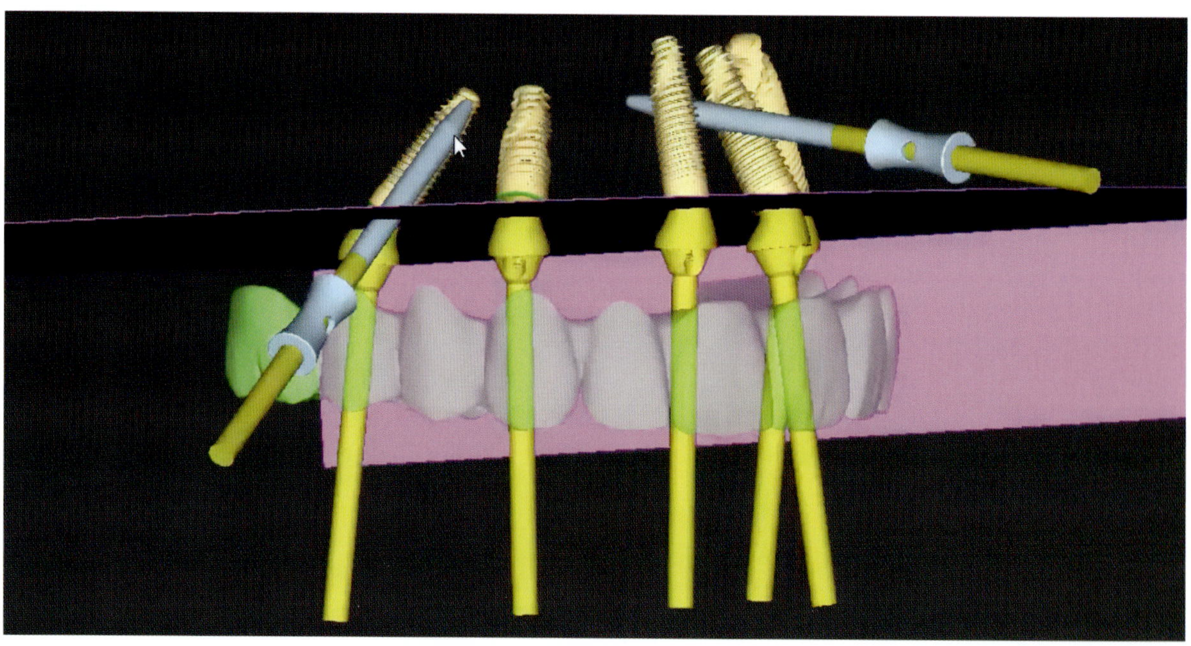

Figure 5.20 **Screen capture showing virtual placement of the fixation pins for securing the foundation guide.**

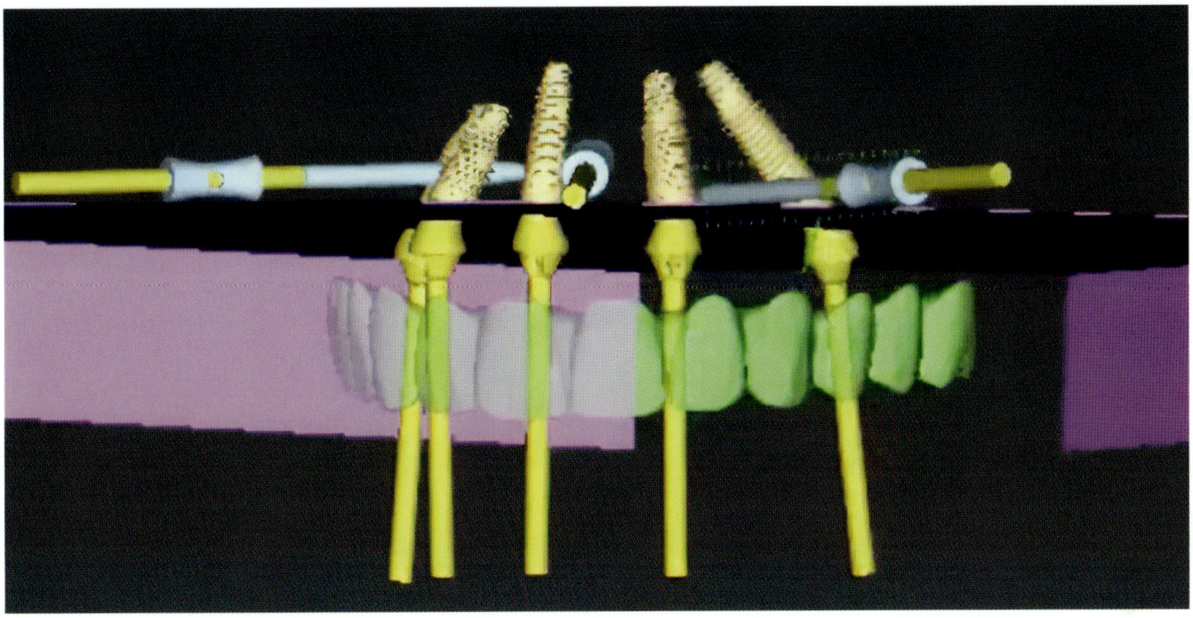

Figure 5.21 **Screen capture showing three fixation pins placed virtually. Note that the pins can be angled in a manner that allows for accessibility and appropriate space between implants.**

Wrap-up and approval of the case design

Once you have completed the design of the case, your planner will want approval from you to begin production of the stackable surgical guide. Confirm the date of the surgery and the date you would like the case to arrive in your office. Choose the material you would like the guide created from. There are several acceptable materials to choose from, as covered in Chapter 4. For the foundation guide, my current choice is a carbon-fiber reinforced material, milled titanium, or cobalt-chrome if either of those is unavailable. Verify any other pertinent patient details as well as the shade selected for the interim prosthesis, and inform the laboratory whether or not you want an emergency backup denture. You should also be able to have the laboratory list and send you and your team the implants and components that will be needed during the surgery. Do not forget to order any additional items you may need, such as pins, screws, drills, or other parts or tools that the lab is responsible for getting to you for the surgery.

SURGERY PREPARATION

- Surgical suite
- Implants and Implant components (The Inventory Effect)
- Biologics
- Medications and Gases
- Hemostasis
- Instrumentation/Materials
- Surgical reports

SURGICAL WORKFLOW

- Roll call
- Anesthesia/Throat pack

GUIDED IMPLANT PLACEMENT USING STACKABLE SURGICAL GUIDES

- Indexing aligner
- Flap placement
- Foundation guide
- Extractions
- Bone reduction
- Osteotomy guide/Implant placement
- Carrier guide/Abutment aligner

GUIDED CONVERSION

- Interim prosthesis pick-up
- Replica appliance
- Closure/Suturing
- Delivery of interim prosthesis
- Postsurgical/Postoperative management

THE FIXED FULL-ARCH GUIDED IMPLANT SURGICAL PROCESS

SECTION IV

SURGERY PREPARATION

CHAPTER **6**

Commitment: Learn from those who have gone before you and implement what you learn.

I am a big believer in learning from others' mistakes and following the example of those who have succeeded. More importantly, we must implement what we have learned by taking action.

There is an old adage, "fail to plan, plan to fail." An important aspect of planning for the surgical phase of fixed full-arch implant dentistry is having the appropriate armamentarium organized and available. This starts with having a well-trained assisting team that coordinates and prepares the setup. In our practice, I have delegated this responsibility to our lead surgical assistants. They are responsible and accountable for making sure that everything we need to provide the guided surgery and conversion is ready and available. This is vital to efficiency, provides peace of mind, and ensures a smooth surgical process. This chapter presents an overview of the physical space and armamentaria you will need to prepare for surgery.

SURGICAL SUITE

I have the luxury of using an operating suite in my practice. It is large enough to accommodate everything I need to make the surgery comfortable for my patient, my team, and myself. The room dimensions are 17' × 11'. Your operatory need not be this spacious, but it must be large enough to accommodate the patient, you, two or more assistants, and ideally an anesthesia provider. Typical dental operatories that might be appropriate for restorative dentistry do not always provide adequate space for fixed full-arch implant surgery.

Before you attempt your first fixed full-arch implant surgery, be sure that you have planned out your space, know where everything is located, assembled your team, and determined if the room will be accommodating. In addition to the space considerations, you should also have emergency equipment as well as an automated external defibrillator (AED) close by. Typically, I recommend conducting a practice run before the day of surgery if it is your first time (Figs. 6.1, 6.2).

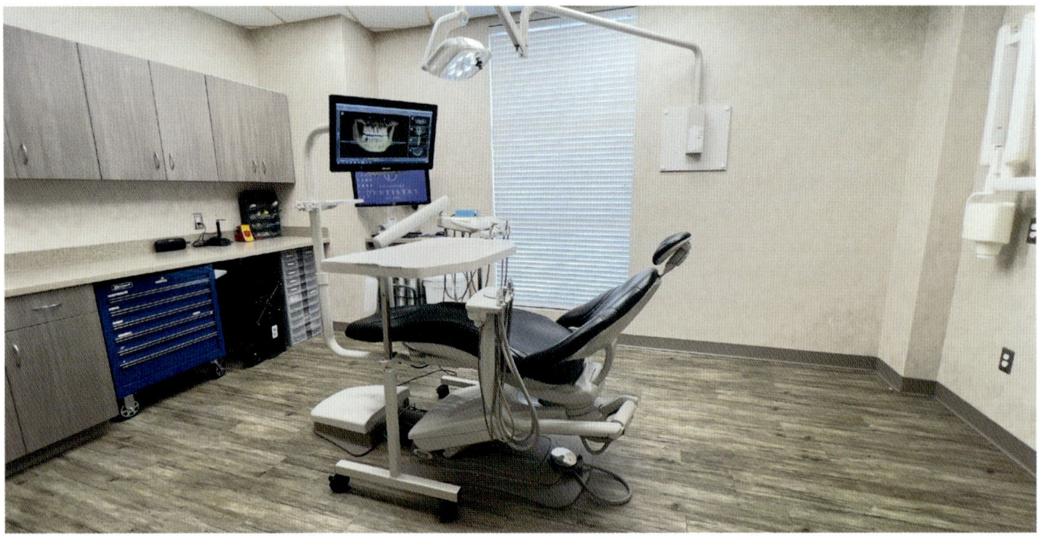

Figure 6.1 The surgical suite in the author's practice.

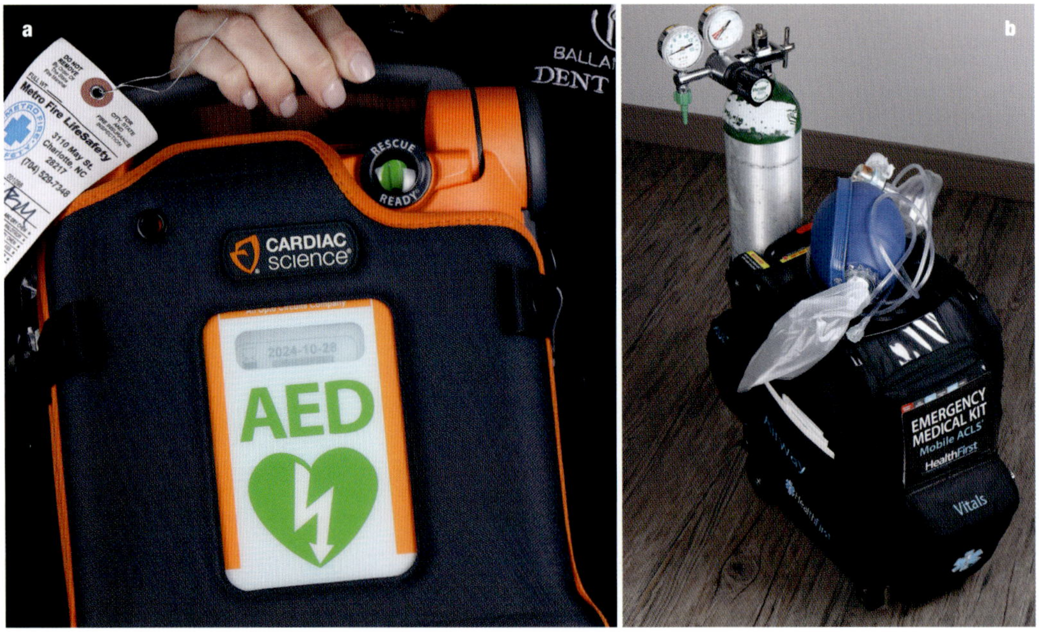

Figure 6.2 (a) An automated external defibrillator (AED) and (b) an emergency equipment and medical kit are vital to providing a safe surgery. This equipment should be tested, monitored, and reviewed frequently.

IMPLANTS AND IMPLANT COMPONENTS

Because the implant brand, implant sizes, and specific multiunit abutments (MUAs) that will be used at surgery have already been selected, all that remains is to make sure these implants and parts were ordered and are in your stock. In addition to the implants and MUAs, make sure you have the following instruments and components:

- Temporary titanium cylinders or copings
- Healing caps or protection cylinders for the MUAs
- Implant cover screws and healing abutments
- Guided surgical kit with drivers
- Drills, pins or screws, and other components used with the stackable surgical guide system

Depending on the implant system you are using, there may be other accessories available that could help you during your surgery. Spend the time to become familiar with the system you are using and its nuances. I recommend working with an implant company that has a local representative who can walk you through how their system works with guided full-arch implant cases and an implant that is designed to be used in full-arch rehabilitation.

THE INVENTORY EFFECT

Obviously, you need to have implants accessible during your surgery, but I often hear stories, and have been present during surgeries, where the procedure does not go as planned. Sometimes the case must be cancelled or cut short because the right dental implant(s) is not on hand. My solution to this problem, which I refer to as the "inventory effect," is to have access to implants and their components in a variety of diameters and lengths for maximum flexibility. You may be encouraged to order the implants you planned during case engineering and assume that is adequate. However, if any unexpected changes must be made during the surgery and the only implants on hand are the ones planned for the case, you may not be able to complete the surgery. I recommend one of the following courses of action:

- Contact your implant company representative and ask if the company offers any financial incentives for placing a bulk order of dental implants and components in varying sizes. Even if they do not, this is worth the investment because it will give you an inventory of implants to choose from if or when you happen to need a different implant or component during your surgery than the ones you planned to use.

- Discuss the option of implant consignment with your dental implant company. Consignment allows you to have a dental implant inventory without having to pay up front for the stock. As you use the implants, the company will charge you for them and restock accordingly.

Negotiating with your implant company is worthwhile if you plan to provide fixed full-arch implant dentistry in your practice on a regular basis. In my practice, I have chosen a combination of these options. Purchasing a bulk order of dental implants lets the implant manufacturer know you are serious about placing implants, and over time the company may be willing to allow you to accrue a consignment package from them (Fig. 6.3).

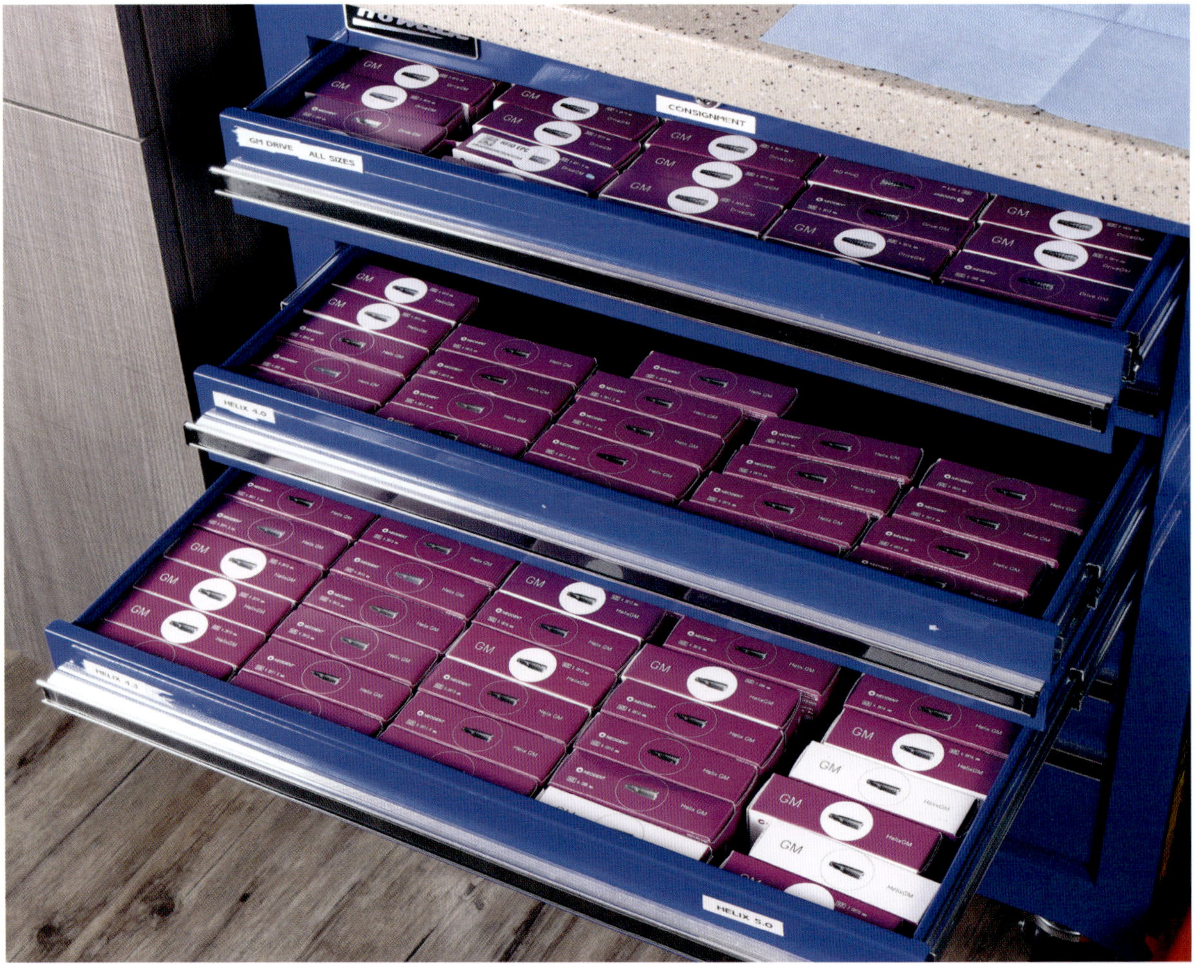

Figure 6.3 **The "inventory effect": having access to implants and their components in a variety of diameters and lengths for maximum flexibility. This is a consignment of dental implants in the author's practice.**

BIOLOGICS

I use the term *biologics* to describe the various materials used during surgery to preserve and regenerate bone and soft tissues, which is often referred to as *guided bone regeneration* (GBR). Thus, biologics might include different types of bone grafts or substitutes, membranes, wound dressings, and platelet-rich fibrin (PRF). If you elect to use these during your surgeries, which I recommend, make sure you have them in your stock. Although sutures may not be considered biologics, you will also need to have a variety of these at your disposal as well.

MEDICATIONS AND GASES

There are several medications you should be familiar with and have access to on the day of surgery. Before each surgery, check and make sure you have suitable amounts on hand:

- Local anesthetics
- Oral/intramuscular/intravenous medications: sedatives, opioids, antiemetics, corticosteroids, anti-inflammatory agents, antibiotics, etc.
- Oxygen, nitrous oxide, and any other anesthetic gases
- Emergency drugs required for advanced cardiac life support

HEMOSTASIS CONTROL

Hemostasis naturally occurs in the body through vasoconstriction, platelet plug formation, and coagulation. However, full-arch implant surgery can be bloody, and controlling hemostasis can be especially challenging in some patients. Remember that a patient's medical conditions and social history, in addition to their medications and use of supplements, play a role in how much bleeding takes place during surgery. Having an anesthesiologist or certified registered nurse anesthetist (CRNA) present during surgery can be beneficial because they can reduce the patient's blood pressure by administering medications during intraoperative bleeding.

However, you will also need to be prepared with a few other helpful items. To control bleeding during surgery, have plenty of 4 × 4 gauze, Surgicel® (Ethicon), bone wax, and/or gelatin sponges on hand. These will enable you to control most of the minor venous bleeding episodes you encounter. You will occasionally need to control arterial bleeding as well. To be prepared, consider investing in a diode or CO_2 laser and/or an electrosurgery device (monopolar or bipolar). In addition, it is helpful to understand techniques to control hemostasis by ligation with suturing or by using a handpiece and a Thermacut® bur (Dentsply Sirona) without water.

Be sure you are comfortable with the fundamentals of hemostasis during oral surgery before attempting your first fixed full-arch implant case. The last thing you need is for a patient to have bleeding during your surgery that you cannot control.

INSTRUMENTATION AND OTHER MATERIALS

Figures 6.4 and 6.5 show a basic instrument setup that can be used to complete fixed full-arch implant surgery. If you perform implant surgery in your practice and have a surgical instrument setup that you are comfortable with, you do not necessarily need to make any additions to it. It is likely that you have a few favorite instruments or accessories that do not appear in my setup. I prefer to use Berman dental instruments when I can because they are high quality and cost effective.

In addition to surgical instruments, you will also need a straight surgical handpiece with a surgical motor and surgical burs as well as prosthetic burs to be used in the laboratory and when making prosthetic adjustments. I have developed a prosthetic and surgical bur kit that is simple and efficient to use and can be ordered directly from Komet USA **(Fig. 6.6)**.

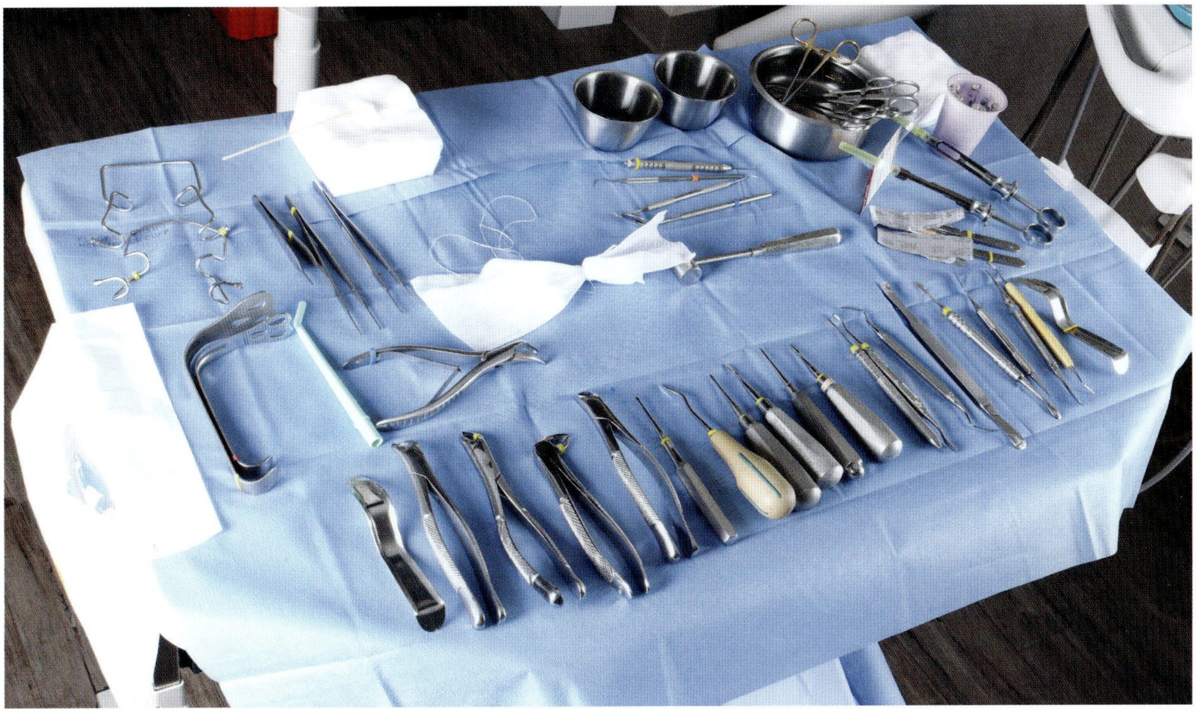

Figure 6.4 The author's surgical instrumentation setup with instruments from Berman Dental.

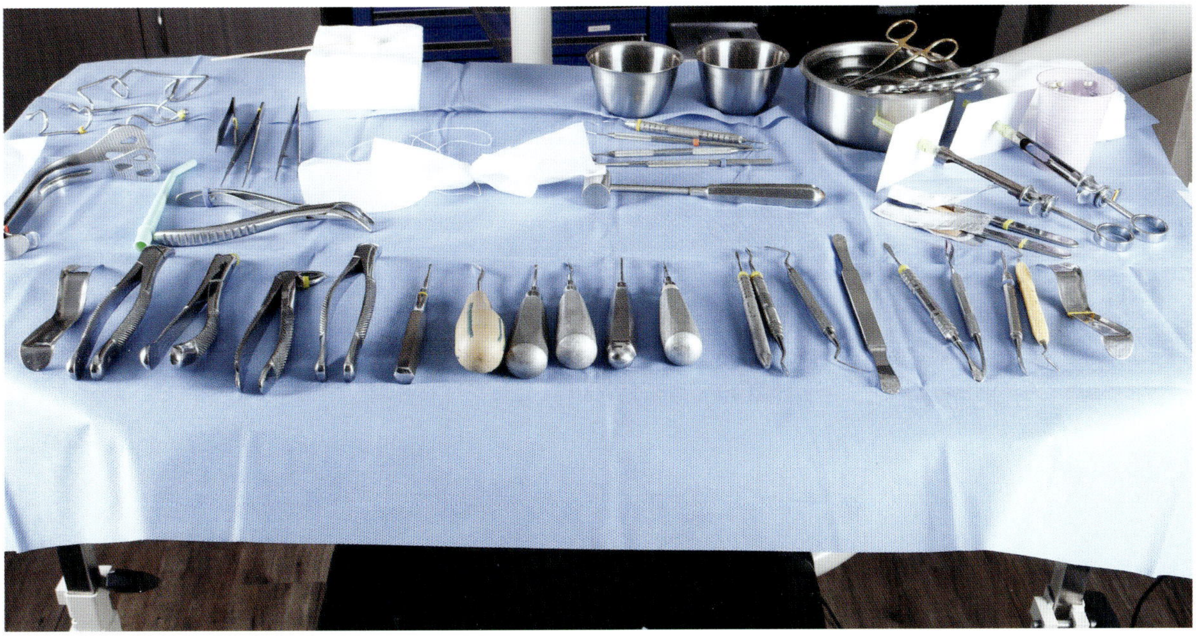

Figure 6.5 Berman Dental instrument setup for surgery.

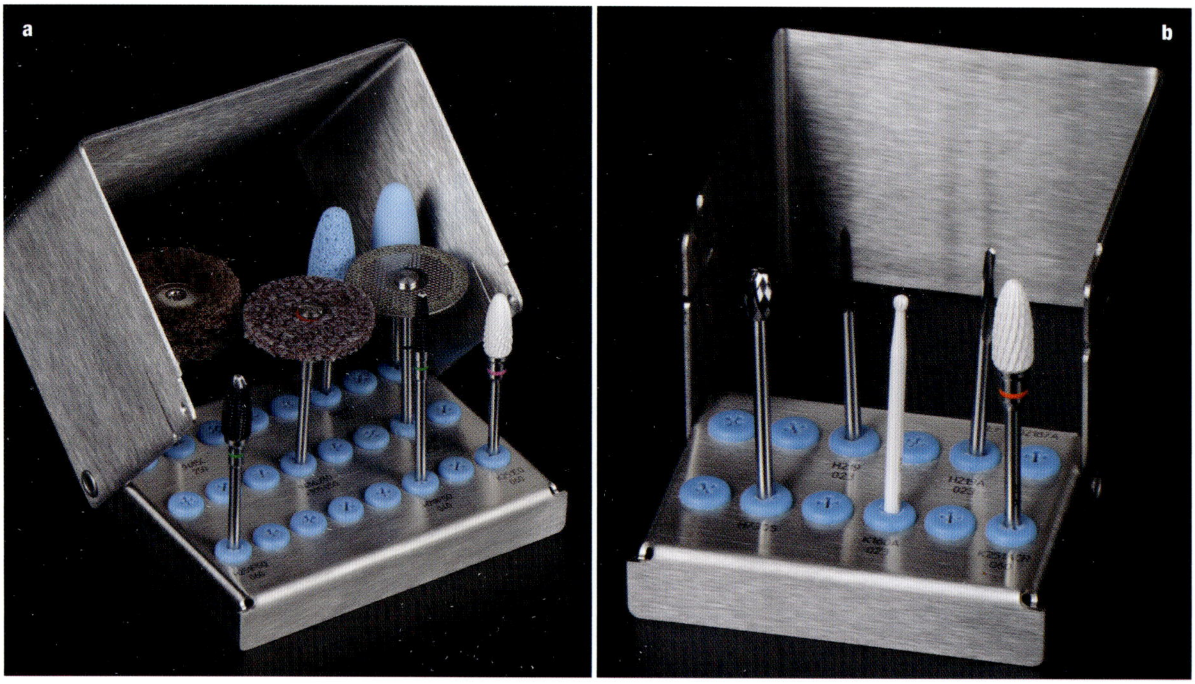

Figure 6.6 (a) **Prosthetic and** (b) **surgical bur kits for fixed full-arch implant dentistry (Komet USA).**

Checklist of the author's instrument and material setup for fixed full-arch implant surgery

Table 1

- 2x Syringe
- 2x Scalpel
- 2x Minnesota
- 2x #9 periosteal elevator
- 2x Straight and angled periotomes
- 1x #301 elevator
- 1x #34 elevator
- 1x B elevator
- 1x 150 forcep
- 1x 151 forcep
- 1x Ash forcep
- 1x cowhorn forcep
- 1x Curette
- 1x Selden
- 1x Prichard
- 2x Mirror
- 1x Explorer
- 1x Perio probe
- 1x Spear
- 1x Bone file
- 1x Small mallet
- 1x Cotton plier
- 1x Small pick up
- 1x Large pick up
- 1x Wire driver
- 1x Gold handle Hemostats
- 1x Dean scissors
- 1x Rongeurs
- 2x Bite block
- 1x Small Sweetheart
- 1x Large Sweetheart
- 1x Small lip retractor
- 1x Regular lip retractor
- Throat sponges
- Fixation Pins and or screws
- 4x4 Gauze
- 2x Large bowl
- 2x Small bowl
- 4x 3.0 Chromic Gut Sutures
- 4x 3.0 PGA Sutures
- Local Anesthetic (Marcaine, Lidocaine, Articaine)
- Tatum serrated curettes
- Extra suction tips
- Mouth prop
- High speed handpiece
- Straight handpiece
- Komet surgical & prosthetic kits
- Surgical 557

Table 2

- Implant motor
- Implant tubing and sodium chloride
- Straight and angled implant handpiece
- Guided implant placement kit
- Salvin angled torque wrench
- Laser
- Hand driver and latch attachment
- Versa osseodensification burs

Table 3

- Stellar DC and tips
- Rubber dam
- Curing light
- Appliances and guides
- Implants
- Multiunit abutments
- Tissue caps
- Temp Cylinders
- Heavy body impression material fast set and tips
- Articulating paper
- Vaseline
- PRF red and white tubes
- Blood collection setup
- Alcohol gauze
- 2x2 and tape
- Tourniquet
- Fibrin compressor
- Biologics

SURGICAL REPORTS

Surgical reports are 2D or 3D visualizations of the full-arch implant surgery case based on the plan that you and your digital planner have put together. Think of them as your surgical map. They can be in print or digital format, but the latter will require you to use the software in which the case was planned to visualize it. Having access to 3D digital surgical reports during surgery is helpful, especially if changes need to be made. A 2D printed surgical report is generally all you will need to guide you and your team through the surgery.

Surgical reports are a good way to get organized and re-familiarized with the details of the case (Figs. 6.7, 6.8). In our practice, surgical reports are reviewed, printed, and then posted in the surgical operatory. I have them taped to a wall or posted beside me so I can refer to them while I am working. A good rule is to review these reports at least once before the surgery, but do not wait until just before the surgery to make sure things are in order. We generally prepare and review everything we need for surgery the evening before the surgery takes place.

a

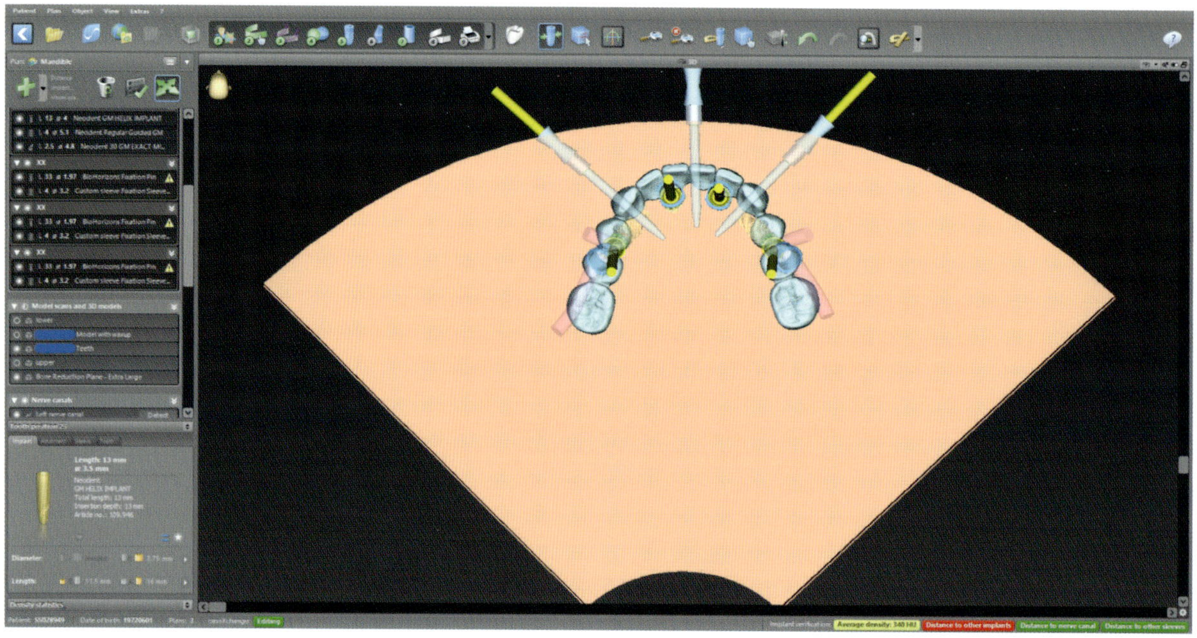

b

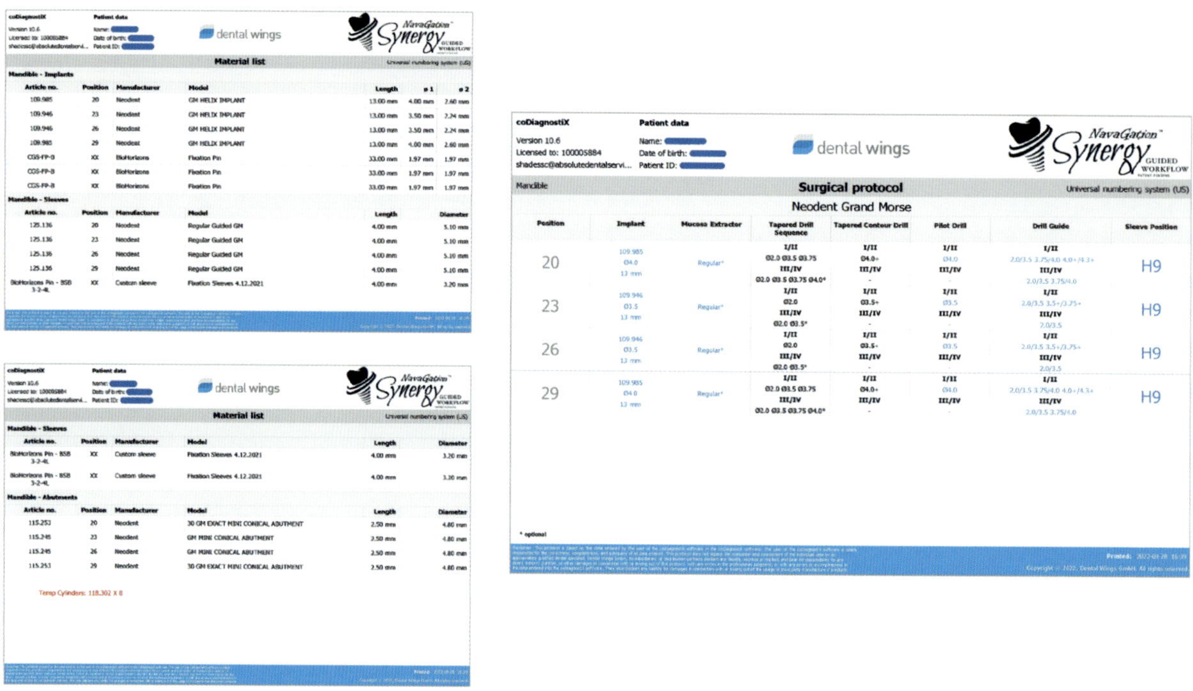

coDiagnostiX
Version 10.6
Licensed to: 100005884
shadessc@absolutedentalservi...

Patient data
Name: [redacted]
Date of birth: [redacted]
Patient ID: [redacted]

dental wings

NavaGation Synergy GUIDED WORKFLOW

Material list — Universal numbering system (US)

Mandible - Implants

Article no.	Position	Manufacturer	Model	Length	ø 1	ø 2
109.985	20	Neodent	GM HELIX IMPLANT	13.00 mm	4.00 mm	2.60 mm
109.946	23	Neodent	GM HELIX IMPLANT	13.00 mm	3.50 mm	2.24 mm
109.946	26	Neodent	GM HELIX IMPLANT	13.00 mm	3.50 mm	2.24 mm
109.985	29	Neodent	GM HELIX IMPLANT	13.00 mm	4.00 mm	2.60 mm
CGS-FP-B	XX	BioHorizons	Fixation Pin	33.00 mm	1.97 mm	1.97 mm
CGS-FP-B	XX	BioHorizons	Fixation Pin	33.00 mm	1.97 mm	1.97 mm
CGS-FP-B	XX	BioHorizons	Fixation Pin	33.00 mm	1.97 mm	1.97 mm

Mandible - Sleeves

Article no.	Position	Manufacturer	Model	Length	Diameter
125.136	20	Neodent	Regular Guided GM	4.00 mm	5.10 mm
125.136	23	Neodent	Regular Guided GM	4.00 mm	5.10 mm
125.136	26	Neodent	Regular Guided GM	4.00 mm	5.10 mm
125.136	29	Neodent	Regular Guided GM	4.00 mm	5.10 mm
BioHorizons Pin - BSB 3-2-4L	XX	Custom sleeve	Fixation Sleeves 4.12.2021	4.00 mm	3.20 mm

coDiagnostiX
Version 10.6
Licensed to: 100005884
shadessc@absolutedentalservi...

Patient data
Name: [redacted]
Date of birth: [redacted]
Patient ID: [redacted]

dental wings

NavaGation Synergy GUIDED WORKFLOW

Material list — Universal numbering system (US)

Mandible - Sleeves

Article no.	Position	Manufacturer	Model	Length	Diameter
BioHorizons Pin - BSB 3-2-4L	XX	Custom sleeve	Fixation Sleeves 4.12.2021	4.00 mm	3.20 mm
BioHorizons Pin - BSB 3-2-4L	XX	Custom sleeve	Fixation Sleeves 4.12.2021	4.00 mm	3.20 mm

Mandible - Abutments

Article no.	Position	Manufacturer	Model	Length	Diameter
115.253	20	Neodent	30 GM EXACT MINI CONICAL ABUTMENT	2.50 mm	4.80 mm
115.245	23	Neodent	GM MINI CONICAL ABUTMENT	2.50 mm	4.80 mm
115.245	26	Neodent	GM MINI CONICAL ABUTMENT	2.50 mm	4.80 mm
115.253	29	Neodent	30 GM EXACT MINI CONICAL ABUTMENT	2.50 mm	4.80 mm

Temp Cylinders: 118.302 X 8

coDiagnostiX
Version 10.6
Licensed to: 100005884
shadessc@absolutedentalservi...

Patient data
Name: [redacted]
Date of birth: [redacted]
Patient ID: [redacted]

dental wings

NavaGation Synergy GUIDED WORKFLOW

Mandible — **Surgical protocol** — Universal numbering system (US)

Neodent Grand Morse

Position	Implant	Mucosa Extractor	Tapered Drill Sequence	Tapered Contour Drill	Pilot Drill	Drill Guide	Sleeve Position
20	109.985 Ø4.0 13 mm	Regular*	I/II Ø2.0 Ø3.5 Ø3.75 III/IV Ø2.0 Ø3.5 Ø3.75 Ø4.0*	I/II Ø4.0+ III/IV -	I/II Ø4.0 III/IV -	I/II 2.0/3.5 3.75/4.0 4.0+/4.3+ III/IV 2.0/3.5 3.75/4.0	H9
23	109.946 Ø3.5 13 mm	Regular*	I/II Ø2.0 III/IV Ø2.0 Ø3.5*	I/II Ø3.5+ III/IV -	I/II Ø3.5 III/IV -	I/II 2.0/3.5 3.5+/3.75+ III/IV 2.0/3.5	H9
26	109.946 Ø3.5 13 mm	Regular*	I/II Ø2.0 III/IV Ø2.0 Ø3.5*	I/II Ø3.5+ III/IV -	I/II Ø3.5 III/IV -	I/II 2.0/3.5 3.5+/3.75+ III/IV 2.0/3.5	H9
29	109.985 Ø4.0 13 mm	Regular*	I/II Ø2.0 Ø3.5 Ø3.75 III/IV Ø2.0 Ø3.5 Ø3.75 Ø4.0*	I/II Ø4.0+ III/IV -	I/II Ø4.0 III/IV -	I/II 2.0/3.5 3.75/4.0 4.0+/4.3+ III/IV 2.0/3.5 3.75/4.0	H9

* optional

Figure 6.7 (a, b) A 2D printed surgical report overview for a mandibular arch case displaying the implant sizes, positions, and other pertinent information.

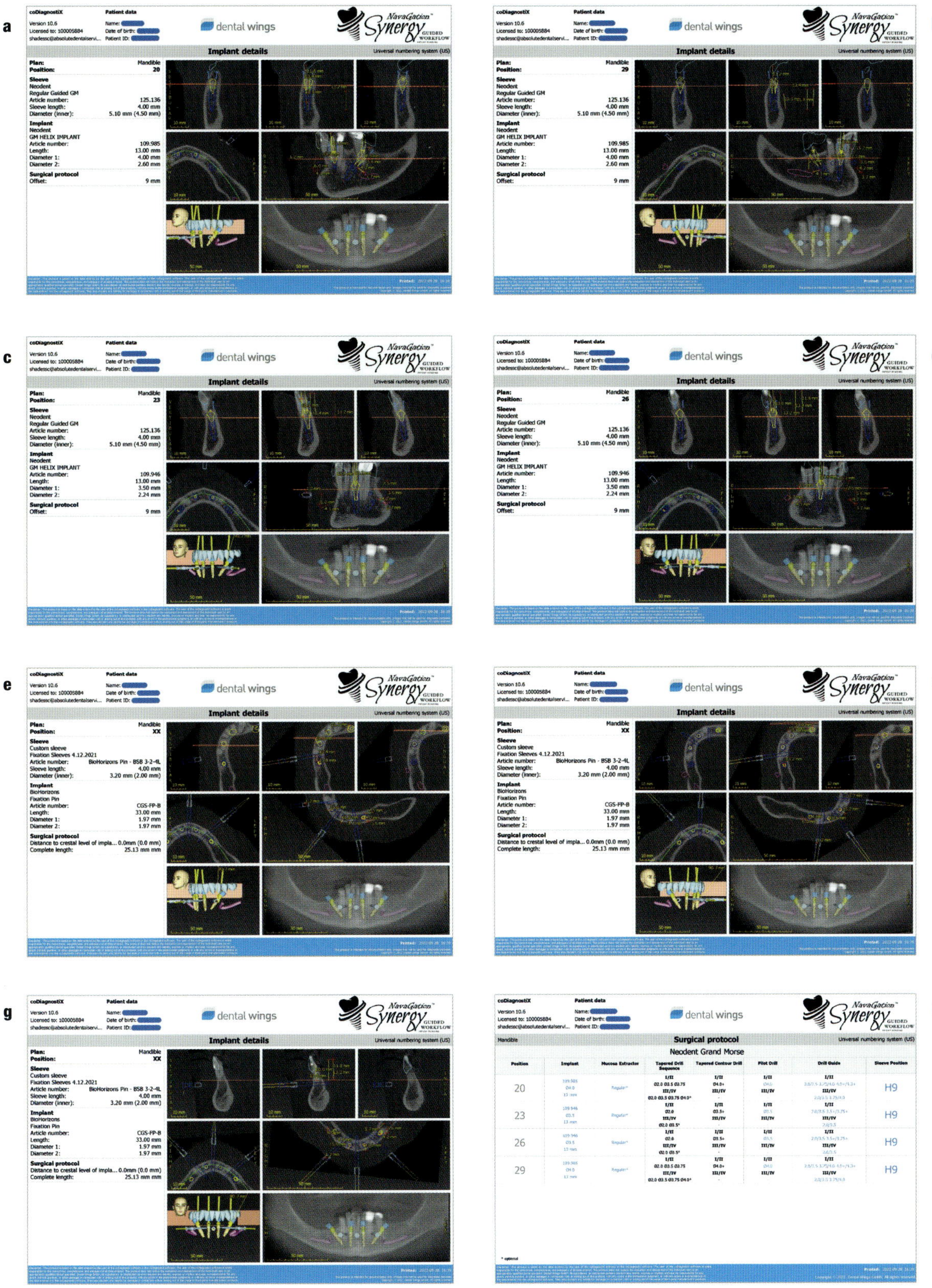

Figure 6.8 (a-h) Surgical case reports for a mandibular arch displaying the details of each implant.

1. ROLL CALL
2. ANESTHESIA AND THROAT PROTECTION
3. VERIFICATION OF INDEXING ALIGNER FIT
4. INCISION AND FLAP ELEVATION
5. FOUNDATION GUIDE PLACEMENT/FIXATION
6. TEETH EXTRACTION (DENTATE PATIENTS)
7. BONE REDUCTION
8. OSTEOTOMY GUIDE AND IMPLANT PLACEMENT
9. CARRIER GUIDE/ABUTMENT ALIGNER AND MUA PLACEMENT
10. INTERIM PROSTHESIS PICK-UP
11. REPLICA APPLIANCE PICK-UP
12. INTERIM PROSTHESIS CONVERSION
13. CLOSING AND SUTURING
14. SEATING OF THE FINISHED INTERIM PROSTHESIS
15. POSTSURGICAL PROCEDURES
16. POSTOPERATIVE APPOINTMENTS

STEP-BY-STEP SURGICAL WORKFLOW

CHAPTER **7**

Commitment: Set your goals, but be patient and don't rush.
Dream a big dream and shoot for the moon. Just understand that Rome wasn't built in a day. Give yourself time to succeed in whatever you endeavor to achieve.

The step-by-step workflow presented in this chapter is based on the stackable surgical guide systems that I have used in my practice. Though most stackable systems are similar, each has variations and nuances that result in slight differences in the surgical steps. I encourage you to read through the surgical workflow in this text and make note of any differences in the stackable guide system you have chosen.

Note: *The surgical photographs in this chapter are drawn from a variety of cases and are intended to demonstrate a broad range of steps, equipment, and instrumentation used in the surgical process.*

STEP 1: ROLL CALL

The day before your surgery case, take the time to verify that you and your team are prepared. All surgical case components should be in the office at least a couple of days prior to your surgery. In my practice, this is all delegated to highly trained dental assistants who are assigned specific responsibilities. If anything pertinent to the surgery is missing or has been overlooked—a piece of equipment, materials, supplies, etc.—it can add significant stress to your procedure. The following is the pre-surgery checklist that we use in our practice.

Guided Full-Arch Pre-surgery Checklist

Make sure the following tasks are completed the day before surgery:

- Patient prescriptions called into pharmacy
- Patient confirmed by phone or text
- Surgical suite is clean and equipment checked
- Surgical instrument kits autoclaved
- Guided surgery implant drill kits autoclaved
- Bur kits autoclaved
- Surgical reports posted
- Stackable surgical guides and case opened; components checked
- Implant and components stocked and inventory checked
- Dental assistants assigned

In addition to reviewing your pre-surgery checklist, confirm that you will have the appropriate clinical auxiliary team support for your case. Guided full-arch surgery requires significant concentration and attention to detail. I generally engage at least two and sometimes three dental assistants to help me (Fig. 7.1), dividing the responsibilities as follows:

- **Surgical dental assistant 1:** Provides suction and retraction
- **Surgical dental assistant 2:** Handles and organizes instruments, guide components, and dental implants/components and manages prosthesis conversion
- **Floater dental assistant:** Take notes, records, and floats, or acts as a "gopher"; steps in if one of the other assistants needs a break
- **Anesthesiologist or certified registered nurse anesthetist (CRNA):** Provides deep conscious sedation or general anesthesia

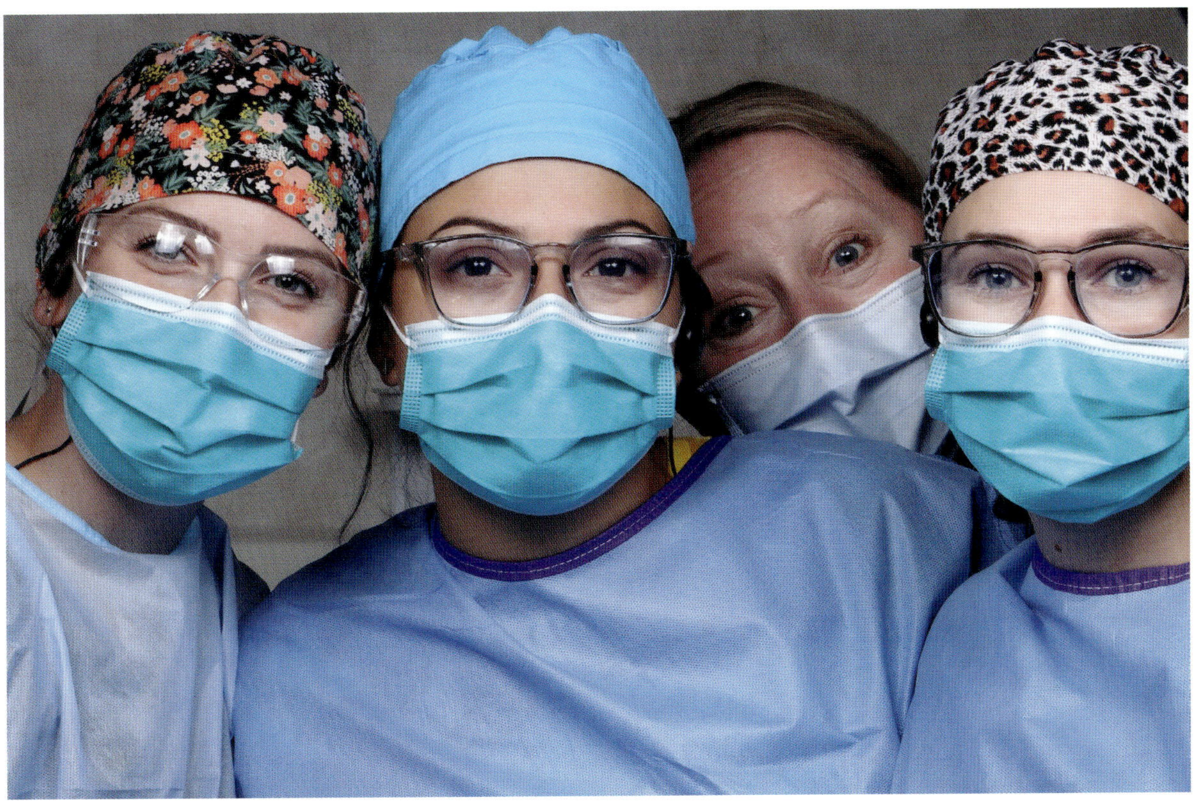

Figure 7.1 Four members of the author's surgical team (*left to right*): Stephanie, Jenni, Dr. Dulin (anesthesiologist), and Bethany.

STEP 2: ANESTHESIA AND THROAT PROTECTION

Full-arch implant surgery cases, especially dual-arch cases, require a significant amount of time and focus. They can be completed without a sedative, but only if excellent local anesthesia is administered, and only with a patient who can tolerate a lengthy surgical procedure. In my practice, the surgery is performed with the patient under deep intravenous sedation or general anesthesia (Fig. 7.2). I have experience with cases where the patient is not sedated or under general anesthesia, and the surgery is far too stressful for the patient as well as the clinician and team. I recommend that you or (ideally) another clinician, such as a CRNA or anesthesiologist, provide sedation or general anesthesia for the patient. When an anesthesiologist or CRNA provides this care, I can focus entirely on the surgery and prosthetic conversion. In my opinion, this is the safest and best approach, especially for an unseasoned clinician.

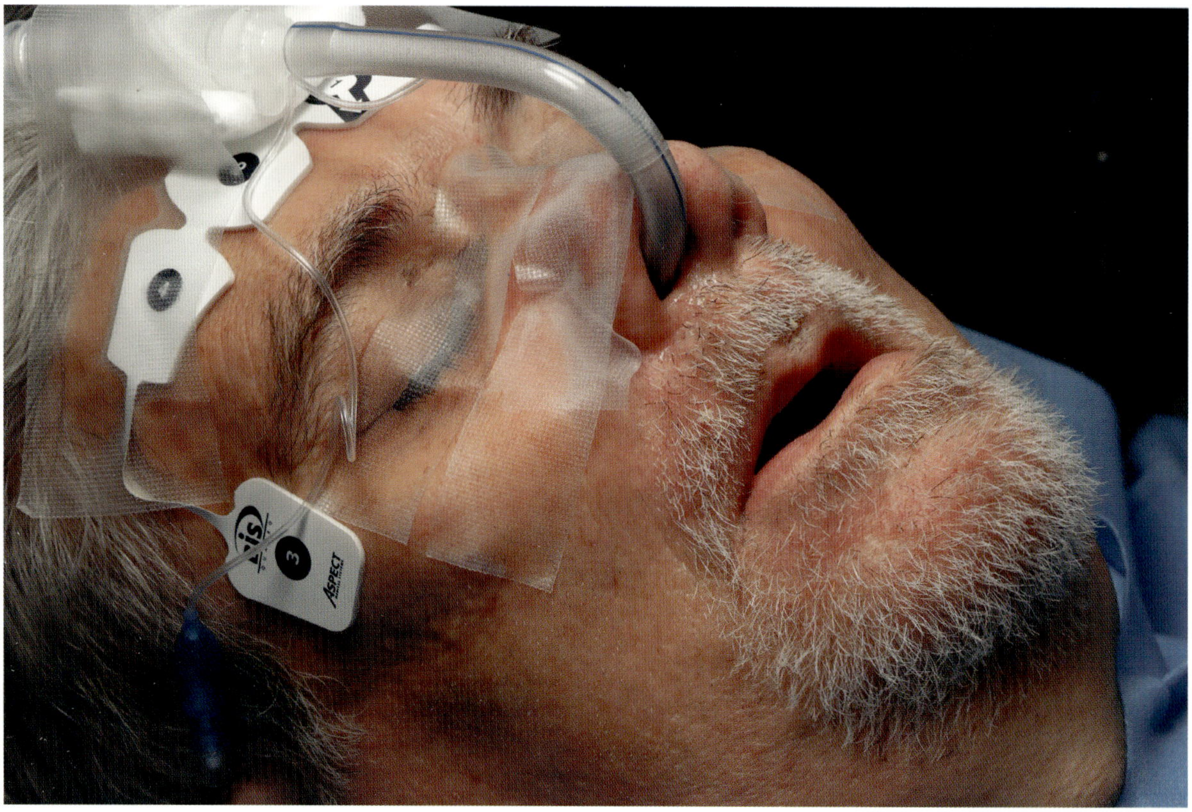

Figure 7.2 **Patient under general anesthesia.**

Once the patient is comfortably sedated, proceed with the following:

A. Place a throat pack or another form of throat protection to prevent aspiration of implants, implant parts, dental devices, and/or debris created during the surgery, and use a cheek retractor for visibility during the procedure (Fig. 7.3).

If the patient is intubated under general anesthesia, a throat pack with a long piece of floss can be tucked behind the tongue, with the floss extending out of the patient's mouth for retrievability (Fig. 7.4). It is crucial that throat packs not get lost or end up being forgotten: *Always* declare "placing throat pack" and "removing throat pack" in front of the surgical team. Make sure the number of throat packs and times they were placed and removed are recorded in the notes. In cases where a lot of bleeding occurs during surgery, consider replacing the throat pack once or even several times. As a rule, I place a throat pack at the beginning of surgery and then again at the midpoint if the case will be longer than 3 hours. If the patient is conscious and nonintubated, place a large piece of gauze or sponge toward the back of the throat, albeit not so far back that it triggers a gag reflex.

PRO TIP: Order of procedures

For dual-arch cases, complete the surgery in the maxilla before moving to the mandible. Some clinicians prefer to complete the surgery in both arches before beginning conversion of the interim prostheses, but I have found that it is more efficient and less risky to complete one arch at a time. With a highly trained team of auxiliaries, you can be working on the mandible while your team is converting the maxillary interim prosthesis.

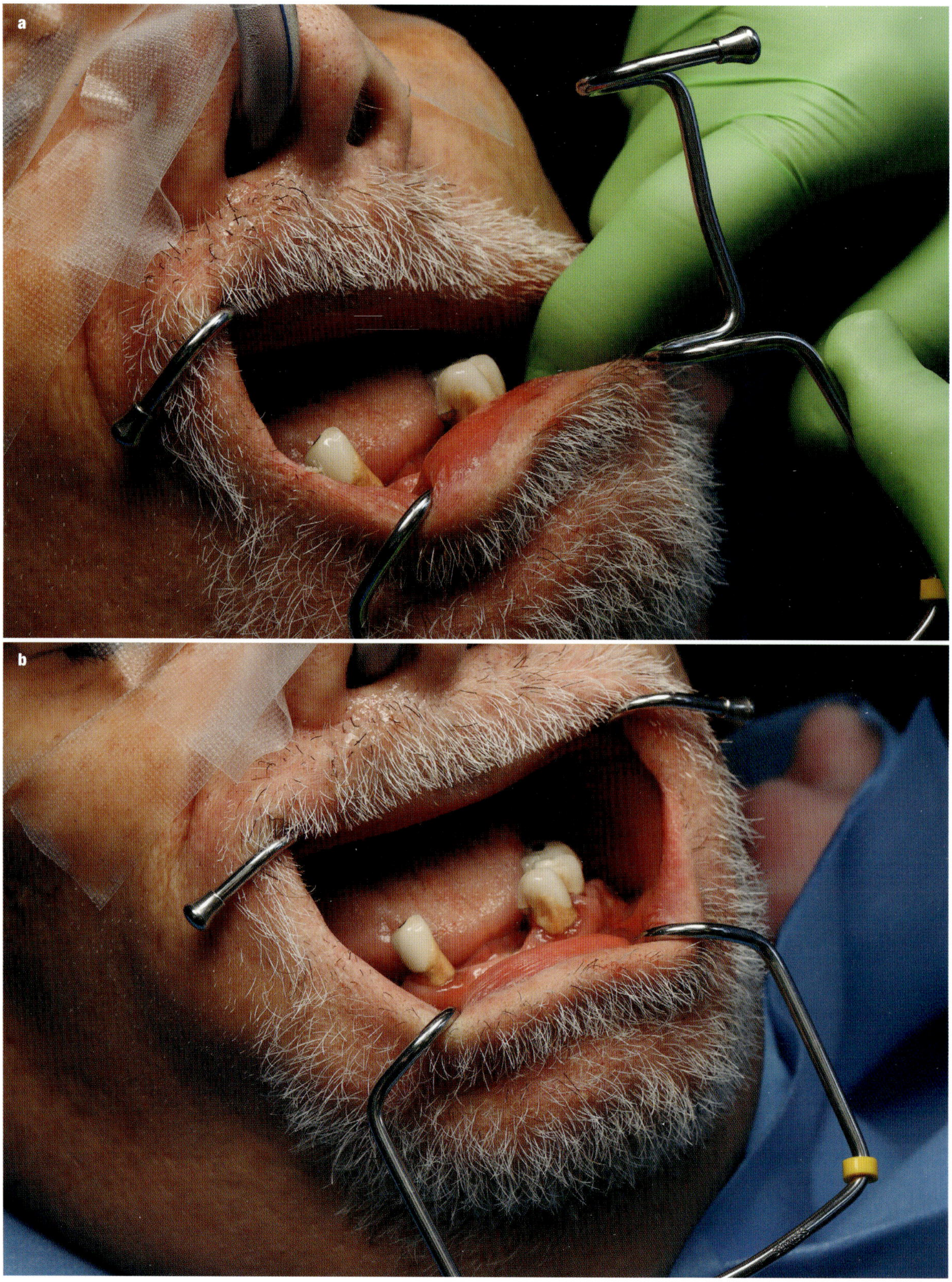

Figure 7.3 (a) Placement of surgical cheek retractor; (b) Surgical cheek retractor in position.

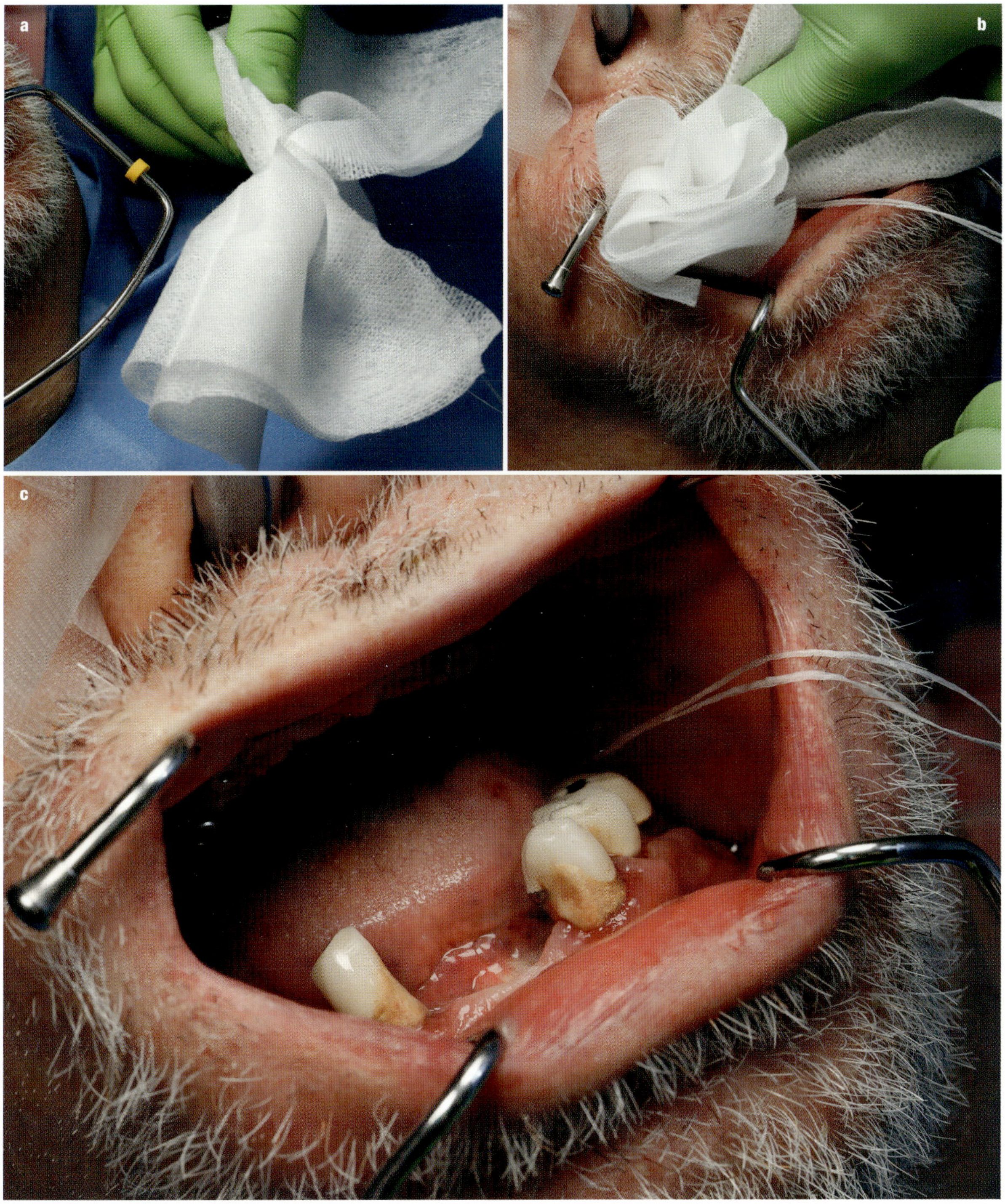

Figure 7.4 (a) Throat pack tied with floss for ease of retrieval; (b) Placement of throat pack; (c) Throat pack in place.

B. Administer local anesthesia.

Providing local anesthesia in full-arch implant surgical cases is more technique-sensitive if the patient is not under general anesthesia, and thus it will take more time. Use whatever techniques are appropriate to achieve profound local anesthesia. In the maxilla, the entire arch and palate should be fully anesthetized. In the mandible, consider blocking both inferior alveolar nerves and buccal nerves and provide lingual anesthesia. Buccal infiltration may also be appropriate. Always record the type and amount of local anesthesia being used (Fig. 7.5).

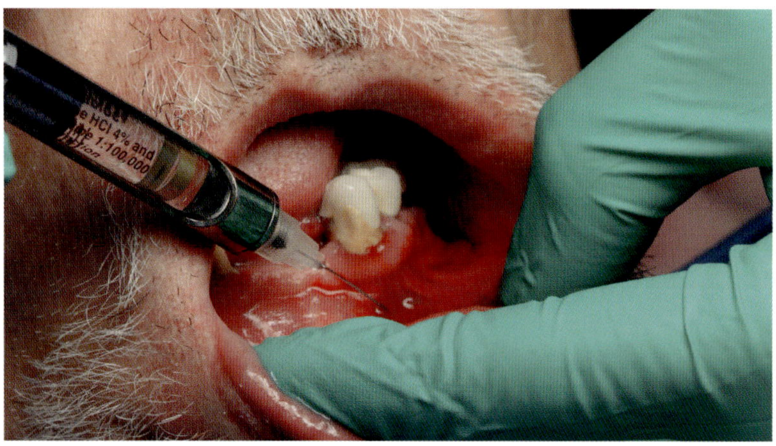

Figure 7.5 Buccal infiltration of local anesthesia (4% articaine HCL with epinephrine 1:100,000) in the mandible.

PRO TIP: Administering local anesthesia

When a patient is under general anesthesia, administer local anesthesia just as you would if the patient were under conscious sedation. Local anesthesia should be given at the beginning and even consider re-anesthetizing toward the end of surgery. If the patient is unconscious, why would it matter you may ask? Dental anesthesiologists have stated that even though the patient will not be consciously aware of pain during surgery, it should be considered for stabilization of vital signs during the surgery as well as a decreased depth of necessary general anesthesia. Local anesthesia helps avoid activation of the deep pain pathways. Patients also tend to recover better and have improved recovery times when local anesthesia is given[1].

STEP 3: VERIFICATION OF INDEXING ALIGNER FIT

A. Place the indexing aligner in the patient's mouth and verify that it seats completely and intimately (Fig. 7.6).

The indexing aligner may index on the teeth and edentulous ridge in partially edentulous patients or on soft tissues in completely edentulous patients (Fig. 7.7). There are also ways to index edentulous cases on maxillary or mandibular boney ridges.

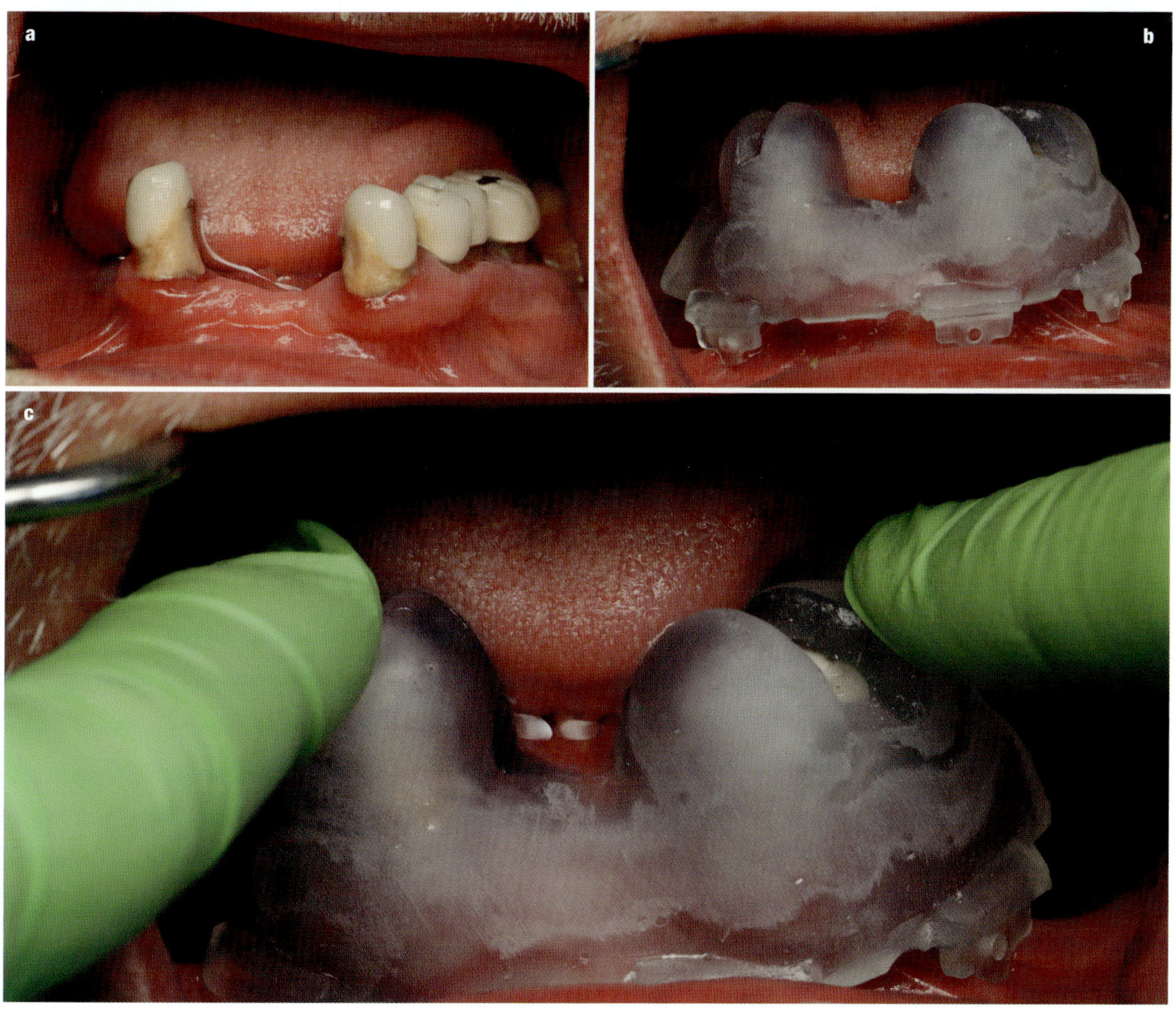

Figure 7.6 Placement of the indexing aligner in a partially edentulous mandible. (a) Preoperative view; (b) Placement of indexing aligner on teeth; (c) Checking the indexing aligner stability and fit using both hands.

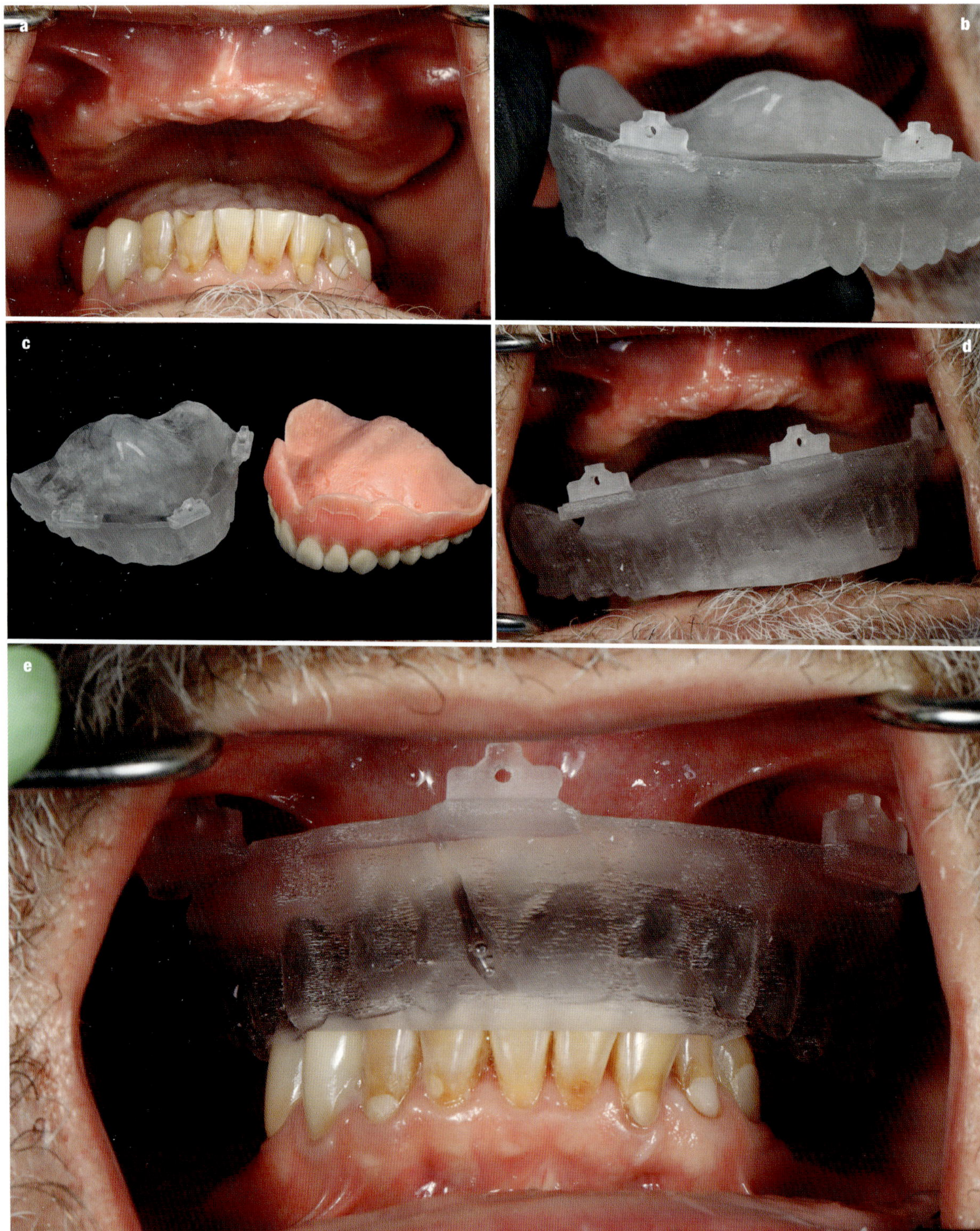

Figure 7.7 Placement of indexing aligner in fully edentulous maxilla. (a) Preoperative view; (b) Soft tissue–borne indexing aligner; (c) Indexing aligner placed beside the patient's full-mouth denture, which was used to create it; (d) Placing the indexing aligner over the edentulous arch; (e) Appearance of the indexing aligner in place and occluding with the opposing arch for stability and to check occlusion.

B. Look through the windows of the aligner and check to make sure there is no space separating it from the teeth, the soft tissues, or the edentulous ridge (Fig. 7.8).

If there is space and the indexing aligner is not seating properly, look carefully to determine what could be holding it up. Consider that a shallow buccal or lingual vestibule may be keeping the aligner from seating. Also confirm that the dentition did not change in the period since the original intraoral scan or impression was taken. Remove the aligner and inspect the intaglio surface for the presence of any debris. It is vital for the indexing aligner to fit well for complete seating of the foundation guide.

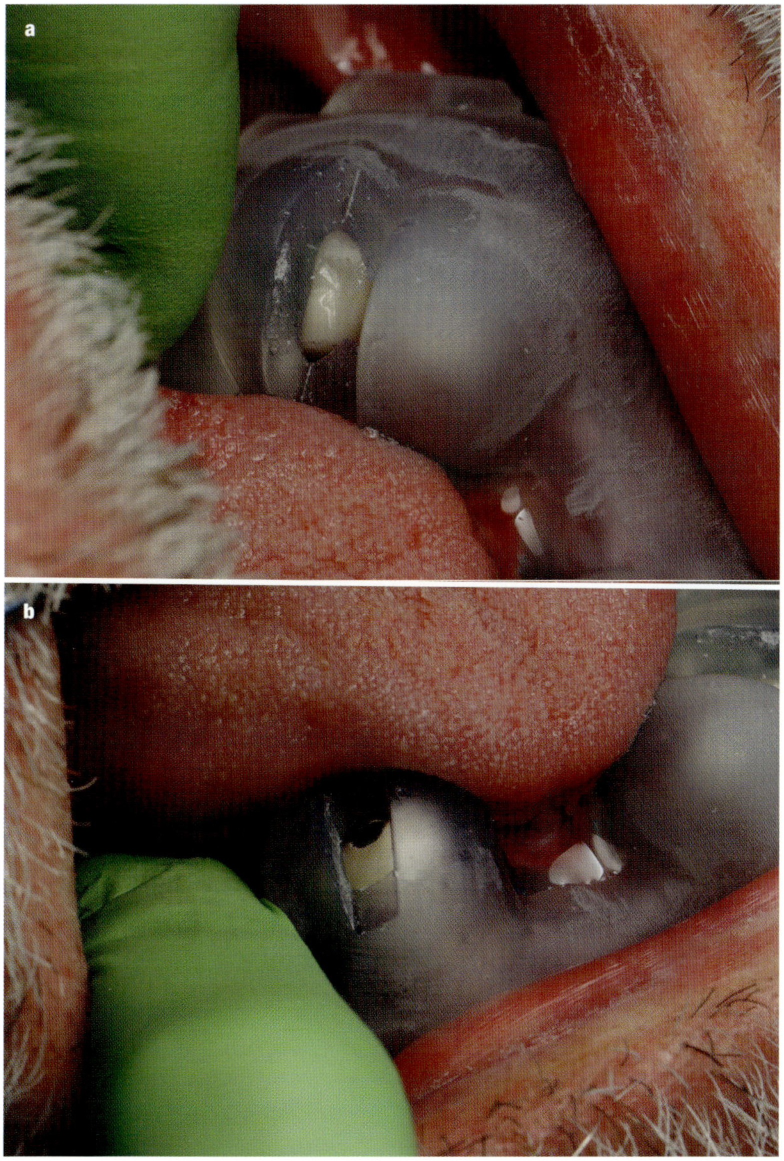

Figure 7.8 (a) Window cut into an indexing aligner; (b) Properly seated indexing aligner, as confirmed by the view through the window showing the teeth.

STEP 4: INCISION AND FLAP ELEVATION

If you are using a floating-style foundation guide, you could delay flap elevation until after you extract the teeth; however, this would require you to remove the guide and then replace it, which I do not recommend (except in cases where there is adequate keratinized tissue in the buccal areas, as shown in Figure 7.9). With an anatomical-style or hybrid floating-/anatomical-style foundation guide, the flap must be elevated on the buccal or facial surface before the teeth are extracted. This is the technique I myself use and recommend for greatest accuracy.

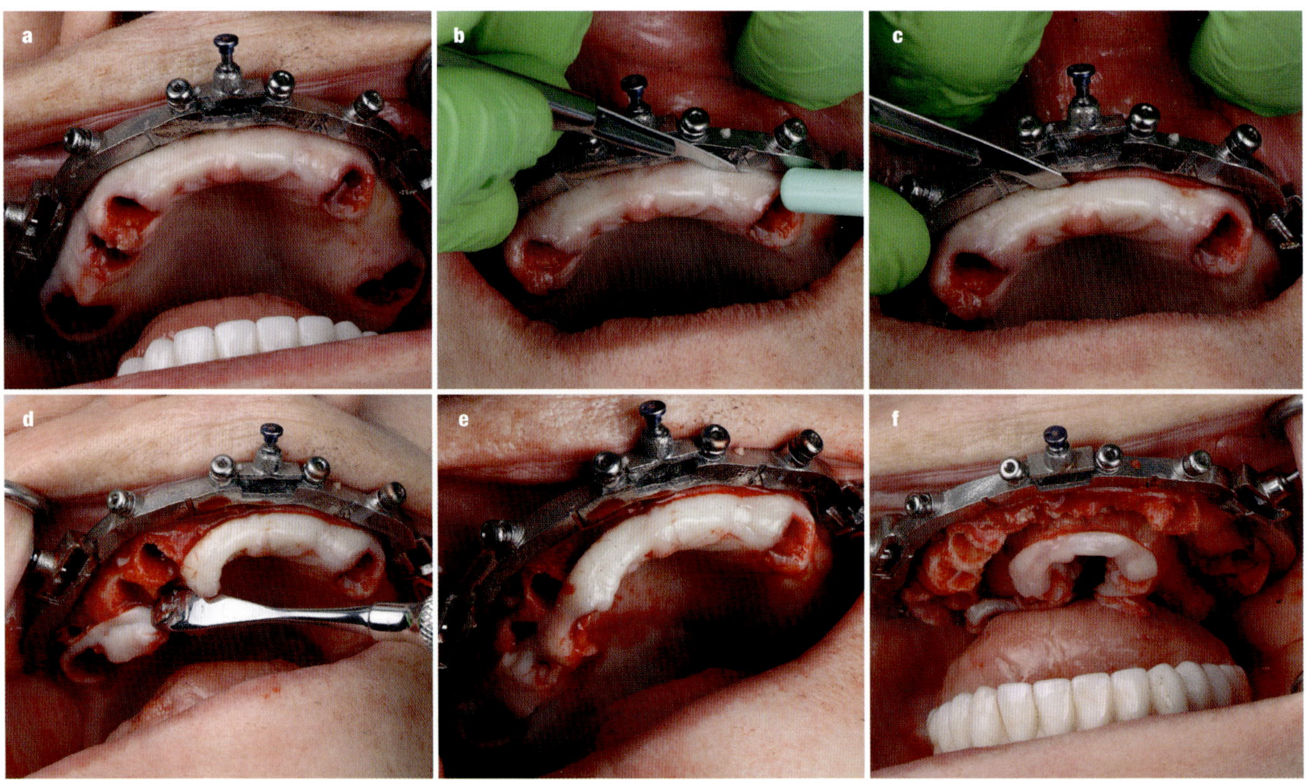

Figure 7.9 (a-f) **Incision and flap elevation after fixation of a floating-style foundation guide in a case with abundant keratinized tissue in the buccal areas of the ridge.**

A. Carefully use a no. 12 curved or no. 15 straight blade (or a combination of the two) to release the interdental papillae around the teeth (if present) and to carry the incision through any edentulous areas (Fig. 7.10). As you do this, try to preserve as much keratinized tissue as possible.

When working in the maxilla in a patient who is fully edentulous or has edentulous areas, place the incision closer to the buccal of the ridge crest, but leave at least 3 mm of keratinized tissue if possible. The reason is that after bone reduction, you may be able to extend the palatal tissue coronally and hitch it over the multiunit abutments (MUAs), using a tissue punch to create circular holes in it. This provides a predictable circumferential band of keratinized tissue around the abutments and allows for initial stability in the flap.

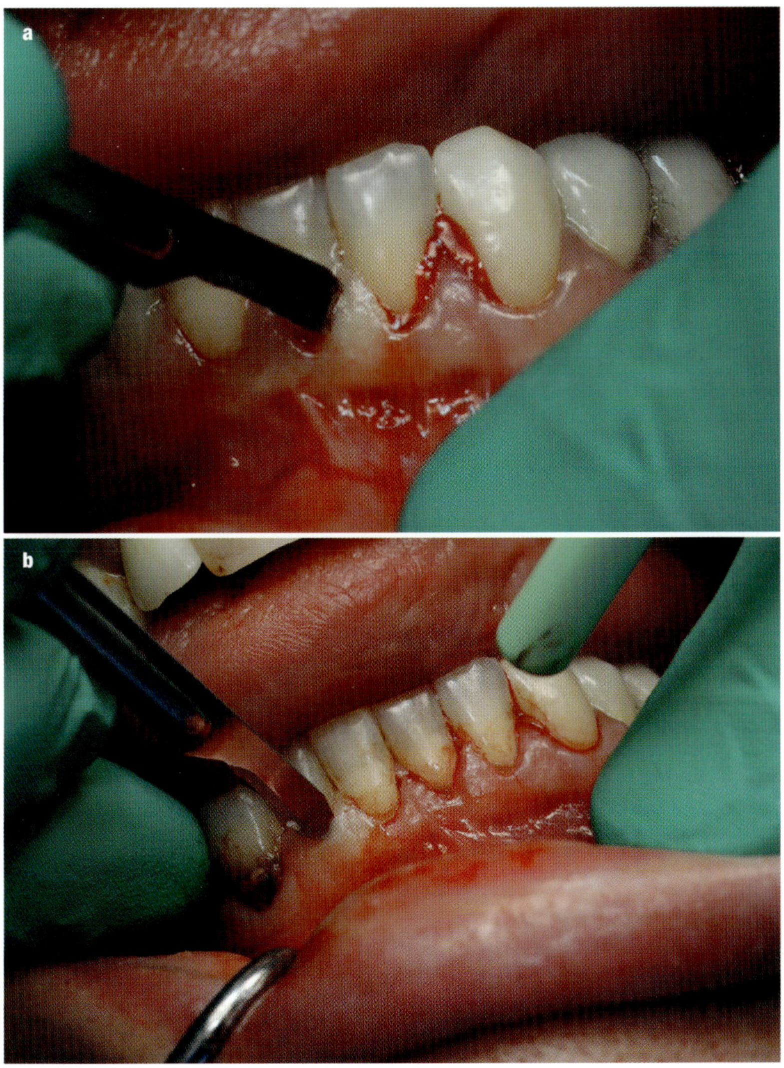

Figure 7.10 (a) Releasing incisions being made around the interdental papillae using a no. 15 straight blade; (b) This technique preserves the keratinized tissue around the necks of the teeth during flap placement.

B. Release the tissue and elevate the flap only on the buccal/facial aspect—not on the lingual/palatal aspect—prior to placing the foundation guide.

You will elevate the flap in those areas after the foundation guide has been placed but before you extract any teeth. By delaying flap elevation on the palatal/lingual aspect, the bleeding and swelling of those tissues is postponed and the indexing may be more stable during placement of the foundation guide.

C. After releasing the tissue, advance a full-thickness buccal flap as far apically as necessary to allow the foundation guide to be placed without impinging on tissue.

Use a Molt no. 9 periosteal elevator and/or a no. 3 Prichard periosteal hollow handle elevator to release the full-thickness flap (Fig. 7.11). Full-thickness flaps optimize visualization and result in less bleeding (Fig. 7.12).

Note: *When elevating and advancing tissue flaps, be aware and identify important anatomical structures such as the mental neurovascular bundles (Fig. 7.13). Also, exercise caution while releasing the tissue on the lingual of the mandible; the lingual flap into the floor of the mouth should be made gently, as the periosteum attached to this area is easily retracted. It is always desirable to start thinking about these issues during the planning stages of your case.*

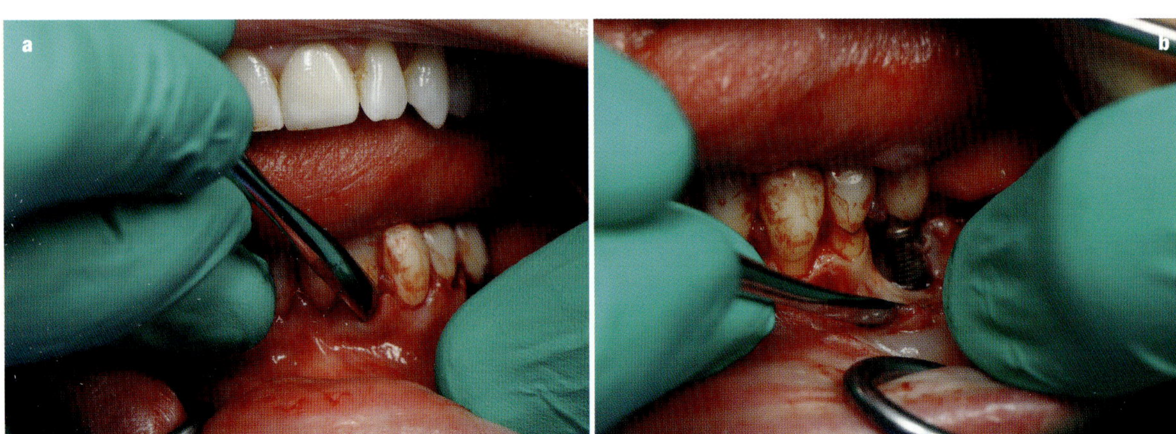

Figure 7.11 (a) Elevation of a full-thickness flap using a no. 3 Prichard periosteal elevator; (b) The same instrument being used to reflect tissue around a failing implant.

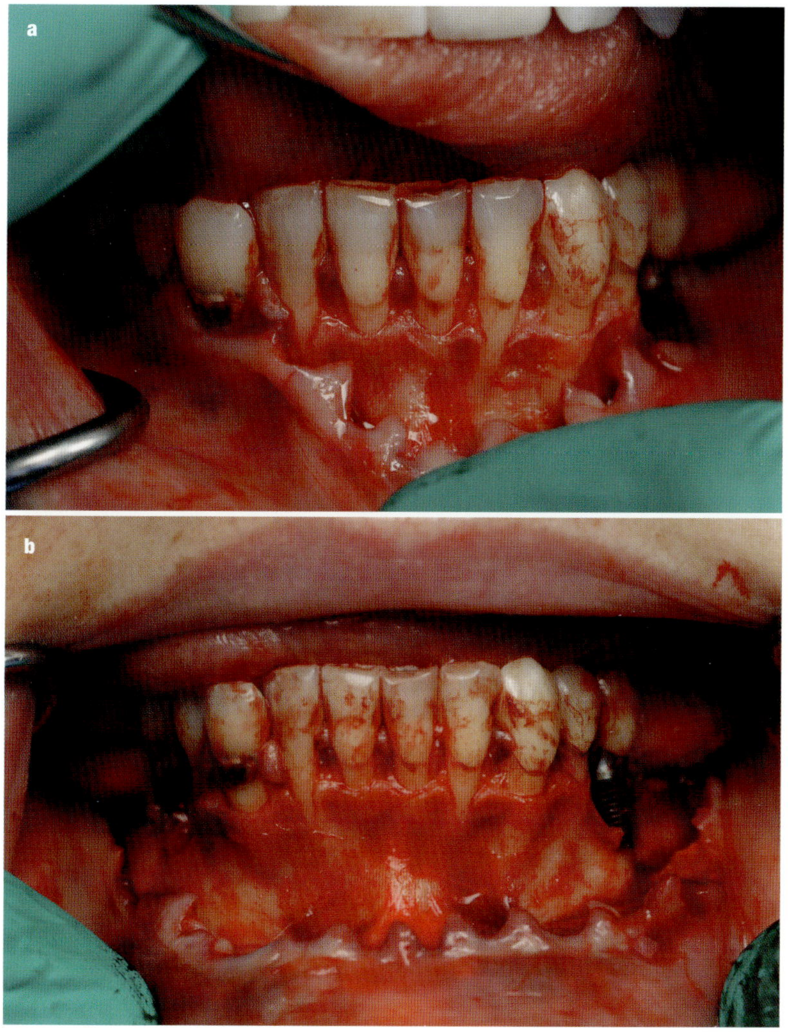

Figure 7.12 (a) Elevation of the full-thickness flap in the anterior mandible; (b) View of anterior mandible following elevation of full-thickness flap in preparation for seating of the foundation guide.

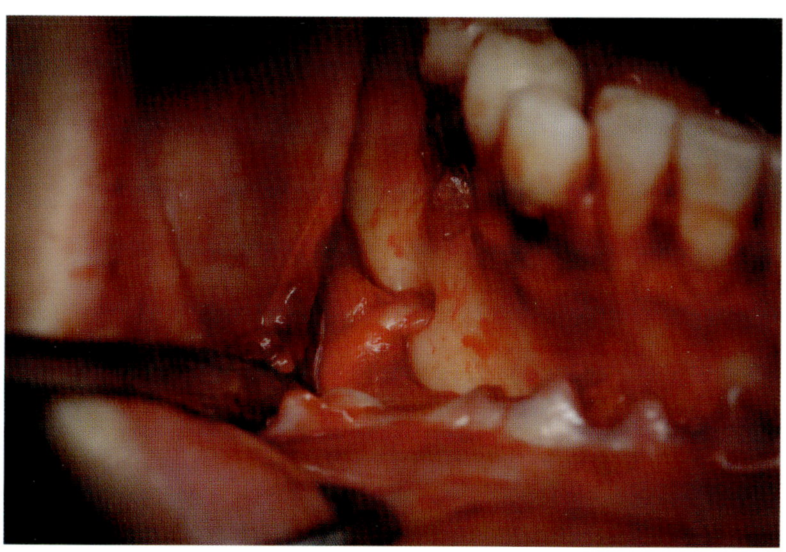

Figure 7.13 View of the mental neurovascular bundle in the right side of the mandible.

STEP 5: FOUNDATION GUIDE PLACEMENT/FIXATION

- **A.** Once the full-thickness flap is released on the buccal/facial aspect and the important anatomical structures are identified, place the indexing aligner with the foundation guide back on the teeth and/or edentulous areas (Fig. 7.14). Re-verify complete seating of the aligner and confirm that the foundation guide is not impinging on bone or any soft tissues.

In some cases, you may be able to fasten the indexing aligner to the foundation guide before seating it, or you may have undercuts that make it necessary to fit each guide separately during positioning. When using a stackable floating-style foundation guide, it should appear that the foundation guide is "floating" just off the bone. When using an anatomical-style (nonfloating) guide, it should fit intimately with the bone. With a hybrid-style foundation guide, it may be partially seated on bone and partially floating. The foundation guide and indexing aligner should be fastened together with some type of attachment system, such as pins or a locking mechanism.

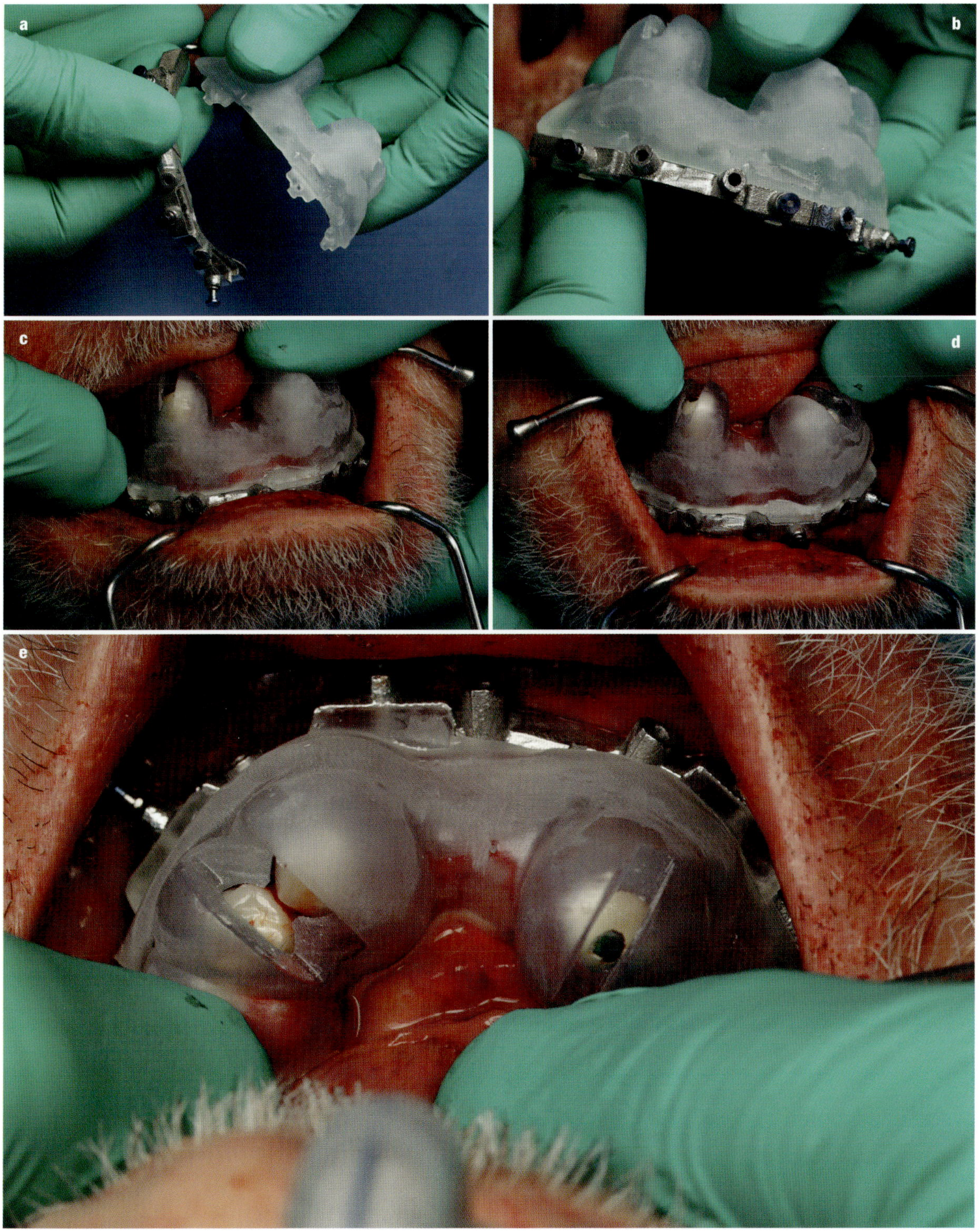

Figure 7.14 (a) Placement of the indexing aligner into a floating-style foundation guide; (b) Indexing aligner seated intimately with the foundation guide and locked in place; (c) Indexing aligner seated with foundation guide over teeth and edentulous ridge areas of mandible; (d) Checking the stability of seated aligner and foundation guide with both hands; (e) Verification of complete seating is accomplished by viewing the teeth through the windows of the indexing aligner.

B. After you have verified proper positioning of the foundation guide, use pins or screws to affix it to the bone (Fig. 7.15).

Some anatomical guides require screws, whereas floating-style guides use pins designed to pass through cylinders in the foundation guide. When placing pins or screws in the foundation guide, make sure the indexing aligner is held securely in place and is always attached and stable. Begin by drilling one pin or screw hole and securing the pin or screw in that hole before moving on, always checking that the indexing aligner remains immobile. If you are using long pins that will perforate not only the buccal/facial cortex, but also the lingual or palatal plate, be watchful of where the pin will end up. In the maxilla, especially, it is wise to drill short. The bone in the maxilla is less dense than in the mandible and may not provide adequate resistance for fixation of the guide. If you drill completely through the facial and palatal plates, you may find that your pins are not adequately stable. After consecutively drilling pin or screw holes and securing the pins or screws, the foundation guide should be securely affixed to the bone.

PRO TIP: Placing the foundation guide, part 1

Prepare the fixation pin holes and place the fixation pins one at a time. If you observe any movement in the indexing aligner or foundation guide during placement, it may be because you have hit a tooth root or other anatomical structure. If this occurs, remove the pin, redrill, and replace the pin.

If you happen to drill into a tooth, do not be overly concerned; continue placing all the other pins in the foundation guide. Once it is secured, remove the pin, extract the tooth and root, and replace the pin in that area.

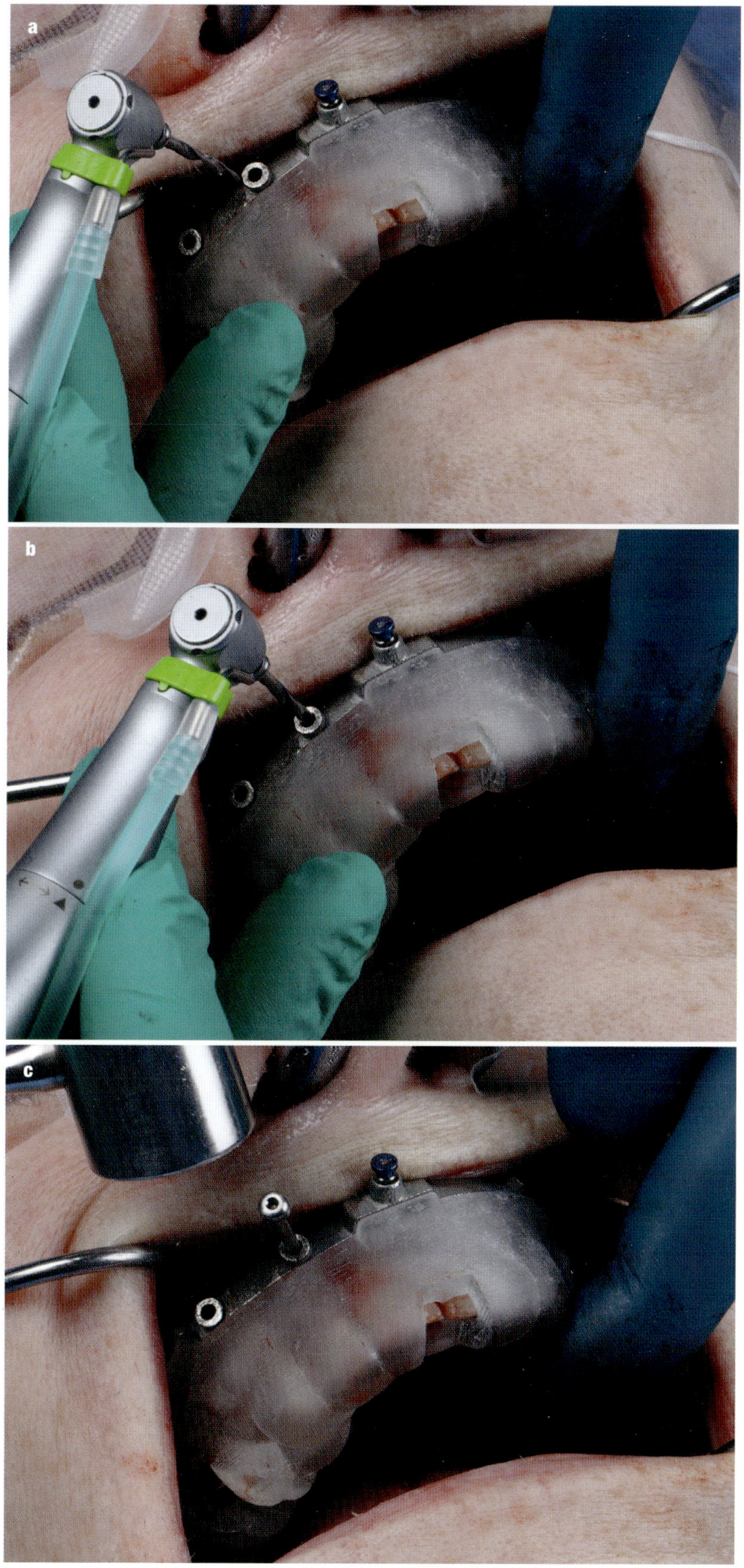

Figure 7.15 Affixing the foundation guide to the bone using the pin or screw channels. (a) Line up the drill with the foundation guide pin channels; (b) Drill into the access channels; (c) Tap a pin into each access channel once drilling is complete.

PRO TIP: Placing the foundation guide, part 2

In the mandible, you might want to avoid drilling the pin holes through the lingual cortex/plate. Instead, you can use shorter pins, tapping them in gently for final placement. This avoids critical anatomy that exists in the sublingual space. To tap in the fixation pins, it can be helpful to use a mirror handle with the mirror part unscrewed. This will prevent you from missing the pin and damaging the patient's lip. It also allows for easier access to the pin for complete seating (Fig. 7.16).

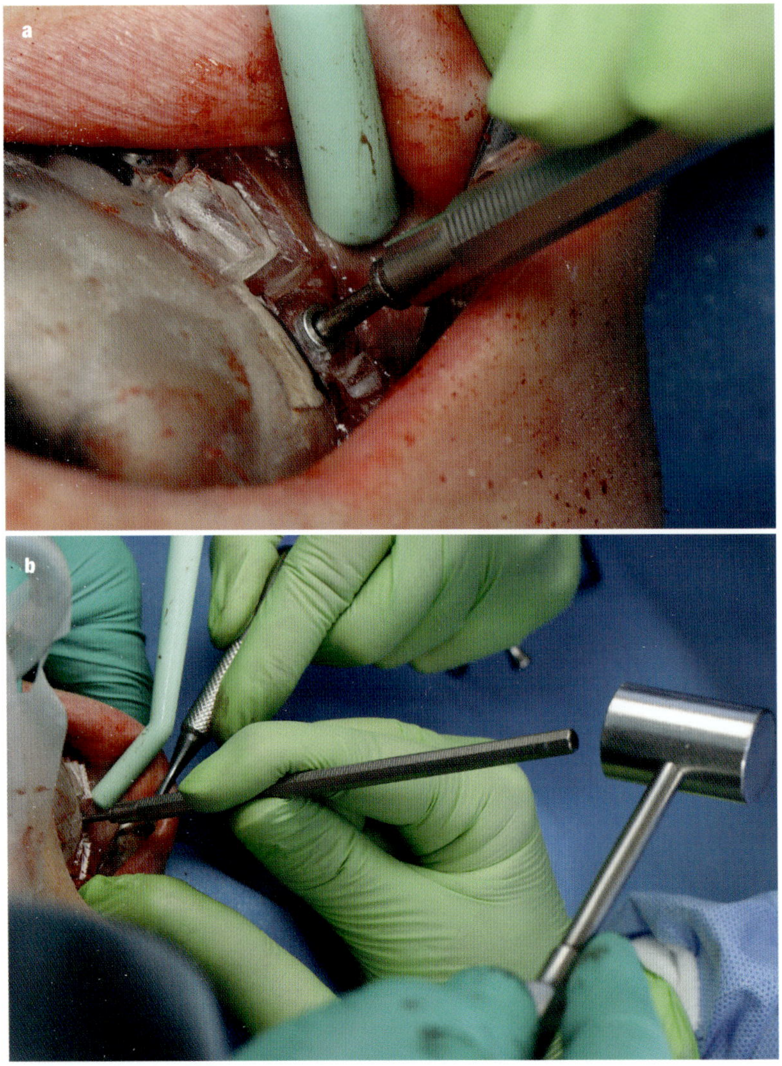

Figure 7.16 Securing the foundation guide in the mandible. (a) Partial pre-drilling, which risks damaging critical anatomy in the sublingual space. Mirror handle used to avoid damage to lips and cheek; (b) Use a mallet to tap the foundation guide pins in place.

C. Gently remove the indexing aligner from the foundation guide and very carefully check for any movement in the foundation guide.

If your foundation guide is made of a flexible resin, use extreme caution when handling or checking it. You want to make sure you will be able to place the other guides and components on the foundation guide without disturbing its position. Foundation guides fabricated from cobalt-chrome, titanium, or carbon-fiber–reinforced materials are stronger and more rigid and therefore less likely to crack if flexing occurs (Fig. 7.17).

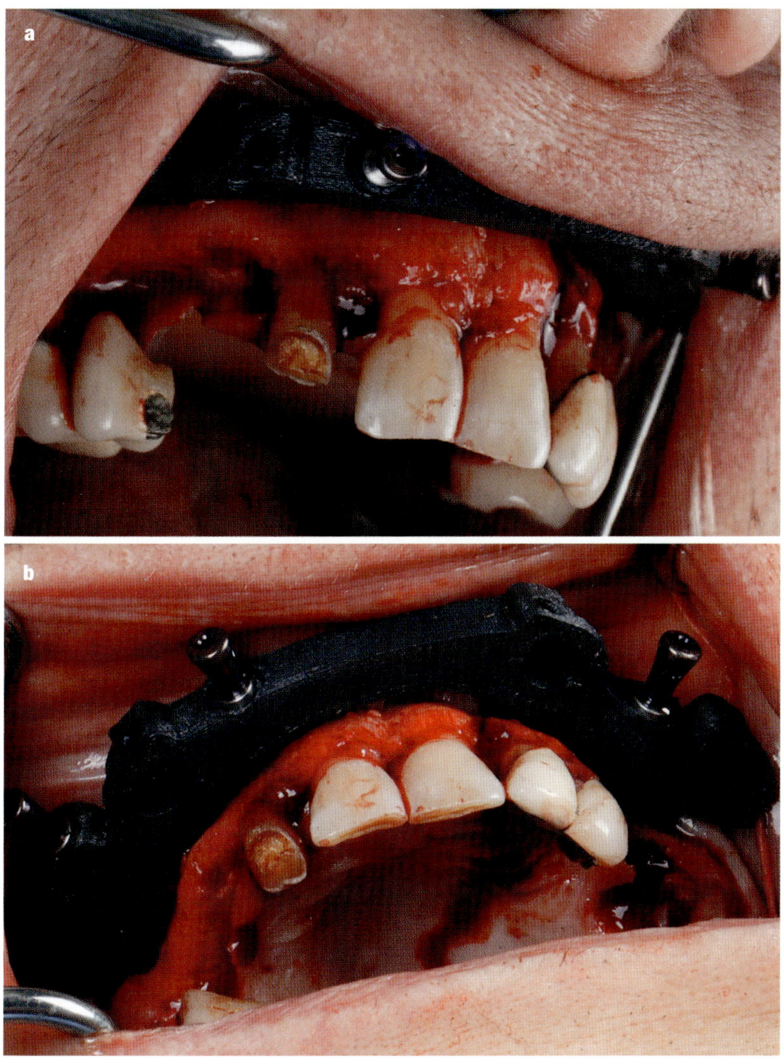

Figure 7.17 (a, b) Removal of indexing aligner from carbon-reinforced foundation guide.

STEP 6: TEETH EXTRACTION (DENTATE PATIENTS)

When your foundation guide is stable, it is time to start extracting the teeth. If your patient is fully edentulous, you may have already placed your foundation guide and elevated your flaps. If there are no teeth to extract, skip to **Step 7**: Bone Reduction.

A. Resume elevating the full-thickness flap, this time working on the lingual/palatal surface.

The palatal flaps are the most challenging and require more effort than the others. Be careful to release the flap just enough to provide adequate visualization and bone reduction. I find it helpful to place a silk suture through the palatal tissue and tie it together, as it allows me to see the maxilla more clearly. This can also be helpful when the subsequent guides are being placed on the foundation guide, to avoid impinging on the tissues (Fig. 7.18).

The lingual tissue of the mandible is easily elevated; often, once the keratinized tissue is retracted, the mucosa and periosteum will pull away with very little effort. When releasing tissue on the lingual, remember to exercise caution so as to avoid the anatomical structures in the floor of the mouth. This area is highly vascularized, and bleeding can be profuse if arteries or veins are pierced.

B. Begin elevating the teeth from their sockets.

You will want to remove the teeth as atraumatically as possible. The key is to avoid inadvertently fracturing bone, even if you have a significant amount of bone reduction planned. The two techniques I employ to remove teeth with the least amount of stress to the surrounding bone are as follows:

1. Use a periotome to release the alveolar crest subgroup of periodontal fibers around the neck and coronal portions of the teeth. This takes some patience, especially if the patient is mostly dentate, but it is worth the effort if you successfully remove the teeth without fracturing off a vital portion of the bone plate. Gently elevate the roots of the teeth with an elevator to loosen them so they can be extracted atraumatically (Fig. 7.19).
2. Using a surgical cutting bur, "score" the bone by carefully drilling through the buccal cortex to the tooth roots just superior to the foundation guide. You can drill deeper interproximally, but avoid going through the lingual (or palatal) plate. I prefer to use the Komet H219 or 219A bur for this purpose (Fig. 7.20).

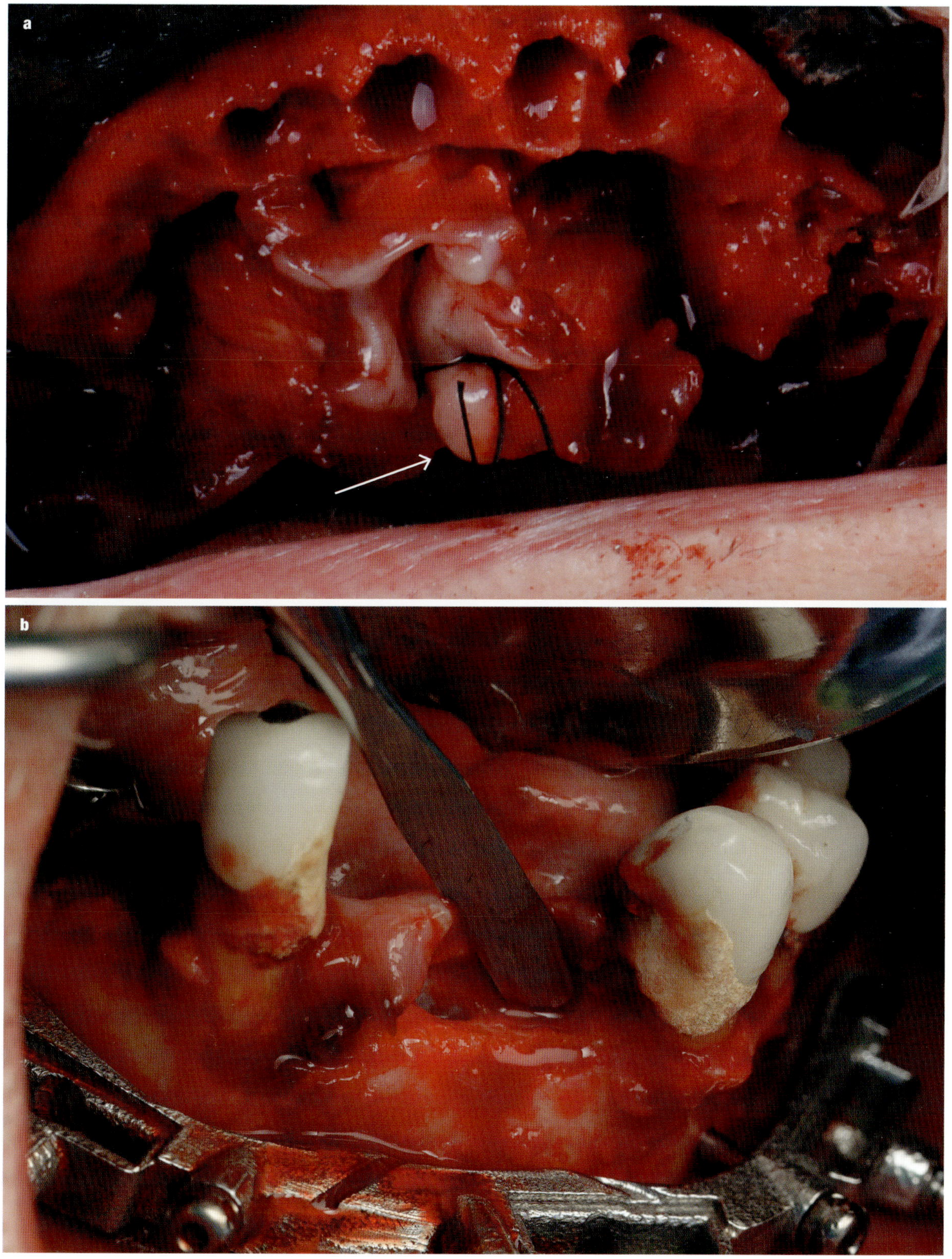

Figure 7.18 (a) Placement of a silk suture (*arrow*) to stabilize the palatal flap for better visibility; (b) Release of the lingual flap after placement of the foundation guide.

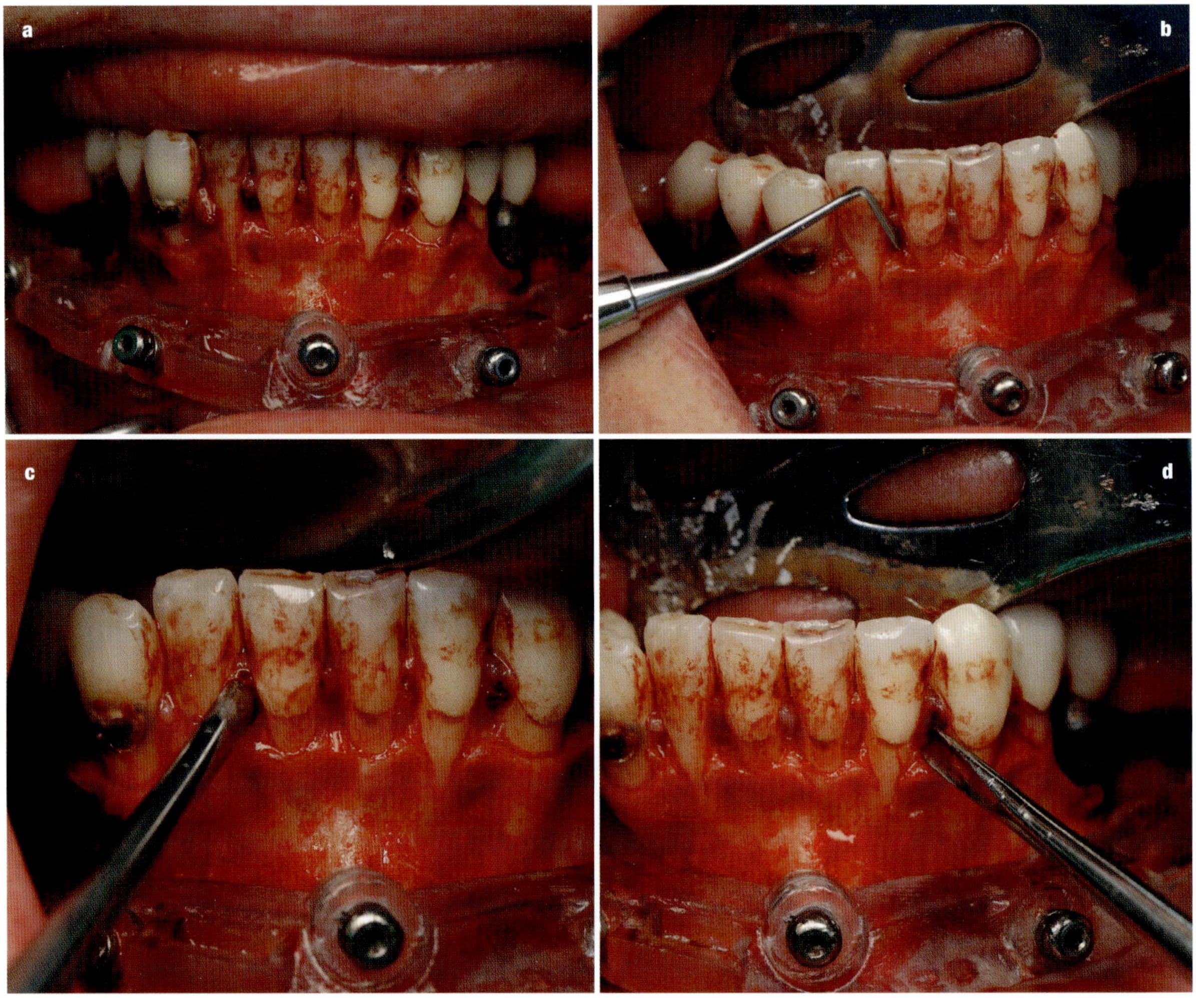

Figure 7.19 (a) Appearance of anterior mandible after completion of flap elevation and bone exposure; (b) Use of a periotome to release the periodontal ligaments around the teeth; (c, d) Use of a surgical elevator to loosen the teeth.

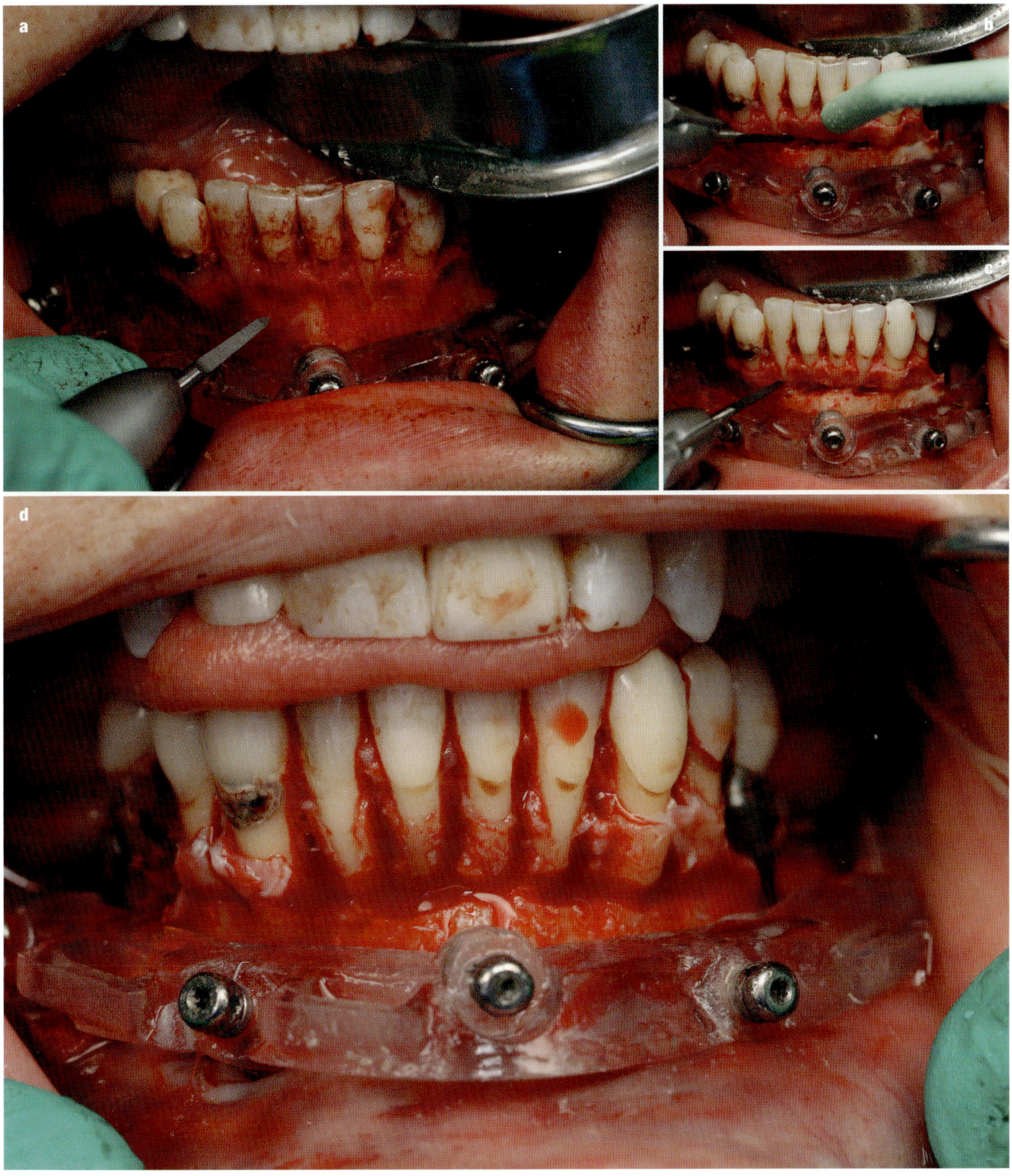

Figure 7.20 (a-c) Scoring the mandibular bone interproximally to release tension prior to tooth extraction. Exercise caution to avoid penetrating the lingual plate; (d) Exposure of the roots of the mandibular teeth after bone scoring along a resin foundation guide.

C. Once you have released an appropriate amount of tension around the teeth, begin extracting them (Fig. 7.21).

I generally start with the anterior teeth because it allows for better visualization, and it is easier to remove the posterior teeth once the anterior teeth are out of the way. Consider using forceps for extraction that you are comfortable with. Sometimes you may find that it makes more sense to section the teeth in the molar regions. If you are comfortable doing so, section the molars and carefully remove the roots. In the maxilla, it is helpful to know where the sinus floor is in relation to these teeth and best to avoid perforation of the sinus. If a perforation does occur, you will need to repair it.

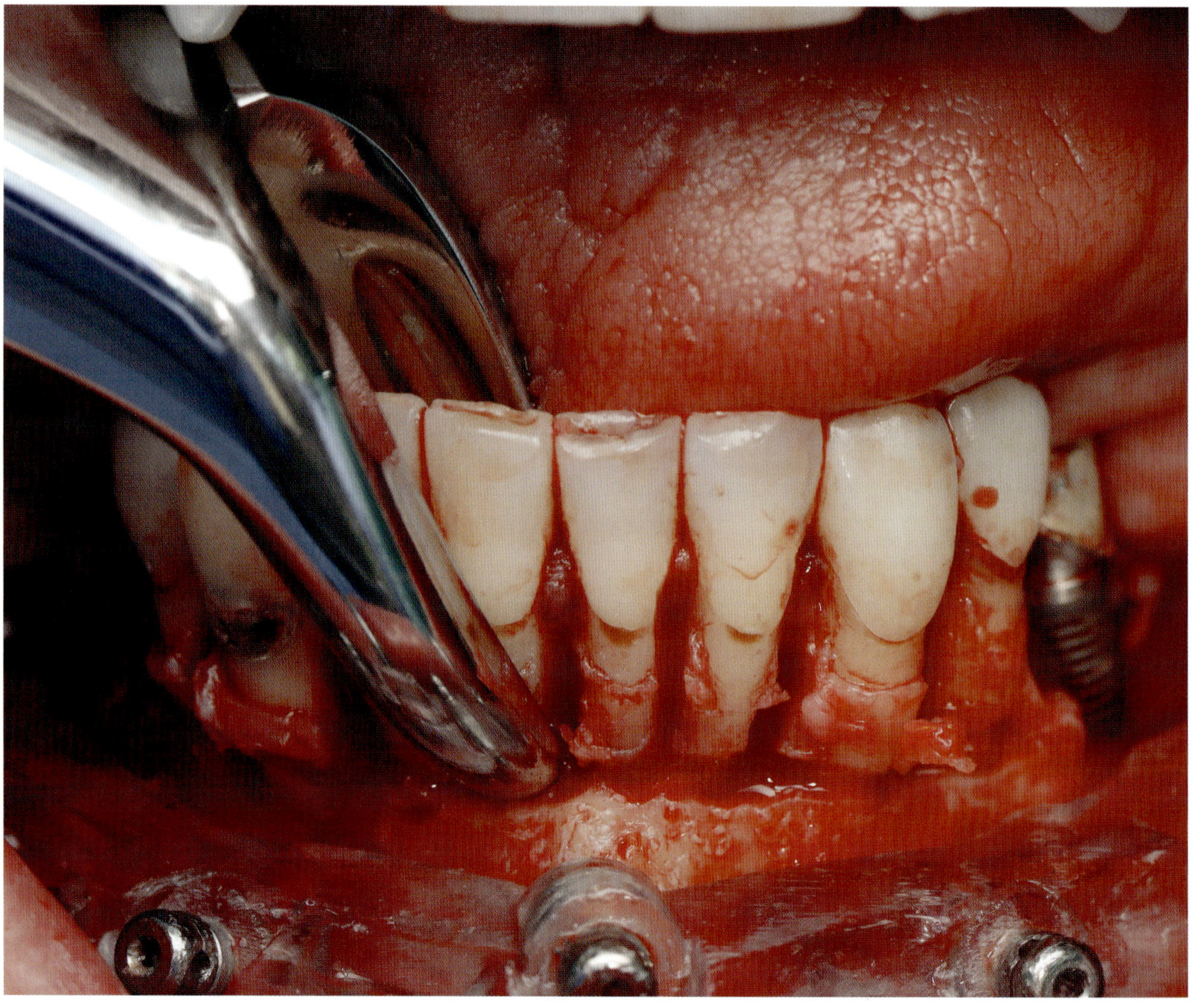

Figure 7.21 **Use of a no. 151 universal forceps to extract the anterior teeth in the mandible.**

D. After extracting the teeth, remember to meticulously curette and debride the sockets to remove any periapical cysts or infection that may be present.

Periapically abscessed teeth are common in terminal dentitions, and identifying these areas on the CBCT prior to the surgery is helpful. We document these areas in the surgical planning phase. If you prefer, you may wait until the next stage and remove these cysts, granulation tissue, and infections after bone reduction has been completed. You do not want to forget, however, because this could compromise healing and the osseointegration of the implants (Figs. 7.22, 7.23).

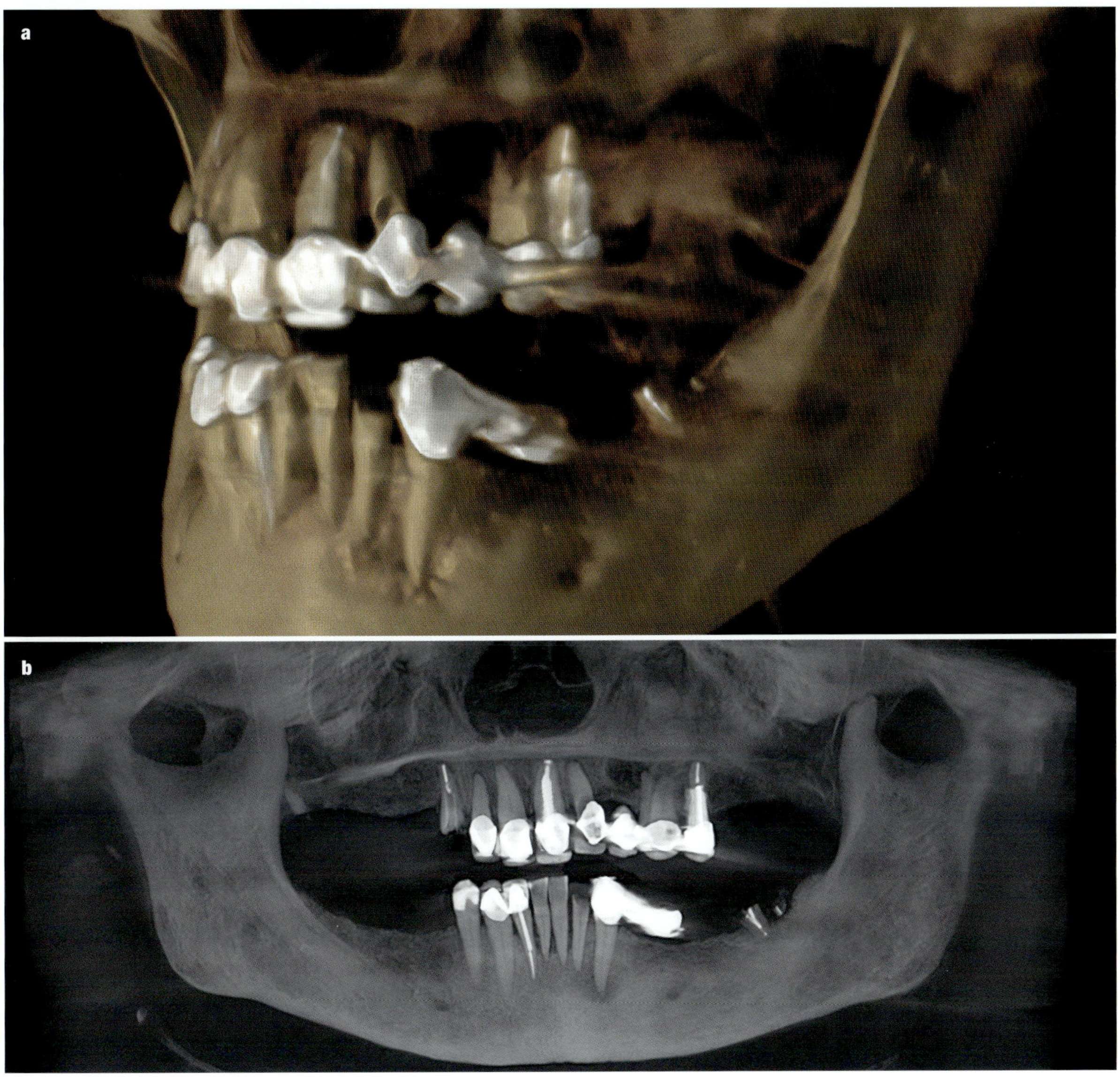

Figure 7.22 CBCT images of suspicious periapical lesions. (a) 3D view; (b) Panoramic view.

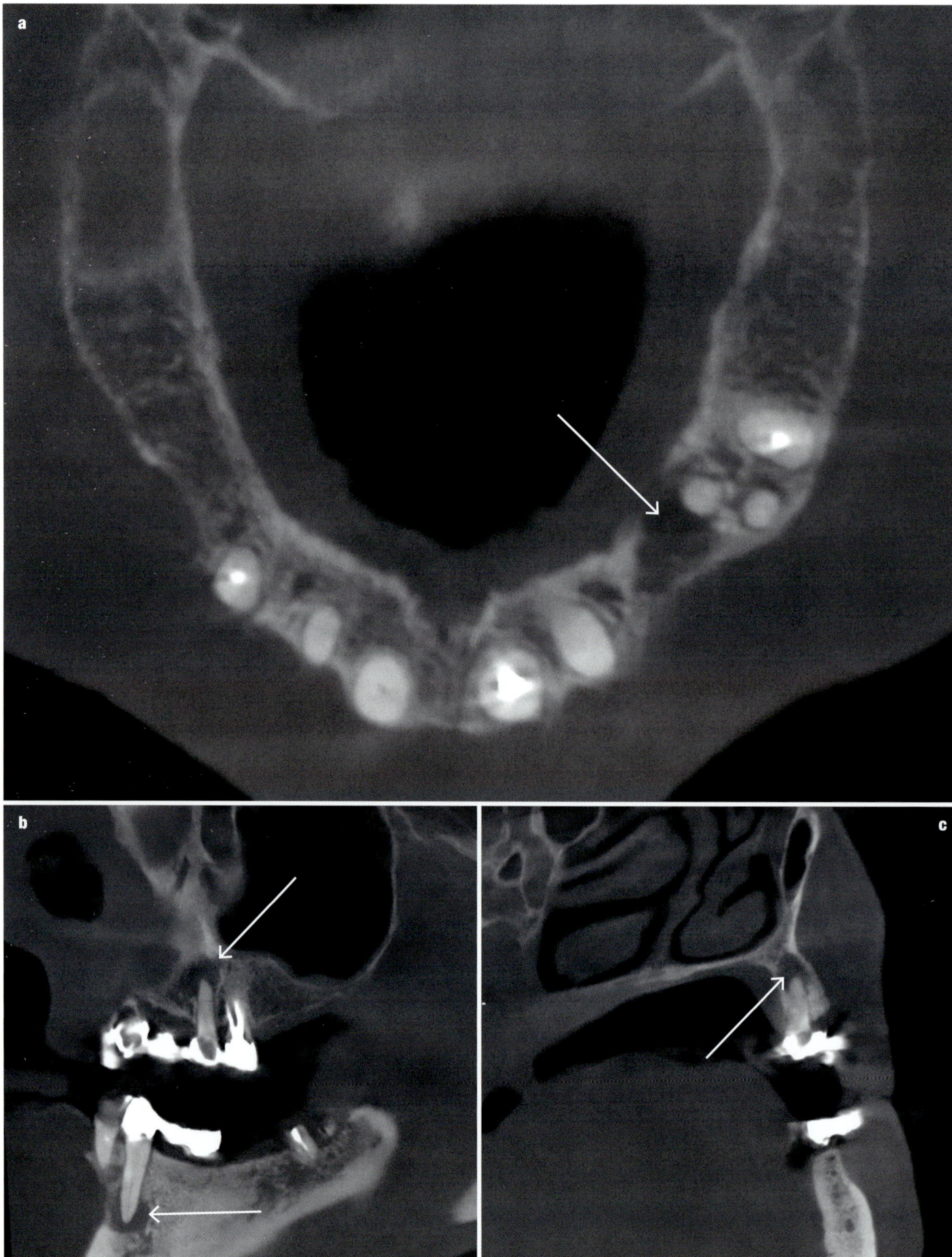

Figure 7.23 CBCT images with *arrows* indicating the locations of periapical lesions. (a) Axial view; (b) Sagittal view; (c) Coronal view.

STEP 7: BONE REDUCTION

Bone reduction is a critical step in the surgical process. Too much reduction can prevent the implants from being guided into crestal or subcrestal positions. To compensate, the implants would have to be placed more apical in the bone, which in turn would change the position of the angled implants in the interim prosthesis. In this scenario, there is also a significant risk of one implant hitting the apex of an adjacent implant or impinging on vital nerve tissue. The alternative, which is not ideal, is to leave the implants supracrestal and perform grafting procedures to cover the exposed threads before closing and suturing.

Conversely, if insufficient bone reduction is carried out, the rest of the stackable guides will not fit appropriately on the foundation guide. Insufficient bone reduction is the most common mistake I see clinicians make during this part of the procedure, probably because it can be just plain scary and general dentists are taught early on that bone is precious and should be reduced as little as possible. This mindset is desirable and necessary during the planning stages of a case but can be problematic if the reduction is not carried out according to the surgical plan.

Bone reduction can be accomplished using various cutting tools, including bone saws, lasers, piezosurgery units, burs, and so forth. In my experience, the straight handpiece with a few select surgical burs accomplishes the job efficiently and affordably. Many clinicians already have a straight surgical handpiece in their armamentarium, so that is the method I prefer to teach and perform myself. Figure 7.24 shows the surgical bur kit alongside the conversion bur kit I use. I developed these kits for Komet USA with assistance from two experienced oral surgeons and Thomas Kuun, MDT. They were designed for simplicity with the minimum number of burs needed to complete procedures.

A. Using a straight surgical handpiece at 800 to 1,200 rpm, begin reducing bone in the anterior regions. Start from a buccal (or facial) approach, placing the bur a few millimeters superior to the foundation guide and perforating through the cortex if necessary.

The surgical assistant should be retracting any soft tissues on the palatal or lingual aspect, especially the tongue. Pay close attention to structures that could be in the path of reduction (Fig. 7.25).

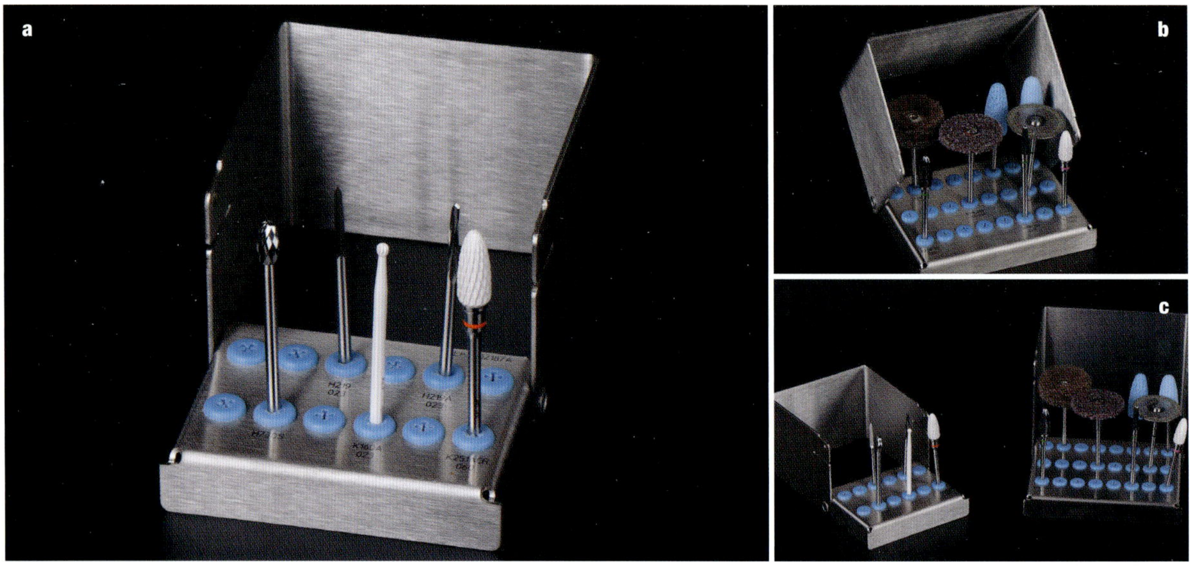

Figure 7.24 (a-c) **Komet surgery and prosthetic kits for fixed full-arch dental surgery.**

PRO TIP: Bone reduction, part 1

During bone reduction, you might inadvertently hit one of the many small blood vessels that run throughout the maxilla and mandible. The first time this happens, do not panic; there are several ways to stop this miniature geyser. First, use a gauze pad and place pressure over the area, and remove it slowly to locate the source of the bleeding. Then, consider one of the following:

- Use a round bur in a straight handpiece and slowly run it in reverse, without irrigation, in the area where the vessel is located. The Komet K160A bur works well for this, or you can use a Thermacut bur (Dentsply Sirona) if you prefer.
- If you have one, use a bipolar or diode laser to cauterize the vessel.
- Use your hemostat to grasp or pinch the vessel; this will often crush it and slow the bleeding.
- Have your assistant hold the vessel with your hemostat and throw a stitch around it to tie it off. You may also use this technique if you run into an arteriole hidden in the soft tissues.

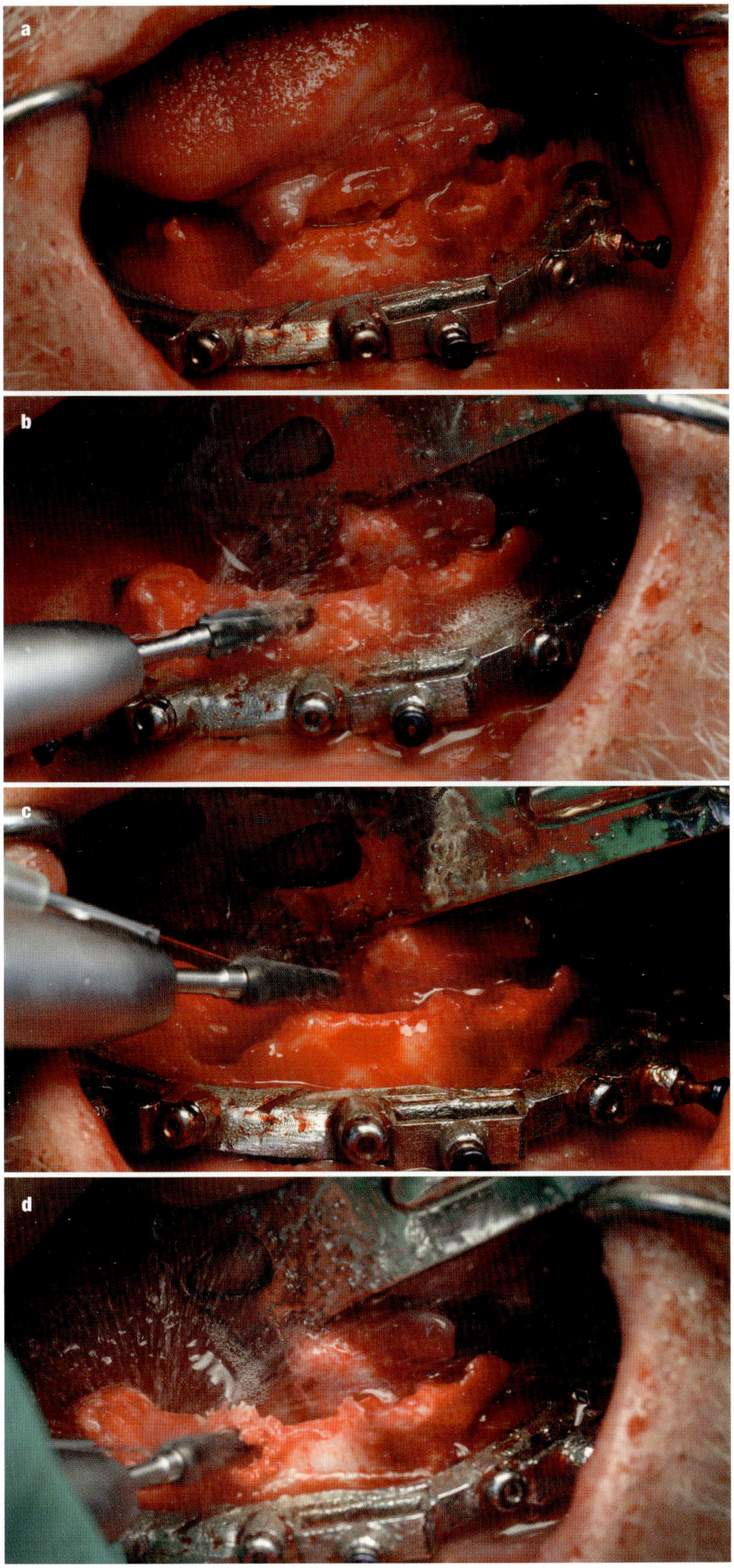

Figure 7.25 Mandibular bone reduction. (a) Appearance of the mandibular ridge with a cobalt-chrome foundation guide prior to bone reduction; (b) Irrigated bur in a straight handpiece preparing for bone reduction; (c) Initial bone reduction in the anterior of the edentulous ridge; (d) Irrigation and careful retraction of the tongue during bone reduction.

B. Move the bur with a horizontal cutting motion, keeping it as parallel to the foundation guide as possible, and avoid binding the bur in the bone.

You may have to make several cuts horizontally to complete this process, which should only take a few minutes. Be sure to move at a speed that allows your surgical assistant to keep up with you and remember to use adequate irrigation through the handpiece or saline streaming into the reduction area from a large-barrel syringe. Irrigation is vital for preventing bone necrosis.

C. Once you have achieved most of the gross bone reduction, you can begin to smooth out the remaining bone.

Continue to irrigate and visually inspect the areas to avoid overreduction. Smoothing the bone will generally eliminate any periosteum that might be present and provide an even platform for the implants (Fig. 7.26).

PRO TIP: Bone reduction, part 2

During bone reduction in the maxilla, pay careful attention if your plan involves the area near the maxillary sinuses. Avoid perforating the sinus membrane with your burs, but if you do perforate it, you will have to repair it.

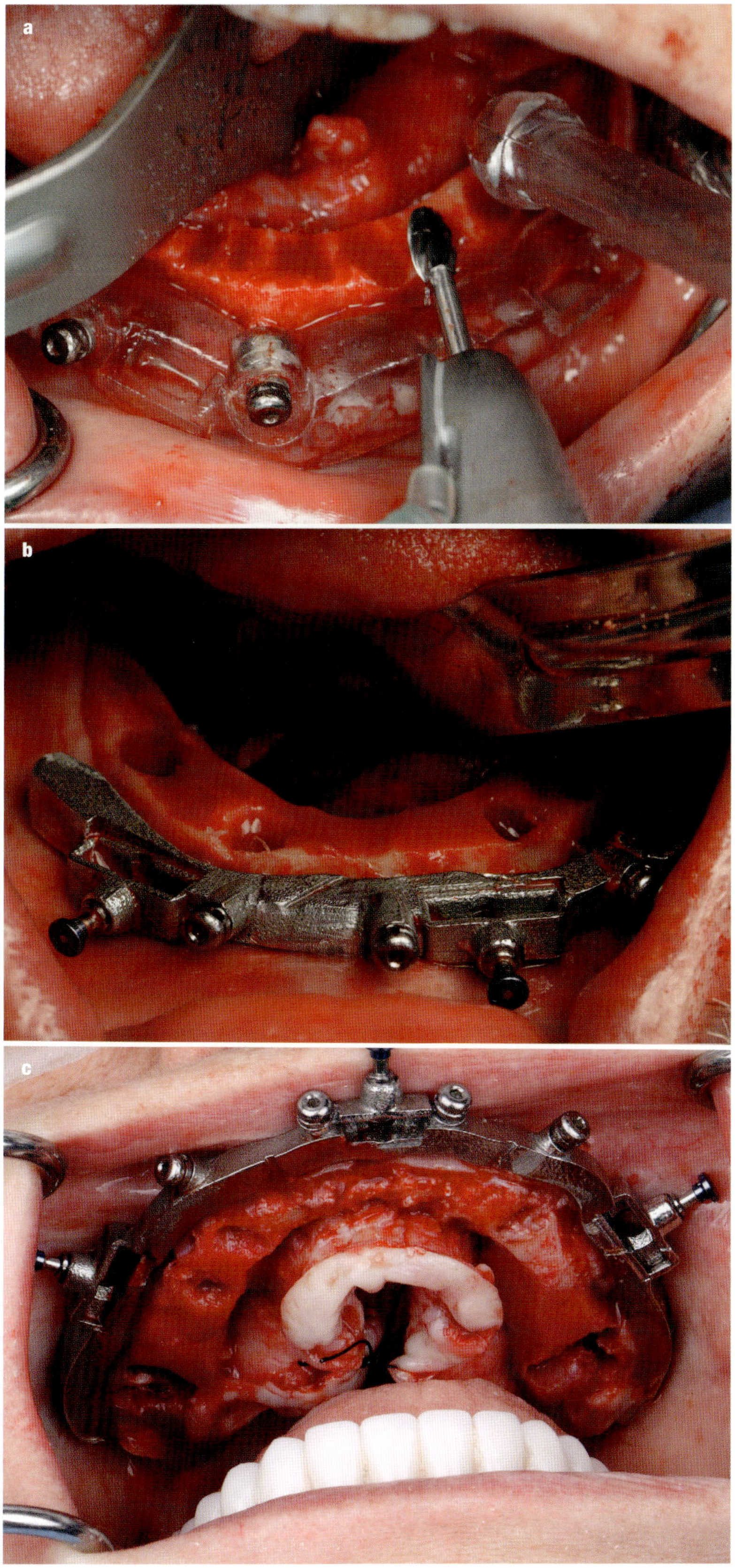

Figure 7.26 Appearance of smoothed and leveled ridges after bone reduction. (a) Reduction and smoothing of anterior mandible around resin foundation guide; (b) Finished and smoothed mandible after bone reduction; (c) Finished and smoothed maxilla after bone reduction.

- **D.** When you think you have achieved the appropriate amount of bone reduction, place the carrier guide or abutment aligner on the foundation guide and determine whether the amount that was planned has been completed.

These guides should fit passively and completely. You should see no gaps or space between the carrier guide or abutment aligner and the foundation guide (Figs. 7.27, 7.28).

- **E.** If the arch you are treating will be occluding with the existing dentition in the opposing arch, check the occlusion of the interim prosthesis by placing it on the carrier guide or into the foundation guide (Fig. 7.29).

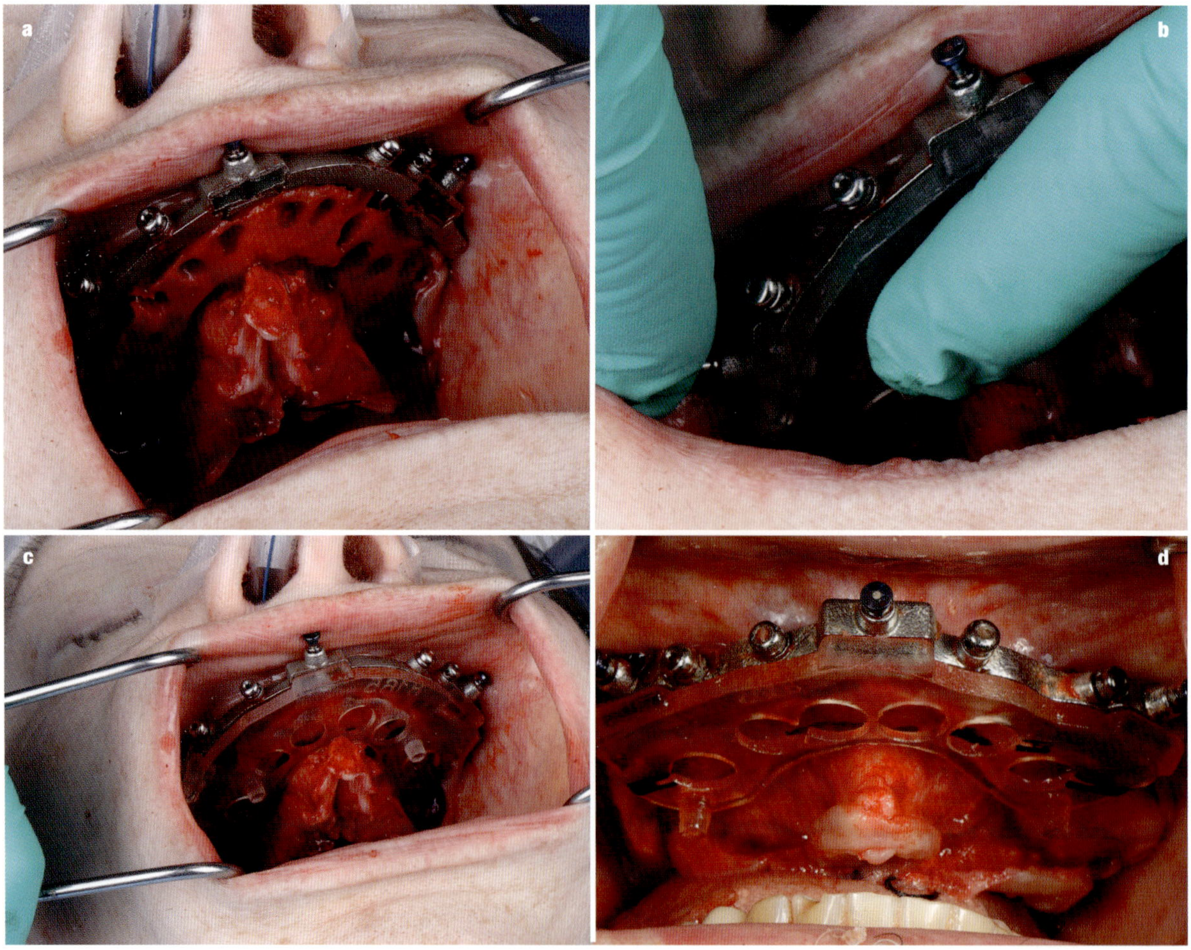

Figure 7.27 Placement of carrier guide on foundation guide after the initial bone reduction. (a) Appearance of smooth and level maxillary bone with foundation guide still in place; (b) Positioning of carrier guide on foundation guide; (c) Carrier guide in place and affixed to foundation guide; (d) Close-up view of the carrier guide on the foundation guide. Note the intimate fit and lack of space between the two guides.

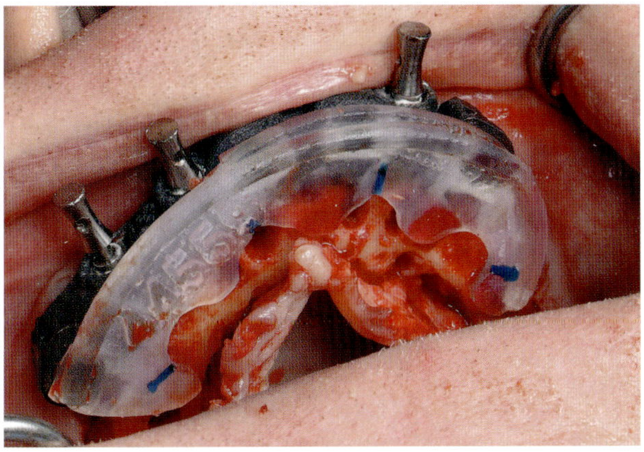

Figure 7.28 Placement of an abutment aligner on a carbon-fiber–reinforced foundation guide after bone reduction.

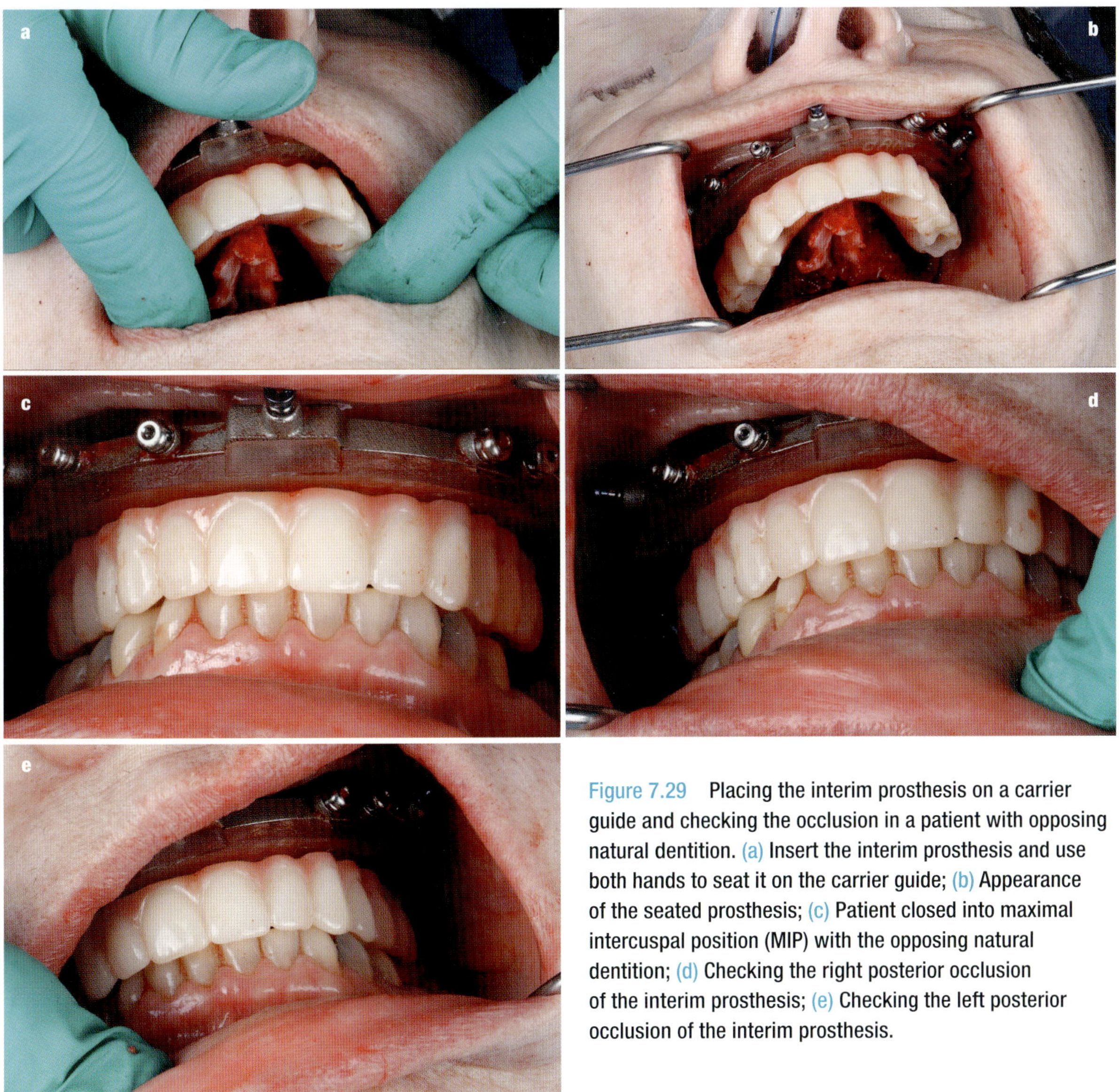

Figure 7.29 Placing the interim prosthesis on a carrier guide and checking the occlusion in a patient with opposing natural dentition. (a) Insert the interim prosthesis and use both hands to seat it on the carrier guide; (b) Appearance of the seated prosthesis; (c) Patient closed into maximal intercuspal position (MIP) with the opposing natural dentition; (d) Checking the right posterior occlusion of the interim prosthesis; (e) Checking the left posterior occlusion of the interim prosthesis.

If the occlusion looks good, proceed to **Step 8**.

If the occlusion is not as precise as you would like and you are certain the carrier guide and interim prosthesis are seated completely and accurately, consider where you will need to make adjustments in the interim prosthesis and/or opposing arch. Also consider the possibility that your foundation guide was placed incorrectly, which could result in your implants being placed in the wrong locations. Remove the prosthesis and/or carrier guide from the foundation guide and proceed with the next step (Fig. 7.30).

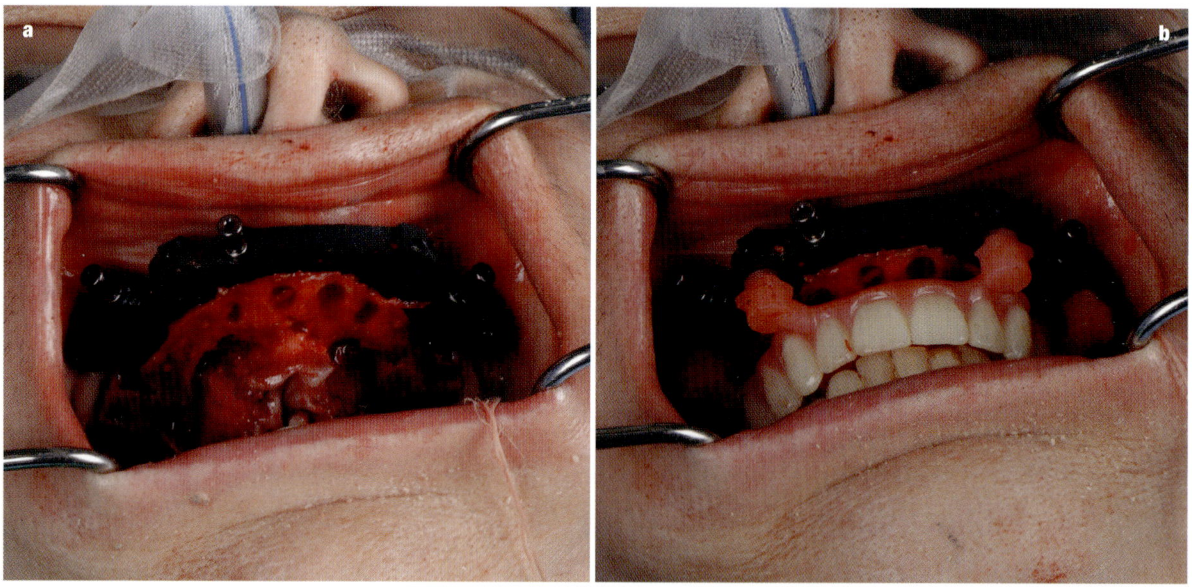

Figure 7.30 (a, b) **Placement of an interim prosthesis on a foundation guide designed for an abutment aligner.**

PRO TIP: Bone reduction, part 3

During surgery in the maxilla, you may have to navigate around the incisive canal and neurovascular bundle. Currently, there is no consensus about the importance of this anatomical structure[2]. Many clinicians have achieved satisfactory surgical results whether they excise it or work around it. I have used the incisive canal as an osteotomy site for a bail-out implant and had good success (Figs. 7.31-7.33).

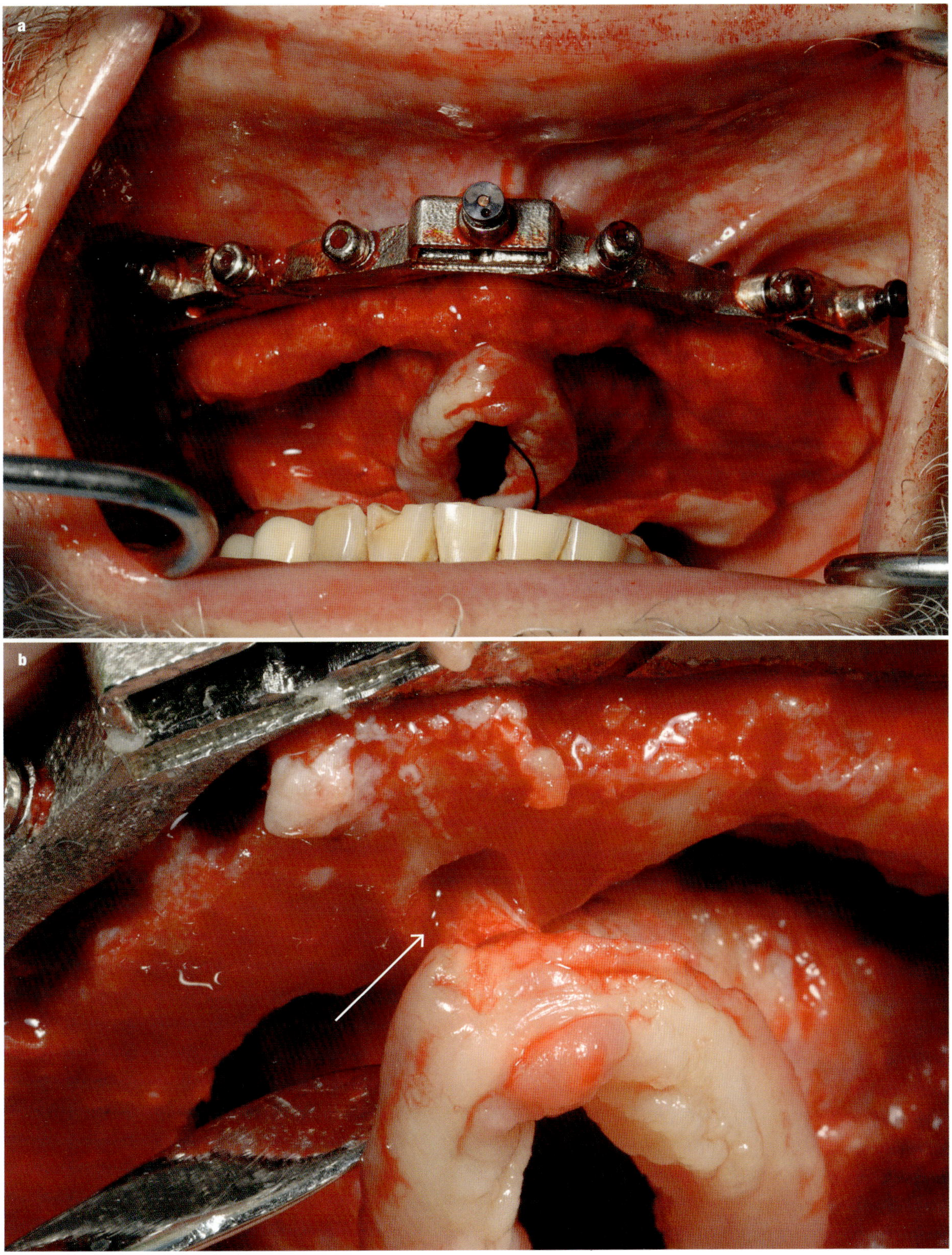

Figure 7.31 (a) Appearance of edentulous maxilla prior to bone reduction; (b) After bone reduction. Note the incisive canal and neurovascular bundle (*arrow*).

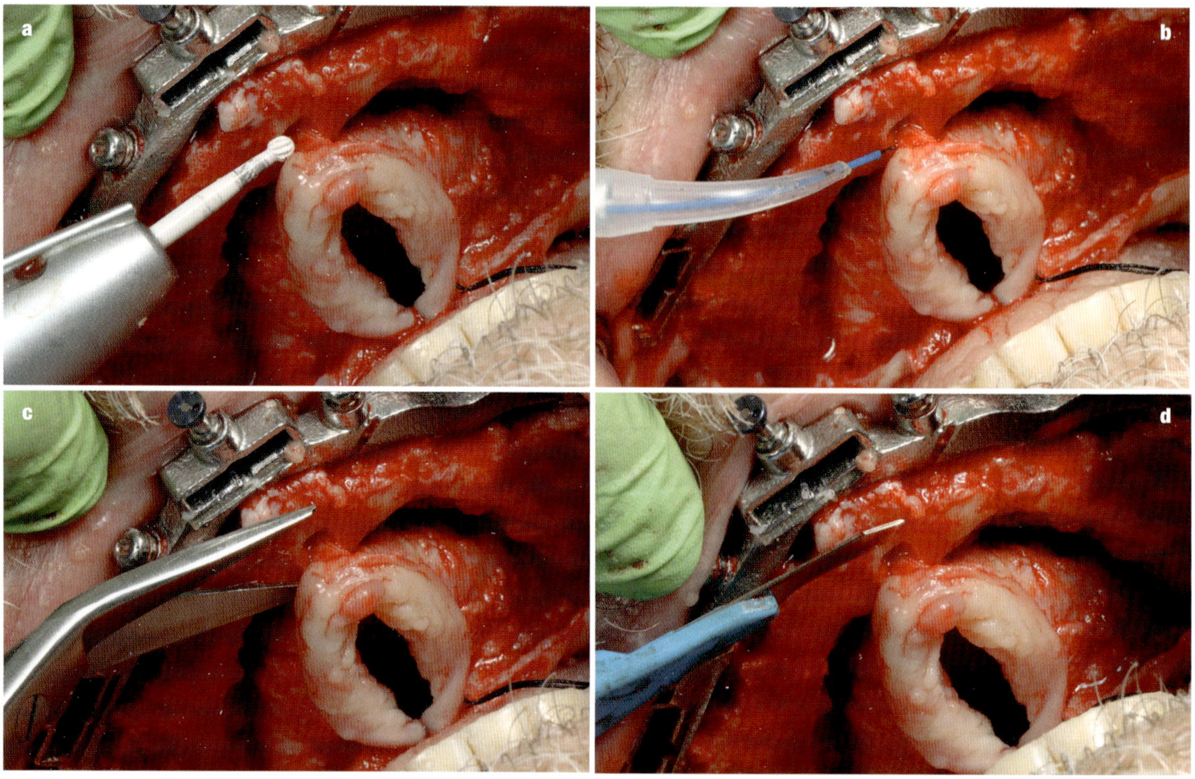

Figure 7.32 Instrumentation for removing or detaching the incisive neurovascular bundle: (a) Bur; (b) Laser; (c) Scissors; (d) Scalpel.

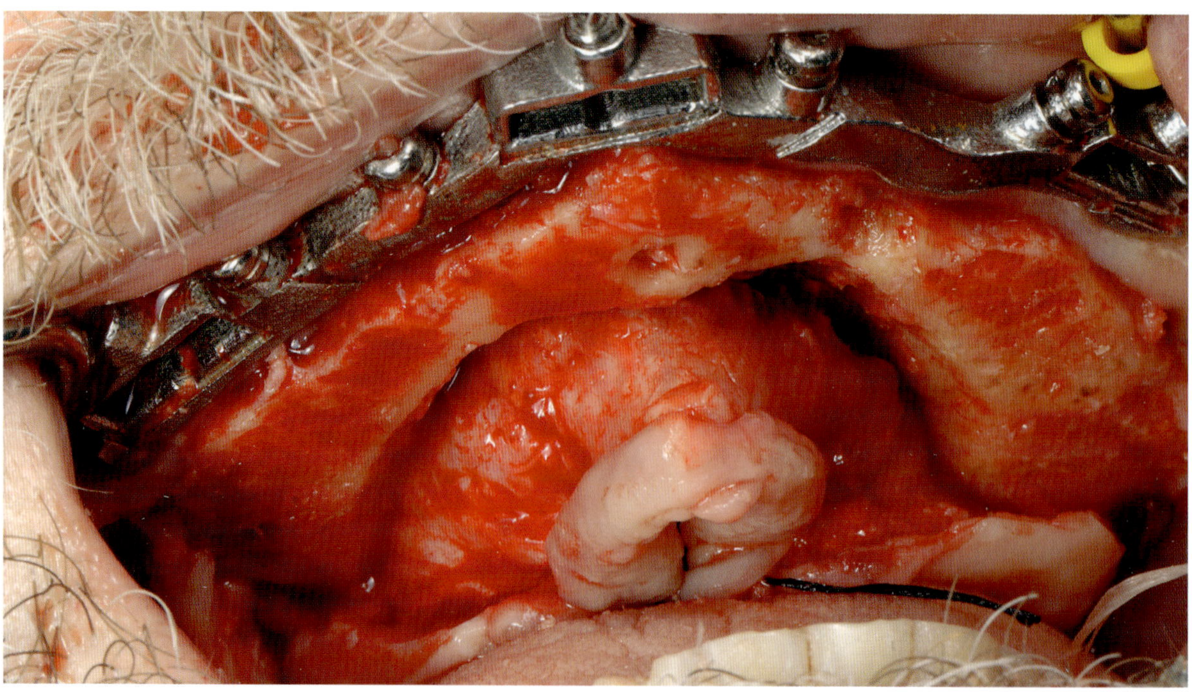

Figure 7.33 Appearance of maxilla after bone reduction and removal of incisive canal neurovascular bundle.

STEP 8: OSTEOTOMY GUIDE AND IMPLANT PLACEMENT

Before you begin to make your osteotomies and place your implants, make sure you have removed any granulation tissue, periapical cysts, or periosteum from the bone where your implants will be placed. As mentioned previously, extraction sites and bone surfaces that have not been debrided and disinfected can be detrimental to the osseointegration of the implants (Fig. 7.34a).

A. Place your osteotomy guide into the foundation guide and make sure it has a passive fit and that the osteotomy guide is fully seated. Then use pins, locks, or another mechanism to stabilize it in the foundation guide.

I prefer a guide that provides strength and allows for adequate vision of the drills and implants and good irrigation in and on the bone (Figs. 7.34b, 7.35, 7.36).

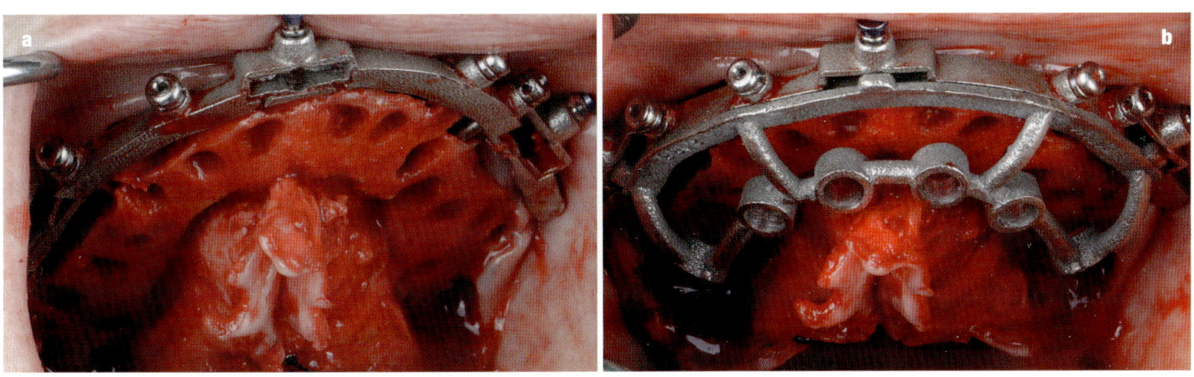

Figure 7.34 (a) Appearance of maxilla after completion of bone reduction and removal of granulation tissue in preparation for placement of the osteotomy guide; (b) Cobalt-chrome osteotomy guide locked into the foundation guide.

PRO TIP: Osteotomy guide, part 1

If the osteotomy guide does not seat completely or the pins or locks cannot be inserted, check the pinholes and the locking chamber for debris that might be obstructing them.

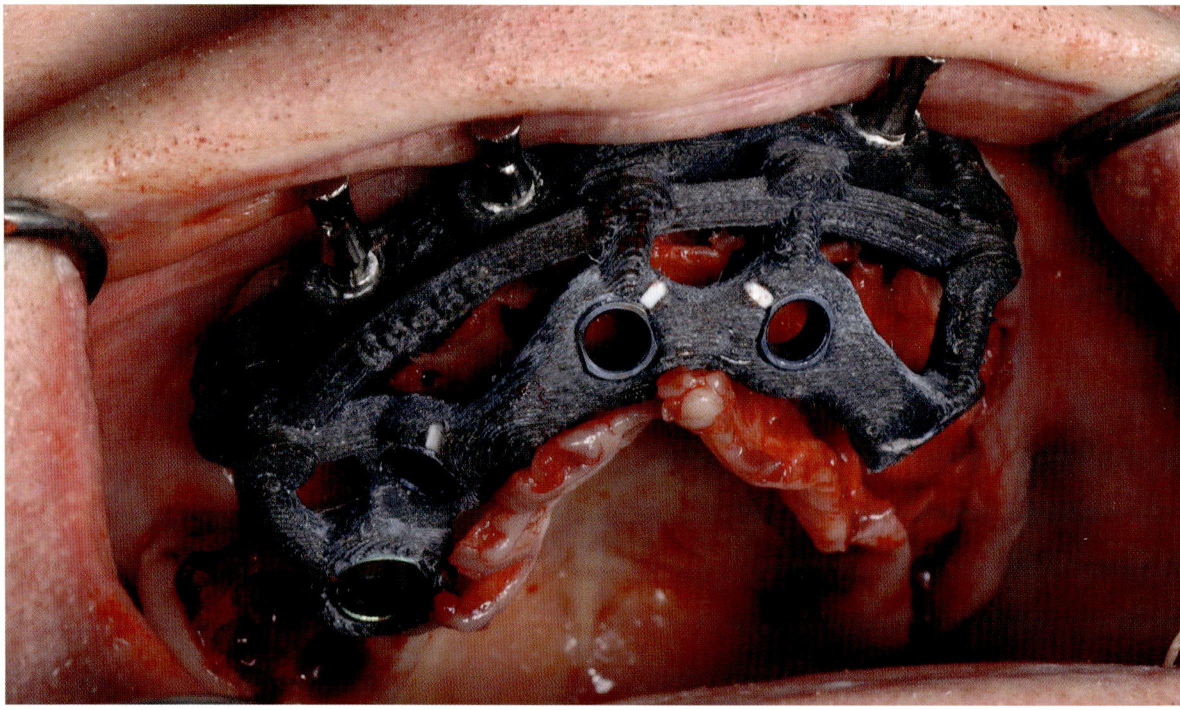

Figure 7.35 Carbon-fiber–reinforced foundation and osteotomy guides fitted together.

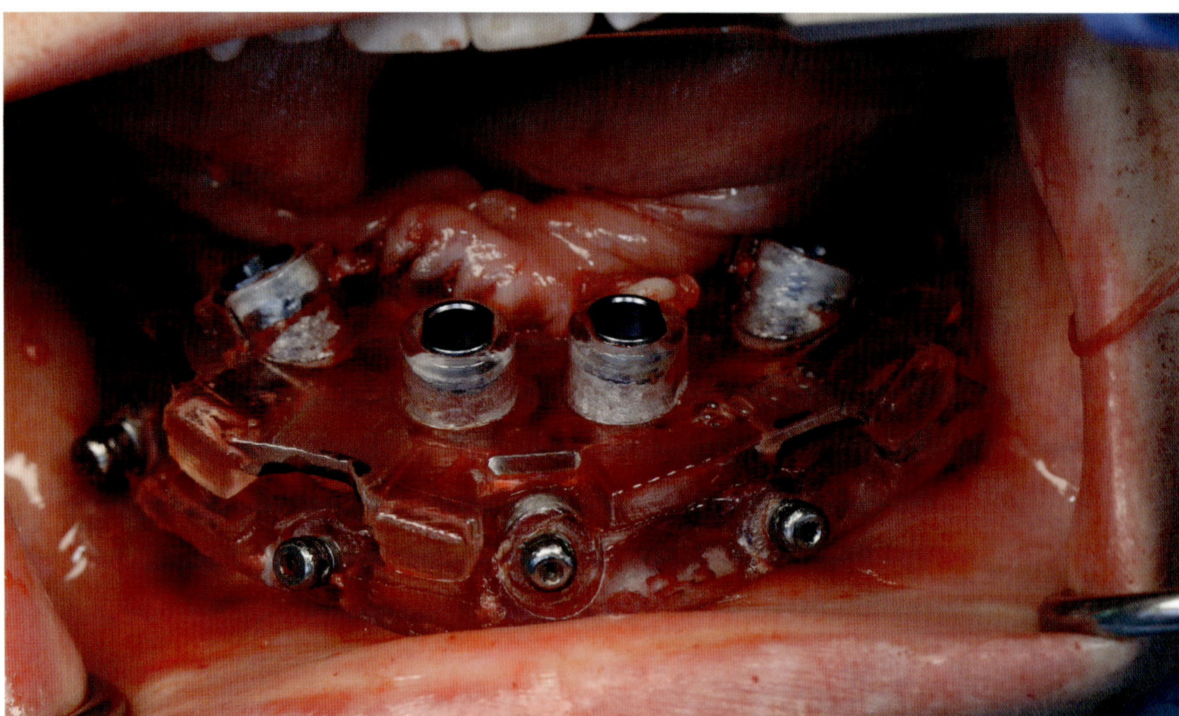

Figure 7.36 Resin osteotomy guide with friction fit on resin foundation guide. Note that visualizing the bone beneath the osteotomy guide and irrigating it during implant placement may be difficult with this type of system.

B. Visualize the bone through the drill guide rings to verify that you are within the boundaries of the maxillary or mandibular ridge.

In the posterior areas, it can be difficult to see through the drill guide rings because of the angles at which the terminal implants are often planned. Note any orientation marks on your guide for implants that will be placed at significant angles and thus require corrective angulated MUAs. If you are using a system that is fully guided, you will be able to drill as well as place your implants through the osteotomy guide rings.

Start with a 2.0-mm pilot drill, perforation drill, or Lindemann bur (depending on bone density), and use the technique you are most comfortable with to make the initial pathway into the bone. If you have any concern about the location of the osteotomy, drill only a few millimeters into the bone. You may have to remove the guide to double check where the osteotomy site is if you cannot view it through the guide. Once you are certain that your osteotomy sites are located correctly, drill with your pilot drill to depth (Fig. 7.37).

PRO TIP: Osteotomy guide, part 2

Always drill to final depth with your pilot drill. Even if you plan to underprepare your osteotomy in the drilling sequence by reducing the final drilling length or diameter, you should still drill to depth with the pilot drill.

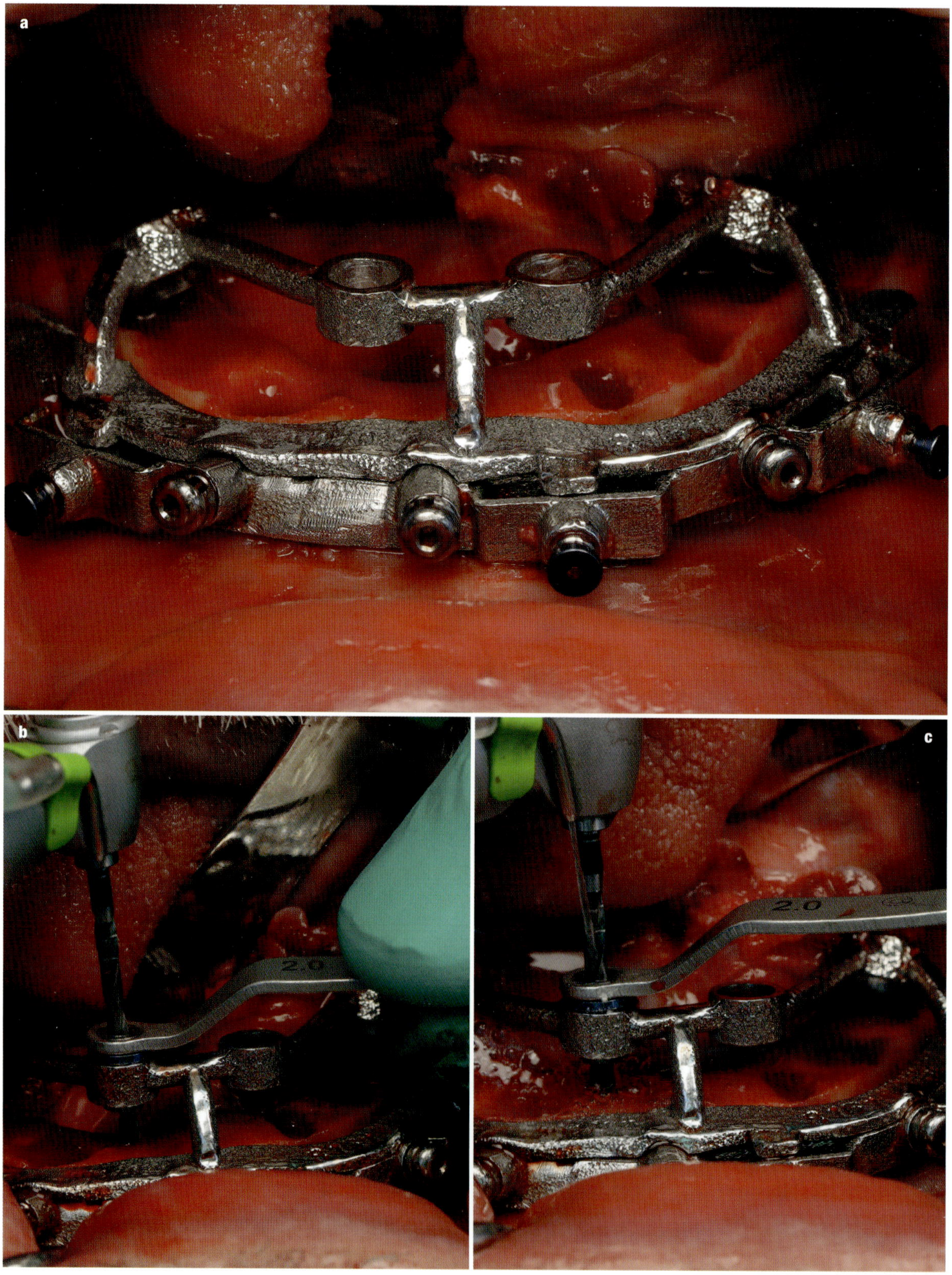

Figure 7.37 (a-c) Preparation of the initial osteotomy site with a 2.0-mm pilot drill using a key placed in the osteotomy guide.

C. As you prepare your osteotomies with the pilot drill, pay attention to your tactile sensation and what it tells you about the quality and density of the bone. If the tactile feedback you are getting indicates a lack of density, you may want to consider one or more of the following options:

- **Use osseodensification burs.** Densah® burs (Versah) are one way to improve the density of the bone in your osteotomy. An entire protocol has been developed using these burs to improve the odds of achieving appropriate implant stability. I added this system to my personal surgical protocols several years ago and have been able to stabilize implants that otherwise would have to be removed due to insufficient torque (Fig. 7.38).
- **Underprepare your osteotomy.** An underprepared osteotomy may allow you to achieve better implant torque levels in lower-density bone. This technique is widely practiced, but it requires early detection of the bone quality; the larger your osteotomy, the lower your chances are of being able to use this method. You can underprepare the diameter as well as the length of your osteotomy if you have achieved sufficient length with your pilot drill.
- **Consider changing the diameter and/or length of the implant in the osteotomy.** This is the option I would consider last, and only if there is an abundance of bone and space for the implant. Otherwise, it is wiser to stick to the original plan. In cases where I do have sufficient width and/or length, I will almost always attempt to engage the denser cortical bone in the nasal floor or sinus walls in the maxilla and the cortical bone surrounding the mandible. These factors should have been taken into consideration at the time of planning the case but sometimes are overlooked.

PRO TIP: Osteotomy guide, part 3

If you encounter bone density that is lower than you expected and decide to apply one of the methods described in this section to increase it, consider placing just one implant before preparing all the osteotomy sites. Focus on figuring out which technique works best for the first implant site, then replicate it around the arch. If you were to prepare all the osteotomy sites prior to placing a single implant, you may be left with fewer options.

If your tactile feedback tells you that the bone is denser than you expected, consider using a slower pumping motion with plenty of irrigation to create your osteotomies. You may also want to check that your implant burs are sharp and do not need to be replaced. Having an extra surgical kit or burs is helpful. Another option is to use the Densah burs in a clockwise motion, to efficiently cut bone as opposed to densifying it. You are most likely to encounter this denser type of bone in the mandible and anterior maxilla. Some implant systems include "plus" drills that increase an additional fractional amount in diameter.

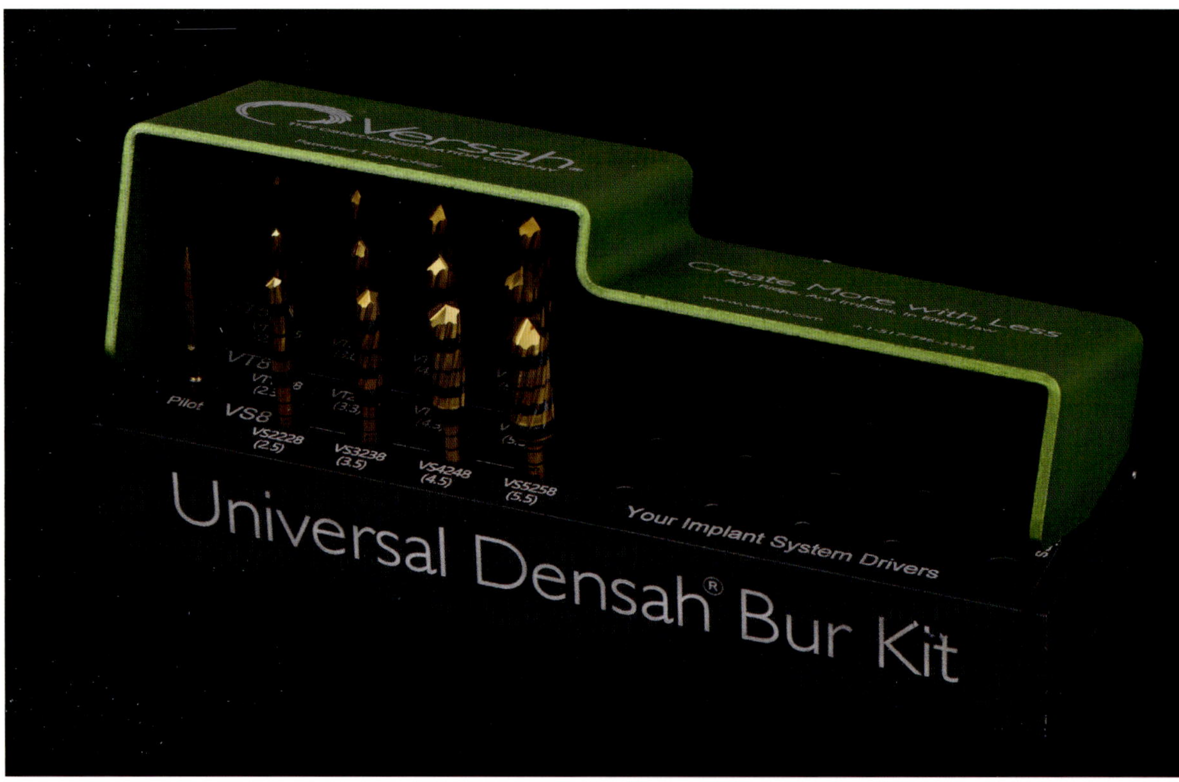

Figure 7.38 **Densah® bur kit (Versah) with osseodensification burs. Although not designed specifically for guided surgery, this is the kit the author prefers. Versah also markets a guided surgery osseodensification kit as well.**

D. Assuming you are comfortable with your drilling protocol and have created the osteotomies, it is time to place the implants (or remaining implants).

Although it may be most efficient to place them in order, I place the implants where I feel best about the chances of achieving the appropriate torque if I have any concerns.

PRO TIP: Osteotomy guide, part 4

Guided implant systems vary in their design and how drill length is determined. Some systems require a key when stepping up to the next drill size. If you have planned the case correctly and are using a system designed for guided surgery, you should feel confident that the osteotomy rings will help you accurately place your implants. However, it is always wise to check your drills or keys before surgery to make sure they fit well into the osteotomy rings in your guide, with no binding of the drills. Using OEM (original equipment manufacturer) ring sleeves should prevent this potential problem but is not always necessary.

E. As you are placing the implants, use 30 to 35 Ncm of torque and carefully guide the implants through the guide sleeves (Fig. 7.39).

When the head of the implant is about 3-5 mm above the guide sleeve, it can be manually torqued in place (Fig. 7.40). Using this technique, you will have a better idea of what your torque value is at the top of the sleeve. If your implant will have an angled MUA, then pay attention to the orientation mark that should be present on the sleeve or guide and the implant driver. Align the implant driver markings with this sleeve marking to attain the appropriate final torque and orientation of your implant (Figs. 7.41, 7.42). Once your implants have been torqued, you can remove the osteotomy guide (Fig. 7.43).

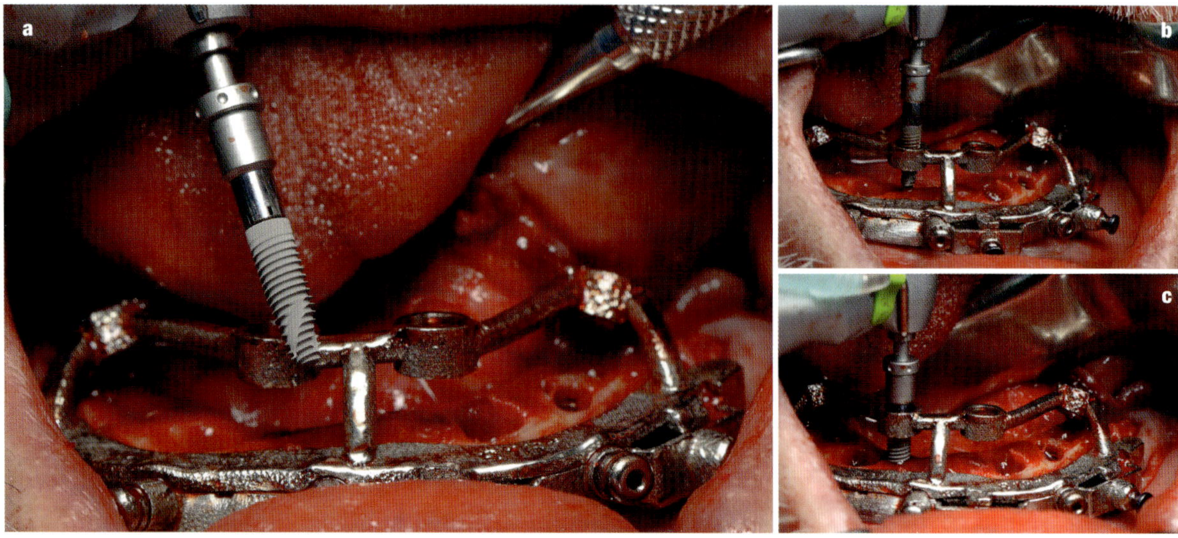

Figure 7.39 (a-c) Implant placement through the osteotomy guide sleeve without the use of a key.

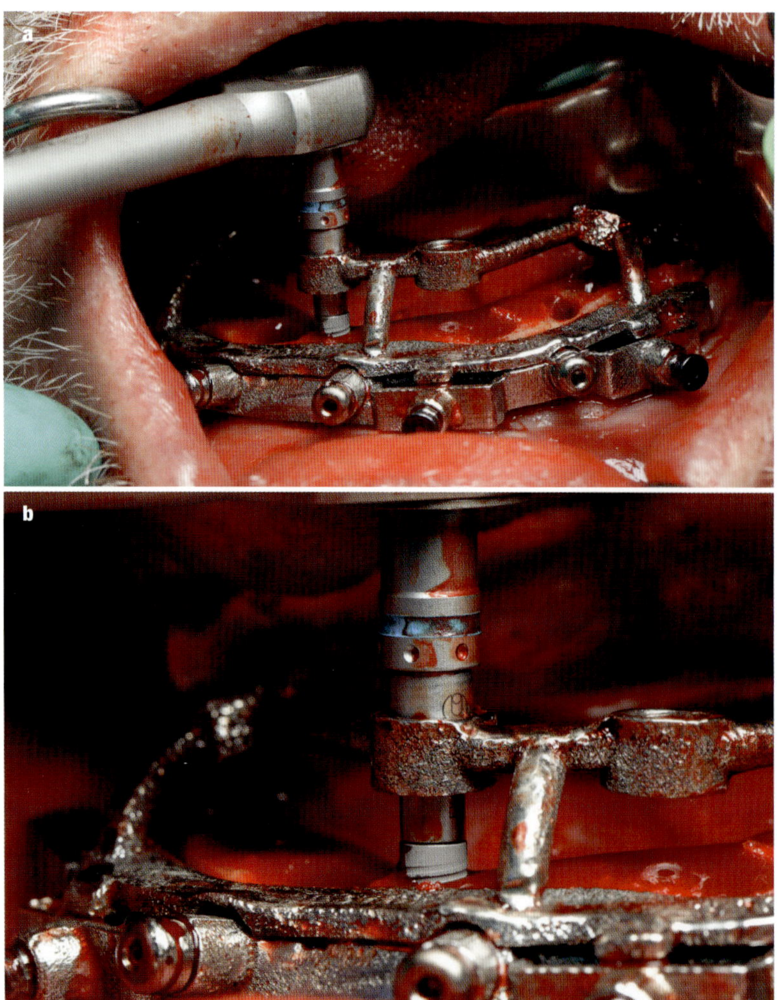

Figure 7.40 (a) Use of a torque wrench to finalize placement of the implant through the osteotomy guide; (b) Close-up view of the implant driver in the torque wrench as it is used to complete the implant placement.

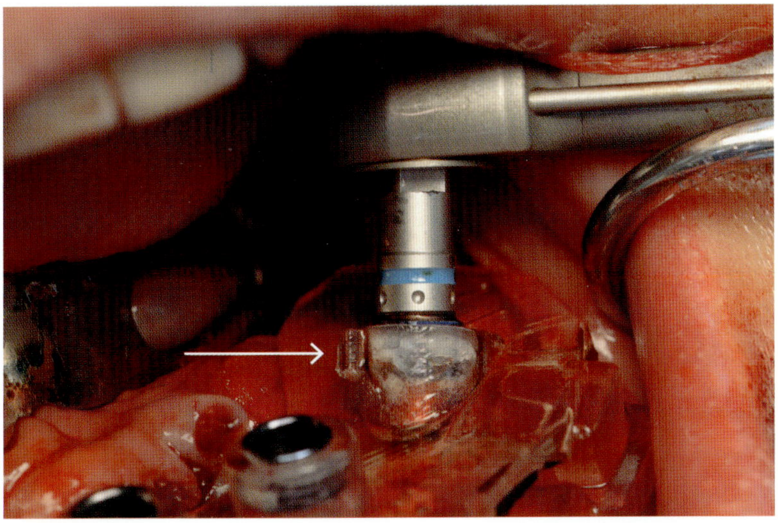

Figure 7.41 Note the orientation button on the guide sleeve (*arrow*) and the dimples on the implant driver. These markings need to be aligned when an angled multiunit abutment (MUA) is used.

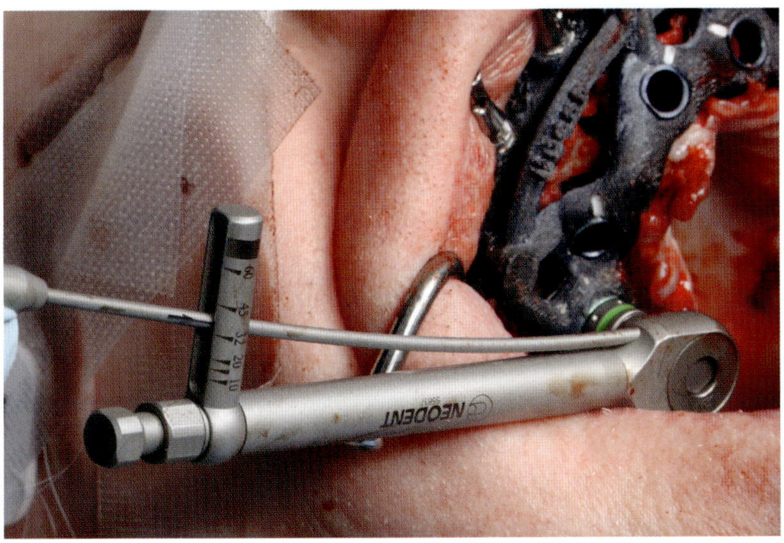

Figure 7.42 Use of a torque wrench to reach final torque value on the implant.

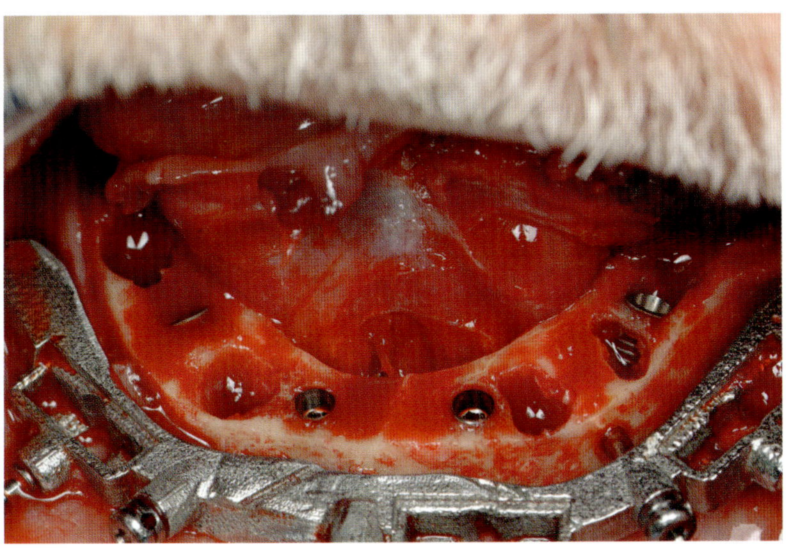

Figure 7.43 Removal of the osteotomy guide from the foundation guide after the placement of mandibular implants.

Implants and torque values

In courses I have attended and during conversations with other surgeons, I have consistently heard that there should be a minimal amount of total torque achieved throughout the arch to safely load the implants with an interim prosthesis. In addition, many implant systems have their own guidelines on minimum and maximum torque values needed to achieve fixation and stability. I have used the following guidelines successfully for hundreds of fixed full-arch implant cases.

- Torque value of each implant: 25-65 Ncm
- Torque value across the arch (torque of all implants combined): 150 Ncm

Implant stability quotient (ISQ) is a quantitative measure of implant stability using a device that displays a value between 1 and 100. Higher ISQ values denote higher primary stability, and there is evidence that ISQ numbers below 60 suggest low implant stability. Devices that measure ISQ can be used during and after surgery. Although I have not used one of these devices at the time of surgery, you may prefer to use one for determining whether to immediately load your interim prosthesis. If so, follow the guidelines established by the manufacturers of these devices. If you prefer using torque values, then you may apply the principles that follow.

I. If you do not get torque of 25 Ncm or greater on an implant, consider placing one or more "rescue" implants:

- Remove the implant and replace it with an implant one size larger in diameter. (As I explained in Chapter 6 [see The Inventory Effect], it is imperative to have extra implants on hand.) Before doing this, be sure to evaluate the amount of bone available as well as the spacing between your implants.
- Remove the implant and replace it with a longer implant. Only do this if the increased length will not impinge on an adjacent implant and if you can engage denser cortical bone.
- Remove the implant and place a larger-diameter implant that also has greater length.

Again, check your printed or digital surgical reports and/or the CBCT for confirmation of available bone, and avoid anatomical "land mines" such as the inferior alveolar nerves, mental nerves, lingual artery, and sinus and nasal cavities.

PRO TIP: Osteotomy guide, part 5

For indexing with angled MUAs, remember that placing an implant in a different vertical position than originally planned will require a change in the horizontal location of the screw access channel in the interim prosthesis. Submerging an implant deeper than planned will cause the access channel in the MUA to be more anterior, whereas placing an implant more coronal than originally planned will cause the access channel to be more posterior.

II. If you do not get a torque of 150 Ncm or greater across the arch:

- Follow the previously mentioned steps for one or more implants until 150 Ncm is achieved.
- Consider careful nonguided placement of additional implants until 150 Ncm or more is reached.
- Consider delayed loading of the case.

PRO TIP: Insufficient torque

For cases in which the implants cannot be loaded immediately (for whatever reason), you can save a lot of time by indexing the interim prosthesis or a replica appliance off of two or more MUAs to use in a future pick-up procedure. Once the implants have osseointegrated and are uncovered, you will spend less time converting to a fixed prosthesis. Always be prepared to place cover screws on the implants and close. This is when that back-up denture you ordered will come in handy.

Note: *If you are just beginning your journey into implantology, it is advisable to perform and be comfortable placing single implants without a guide. This may seem to contradict the overall message of this book, but it does not. Guided full-arch dental implant surgery is the most predictable way for most general dentists and specialists to achieve the best results for most patients. However, having the skill to place a single implant without the help of a guide can be a great advantage when something goes wrong (as it eventually will). Most experienced implantologists would agree that using guides as a "crutch" is not a good idea. Knowing how and being able to practice the fundamentals of nonguided surgery is important and strongly advised.*

III. If you do not get at least 25 Ncm of torque on one or several implants but have 150 Ncm or more total torque across the arch:

- Use your best judgment and consider all the potential implications.

Occasionally, I have an implant that does not torque above 25 Ncm. If the implant is stable at around 20 Ncm, I will generally put this implant to "sleep"—that is, place a cover screw in it and bury it. I then test and load that implant in a few months during the prosthetic phase of treatment. The success of this strategy depends on the location of the implant and the anteroposterior (AP) distance between it and other implants. If the implant is a terminal support of the prosthesis, then the cantilever of the prosthesis must be reduced based on the guidelines presented in Chapter 5. If that results in too much distance between loaded implants, or if the interim prosthesis is imbalanced in terms of support because of this loss of support, the interim prosthesis may flex, break, and/or become loose. Again, sometimes it is safer, and in the patient's (and your) best interests, to choose delayed loading in such cases.

STEP 9: CARRIER GUIDE/ABUTMENT ALIGNER AND MUA PLACEMENT

Once all the implants are torqued and stable and you are satisfied with their positioning, the MUAs can be placed. It is helpful if your assistant has all the abutments lined up and ready, as this makes the process of placing them more efficient. Because the case was planned and your implants have been rotated into the appropriate positions, placing the abutments in the correct positions is much easier than in surgeries planned in an analog environment.

Note: *Some stackable guide systems do not use a carrier guide or abutment aligner. In such cases you may have to visualize the MUA placement using the interim prosthesis.*

A. Place the carrier guide or abutment aligner on the foundation guide as you did after bone reduction and verify again that it is passive and not impinging anywhere. Use whatever locking mechanism is provided to fasten it in place (Fig. 7.44).

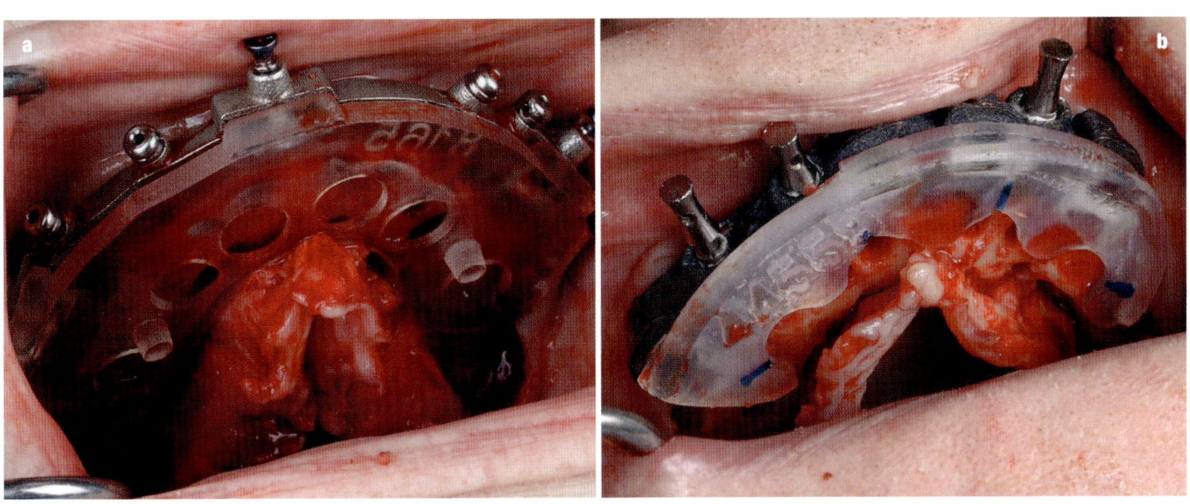

Figure 7.44 (a) Carrier guide seated and secured on a cobalt-chrome foundation guide; (b) Abutment aligner placed on a carbon-fiber–reinforced foundation guide.

- **B.** Verify that the implants are visible and that the holes in the carrier guide (if your system uses one) allow room for proper positioning of the MUAs.

- **C.** Like the osteotomy guide, the carrier guide or abutment aligner should have markings that allow you to see how the angled MUAs should be oriented. These markings indicate where the screw access channels are located so that your driver will match up with them. Straight abutments do not have (or need) markings on the carrier guide.

- **D.** Place the multiunit abutments along the arch as specified in the surgical plan (Fig. 7.45a).

As has been discussed, there are several types of angled abutments. In the implant systems I use, the most common are 17 and 30 degrees, but there are others out there. Also, the heights of the abutments vary but are generally 1-4 mm.

- **E.** Torque the abutments to the specification set by the implant system you are using.

As you torque the MUAs, pay attention to any rotational movement of your implant. If the implant rotates, it may be necessary to consider using a "rescue implant" because you may no longer have enough initial stability to load the implant. This will happen occasionally if the torque on your implant is borderline (usually below 25 Ncm). If you have reached the appropriate torque on the MUA and you notice only a slight movement, you may consider not replacing it. This might be acceptable if there are stable implants adjacent to the implant that rotated slightly. I have found that there is less risk of losing minimally torqued implants when they have neighboring implants that are well anchored and have initial stability. Different implant systems recommend different torques for the MUAs. Follow the manufacturer guidelines for final torque (Fig. 7.45b).

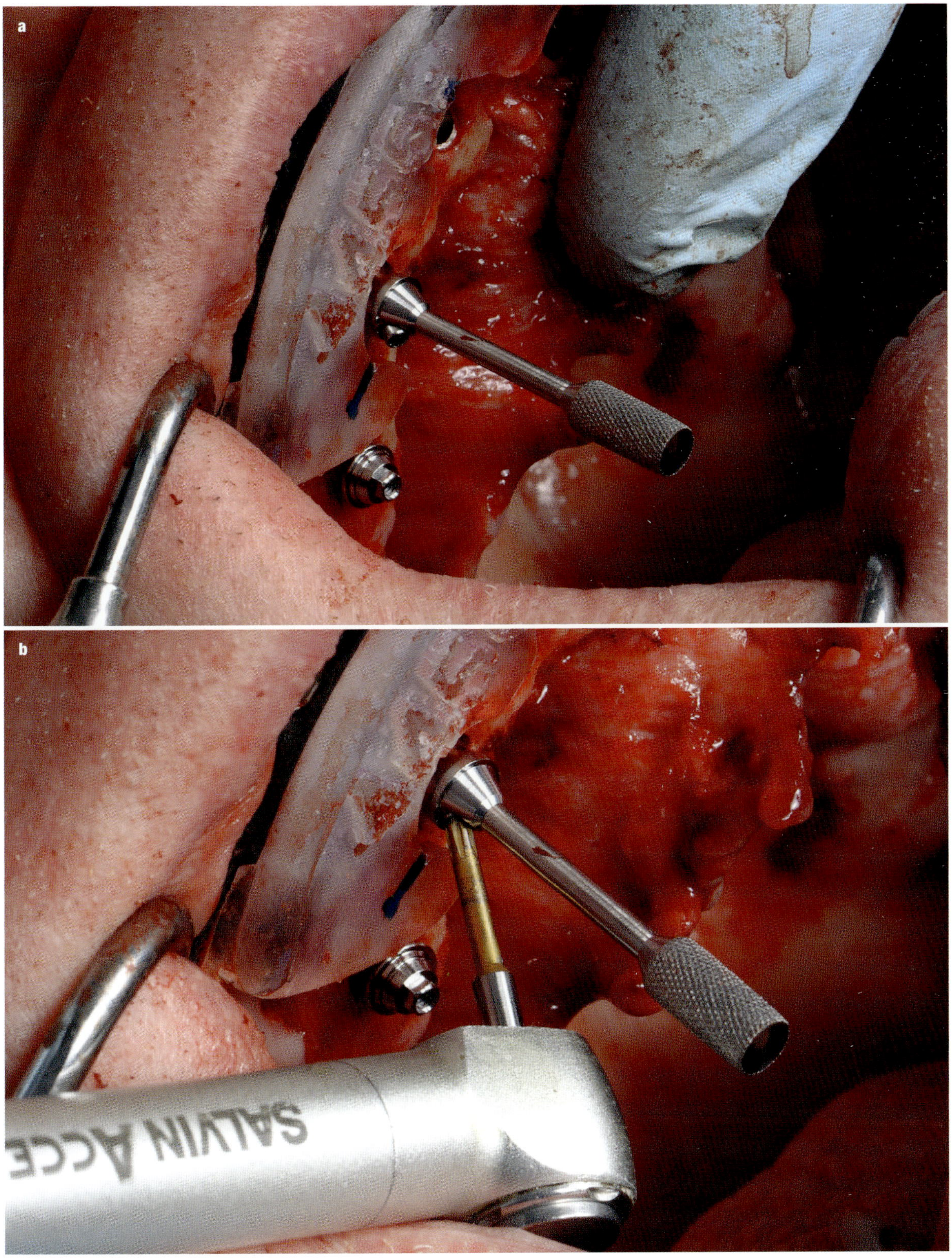

Figure 7.45 (a) Placement of a 17-degree MUA using an abutment aligner. Note the alignment of the abutment screw with the mark on the abutment aligner; (b) Torquing the MUA to the specification provided by the implant manufacturer.

F. As you place the MUAs, you may observe differences in their heights. This can be a variable factor based on the depth at which the implants were placed. If the position of an implant is acceptable but the MUA is either too short or potentially too tall, keep in mind that you may be able to change it during the definitive prosthetic phase.

Many clinicians I have spoken to agree that 1.5- to 2.5-mm abutments work well if your implant is placed just below or at the crest of the ridge. It is preferable to have the MUA shorter rather than taller if it is not impinging on bone and the abutments are aligned throughout the arch (Fig. 7.46).

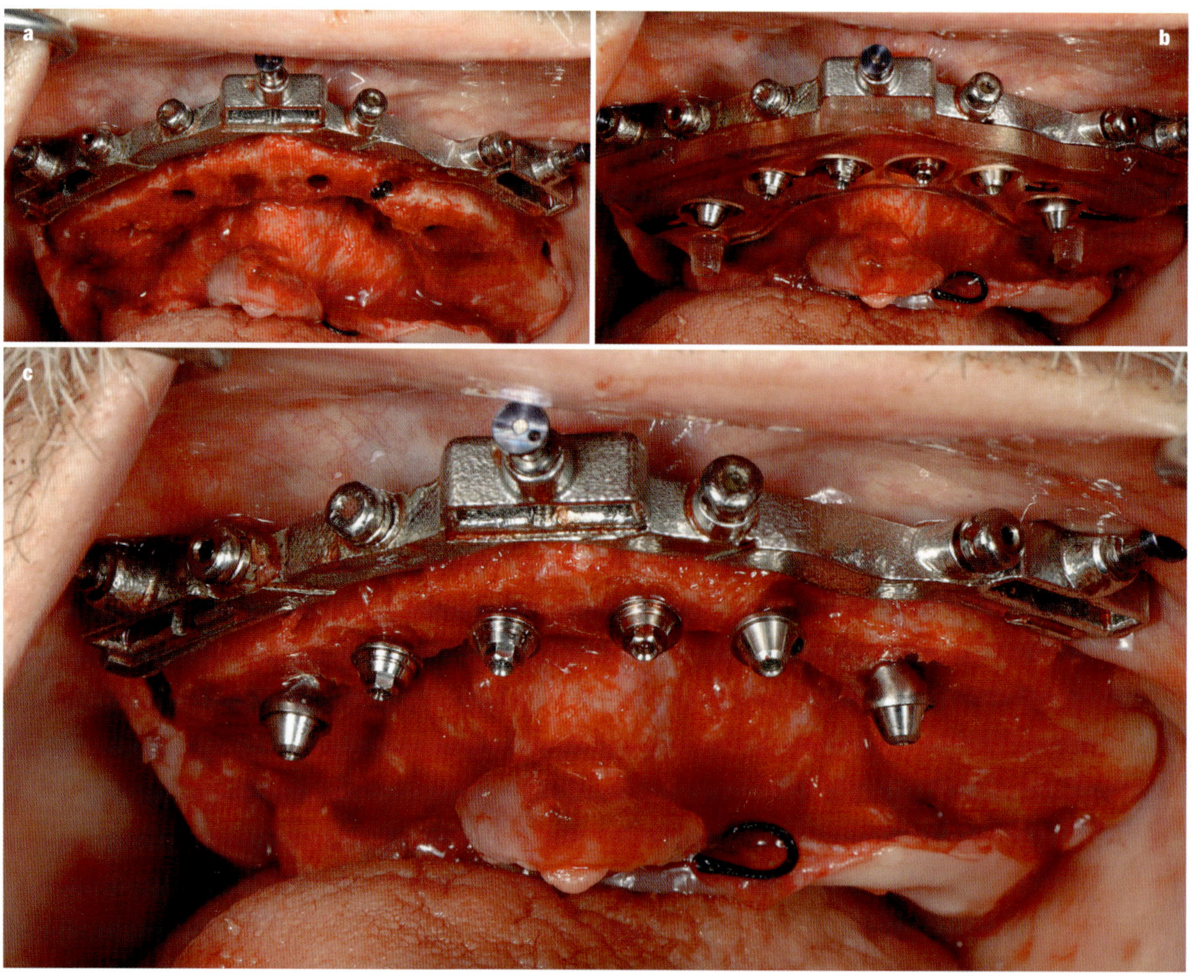

Figure 7.46 Placement of MUAs using a carrier guide. (a) Implants in the maxilla prior to placement of the MUAs; (b) Placement of MUAs through the carrier guide; (c) MUAs after removal of the carrier guide. Note the relatively uniform alignment of the MUAs.

Note: *If you use a carrier guide during placement of the MUAs, it may prevent visualization of the implant or impinge on the MUA. If this is the case, you can always remove the carrier guide and use it merely as a reference. The holes in the carrier guide can also be enlarged with a handpiece and bur to accommodate visualization and access.*

G. Once the MUAs are appropriately torqued, make sure the carrier guide (if your system uses one) is in place, because the next steps will require the interim appliance to be seated on it. If your system uses an abutment aligner, it should be removed to make room for the interim prosthesis, which will attach to the foundation guide (Figs. 7.47, 7.48).

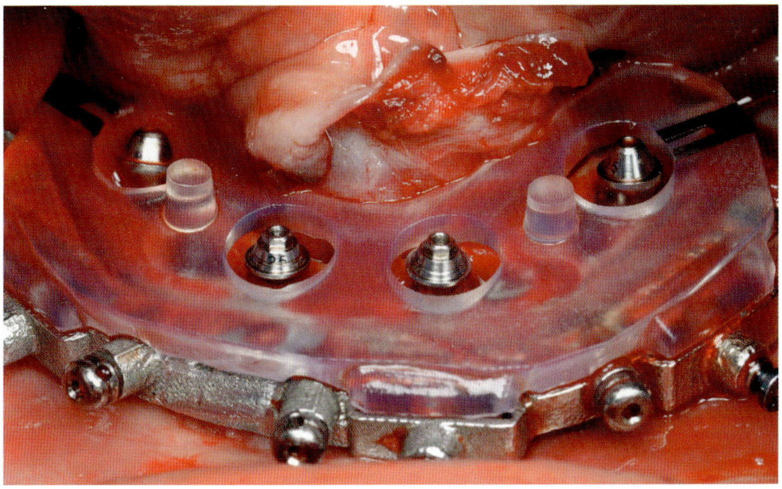

Figure 7.47 Carrier guide on a cobalt-chrome foundation guide, with MUAs in place.

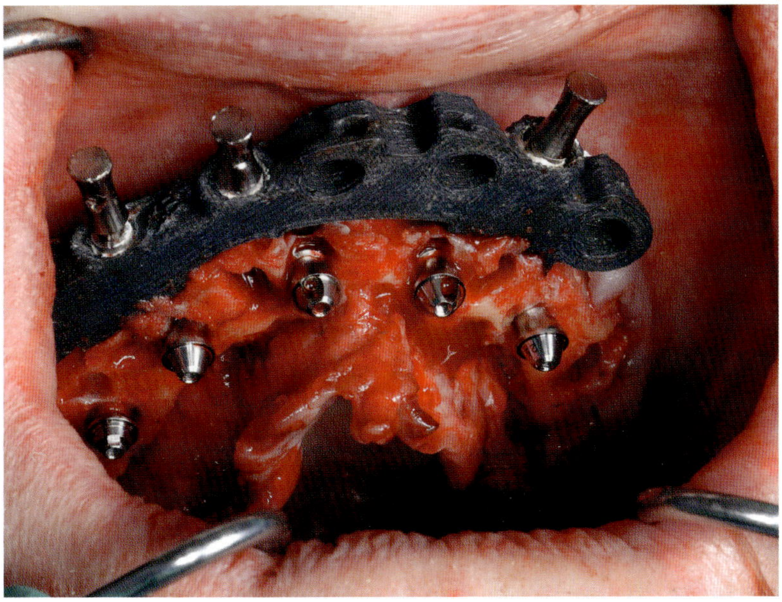

Figure 7.48 Appearance of a carbon-fiber–reinforced foundation guide immediately after removal of the abutment aligner, in preparation for the interim prosthesis pick-up.

STEP 10: INTERIM PROSTHESIS PICK-UP

Many full-arch stackable surgical guide systems approach the interim prosthesis pick-up in a similar fashion. However, there are some notable differences. I will review the process that has worked best for me in terms of efficiency and the ability to delegate to team members. Many of the steps that follow can be delegated to a highly trained dental assistant or a lab technician with some clinical experience. When you are first getting started, I would recommend doing all of these steps yourself, so you have a clear understanding of how everything works. That way if your team has any issues, you are familiar with the process and can help problem solve. If you are a general practitioner and are doing the surgery as well as the prosthetic pick-up, this may be the easiest route to take at first.

A. Place block-out material such as a small piece of rubber dam around each of the temporary titanium cylinders.

You also may want to air abrade or roughen the surface of the cylinders with a bur or disc. Some manufacturers place retention grooves on their temporary cylinders, which will also be sufficient.

B. Before placing the temporary cylinders, confirm that the MUAs are in the proper orientation for pick-up by placing the interim prosthesis on the foundation guide or carrier guide and looking through the access holes in the prosthesis (Figs. 7.49, 7.50).

PRO TIP: Interim prosthesis

If you see that an MUA is not in an ideal position for pick-up (see Fig. 7.50), consider removing the prosthesis and using a straight handpiece and appropriate bur to carefully increase the diameter of the access hole. If the MUA is off by a considerable amount, you may need to reposition the MUA, or—in more extreme situations—rotate the position of the implant. Also confirm that your MUA is the correct size/angulation and that your prosthesis is seated completely on the carrier or foundation guide.

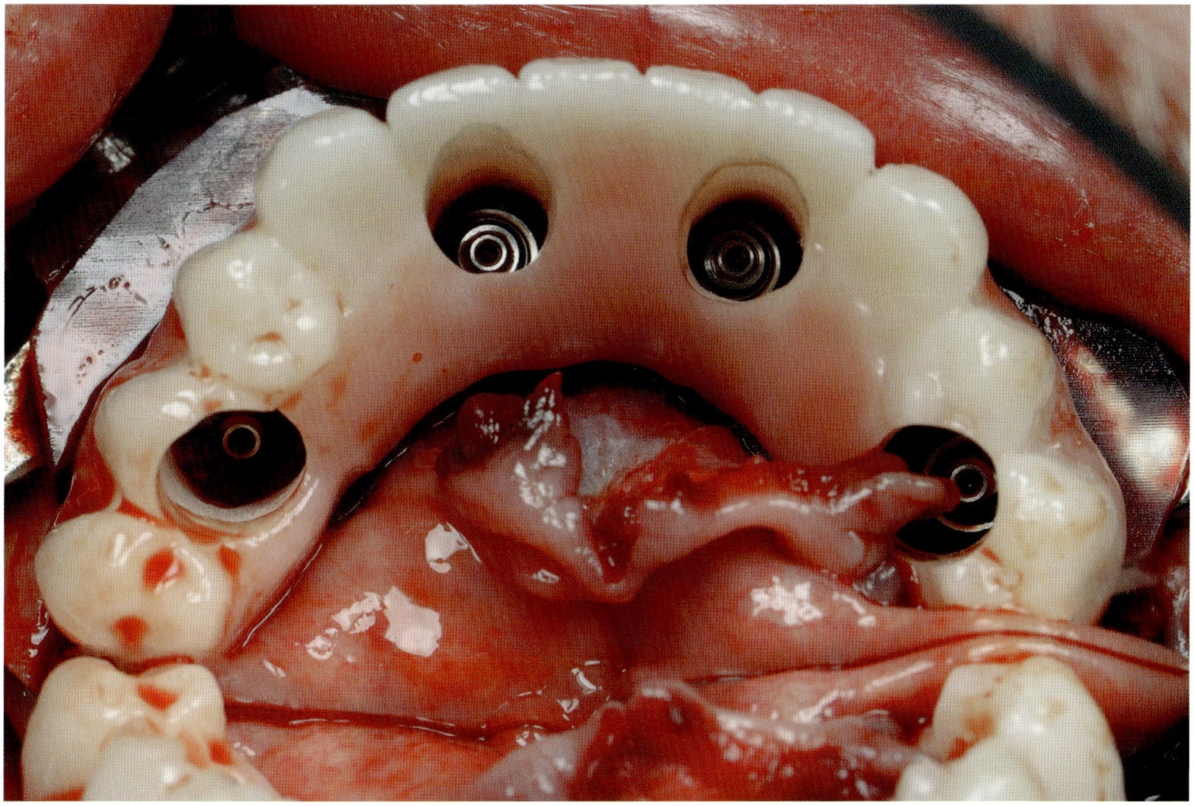

Figure 7.49 Direct visual confirmation of MUA positions through the interim prosthesis.

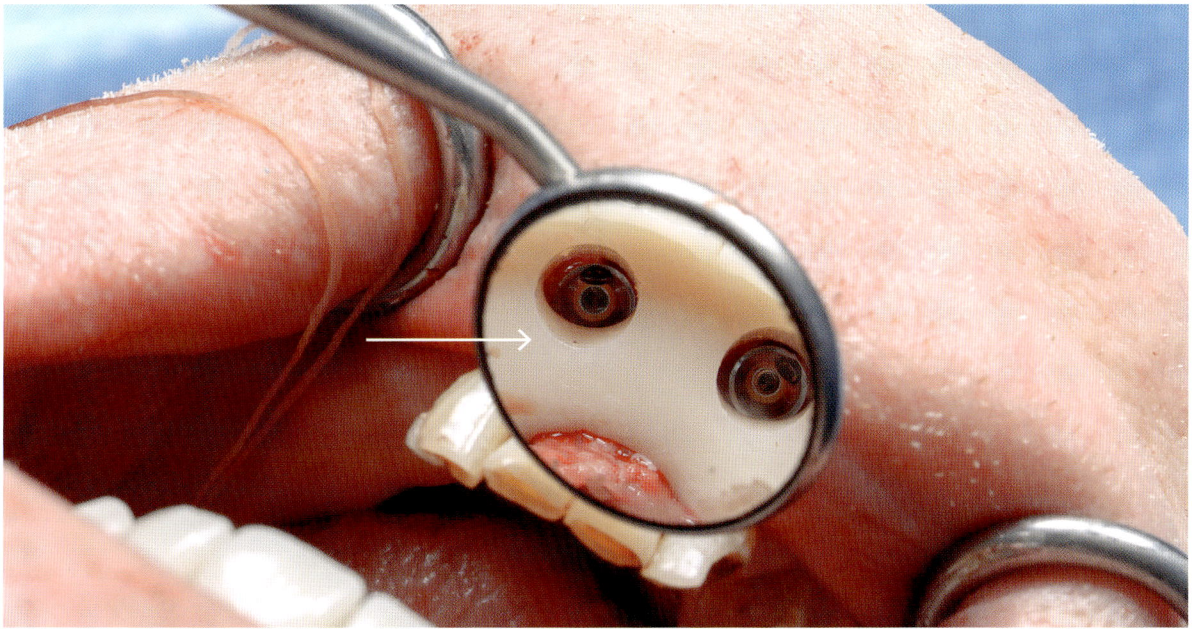

Figure 7.50 Indirect visual confirmation of MUA positions (via a mirror), which reveals that the prosthesis requires slight modification on the lingual (*arrow*) to accommodate the temporary cylinder.

▸ **C.** Starting in the posterior, place the temporary cylinders over the MUAs and loosely screw them in, leaving a little play in the temporary cylinders. This will allow some flexibility that you may need when placing the interim prosthesis if your MUAs are not completely parallel (Figs. 7.51-7.53).

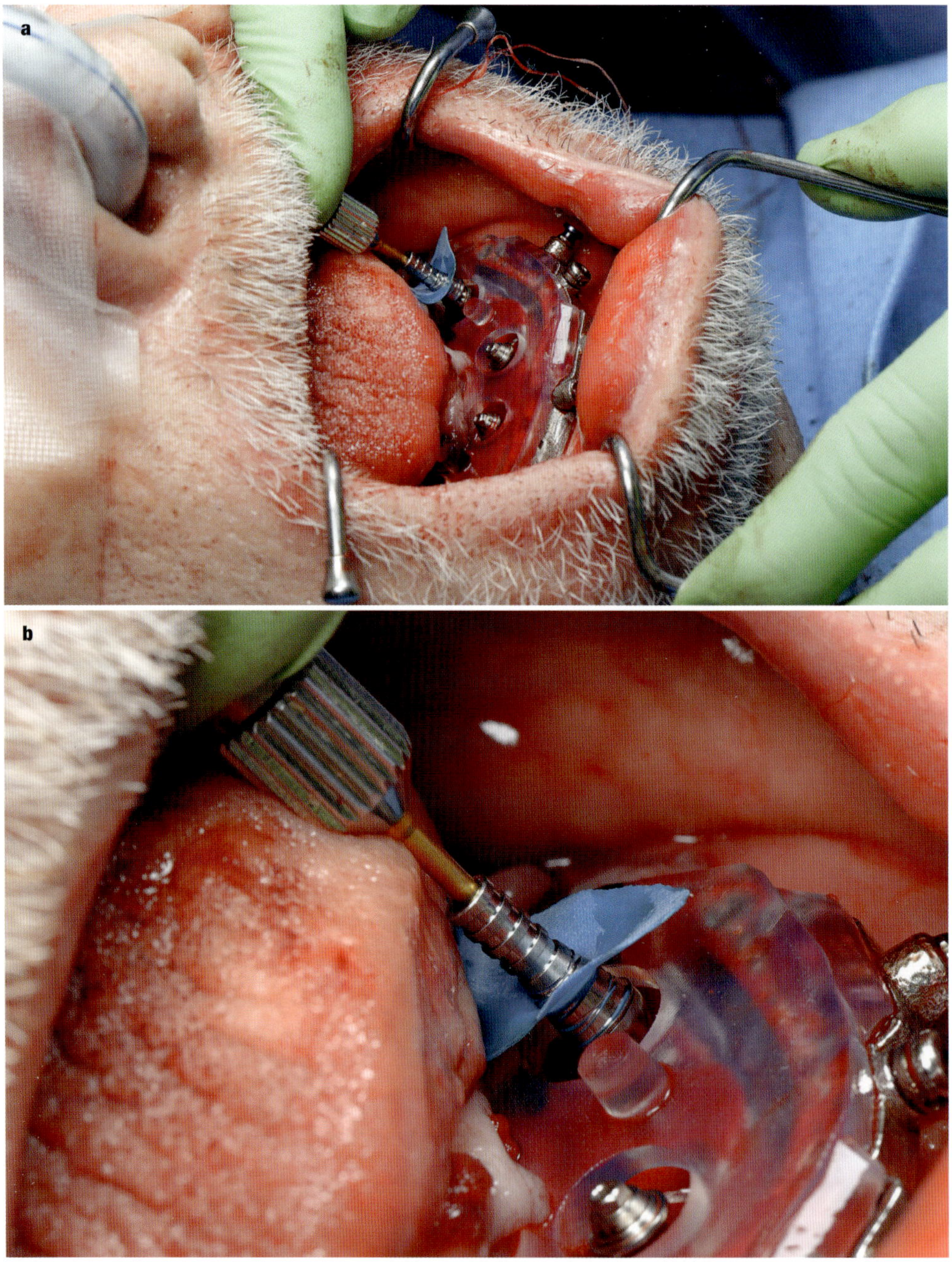

Figure 7.51 (a) Placement of a temporary cylinder (with rubber dam) on an MUA through the carrier guide; (b) Close-up view of the driver used to loosely screw in a temporary cylinder through the carrier guide.

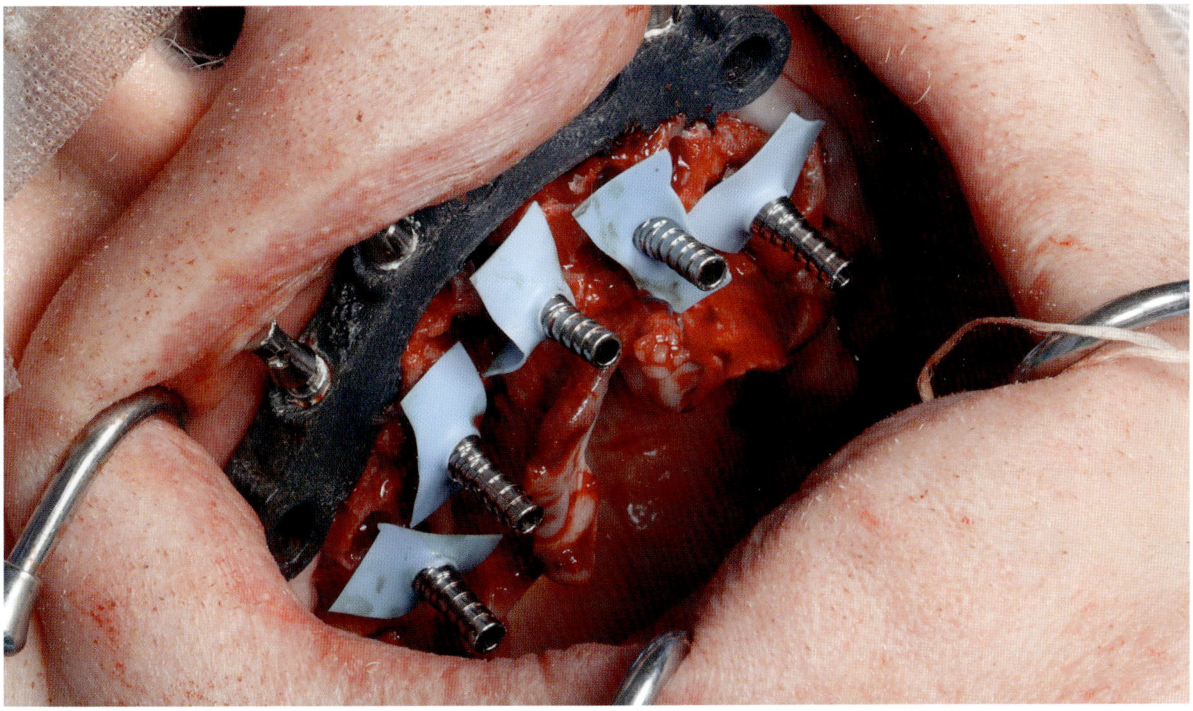

Figure 7.52 Five temporary cylinders placed on MUAs in the maxilla using a stackable guide system that does not require a carrier guide.

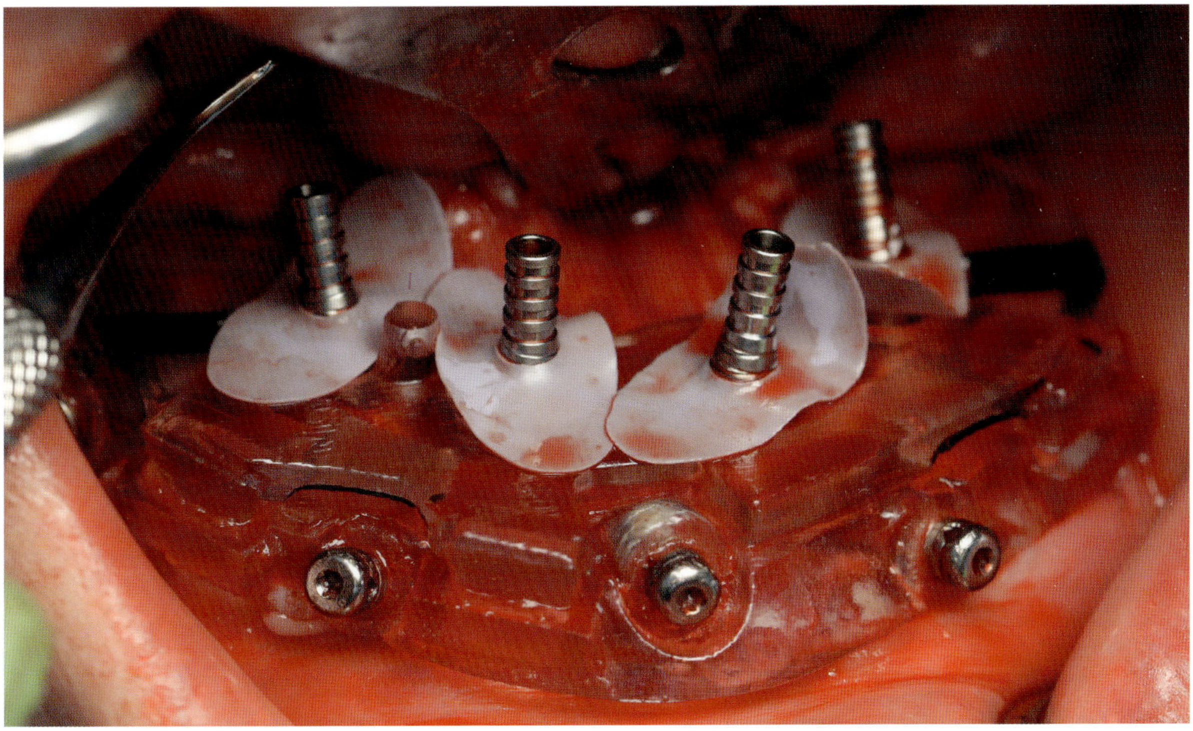

Figure 7.53 Four temporary cylinders placed on MUAs in the mandible through a carrier guide, in preparation for the interim prosthesis pick-up. Rubber dam material is used to block out the pick-up material.

D. Once the temporary cylinders are in position, seat the interim prosthesis on the carrier guide or foundation guide (whichever is relevant to your system). If you are not using a carrier guide, fasten your interim prosthesis to the foundation guide using the mechanism provided by the system (pins, screws, friction fit, etc.) (Fig. 7.54).

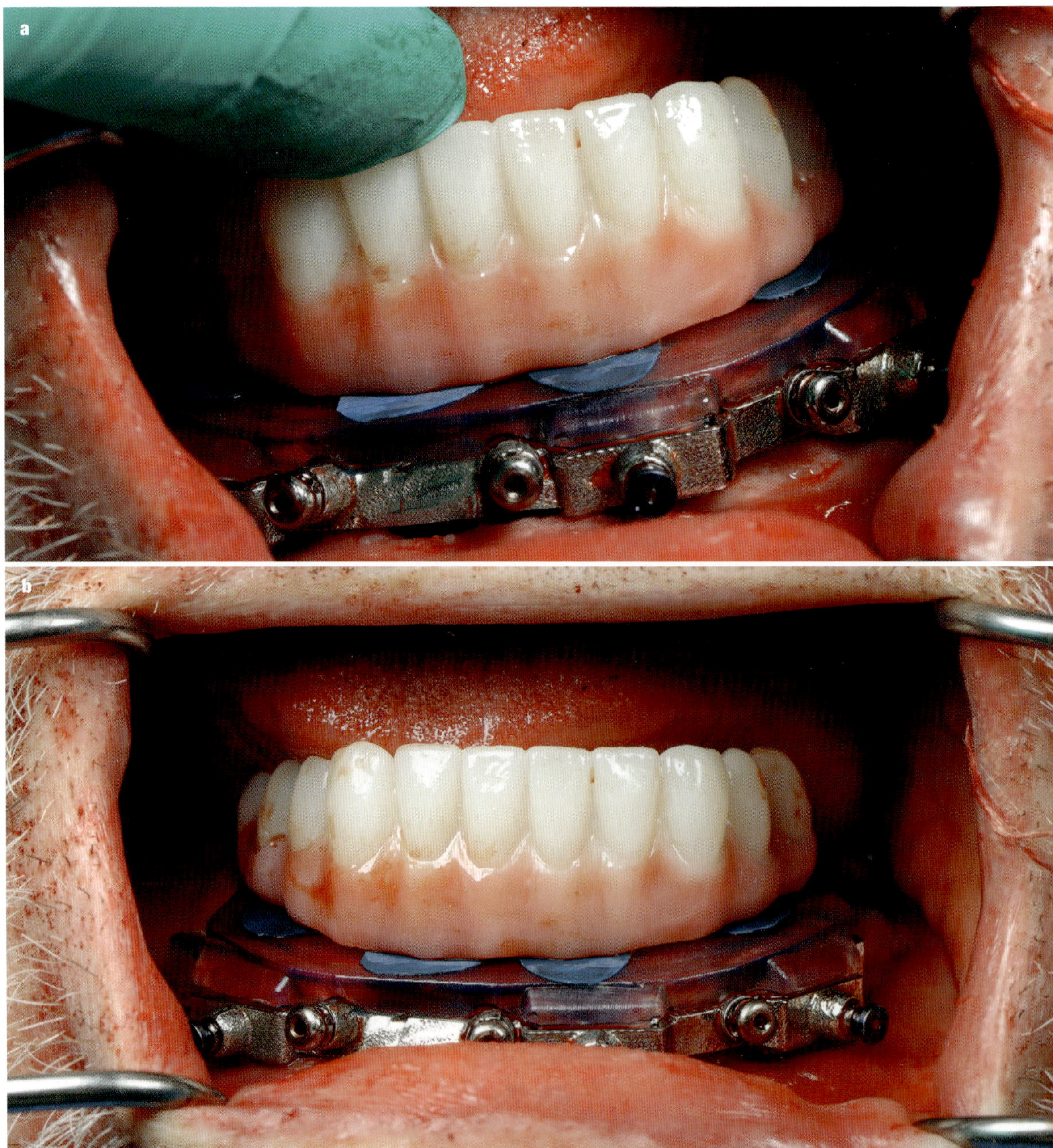

Figure 7.54 (a) Try-in of the interim prosthesis over the temporary cylinders on the carrier guide; (b) Confirmation of passive fit of the interim prosthesis fully seated on the carrier guide.

- **E.** If the prosthesis does not fit passively over the loosely attached temporary cylinders, identify and remove the cylinder(s) that is impinging on the prosthesis and replace it through the access hole in the prosthesis. (Do not forget to place the rubber dam material through the access hole in the prosthesis as well.) If the interim prosthesis still fails to seat passively, remove it and enlarge the relevant access hole(s) slightly.

- **F.** Once the prosthesis fits intimately on the carrier or foundation guide, manually tighten the temporary cylinders or torque them to 10 Ncm. Use direct or indirect vision to peer into each access channel and confirm that it has adequate space circumferentially for pick-up material to flow around the temporary cylinder.

- **G.** Block out the screw access channels in the temporary cylinders.

Of the many materials that can be used for this (e.g., PVS, plumber's tape, and a variety of others), I prefer disposable custom plastic block-out pins. These pins, which are included with some guided systems but also can be purchased separately, are inserted into the temporary cylinders to prevent pick-up material from overflowing into the screw-access openings (Figs. 7.55, 7.56).

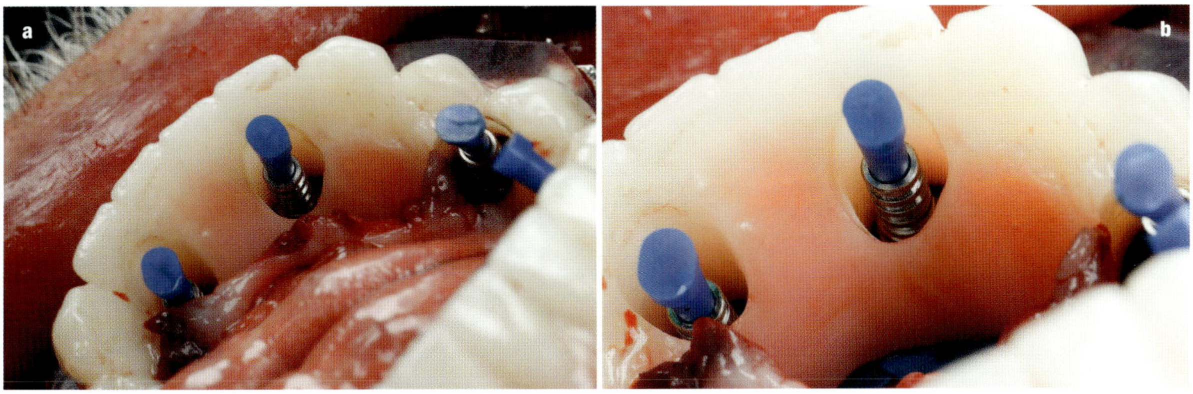

Figure 7.55 (a) Custom block-out pins inserted in the temporary cylinders; (b) Close-up view showing that there is adequate space for acrylic resin pick-up material to flow circumferentially around the temporary cylinders.

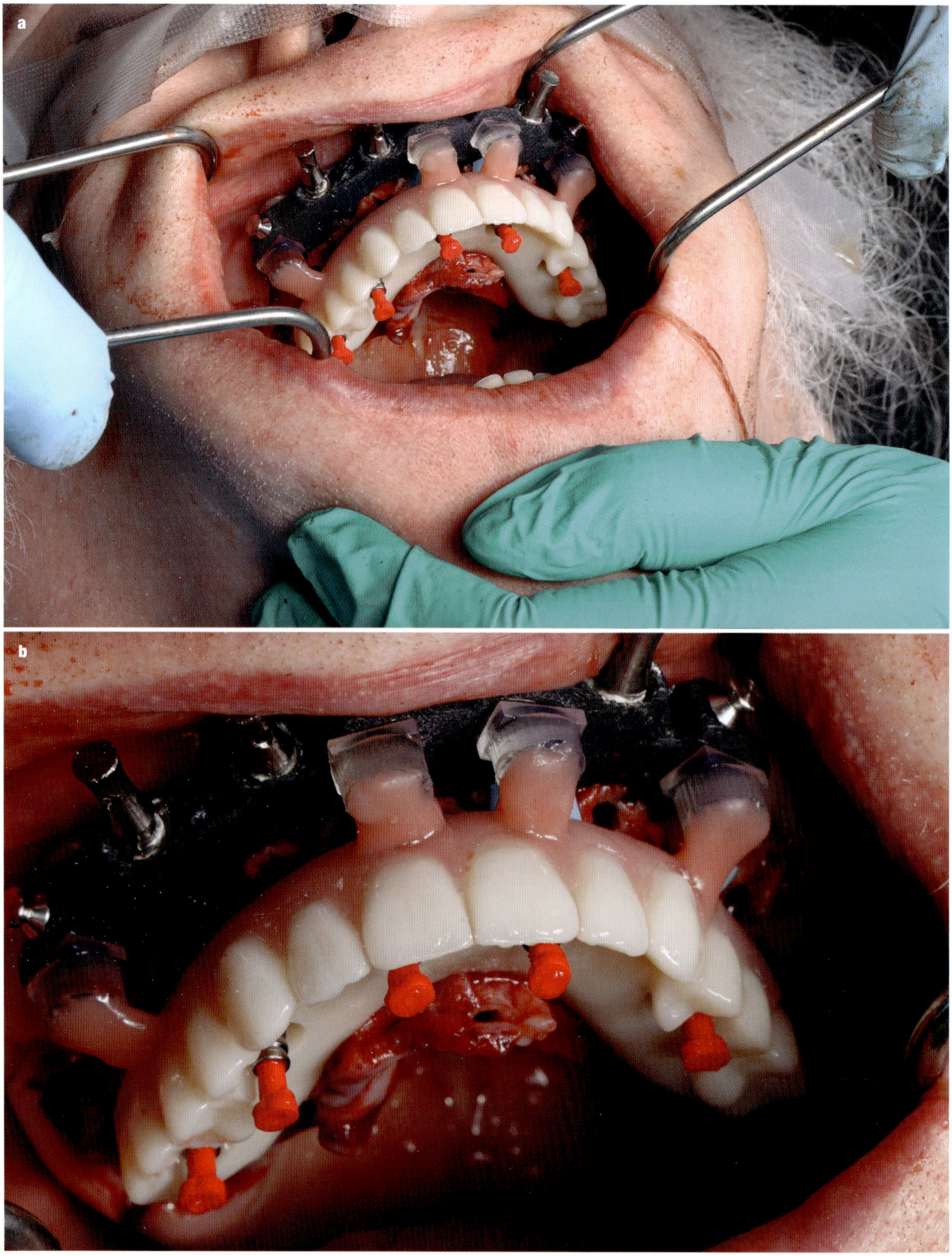

Figure 7.56 (a) Maxillary interim prosthesis secured into foundation guide with block-out pins in place in preparation for pick-up; (b) Close-up view of the temporary cylinders with custom block-out pins ready for pick-up.

H. Irrigate and gently dry the access openings around the cylinders to clear them of any debris or blood, then inject a flowable material into them for the pick-up of the temporary cylinders.

There are several materials that can be used for this, and each has its strengths and weaknesses. The strongest and most predictable material I have found is Stellar DC® acrylic resin (Taub), a flowable dual-cure acrylic that has excellent handling properties and makes efficient use of time. Most importantly, it bonds to both the temporary titanium cylinders and the polymethacrylate (PMMA) interim prosthesis and provides more than adequate strength in a well-designed prosthesis with appropriate occlusal balance. The material can be injected in from the top of the access openings in the prosthesis and light-cured for initial stability. I prefer to fill and then light-cure one opening at a time before moving on to the next one. The goal is to fill each access hole completely. If blood or debris leaks into an unfilled access hole during the process, it can be rinsed and gently dried without affecting the areas that have already been filled. Unlike a self-cure composite or acrylic product that sets up quickly, Stellar DC allows you to take as much time as needed for this process, which helps take pressure off you and your team (Figs. 7.57-7.60).

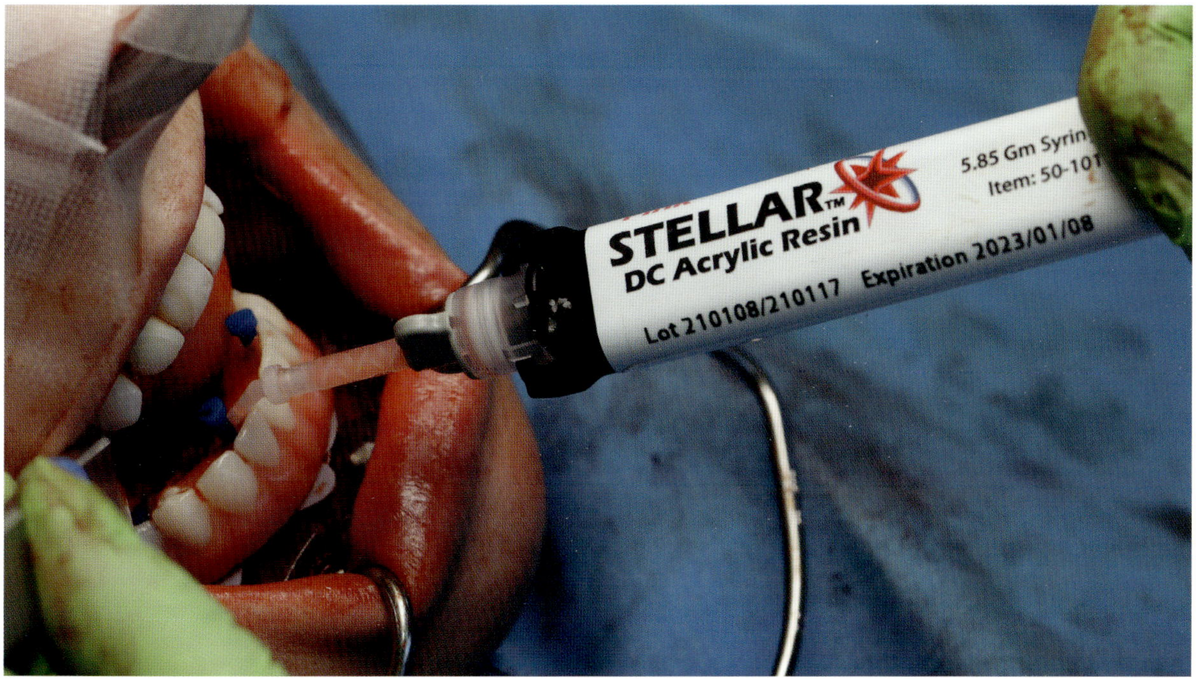

Figure 7.57 Injection of acrylic resin pick-up material in the access holes around the temporary cylinders.

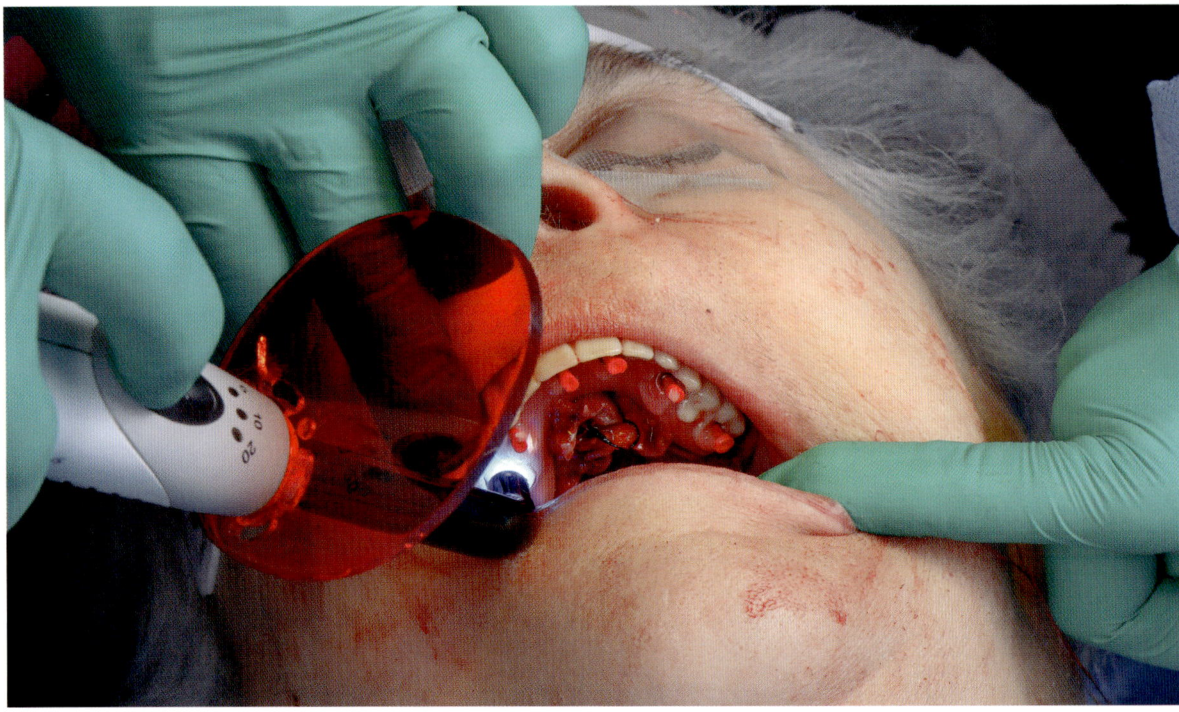

Figure 7.58 Spot-curing of the acrylic resin pick-up material for initial stability of the cylinders.

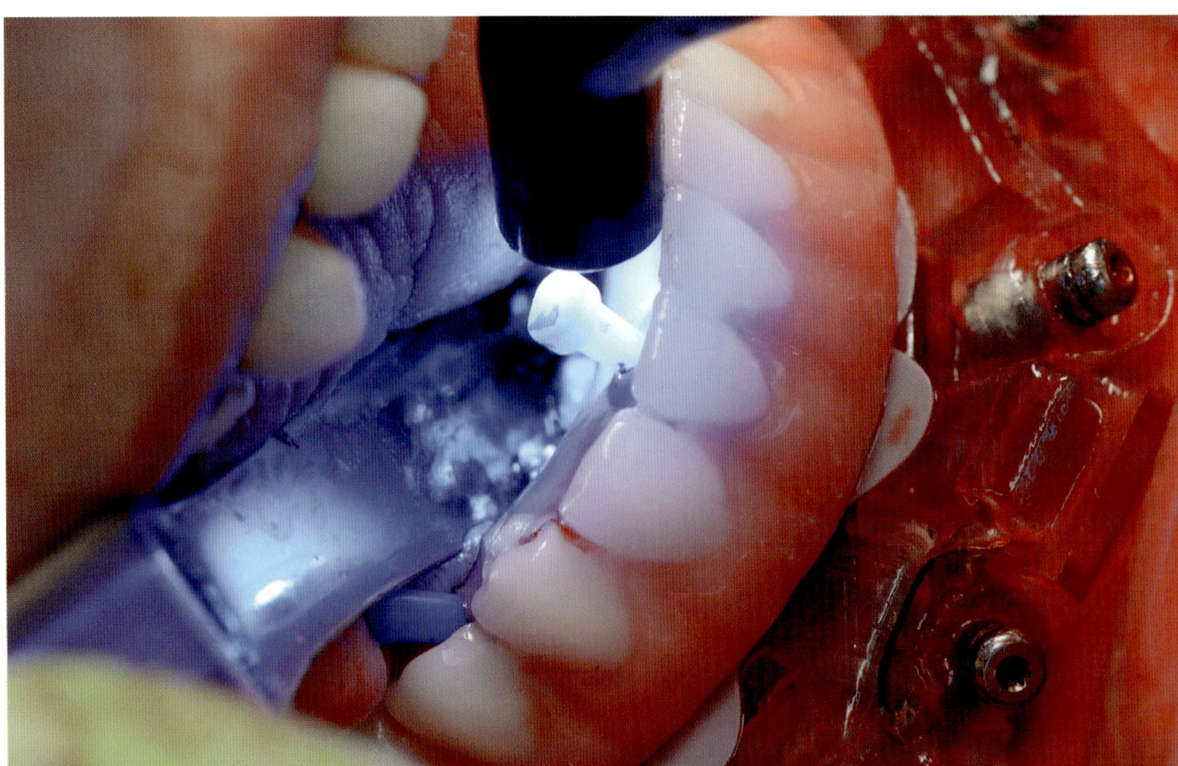

Figure 7.59 Light curing of the pick-up material around a temporary cylinder in the mandible with tongue retracted.

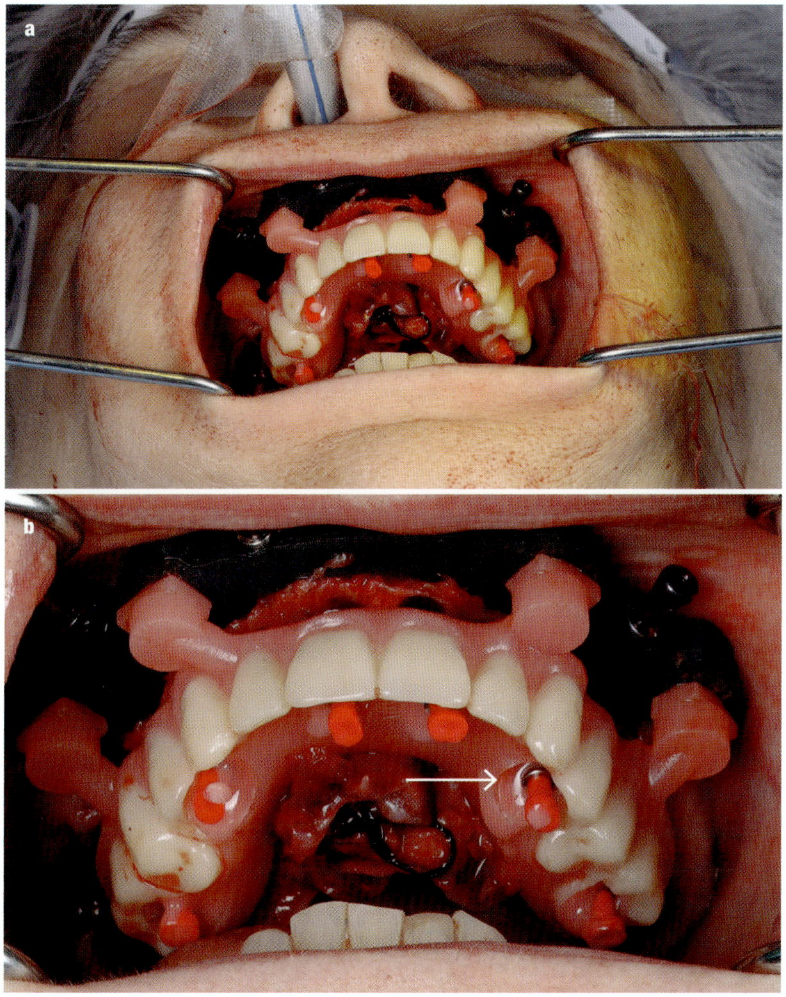

Figure 7.60 (a) Appearance of a maxillary interim prosthesis immediately after injection of acrylic resin into the temporary cylinder access holes; (b) Close-up view revealing incomplete fill around one temporary cylinder (*arrow*). Additional resin should be injected and light-cured before the prosthesis is removed.

I. Begin removing the prosthesis from the MUAs by extracting the block-out material or pins from the screw access channels, and then use a hand driver to remove the prosthetic screws.

If you do not feel some light resistance as you remove the prosthetic screw from each temporary cylinder, it is likely the cylinder was not completely seated. Thus, you should remove it from the prosthesis and repeat the process to pick up that cylinder again.

J. When the interim prosthesis is loose and all prosthetic screws have been removed, lift it off the MUAs. Carefully inspect the intaglio surface for any significant voids in pick-up material and wiggle each cylinder gently with your fingers or an instrument to make sure it is stable in the prosthesis.

If you detect any mobility, remove the temporary cylinder from the prosthesis, clean out that access opening, and repeat the process to pick up the temporary cylinder on that MUA. When doing this, be sure to screw the interim prosthesis back onto the MUAs in all the other (stable) sites so it is completely seated. Once you have confirmed all the temporary cylinders are stable, hand it off to a lab technician or trained team member to do the final clean-up and conversion (Fig. 7.61).

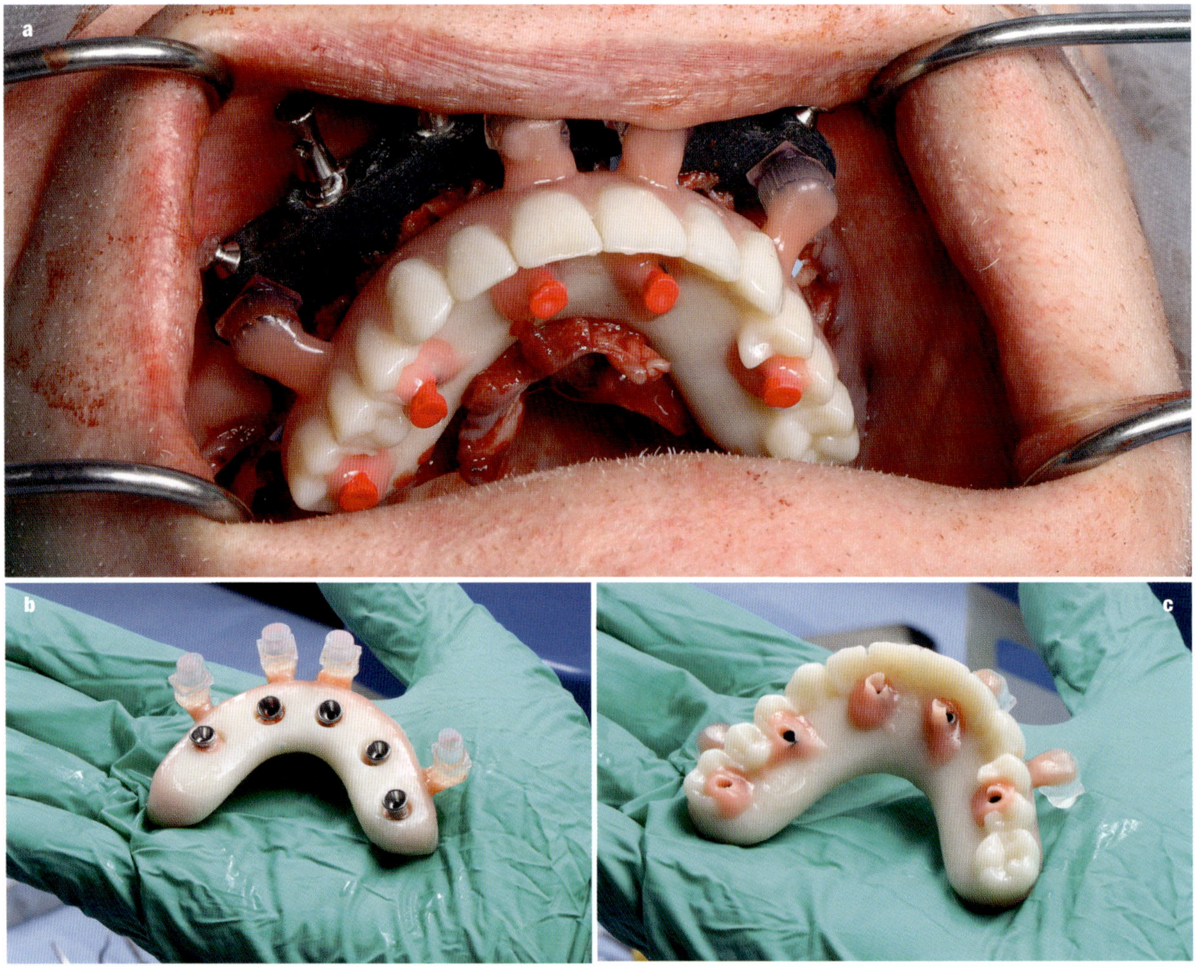

Figure 7.61 (a) Light-cured interim prosthesis ready for removal from the foundation guide; Inspection of the (b) intaglio and (c) occlusal surfaces of the interim prosthesis immediately after removal from the foundation guide.

STEP 11: REPLICA APPLIANCE PICK-UP

The replica appliance can play an important role in the future prosthetic workflow, as discussed in Chapter 4. It eliminates the need for a verification appliance or traditional verification jig, thus reducing the number of future appointments. In addition, it confirms the vertical dimension of occlusion (VDO), teeth position, and occlusion and records the soft tissues surrounding the implants, which can be used for development of the intaglio surface of the definitive prosthesis. During the prosthetic phase of treatment, it vastly improves the clinician's overall efficiency.

A. Employ the technique described in Step 10 for the interim prosthesis pick-up (or use your preferred technique) to complete the replica appliance pick-up.

The steps involved in the replica appliance pick-up are essentially the same as for the interim prosthesis pick-up (Figs. 7.62, 7.63). Whether you use a traditional or a newer, more advanced technique, no further steps are required once you have picked up your replica appliance and confirmed the stability of the temporary cylinders. Simply disinfect the replica appliance and set it aside with the case to be used during the prosthetic workflow phase in a few months.

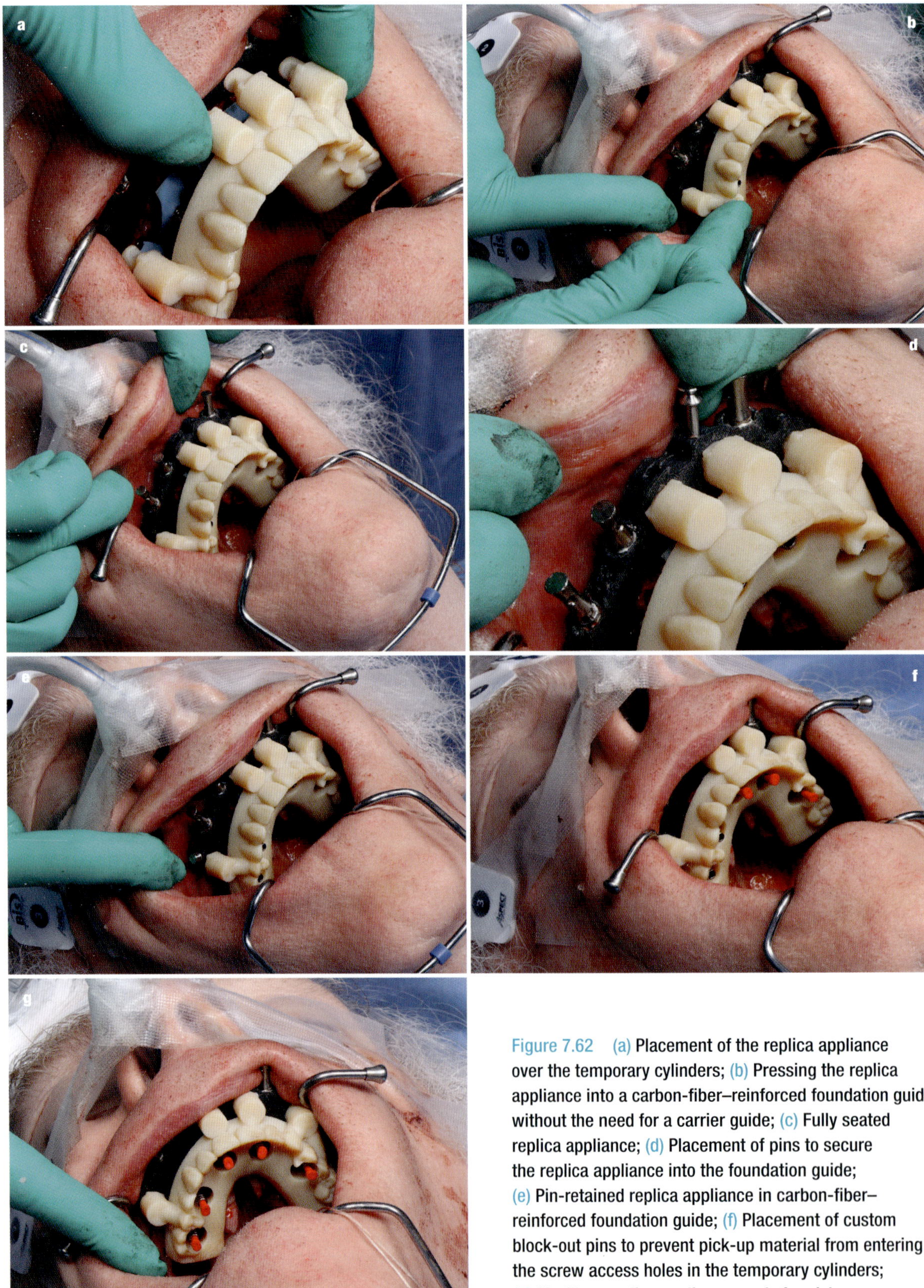

Figure 7.62 (a) Placement of the replica appliance over the temporary cylinders; (b) Pressing the replica appliance into a carbon-fiber–reinforced foundation guide without the need for a carrier guide; (c) Fully seated replica appliance; (d) Placement of pins to secure the replica appliance into the foundation guide; (e) Pin-retained replica appliance in carbon-fiber–reinforced foundation guide; (f) Placement of custom block-out pins to prevent pick-up material from entering the screw access holes in the temporary cylinders; (g) Maxillary replica appliance ready for pick-up.

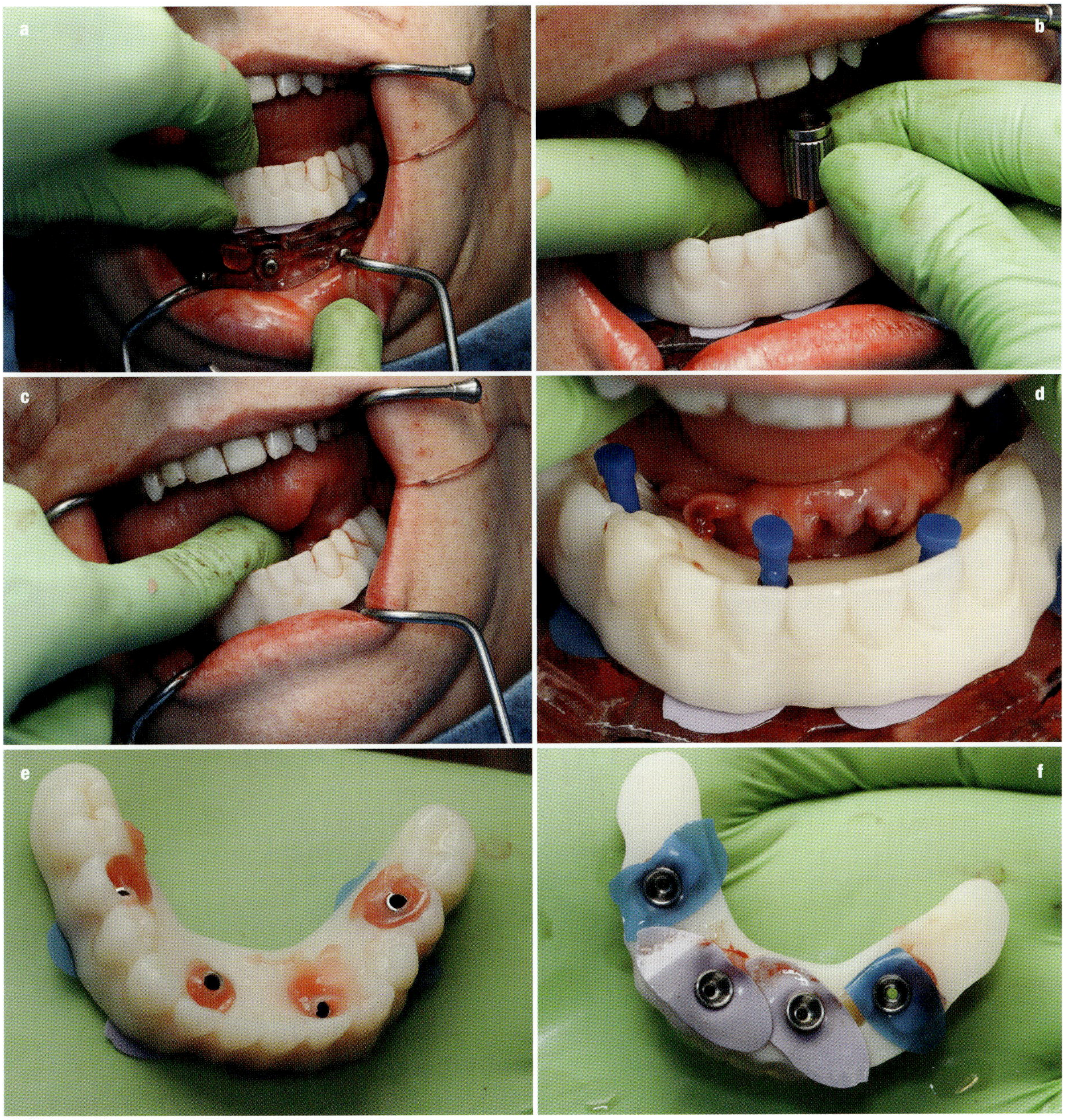

Figure 7.63 Preparations for the replica appliance pick-up using a carrier guide. (a) Placing the replica appliance on the carrier guide; (b) Placing the temporary cylinders through access holes in the replica appliance; (c) Confirming that the appliance is fully seated; (d) Custom block-out pins in place; Inspecting the (e) occlusal and (f) intaglio surfaces of the replica appliance after completing the pick-up and removing it from the carrier guide.

STEP 12: INTERIM PROSTHESIS CONVERSION

For a maximally efficient workflow, have a team member or lab assistant complete the conversion of the interim prosthesis. In our practice, we asked an experienced laboratory technician to teach the final conversion steps to one of our dental assistants, and she in turn trained other dental assistants. The doctor's time should be spent with the patient, wrapping up the surgery or starting surgery on the second arch. For best results and to avoid contaminating the surgical area, complete the conversion in a laboratory setting.

- **A.** Use a cleaning solution to disinfect the prosthesis and then rinse it under running water (Fig. 7.64a).

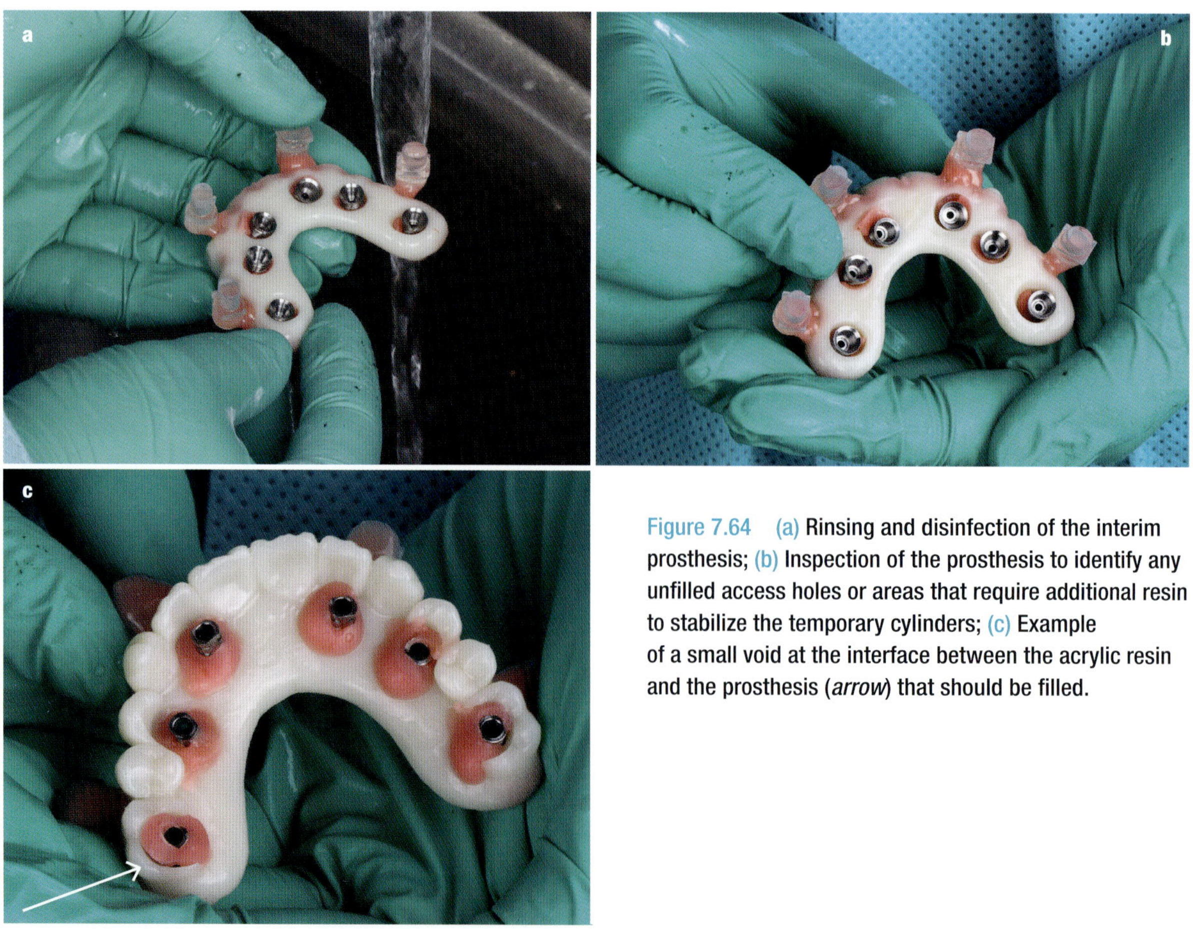

Figure 7.64 (a) Rinsing and disinfection of the interim prosthesis; (b) Inspection of the prosthesis to identify any unfilled access holes or areas that require additional resin to stabilize the temporary cylinders; (c) Example of a small void at the interface between the acrylic resin and the prosthesis (*arrow*) that should be filled.

B. After you dry the disinfected prosthesis, re-check the stability of the temporary cylinders visually and manually using a light touch. If any areas in the prosthesis are underfilled, use Stellar DC or another acrylic resin material to backfill and then cure them.

Take care not to overfill the areas around the cylinders to avoid creating more work for yourself during the finishing steps and to prevent material from flowing into the screw-access channels (Figs. 7.64b, 7.64c).

C. Once you are confident of the stability of the temporary cylinders, continue adding acrylic resin material in other areas where needed and removing any unnecessary material using the appropriate burs.

There are burs designed specifically for acrylic removal and those designed to cut through the temporary titanium cylinders. Using the correct bur will not only enhance the bur's lifespan but also prevent too much heat from being generated, which can deform and/or crack the temporary cylinders or the prosthesis itself (Figs. 7.65, 7.66).

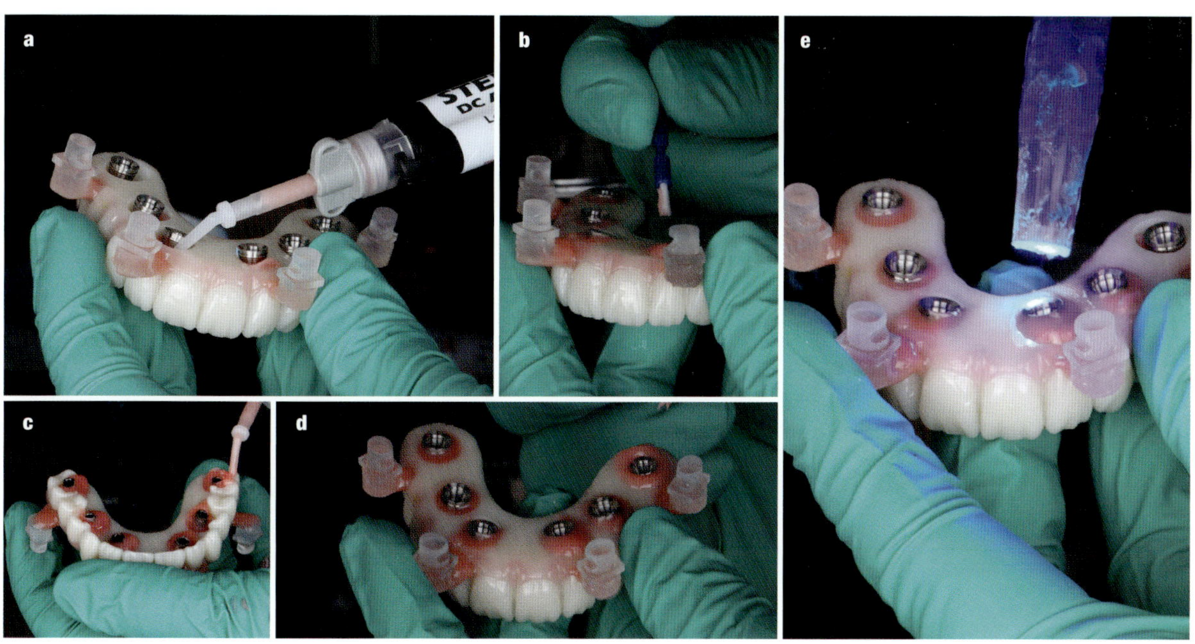

Figure 7.65 (a-e) Injection of Taub Stellar DC acrylic resin into areas of the interim prosthesis, followed by light curing.

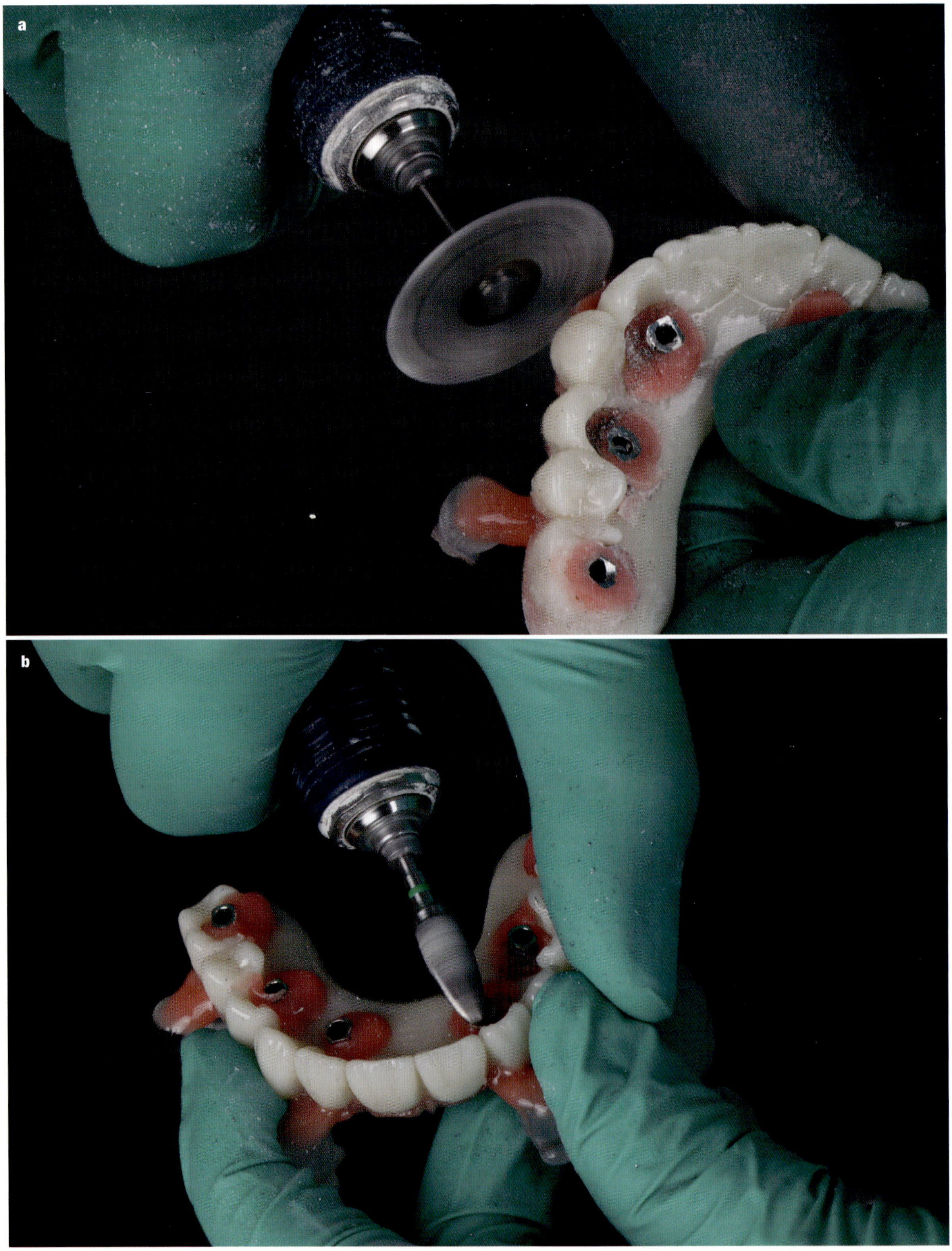

Figure 7.66 (a) Removal of stabilizer feet from the interim prosthesis using a specially designed disc;
(b) Reduction of the temporary cylinders using a Komet H251FSQ 060 prosthetic kit bur designed to cut through titanium.

D. If you use Stellar DC as a pick-up and fill material, consider placing the prosthesis in a warm water bath under pressure to strengthen the acrylic fill material.

We use a Drufomat Scan® pressure machine (Dentsply Sirona) in our office that applies pressure and heat at the same time. This strengthens the bond between the prosthesis and the pick-up material and hardens the Stellar DC as well (Fig. 7.67).

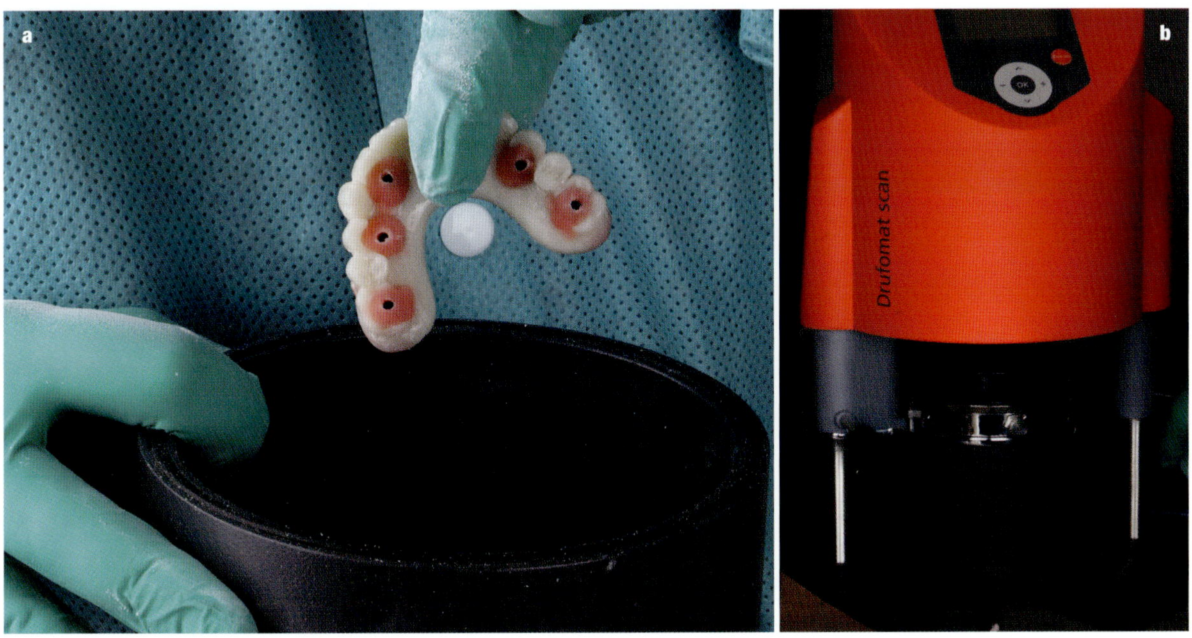

Figure 7.67 (a, b) Placement of the unfinished interim prosthesis into a warm water bath (Drufomat Scan® pressure machine [Dentsply Sirona]) to strengthen it under heat and pressure.

PRO TIP: Interim prosthesis conversion

When modifying the interim prosthesis, reduce the length of the cantilevers posterior to the screw access channels of the terminal implants. I generally try to limit cantilevers to no more than one tooth-length distal to the terminal temporary cylinder. This prevents accidental breakage when the patient is chewing, bruxing, or engaging in other parafunctional habits. For the definitive prosthesis, which is more resistant to flexing and breakage, different rules apply.

- **E.** Once you are satisfied with the strength and durability of the prosthesis, use the burs in the Komet prosthetic kit to contour, finish, and polish it. As a final touch, I like to apply a glaze to the prosthesis that I paint on and then cure (Figs. 7.68a-7.68c).

A laboratory light-curing unit is much more efficient than the handheld curing lights used during clinical procedures (Fig. 7.68d).

- **F.** After adjusting, finishing, polishing, and glazing the interim prosthesis, perform a final inspection and then return it to the surgical suite (Figs. 7.68e-7.68h).

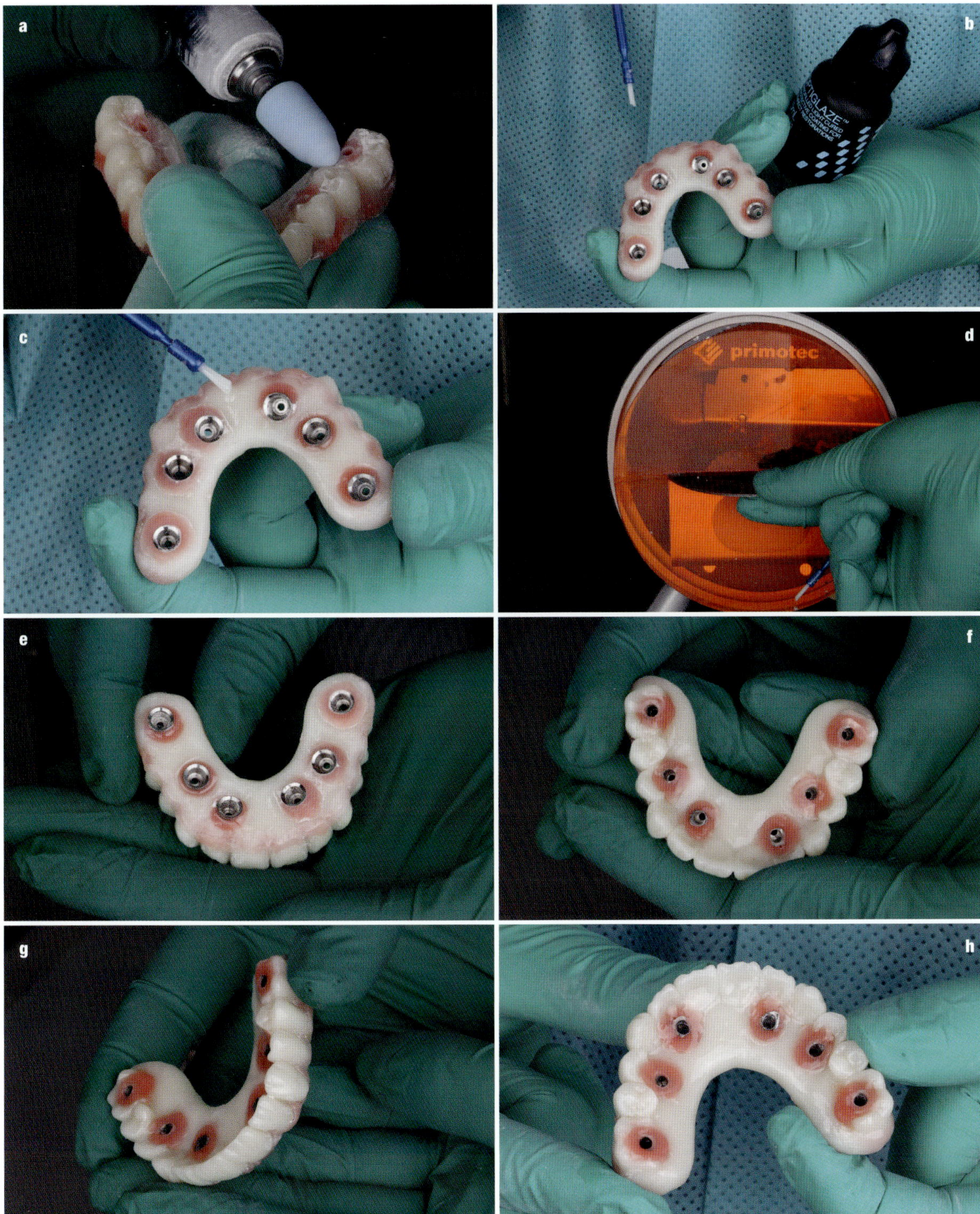

Figure 7.68 Final steps in the prosthesis conversion process. (a) Polishing the interim prosthesis; (b) Applying a glaze (Optiglaze® [GC America]) over the interim prosthesis; (c) Close-up view of glaze application to the intaglio surface of the interim prosthesis; (d) Using a laboratory light-curing system to finalize the glazing process of the interim prosthesis; (e-g) Performing the final inspection of the interim prosthesis after glazing; (h) Appearance of the interim prosthesis once it is ready for intraoral placement.

STEP 13: CLOSING AND SUTURING

The final surgical step is closing and suturing. During this step you will also proceed with any procedures such as bone grafting and/or placing membranes, platelet-rich fibrin (PRF), or any other biologics.

A. If you are confident of the accuracy of the pick-up of the interim prosthesis and/or replica appliance, release the foundation guide from the bone by removing the pins or screws used to secure it.

Remember that once you have removed the foundation guide and closed the tissues, putting it back in place can be difficult and may not be accurate. I usually begin this process immediately after the interim prosthesis has been taken to the laboratory for conversion and I have finished the pick-up of the replica appliance (Figs. 7.69a-7.69e).

B. Place the healing caps on the MUAs and manually tighten them.

Healing caps help you avoid overtightening the sutures and make delivering the interim prosthesis much easier (Figs. 7.69f, 7.69g).

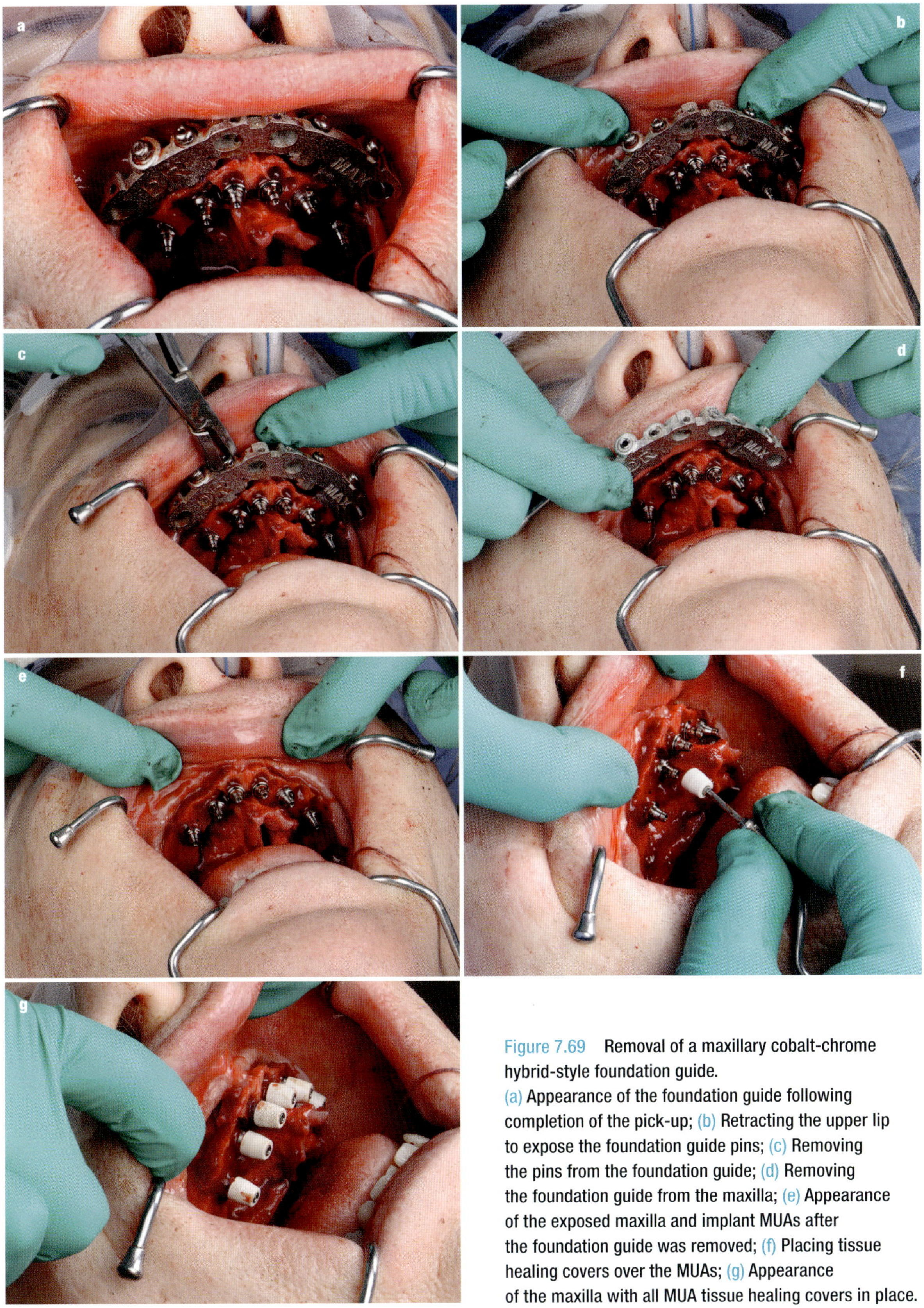

Figure 7.69 Removal of a maxillary cobalt-chrome hybrid-style foundation guide.
(a) Appearance of the foundation guide following completion of the pick-up; (b) Retracting the upper lip to expose the foundation guide pins; (c) Removing the pins from the foundation guide; (d) Removing the foundation guide from the maxilla; (e) Appearance of the exposed maxilla and implant MUAs after the foundation guide was removed; (f) Placing tissue healing covers over the MUAs; (g) Appearance of the maxilla with all MUA tissue healing covers in place.

C. Carefully examine the arch, looking for any areas that would benefit from grafting and/or membrane/PRF placement. Also, perform socket preservation if necessary and/or graft around any implants that require it (Figs. 7.70-7.72).

Note: *If you plan to use PRF or other biologics that take time to prepare, consider preparing them earlier in the workflow. In our practice, we usually draw blood and begin preparation while doing the pick-up for the interim prosthesis and replica appliance.*

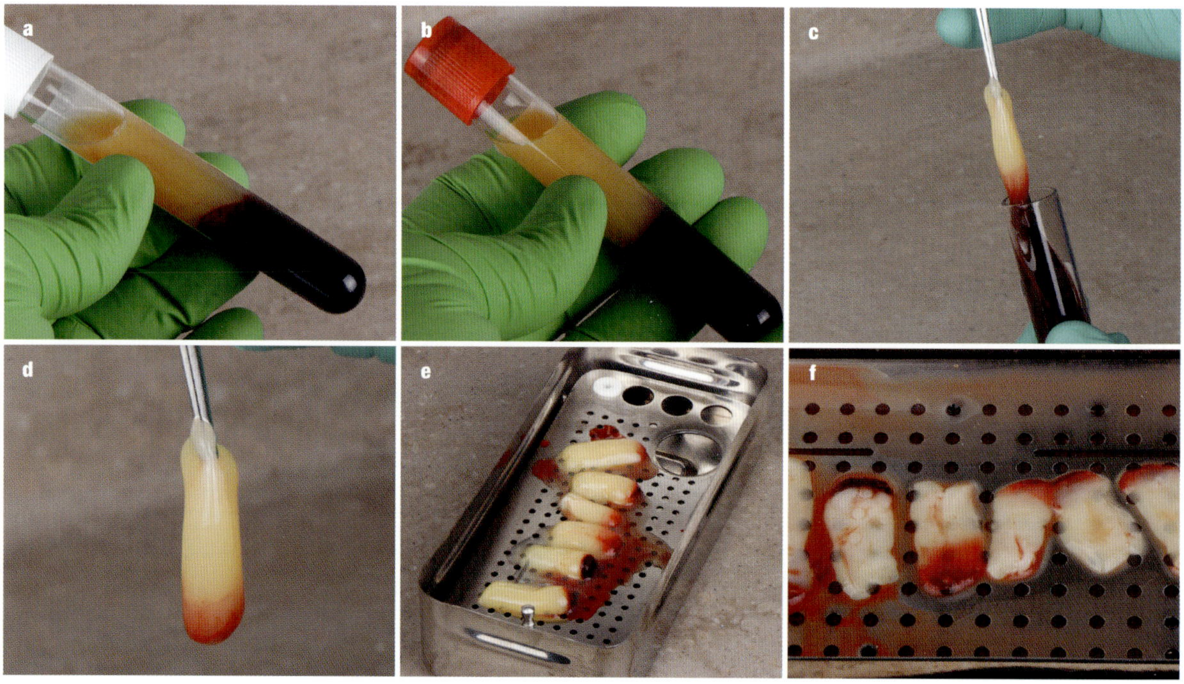

Figure 7.70 Preparation of platelet-rich fibrin (PRF) and PRF membranes. (a) The white-top test tube contains patient blood that has been centrifuged to create PRF liquid; (b) The red-top test tube contains patient blood that has been centrifuged and allowed to clot; (c) Tweezers are used to extract a fibrin clot from the red-top test tube; (d) Close-up view of the fibrin clot, which contains a concentration of platelets and growth factors; (e) Six fibrin clots placed in a PRF membrane box that is used to compress them into membrane configuration; (f) Appearance of the PRF membranes ready for placement.

PRO TIP: Closing and suturing, part 1

I am a big fan of platelet-rich fibrin (PRF) membranes and liquid and its applications in full-arch surgery. If you utilize PRF in your practice, use a tissue punch to hold PRF membranes more securely in place over implants and ridges. Punch a hole in the PRF membrane, then place it over the MUA healing cap and cover the ridge and any grafting material or other membranes that are being used. This punch technique works to stabilize most other membrane materials as well. PRF can also be used to create sticky bone, which is an excellent adjunct for bone grafting.

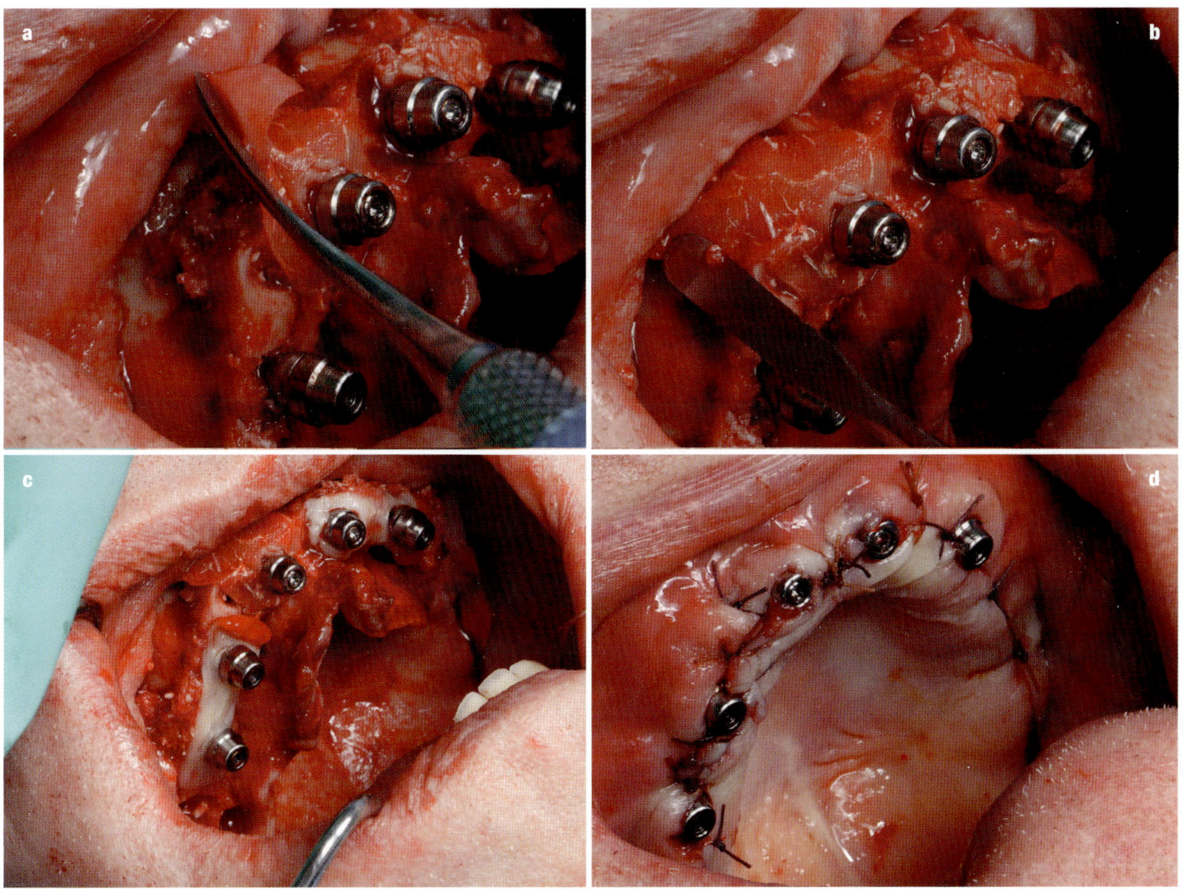

Figure 7.71 Guided bone regeneration (GBR) procedure performed after placement of implants and MUAs in the maxilla. (a) Particulate bone grafting; (b) Placing a resorbable collagen membrane (Striate+® [Orthocell]); (c) Placing PRF membranes over defects; (d) Final suturing and closure.

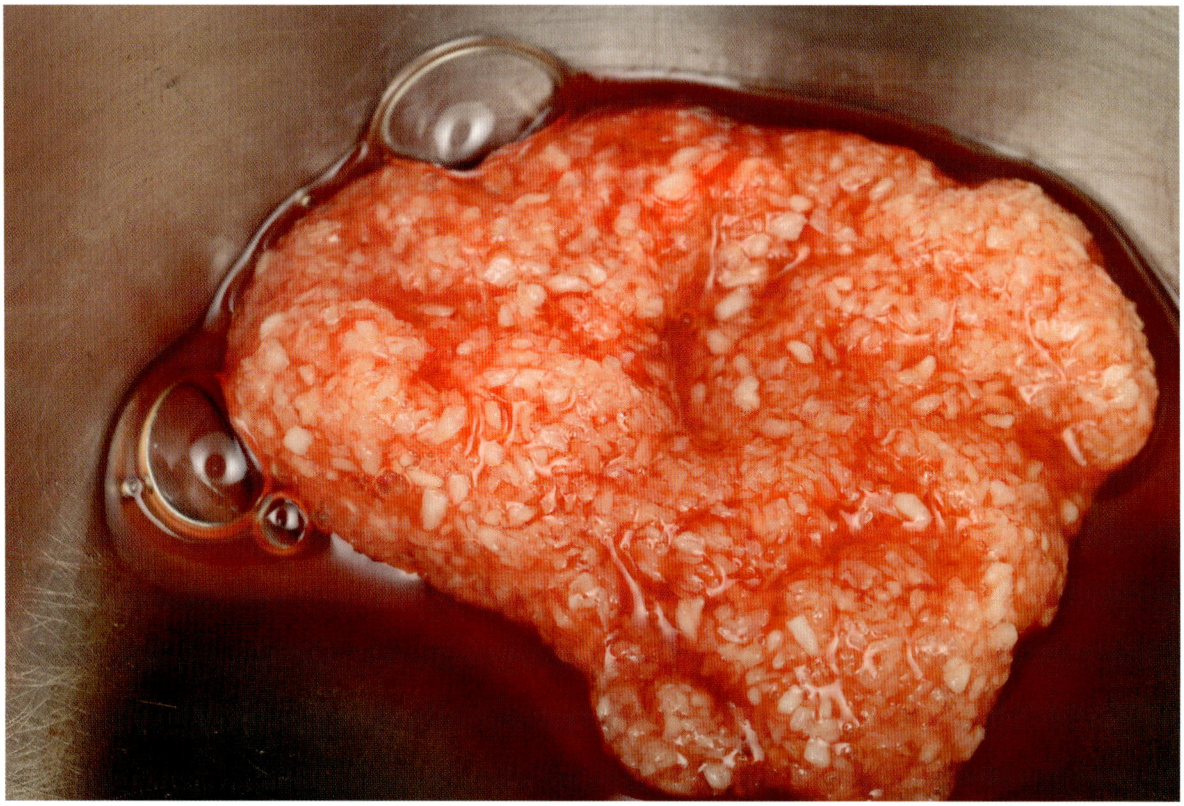

Figure 7.72 **Composite bone graft known as sticky bone, consisting of bone allograft, PRF liquid, and PRF fibrin clots, often used in full-arch implant cases to fill larger defects and for socket preservation.**

D. After advancing the flap over the ridge (and any grafting or membrane materials used), begin suturing the keratinized tissue to obtain primary closure. Use your preferred technique or the one you deem most appropriate for the case, but avoid over- or undertightening the sutures.

Generally, I begin with an interrupted suture technique using a synthetic absorbable material such as polyglycolic acid (PGA) and suturing the PRF into the keratinized tissue of the flap. This can be done efficiently and provides an adequate amount of stability. I then use chromic gut sutures to repair any small tears in the tissues or to close areas in the posterior regions not covered by the interim prosthesis (Figs. 7.73, 7.74).

Often, the amount of attached keratinized tissue in the mandible is insufficient. Keratinized tissue is precious, and each MUA should be surrounded by as wide a band as possible. If your abutments have a deficient amount of keratinized tissue around them after healing, you may

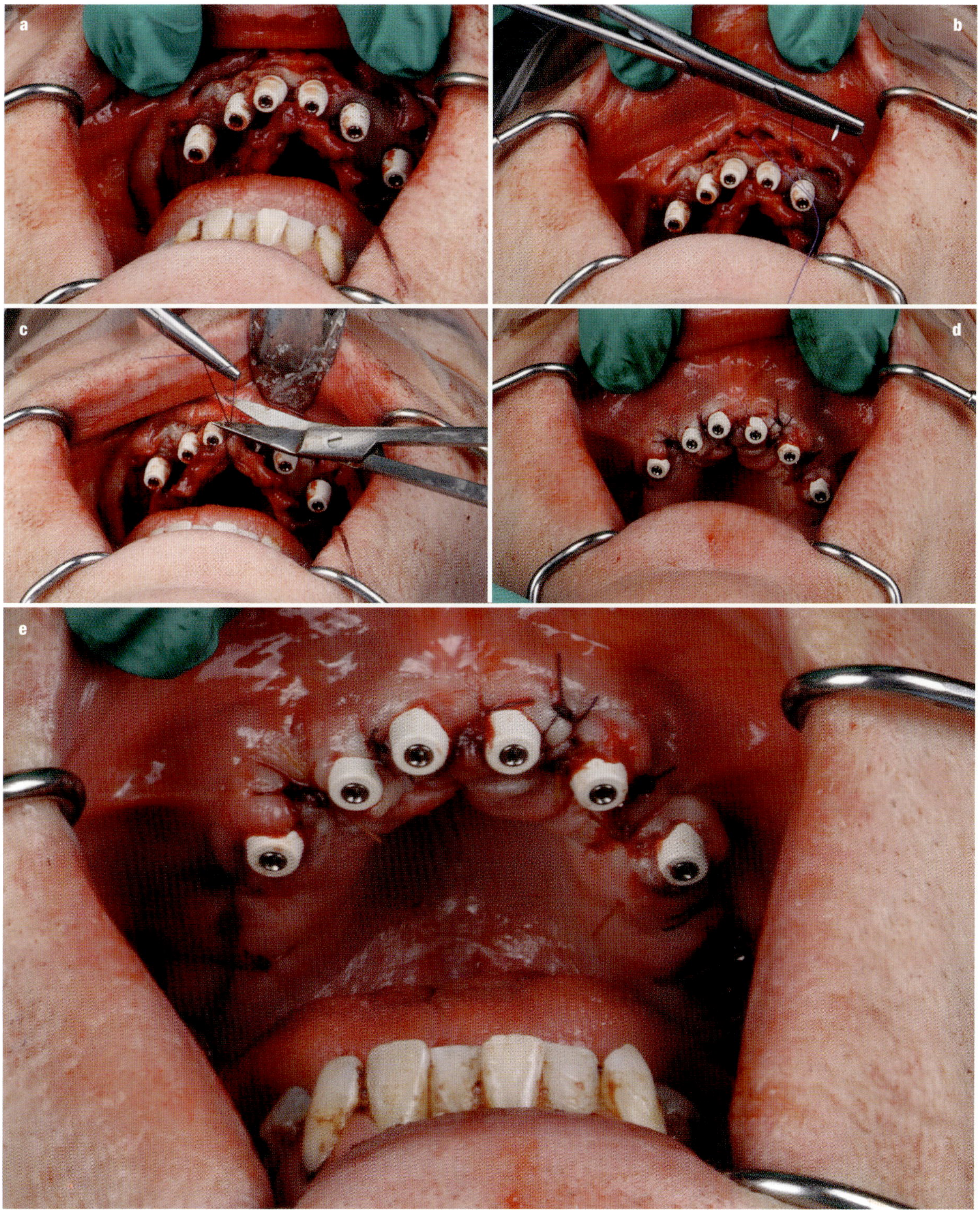

Figure 7.73 (a) Tissue healing covers placed over MUAs, holding PRF membranes in place in the maxilla; (b) Primary closure of the keratinized tissue over the membranes using polyglycolic acid (PGA) suture material and an interrupted suturing technique; (c) The upper lip is carefully retracted to avoid injury when cutting suture tails; (d) Appearance of maxilla after suturing around the MUAs is completed; (e) Close-up view of completed suturing showing a combination of interrupted PGA and chromic gut sutures.

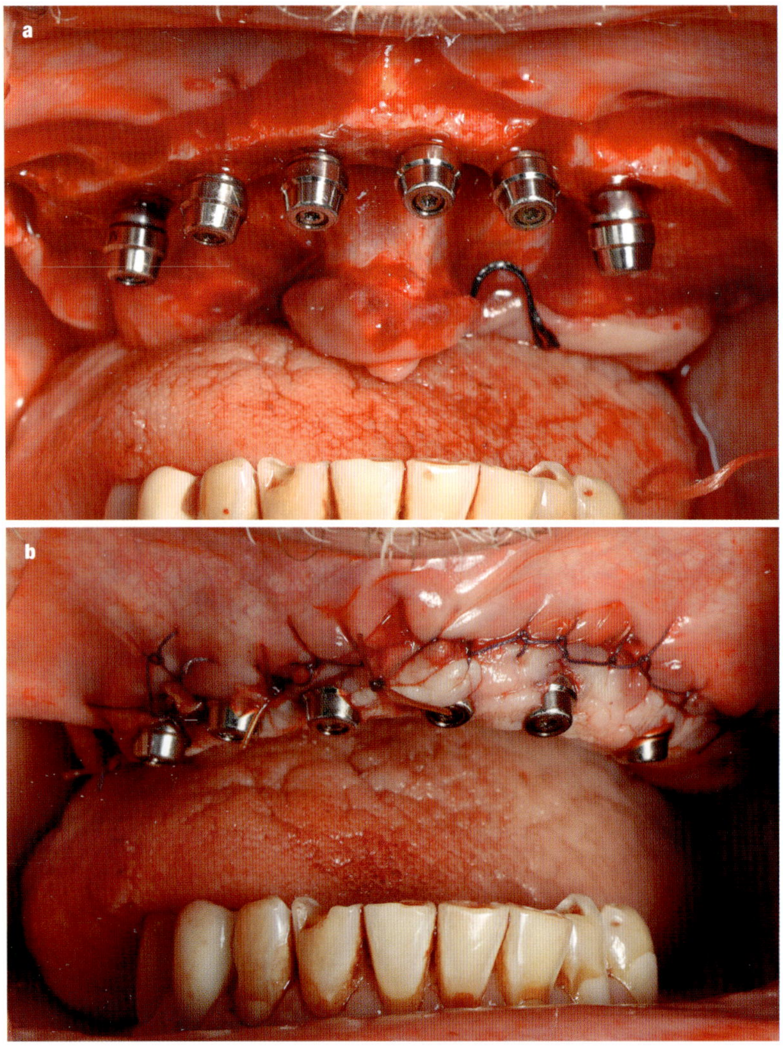

Figure 7.74 (a) Appearance immediately before suturing to close tissue in the maxilla with healing caps in place; (b) After tissue suturing with PGA and chromic gut sutures to achieve primary closure.

have to discuss the need for additional grafting with your patient to ensure the longevity and health of the implant(s). According to Dr. Pamela S. Ray, a board-certified periodontist whom I consulted, preserving the attached keratinized tissue on the lingual or palatal aspect is recommended in situations where keratinized tissue is limited and soft tissue grafting is indicated (Ray PS, personal discussion, 2021). This is because soft tissue grafting on the buccal or facial aspect is easier and more predictable (Fig. 7.75). In dual-arch cases, excess keratinized tissue can sometimes be harvested from the maxilla at the time of surgery and used to graft around deficient areas in the mandible. Keep this in mind as one possible strategy to avoid the need for additional surgical procedures in the future.

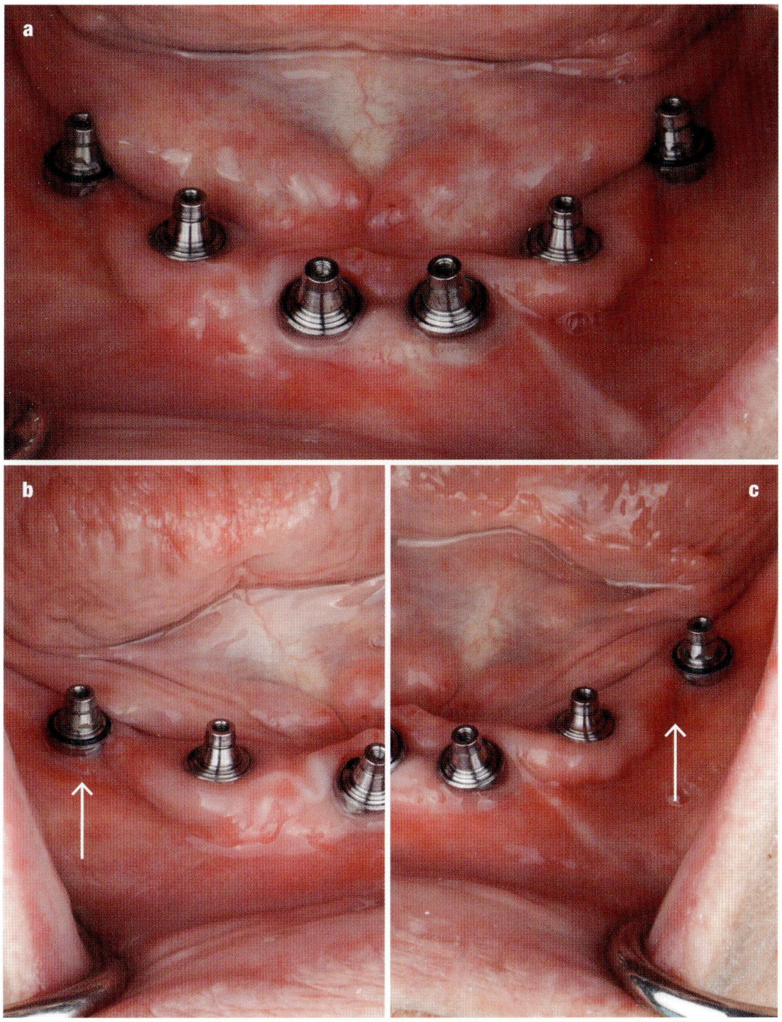

Figure 7.75 (a) Appearance of the implant MUAs at the end of the healing period; (b, c) Close-up views showing the inadequate amount of keratinized tissue around the two terminal MUAs (*arrows*).

PRO TIP: Closing and suturing, part 2

After bone reduction in the maxilla, there is often an excess amount of palatal tissue present. As noted in Step 4, this tissue can often be stretched anteriorly and, using a tissue punch, suspended over the MUAs, similar to the technique described in "PRO TIP: Closing and suturing, part 1".

STEP 14: SEATING OF THE FINISHED INTERIM PROSTHESIS

A. Carefully inspect and then remove the healing caps from the MUAs (Fig. 7.76).

Complete this step as quickly as possible so the tissue does not have time to relax over the MUAs. To increase the visibility of the MUA, it might be helpful to apply pressure to the tissue immediately after a healing cap is removed using a moistened 4 × 4 gauze.

B. Place the interim prosthesis over the tissue and MUAs and press down until you feel the prosthesis seat. Using both hands, check for any rocking or instability of the prosthesis on the MUAs.

If one area of the prosthesis does not seat completely, it is possible that a temporary cylinder was not picked up correctly and will need to be removed and picked up again. However, it is more likely that the prosthesis pick-up was accurate but the soft tissue is creating some resistance.

It is not unusual to encounter resistance from excess tissue when placing the interim prosthesis over the MUAs and ridge, especially in the maxilla. However, the solution is not to force the prosthesis in place by putting excessive pressure on the tissue, which can lead to tissue necrosis during healing. Some of the excess tissue around the MUAs may need to be removed to allow for complete seating, but be careful to preserve a keratinized band around them. In time, the tissue will readhere to the bone and shrink, so do not try to thin it too much. If you are patient, in most cases you will be able to secure the prosthesis to the MUAs.

C. Place prosthetic screws into the reduced temporary cylinder openings in the interim prosthesis and manually tighten each one on the MUAs.

I recommend doing this in a cross-arch pattern instead of tightening the screws on each MUA consecutively. Once all the screws have been hand-tightened, go back and torque each screw to the appropriate value for your implant system (Fig. 7.77).

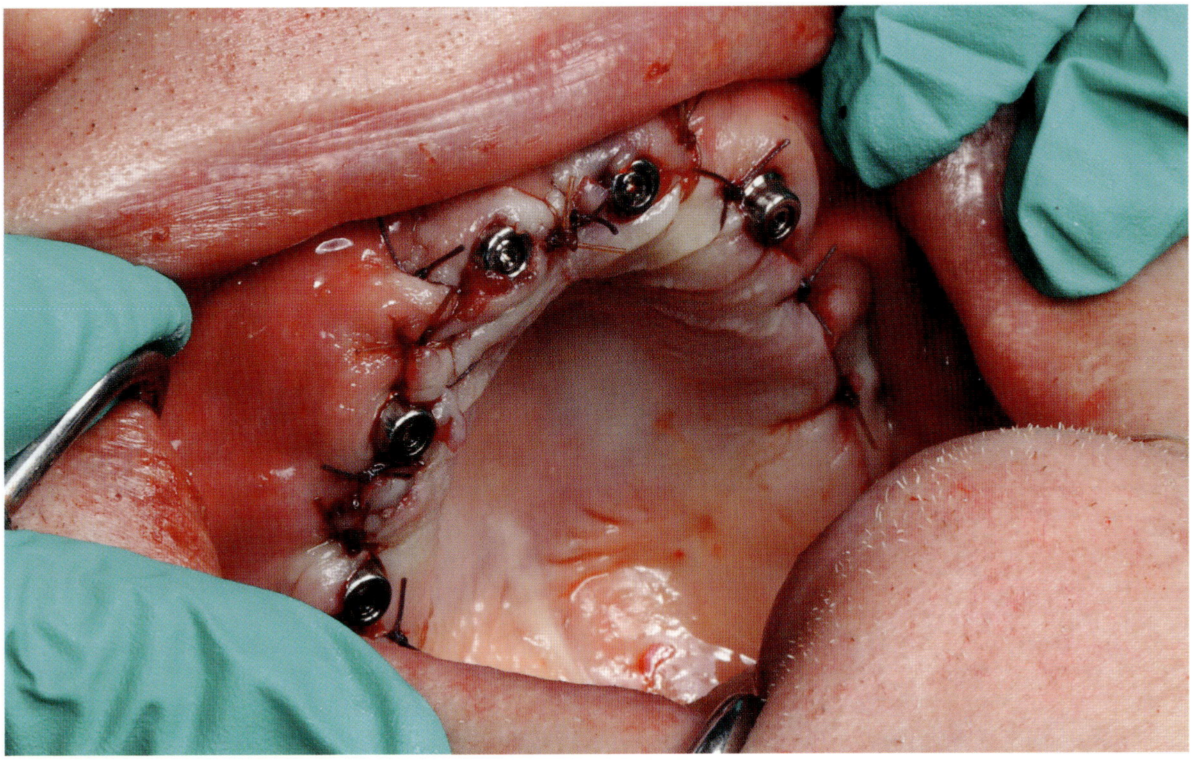

Figure 7.76 **Sutured maxillary tissue around healing caps that are ready to be removed.**

PRO TIP: Interim prosthesis, part 1

If the prosthesis will not seat completely, the problem might be that the tissue is creating too much resistance. The interim prosthesis should not overcompress or cause the tissue to blanch. To prevent future discomfort for the patient as well as tissue necrosis and other possible complications, consider the following steps:

- Apply firm pressure on the tissue for several minutes with the prosthesis, then identify any areas where the tissue prevents it from fully seating. Carefully thin the tissue in that area or remove it from around the MUA(s) with a tissue punch or scalpel. If that does not allow the prosthesis to seat properly, consider the next step.
- Remove the prosthesis and create more space on the intaglio surface of the prosthesis in areas where the compression is occurring. After making these adjustments, polish and re-glaze.

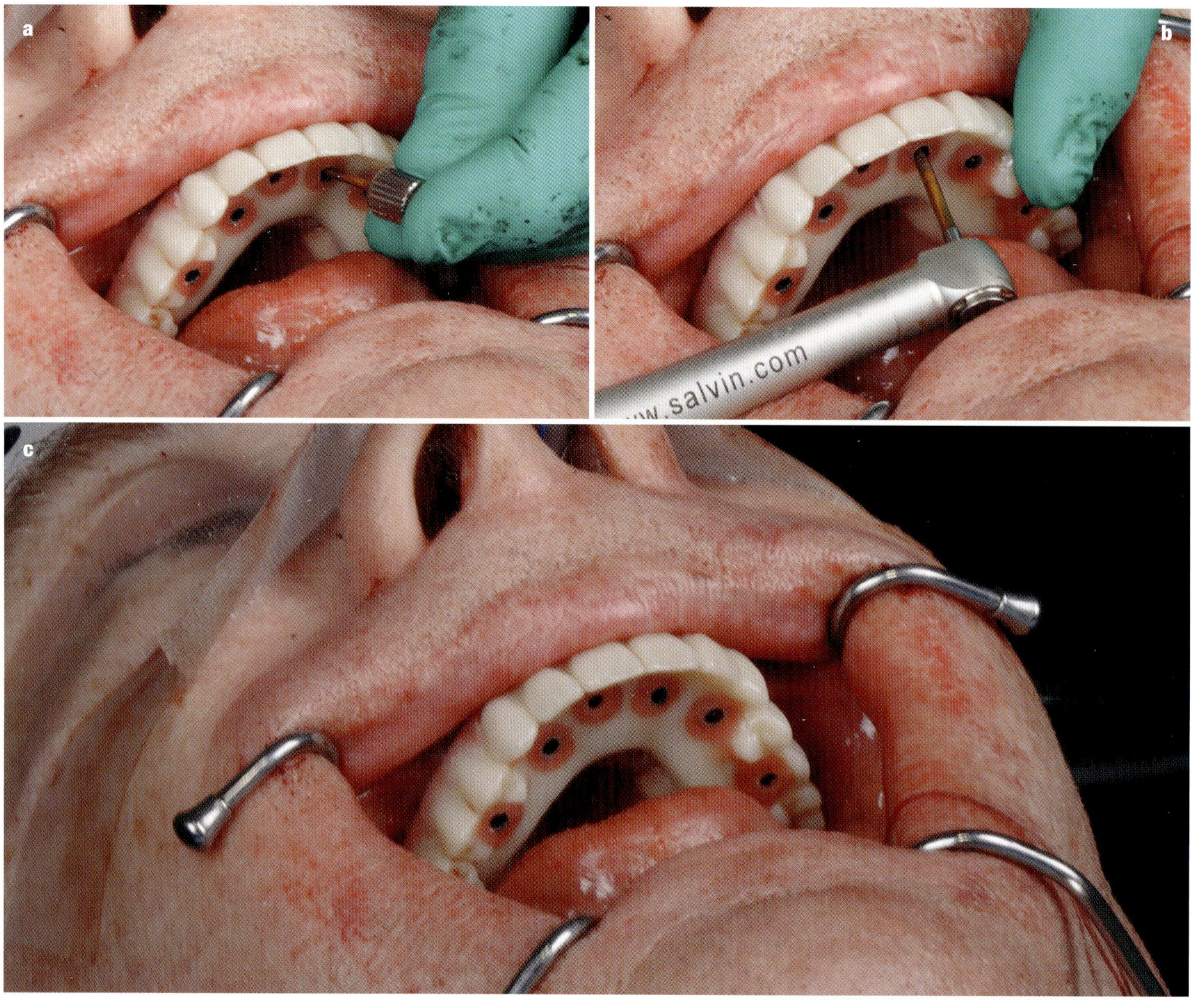

Figure 7.77 (a) Hand driver used to hand tighten prosthetic screws in interim prosthesis; (b) Final torquing of prosthetic screws through the interim prosthesis; (c) Interim prosthesis fully seated and torqued in place over the MUAs.

D. Once the prosthetic screws are in place and there is no longer a choking hazard, remove the throat pack and/or any other throat protection used.

If the patient is under general anesthesia, be sure to alert the anesthesiologist or CRNA and the rest of the team by declaring this out loud and documenting it (Fig. 7.78).

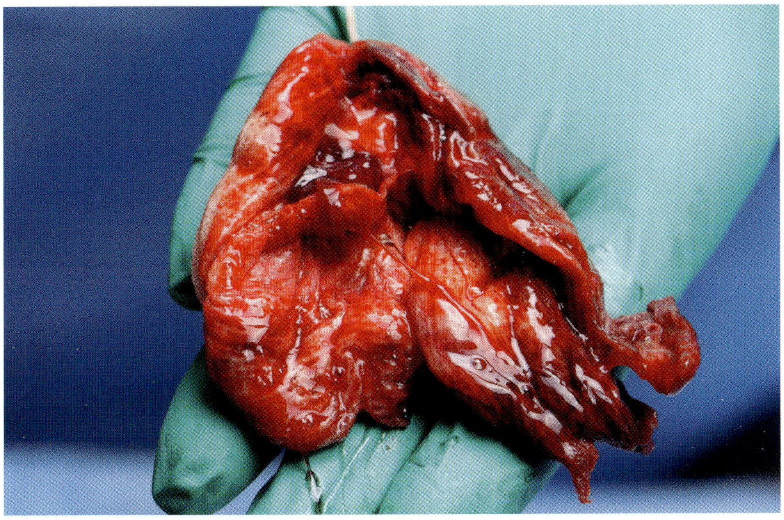

Figure 7.78 Appearance of throat pack upon removal, demonstrating the amount of blood and debris it blocks, thus preventing aspiration or ingestion of these materials and reducing postoperative nausea and vomiting.

E. With the interim prosthesis torqued in place, close the patient into maximal intercuspal position (MIP) (Figs. 7.79-7.81). If necessary, make slight adjustments to the prosthesis or the opposing arch.

The occlusion of the prosthesis against the opposing arch is an important consideration and requires some balance. In some cases where the VDO is opened, this may result in more of a Class II type of occlusal relationship, with a slight anterior open bite. Usually this can be compensated for during the planning stages. Fine-tuning of the patient's occlusion will be carried out during the postoperative phase and follow-up appointments.

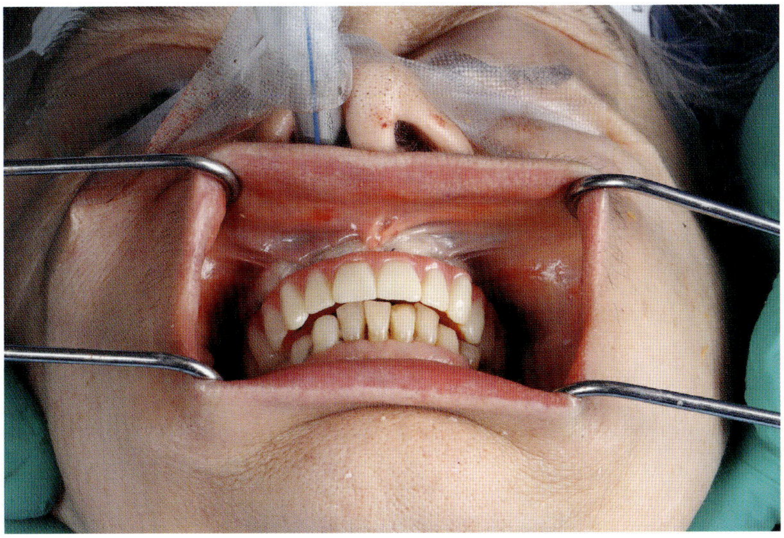

Figure 7.79 Closing patient into MIP.

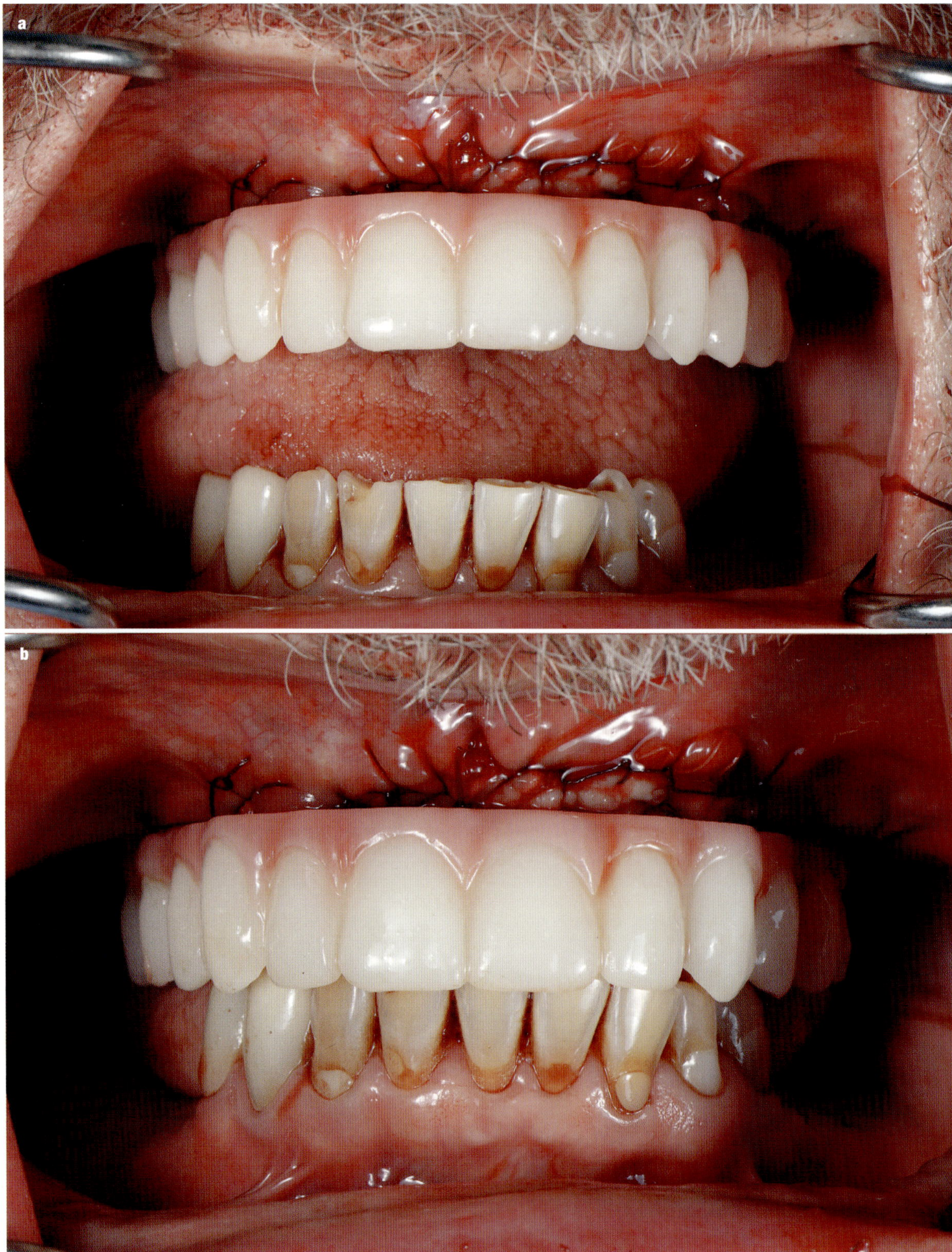

Figure 7.80 Close-up view of the patient's occlusion after placement of the interim prosthesis. (a) Seating of maxillary interim prosthesis; (b) Closing the patient into MIP.

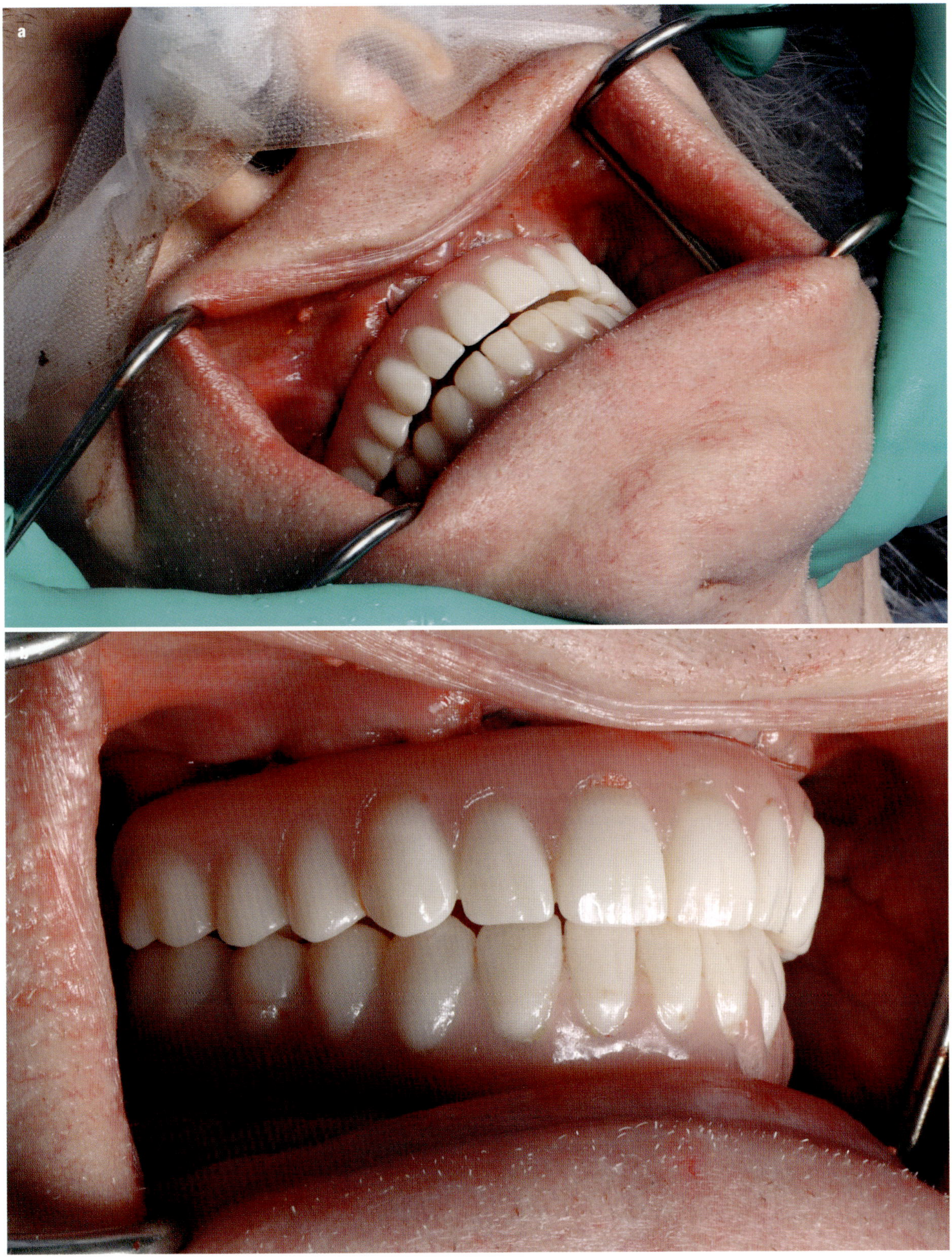

Figure 7.81 (a, b) Checking the occlusion of maxillary and mandibular prostheses in a dual-arch case.

F. To seal the access channels, inject a medium- to heavy-body PVS material over the screws and wipe away any excess (Fig. 7.82).

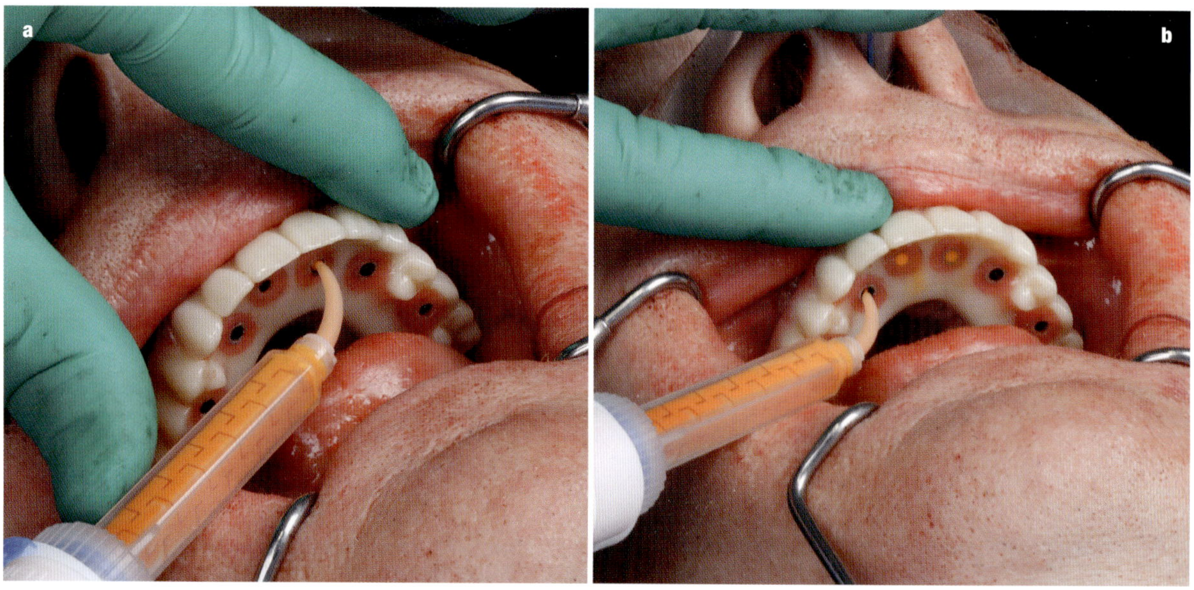

Figure 7.82 (a, b) Injection of heavy-body PVS impression material into screw access channels.

PRO TIP: Interim prosthesis, part 2

In the rare instances when the occlusion or esthetics of the interim prosthesis are considerably off target, the laboratory can remake the prosthesis quite easily. During the surgical visit or at a postoperative appointment, use the replica appliance to obtain a correct vertical dimension of occlusion (VDO). Take a digital or analog impression of the opposing arch and a maxillomandibular relationship record. Send the replica appliance and other data to the lab and ask them to create a new interim prosthesis with the appropriate occlusion. Note that this happens very infrequently in my practice and is almost always a result of improper placement of the foundation guide or inadequate bone reduction in the posterior regions. It may also be a consequence of poor case engineering and planning. Always check for passivity of fit in your interim prosthesis and replica appliance on the foundation or carrier guide.

STEP 15: POSTSURGICAL PROCEDURES

After the surgery, your patient should be placed in recovery. If the patient was sedated or received general anesthesia, as is often the case in my practice, you will have some time to clean up. It is desirable to have the patient in a comfortable resting position in a clean operatory when they come out of recovery. To complete the patient's visit, I recommend the following:

A. Check and record postoperative vital signs and follow the postoperative discharge paperwork.

Our patients generally arrange to have a family member or friend drive them home and help them get settled. Because patients may not remember everything you tell them on the day of surgery, it is best to give written postoperative instructions to the patient before the surgery, along with any prescribed antibiotics, postoperative pain medications, etc. These can be brought to surgery and started immediately or taken on the way home.

B. Consider giving the patient a kit or gift bag of items to take home that will make their experience more comfortable.

Providing a kit or gift bag creates a lasting impression and may set your practice apart from your competitors. In our practice, we include the following:

- Additional postoperative and hygiene instructions
- Ice packs
- A water flosser unit and an extra-soft toothbrush
- A nutritional protein drink
- A VEGA® Oral Care Recovery Kit (StellaLife) and/or an Implant Post-Op Care System (Ora-Care) to reduce the need for narcotic pain medications and steroids as well as to promote healing after surgery.

C. Schedule and/or confirm the first postoperative appointment.

We arrange this to occur within 1 week of the patient's surgery. I usually give the patient 3 to 5 days to recover at home before having to travel back to the office for what could potentially be an uncomfortable visit. Usually within 3 days, most of the swelling and postoperative pain are resolved, and the patient is able drive to the appointment without the need for a companion.

D. Once the patient has left, make sure you or your team sets aside the surgical components of the guide as well as the replica appliance(s).

These components should be sterilized and stored in a safe place for future use. We use the lab box in which the case was delivered to us labeled with the patient's name written in permanent marker. It only takes one time for a patient's case to be misplaced to create stress and a less-efficient prosthetic workflow. Have your team get in the habit of organizing your cases in a safe place in the office where they can be retrieved easily in the future.

E. It should go without saying that the surgical room as well as all the instruments should be autoclaved/sterilized or decontaminated after surgery.

Ideally this should be accomplished right after the patient leaves and before the team leaves for the day.

PRO TIP: Postoperative management, part 1

The day after surgery, it is good form for one of your clinical team members to call the patient to check in and offer encouragement. The patient will often have questions about how the surgery went and may need some guidance on their postoperative care. This also provides an opportunity to confirm the date and time of the first postoperative visit. For additional patient-care points, make this call yourself.

STEP 16: POSTOPERATIVE APPOINTMENTS

After a complex surgical procedure, it is important to see your patient for postoperative appointments, although the number of visits and what takes place at each may vary depending on the patient and any complications that arise.

In my practice, I use a systematic approach to postoperative visits not unlike the one I follow in my surgical and prosthetic workflows. These postoperative appointments have been shaped by many years of practice and what I found provided the best results and experience for my patients. Sometimes clinicians teaching fixed full-arch dentistry gloss over postoperative visit details or even skip them entirely. Taking even a little time with patients postoperatively sends the message that you are concerned about their well-being and enables you to detect potential complications after surgery and in a timely manner. Scheduled properly, these visits do not have to consume a lot of valuable time in your schedule, as much of the appointment can be delegated to a properly trained auxiliary team member. In most cases, I do not schedule these appointments ahead of time because some patients require fewer of them than others.

The first two postoperative visits take about 20 minutes each, whereas the others should take 15 minutes or less and most of that is spent with members of your team. Think of these appointments more as a check or exam in hygiene. They are often double-booked in my practice next to other operative and surgical appointments.

In cases where a patient travels a long distance, we may reduce the number of appointments after the first two. In cases where a patient has complications or requires more attention, postoperative appointments may be closer together and/or require more time. Ultimately, how you manage these appointments is up to you. The guidelines that follow are intended as a practical method that enables predictable scheduling.

Timing and sequence

Postoperative visit no. one: 3 to 5 days after surgery

- **Oral and extraoral examination.** At this visit, the patient may still be experiencing mild swelling, pain, and some bruising, but generally patients have "crested the mountain," as I describe it, and are starting to feel better. Pay close attention to whether the patient's sutures are still intact, and look for any signs of infection or abnormal swelling.
- **Intraoral examination of the prosthesis.** Look for cracks or signs of delamination in the prosthesis.
- **Occlusion.** At this point, just try to make the patient comfortable with their occlusion. Due to swelling, changes to the patient's original VDO, and muscle function, the occlusion may continue to change. Use articulating paper to see where contacts are. Adjust as needed, but try to keep the occlusal contacts more toward the canine/premolar areas than in the posterior region and away from cantilevers.
- **Encouragement and reinforcement of postoperative instructions.** Giving the patient verbal encouragement is good for their mental well-being and creates trust. Have a team member review the instructions for using take-home mouth rinses, sprays, and/or gels for tissue management as well as other oral hygiene instructions. Typically, we only have patients brush their teeth very softly with an extra-soft toothbrush. Dietary restrictions should be reiterated; we simplify this by telling patients they should only eat foods they can cut with a plastic fork. We have given patients plastic forks in their take-home kits in the past as a visual reminder. Patients should also be advised to continue postoperative antibiotic therapy until completed.

Because patients may still be experiencing postoperative pain, we generally encourage them to continue using ice packs on the face and under the jaw as needed and to start weening themselves off any opioids they may have been prescribed. Most healthy patients will do well with 500–1,000 mg acetaminophen or paracetamol every 6 hours in addition to 400–600 mg ibuprofen or the equivalent dose of another nonsteroidal anti-inflammatory drug (NSAID).

Postoperative visit no. two: 2 weeks after surgery

- **Oral and prosthetic examination.** After 2 weeks, most patients will have almost no swelling and bruising, and the oral tissues should look far less inflamed. Check the prosthesis for any damage. At this point you will be able to evaluate the esthetics of the interim prosthesis as well as the patient's speech. If the patient's esthetics and phonetics are acceptable but not as expected, reassure the patient that this is only a temporary prosthesis, and changes will be made during the production of the definitive prosthesis to meet their expectations.

- **Postoperative CBCT.** Some clinicians performing nonguided implant surgery in the U.S. prefer to take a CBCT immediately after surgery to confirm implant placement and to obtain a baseline view of their locations. I generally wait until the 2-week postoperative appointment to take a postop CBCT because the patient can usually handle manipulation around their mouth more comfortably, and I am less concerned about the implants being in a precarious position. My international colleagues tell me that the guidelines for when to obtain a postoperative CBCT and the rationale for doing so are different than those in the U.S. Be sure to follow the guidelines set forth by your licensing board and the standard of care in your region.
- **Digital analysis of occlusion.** There are currently two digital devices marketed in the U.S. (that I am aware of) that are designed to objectively locate the points of occlusion in addition to measuring the amount of force being applied at these points: the T-Scan Novus® (Tekscan) and the OccluSense® (Bausch) (Figs. 7.83, 7.84). Both devices provide a much more accurate record of a patient's occlusion than articulating paper. After using both devices in my practice, I will never go back to checking a patient's occlusion any other way. I recommend that you research these devices and decide which is most appropriate for your practice.
- **Continued encouragement and reinforcement of postoperative instructions.** At 2 weeks postsurgery, the patient may have been avoiding their hygiene regimen because of discomfort, and now is a good time to motivate them to be more diligent. They should be following the hygiene and soft tissue routine outlined at visit no. one. Dietary instructions should also be reviewed along with management of any continuing discomfort.

Postoperative visit no. three: 1 month after surgery

- **Oral and prosthetic examination.** At this point, sutures may have dissolved and tissues will be shrinking and remodeling. If the patient is compliant with their home care, the tissue should look healthy and the prosthesis should be in good condition. There should be no fractures or unusual wear patterns. Check for the presence of any movement or rocking in the interim prosthesis. Occasionally, I will remove the PVS plugs covering the screw access channels and retighten the prosthetic screws to ensure that the prosthesis remains firmly in place, even if the patient does not complain of discomfort when biting or that the prosthesis is loose.
- **Digital analysis of occlusion.** Recheck the patient's occlusion to verify that it has not changed since the previous visit. If there are changes, make the needed adjustments to balance the prosthesis.

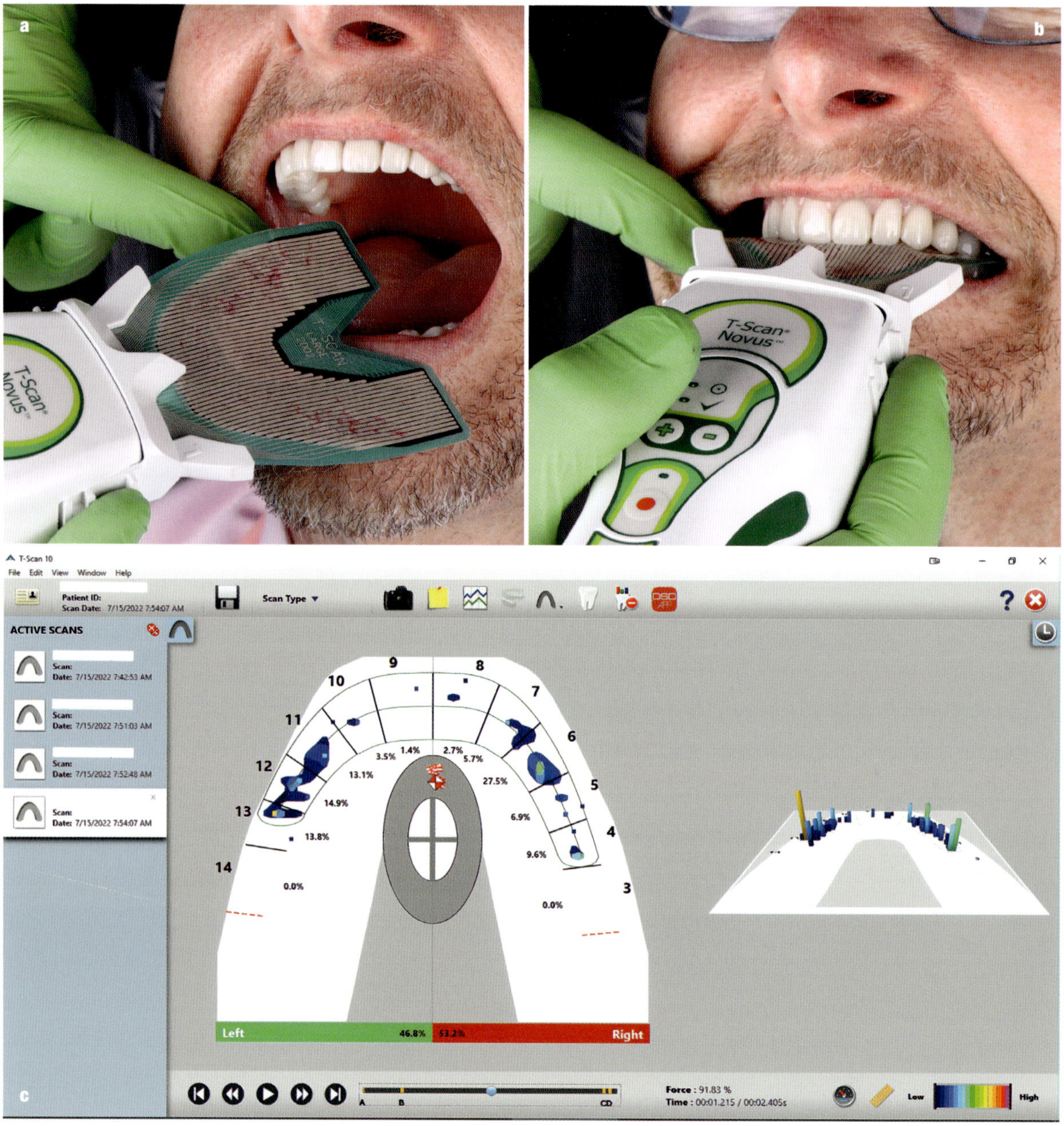

Figure 7.83 (a, b) Use of a T-Scan® device (Tekscan) to measure the patient's occlusion; (c) Screenshot of T-Scan software readout taken while patient is occluding.

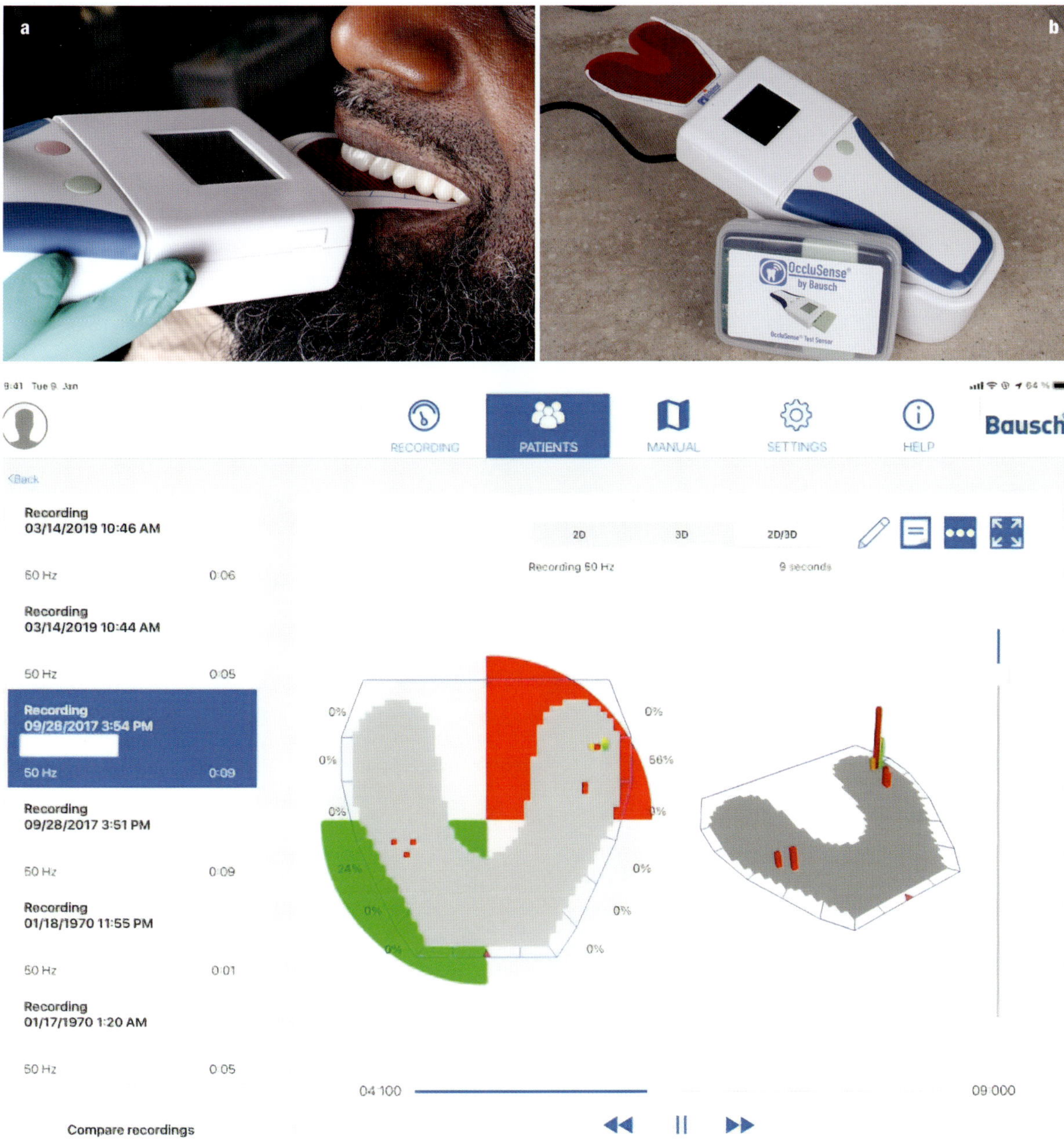

Figure 7.84 (a, b) Checking occlusion with the OccluSense® (Bausch); (c) Screenshot of OccluSense software readout taken while patient is occluding.

- **Hygiene and dietary overview.** Continue to encourage good hygiene. At this point, we like to add water flossing to the patient's daily regimen. We often wait until this appointment to discuss water flossing so patients do not inadvertently delay healing of the soft tissues during the first month after surgery. Remind the patient that it is in their best interest to continue eating softer foods that they can cut with a plastic fork.

Postoperative visit no. four: 2 months after surgery

In my practice, the main purpose of this visit is to check the patient's interim prosthesis. It is not uncommon for the screws in the prosthesis to loosen over time and for the prosthesis to begin rocking or moving during function. This in turn can weaken the prosthesis and eventually result in a fracture.

- **Oral and prosthetic examination.** During this visit, a brief overview of the tissues and prosthesis may be all that is needed. Note any unusual wear patterns in the prosthesis and check stability. I almost always remove the PVS plugs from the screw access channels at this visit and retighten any screws that are not torqued properly.
- **Digital analysis of occlusion.** Continue to analyze the patient's occlusal patterns and manage any areas of significant stress on the prosthesis. Look for balance of occlusal forces rather than a perfect bite.

PRO TIP: Postoperative management, part 2

Occasionally an interim prosthesis becomes loose during the postoperative phase of treatment, prior to the start of the prosthetic workflow. The patient might tell you their prosthesis feels loose, or you may observe this yourself. Another patient might complain of discomfort when biting or chewing. If this happens, remove the PVS plugs covering the screw-access channels and use an implant hand-driver to check whether the screws are still torqued. If any screws are loose, retighten them to the torque specifications recommended by the manufacturer of your implant system. A loose prosthesis can cause a litany of problems as well as failure of implants and other components.

- **Hygiene and dietary review.** Same as postoperative visit no. three.
- **Discussion of prosthetic phase of treatment.** Prepare the patient for the steps and appointments that will be needed to complete the transition from the interim prosthesis to a definitive prosthesis.

Postoperative visit no. five: 3 or 4 months after surgery (optional)

Depending on the case, patient considerations, and even the brand of implants you have placed, you may be ready to proceed with the prosthetic workflow and do not need to schedule a visit at this point. I generally wait 3 to 4 months to begin the prosthetic phase of treatment, but some practitioners start sooner and others later. Use your judgement and understanding of osseointegration, and consider the patient's needs.

- **Oral and prosthetic examination.** Same as postoperative visit no. four.
- **Occlusal examination.** There probably will not be any significant changes to the scheme of the occlusion at this point unless the patient is bruxing or clenching. I simply use articulating paper to verify the distribution of occlusal contacts unless something unusual is noted.
- **Hygiene and dietary overview.** Same as postoperative visit nos. three and four.
- **Discussion of prosthetic phase of treatment.** Prepare the patient for the steps and appointments that will be needed to complete the transition from the interim prosthesis to a definitive prosthesis.

References

1. Townsend JA, Hagan JL, Smiley M. Use of local anesthesia during dental rehabilitation with general anesthesia: A survey of dentist anesthesiologists. Anesth Prog 2014;61:11-17.
2. de Mello JS, Faot F, Correa G, Chagas Júnior OL. Success rate and complications associated with dental implants in the incisive canal region: a systematic review. Int J Oral Maxillofac Surg 2017;46:1584-1591.

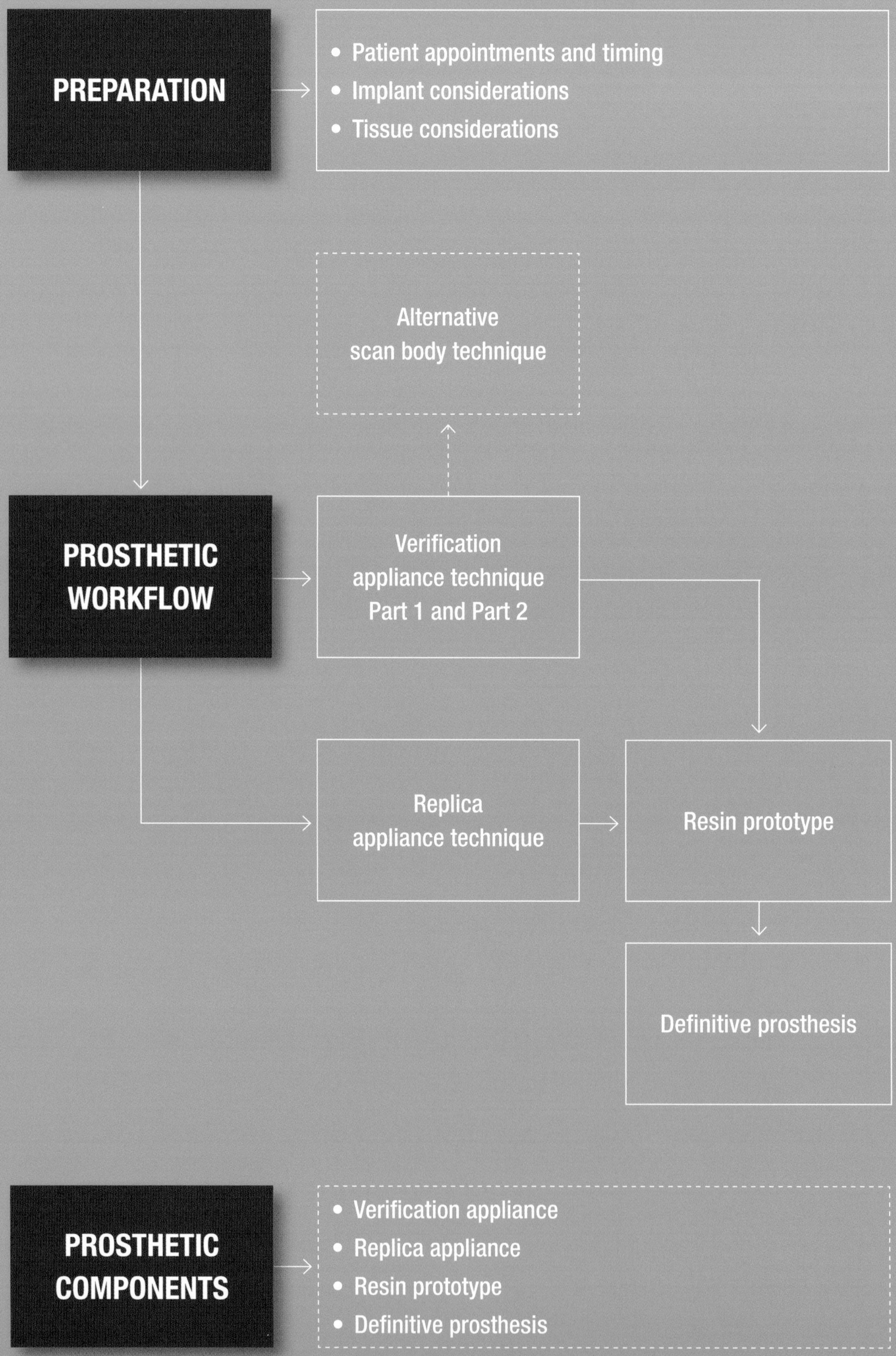
PREPARATION
Patient appointments and timing
Implant considerations
Tissue considerations
Alternative scan body technique
PROSTHETIC WORKFLOW
Verification appliance technique Part 1 and Part 2
Replica appliance technique
Resin prototype
Definitive prosthesis
PROSTHETIC COMPONENTS
Verification appliance
Replica appliance
Resin prototype
Definitive prosthesis

THE PROSTHETIC WORKFLOW

SECTION **V**

PROSTHETIC WORKFLOW PREPARATION AND COMPONENTS

CHAPTER 8

Commitment: Steer clear of addictive behaviors and substance abuse.
Few things can be more damaging to one's life and career than an addiction that is out of control. If you have a problem, admit it and do not be ashamed. There is a way back.

Sometime around postoperative month 3 or 4, most patients are ready to begin the prosthetic workflow. By that time, the dental implants should be osseointegrated and most of the soft tissue healing should be complete. In my experience, much of the prosthetic workflow can be delegated to auxiliary team members; hence, we often double-book patients during these appointments. A well-trained team can increase your efficiency tremendously in this process.

PATIENT APPOINTMENTS WITH TIMING

Generally, there are three to five appointments in the pragmatic prosthetic workflow for restoring patients with fixed full-arch implant prostheses. The appointments vary depending on whether a replica appliance pick-up was performed after the interim prosthesis pick-up procedure. The replica appliance technique provides the fastest and most efficient path to completing the prosthetic workflow, but it is not always an option. For cases in which the surgeon does not pick up a replica appliance or a patient has previously been in a definitive fixed full-arch implant prosthesis, a verification appliance technique can be used. Both workflows are similar in the two final appointments. Becoming familiar with both processes and what they achieve is key to understanding the fundamentals of this workflow. Boxes 8-1 and 8-2 list suggested appointments and times for the verification and replica appliance workflows, respectively, for clinicians who are new to fixed full-arch implant dentistry.

Box 8-1 Suggested appointments and amount of time needed for the verification appliance technique, which is used when a replica surgical appliance is not available or when a patient needs a replacement prosthesis and a digital scan or copy of the original prosthesis is not available

Appointment no., purpose, and timing for verification appliance

No. 1: Verification appliance, step 1; 15–20 minutes per arch

No. 2: Verification appliance, step 2; 30 minutes per arch

No. 3: Digital resin prototype; 30 minutes per arch

No. 4: Delivery; 30 minutes per arch

No. 5: Postdelivery (optional); 20 minutes

Box 8-2 Suggested appointments and amount of time needed for the replica appliance technique, which is used when a replica appliance was obtained at surgery or a master cast from a previous surgery or a digital record of the current definitive prosthesis is available

Appointment no., purpose, and timing for replica appliance

No. 1: Replica appliance verification; 30 minutes per arch

No. 2: Digital resin prototype; 30 minutes per arch

No. 3: Delivery; 30 minutes per arch

No. 4: Postdelivery (optional); 20 minutes

IMPLANT AND TISSUE CONSIDERATIONS

An important first step in preparing for the prosthetic workflow is assessing the stability of the implants, multiunit abutments (MUAs), and soft tissues. Do not underestimate the importance of making sure all the implants in the arch are osseointegrating. Carefully assess whether the MUAs are ideally placed and torqued to specification, and evaluate the quality and quantity of the soft tissues. Skipping these steps can cost time and money if you find that modifications need to be made in the middle of the prosthetic workflow. Worse still would be realizing that modifications need to be made after the definitive prosthesis has been fabricated.

Measuring Implant Stability

There are several methods that can be used to determine whether an implant is integrating. When placing implants, most clinicians rely on torque value to gauge *primary stability*, sometimes also referred to as *mechanical stability*. Later, following a 2- to 4-month healing period, it is important to assess whether the implants have achieved *secondary stability*, especially in fixed full-arch implant cases. Secondary stability, also known as *biologic stability*, is an indication that the implants are undergoing osseointegration. In the past, dentists have relied on subjective methods, including radiographs, auditory percussion testing, and/or their own perception, to assess secondary stability. Today there are several objective ways to determine whether implants in the arch are undergoing osseointegration. One way is to perform a reverse torque test, but this is not recommended as it can be stressful for both patient and clinician and requires removal of the MUAs. Another way is to use a device specifically designed to measure the stability of implants. Several such devices are available, powered by a couple of different forms of technology. The Osstell® (Osstell) and the Penguin® (Aseptico), for example, both use resonance frequency analysis (RFA); they can be employed in the initial stages to assess primary stability and later to assess secondary stability. The AnyCheck® (NeoBiotech), another option, records implant stability test (IST) values. The device I have been using for the past several years is the Periotest M® (Medizintechnik Gulden) (Fig. 8.1). This simple, inexpensive, and easy-to-use device is noninvasive and does not require removal of the MUAs. It uses vibration

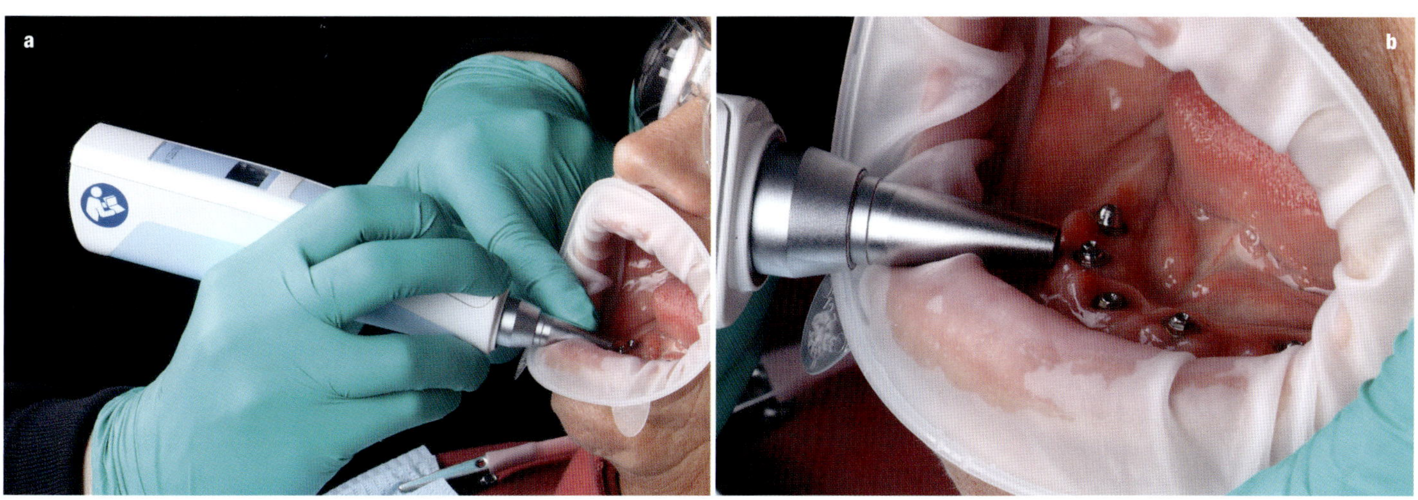

Figure 8.1 (a, b) Use of a Periotest® M (Medizintechnik Gulden) device to test for secondary stability of implants.

analysis to measure the stability of dental implants as well as natural teeth. Although no device can provide absolute verification of secondary (or biologic) stability, a combination of subjective and objective methods can be used by clinicians to evaluate the stability of their implants and avoid expensive and time-consuming errors.

Evaluation of the Tissue

The health of the oral mucosa—particularly the soft tissues surrounding the MUAs—is an important factor in the long-term success of a fixed full-arch implant prosthesis. Oral mucosa consists of attached (nonmobile) and nonattached keratinized tissues as well as nonkeratinized tissue. When the interim prosthesis is removed at the beginning of the prosthetic workflow, it is desirable to have attached, keratinized, nonmobile tissue around the MUAs (Fig. 8.2). If any of the gingiva around an MUA is nonkeratinized tissue, it is potentially more problematic when the nonkeratinized gingiva is located on the lingual aspect of the arch, where grafting is more difficult. This is more common in the mandible due to the natural paucity of attached keratinized tissue in that area.

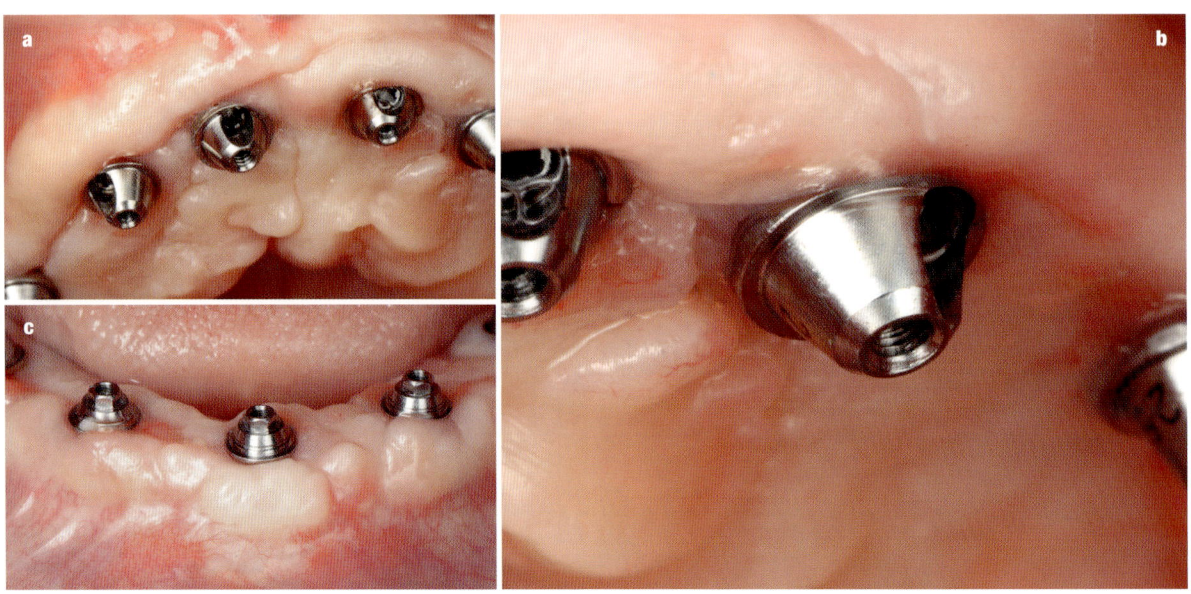

Figure 8.2 **Examples of healthy and abundant attached keratinized tissue around MUAs four months postoperative (a, b) in the maxilla and (c) in the mandible upon removal of the interim prosthesis.**

During the surgical phase of treatment, you should always consider the keratinized tissue precious and preserve as much of it as possible. You can usually achieve this by fine-tuning your surgical approach, although there are times when the tissues around the MUAs are less than ideal no matter how careful you are. An important step in this process of evaluation is to inform patients preoperatively that (*a*) tissue changes can occur, and some areas may be more susceptible to peri-mucositis and peri-implantitis as a result; and (*b*) they may need soft tissue grafting or additional surgical procedures to correct for this. When patient expectations are established ahead of time, it is much easier to have this conversation postoperatively. This also helps patients understand that their participation in the maintenance and hygiene of their new prosthesis (or prostheses) is important to the longevity of its dental implant foundation.

Another aspect of the soft tissues to consider after healing has taken place is the emergence profile of the MUAs—that is, whether the border of each MUA is positioned significantly above or below the collar of the soft tissue. If the border is at or just below the soft tissue collar, the prospects for obtaining an esthetic and hygienic definitive prosthesis are good (Fig. 8.3). MUAs

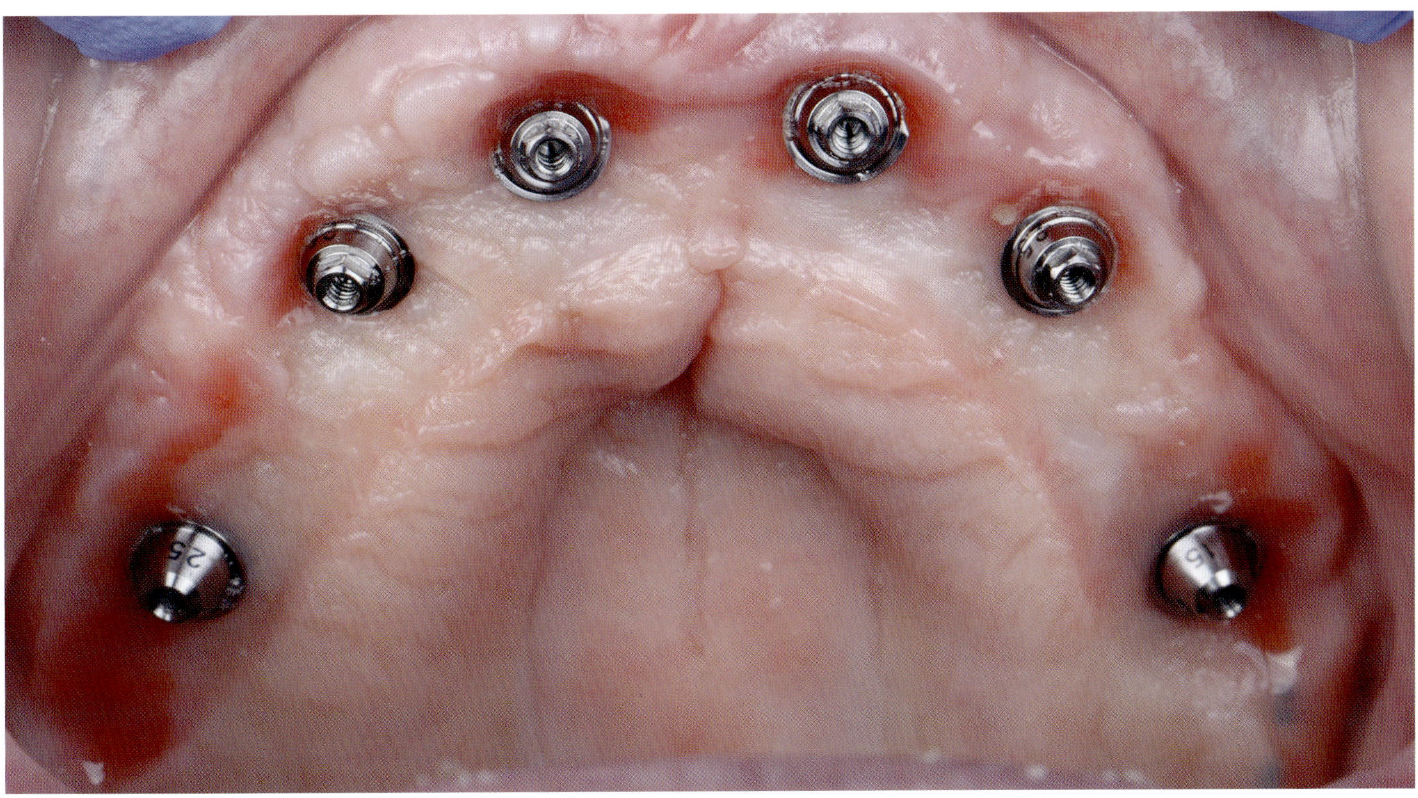

Figure 8.3 **An example of a healed arch with MUAs at the appropriate height and surrounded by sufficient keratinized tissue.**

that are buried significantly below the tissues can be challenging for patients to clean around and require the prosthesis to be beneath the tissue to seal. Conversely, if the border of the MUA is positioned significantly above the collar of the soft tissue, the prosthesis could be esthetically compromised. In addition, the space between the MUAs and the prosthesis can act as a food trap if the intaglio surface of the prosthesis is designed to be hygienic. I have seen several cases over the years in which the clinician attempted to resolve this issue by creating a flange to cover the visible areas. The patient was hygienically compromised as a result, because plaque and biofilm will inevitably collect in the prosthesis and create unhealthy tissue around the MUAs.

At the beginning of the prosthetic workflow is the best time to replace MUAs that are either too tall or too short in relation to the surrounding soft tissue. The process takes only a few minutes and will not require an additional appointment if your practice keeps additional MUAs in stock. Obviously, the interim prosthesis will not fit the same after one or more MUAs are replaced. You must remove the reduced cylinder that fit over the old MUA and pick up a new temporary cylinder on the new MUA. Some implant systems use the same internal sizing for abutments regardless of the diameter of the implant, allowing clinicians who use them to maintain a much smaller stock of MUAs. This is one of the factors I consider when choosing which implant system to use in my practice.

PROSTHETIC COMPONENTS OVERVIEW

There are four components in the prosthetic workflow; each plays an important role in the success of fixed full-arch implant dentistry. I use these components to create a predictable and efficient process in my practice that is easy to follow and simple for team members to grasp. As new technology becomes available, we will be able to remove some of these components and replace them with an entirely digital workflow. I am testing several of these new workflows as I am writing this book.

Verification appliance

The verification appliance is used to achieve three goals: It provides implant verification, confirms the vertical dimension of occlusion (VDO), and records the morphology of the soft tissues for an accurate intaglio surface in the definitive prosthesis.

The verification appliance is a copy of the interim appliance that is printed in resin and then sectioned; each section aligns with an implant MUA by way of a temporary cylinder or a titanium base (Fig. 8.4). The verification appliance technique is my preferred method in cases where a replica appliance was not picked up during the patient's surgery. It can also be helpful to use this appliance for inherited fixed full-arch implant cases where the definitive prosthesis needs to be replaced. Note that once the verification appliance technique is completed, the verification appliance closely resembles the replica appliance.

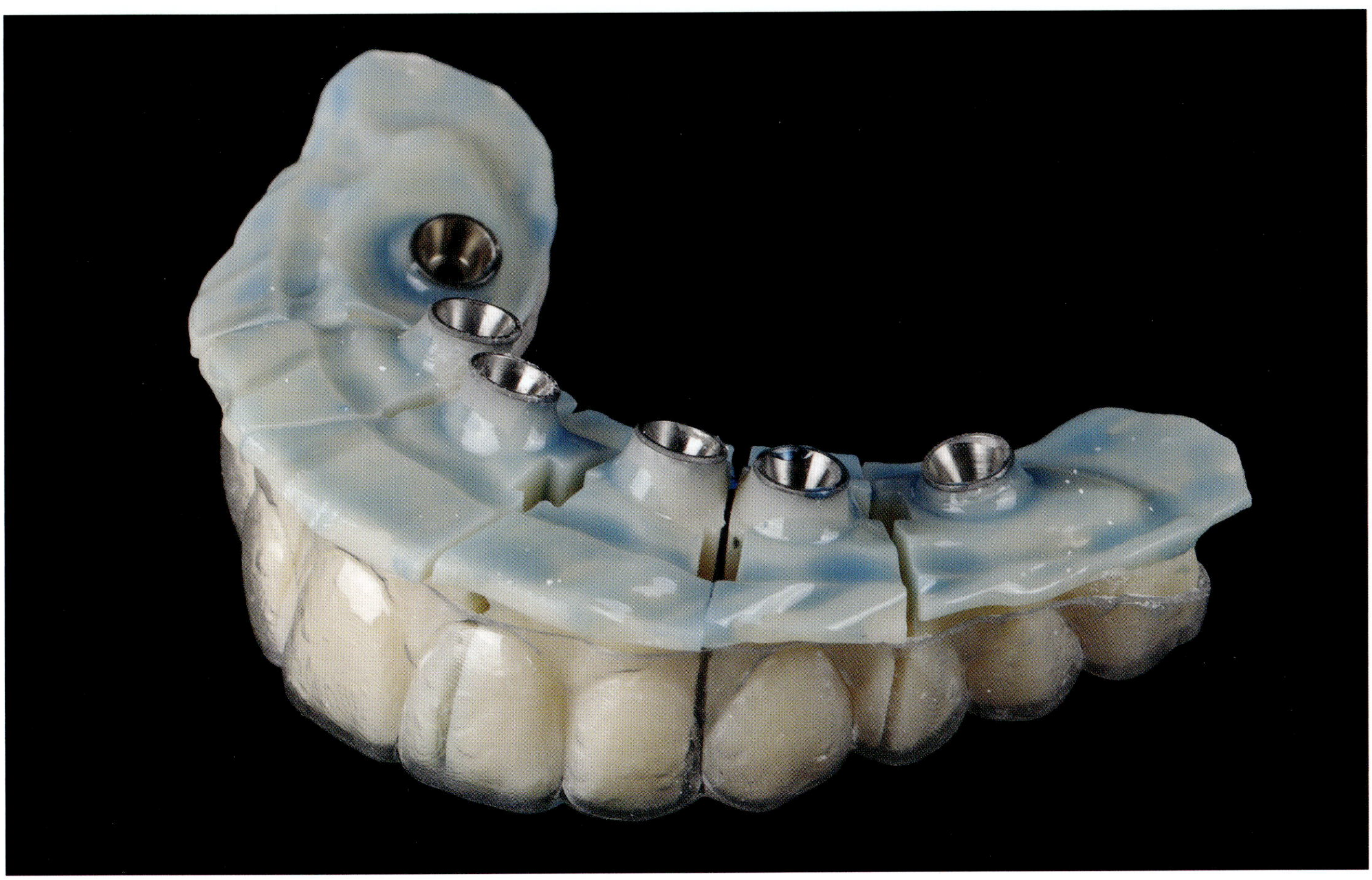

Figure 8.4 **Appearance of a verification appliance that is prepared for indexing with a vacuum thermomold tray.**

Replica appliance

The replica appliance is an exact replica of the patient's original interim prosthesis; accordingly, it can be expected to fit and function in the same way, providing the interim prosthesis did not require substantial occlusal adjustment (Fig. 8.5). Like the verification appliance, the replica appliance can be manufactured from an inexpensive printed or milled material. Some clinicians prefer to use an FDA-approved material that can be worn in the mouth so that it can serve as a back-up interim prosthesis if a patient fractures or has a problem with the original interim prosthesis. The replica appliance technique saves time for the practitioner as well as the patient.

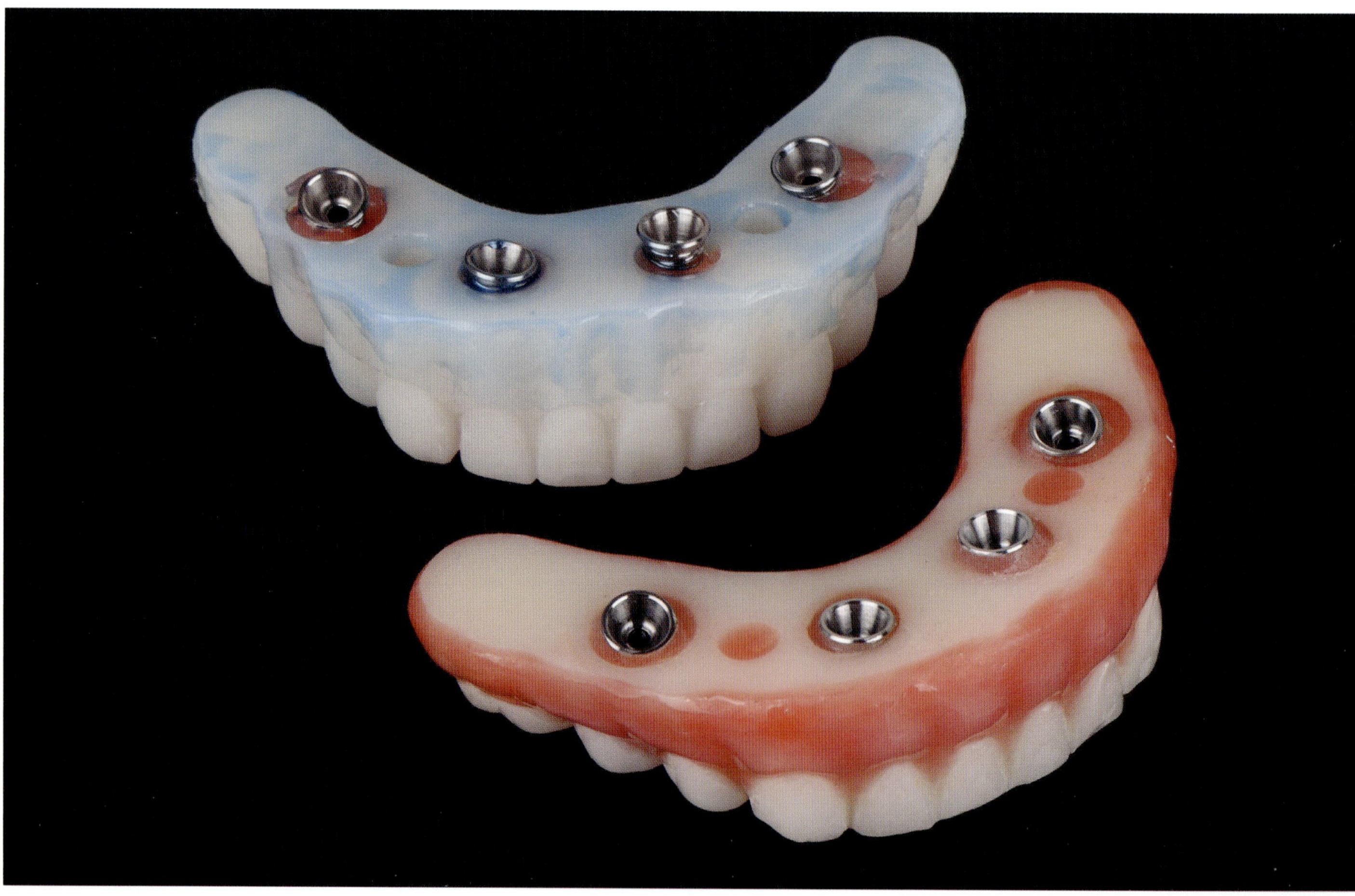

Figure 8.5 Replica appliance (*top*) and interim prosthesis made for the same patient.

Resin prototype appliance

Most dentists are familiar with full-arch try-ins, or proposals, which were traditionally made from wax and used acrylic teeth. Today, with advances in dental technology, printed and milled resin prototypes have become the standard. In my prosthetic workflow, the resin prototype is a modified version of either the verification appliance or the replica appliance (Fig. 8.6). Modifications have been made, with the help of the laboratory, based on patient feedback and clinical assessments to obtain optimal esthetic and functional results. This appliance can help reassure patients that they will have a result they will be happy with. Sometimes it is appropriate to send a patient home with the resin prototype in place to verify comfort and acceptance before moving to the definitive prosthesis. Once the clinician and patient agree on the final changes, it can be sent back to the lab.

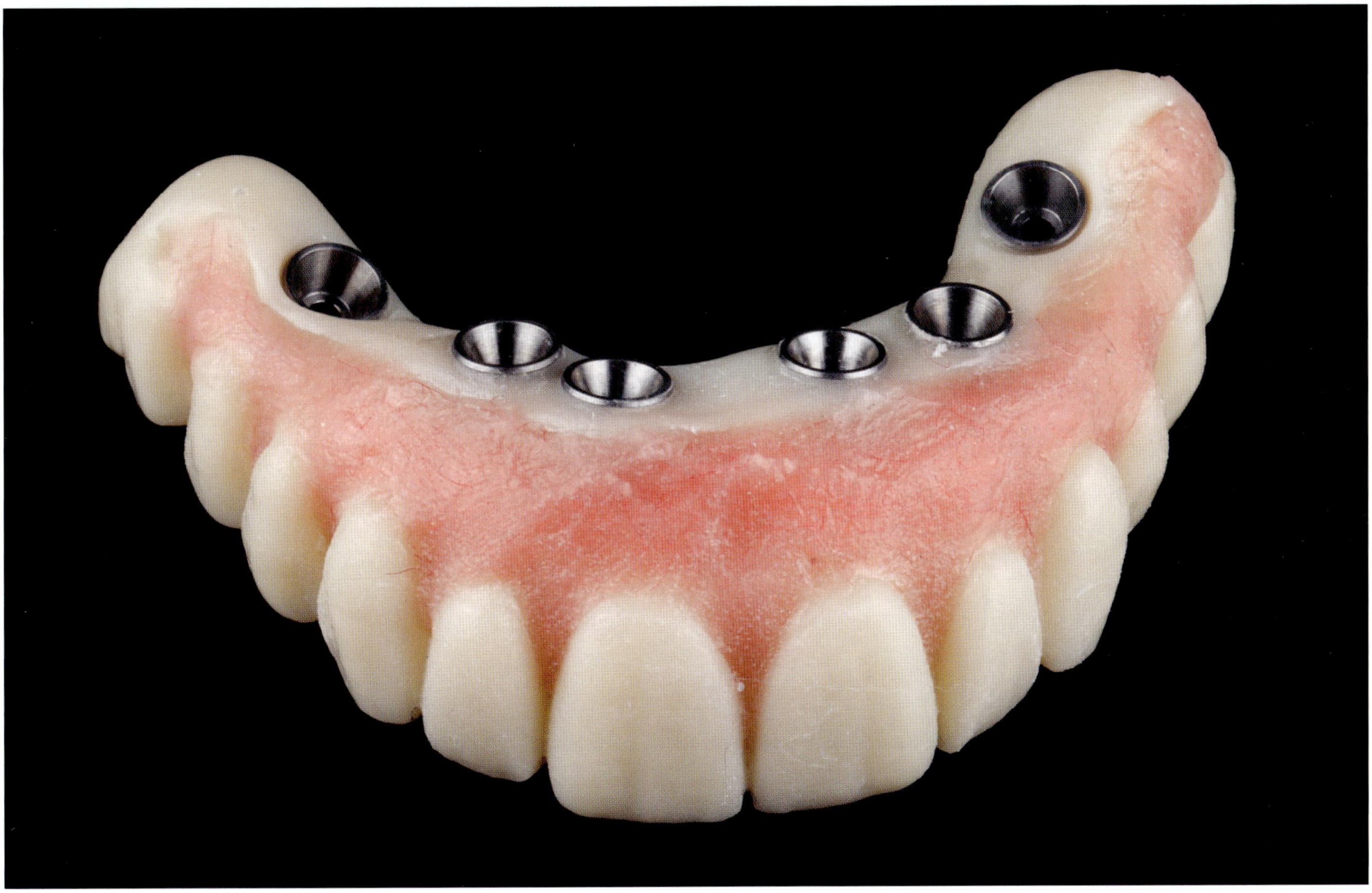

Figure 8.6 **Completed resin prototype appliance with added gingival material.**

Definitive prosthesis

The definitive fixed full-arch implant prosthesis is what patients often refer to as their "permanent" teeth. Over 25 years, I have learned that the term *permanent* should be used very judiciously. In our practice, we generally let patients know that their definitive prosthesis is designed to function and appear as much as possible like their natural teeth, but we cannot guarantee that it will feel just like natural teeth or that it will last forever. There are several different ways to engineer and design these prostheses, and they can be fabricated out of a variety of materials (Figs. 8.7, 8.8).

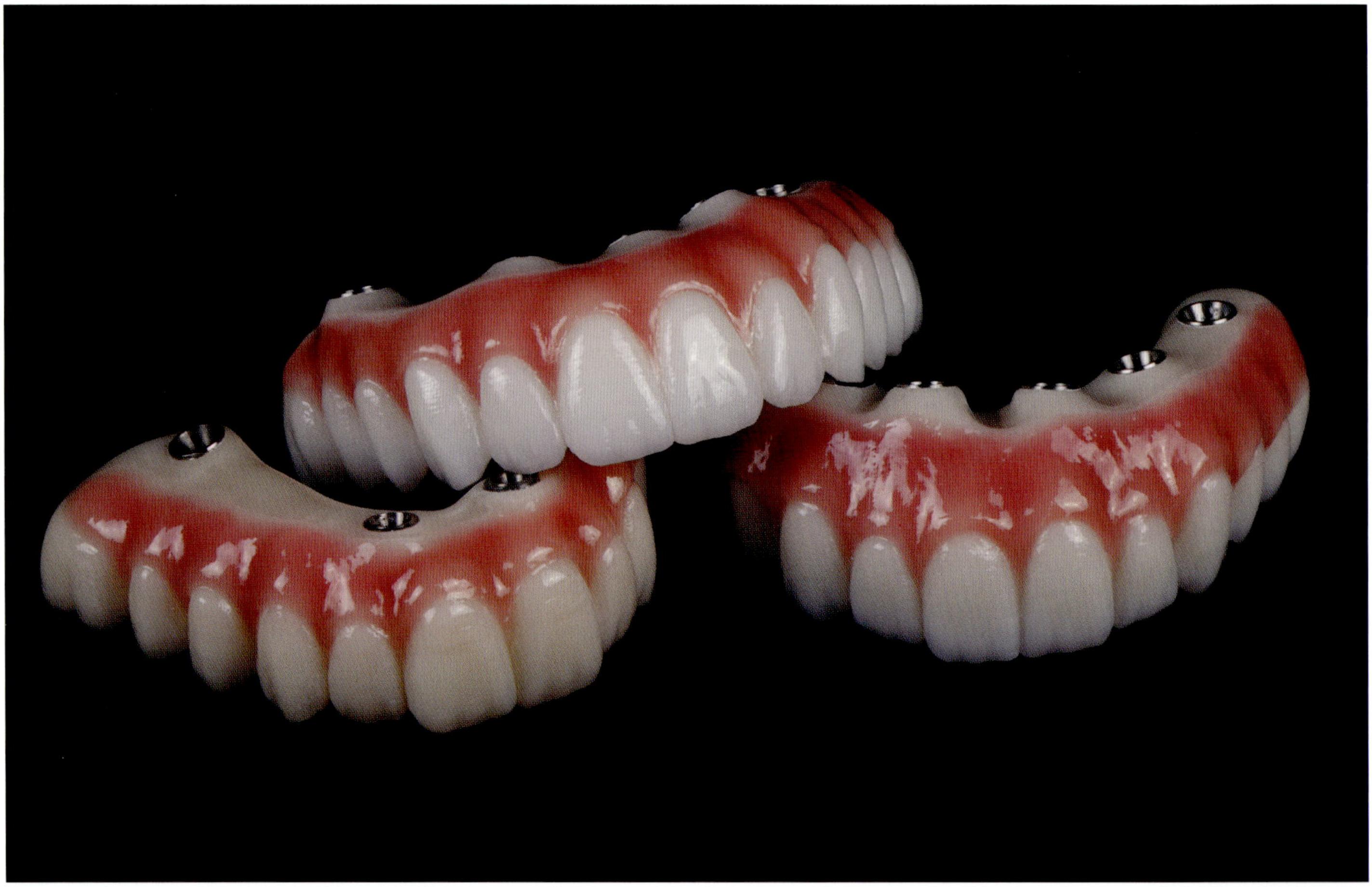

Figure 8.7 **Three definitive prostheses in different shades of monolithic zirconia.**

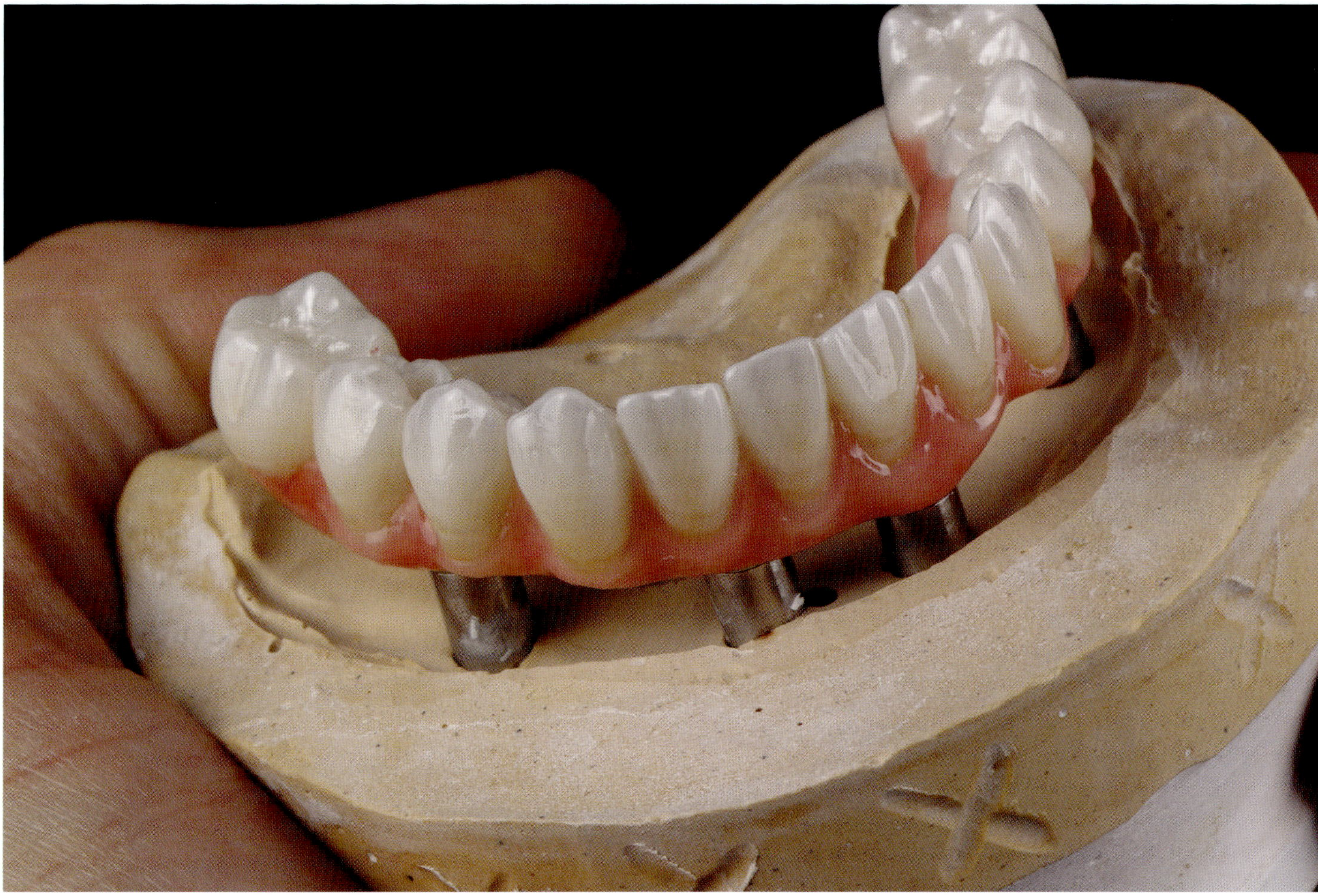

Figure 8.8 Fixed full-arch definitive prosthesis, made of monolithic zirconia with custom staining and glazing, on an index cast.

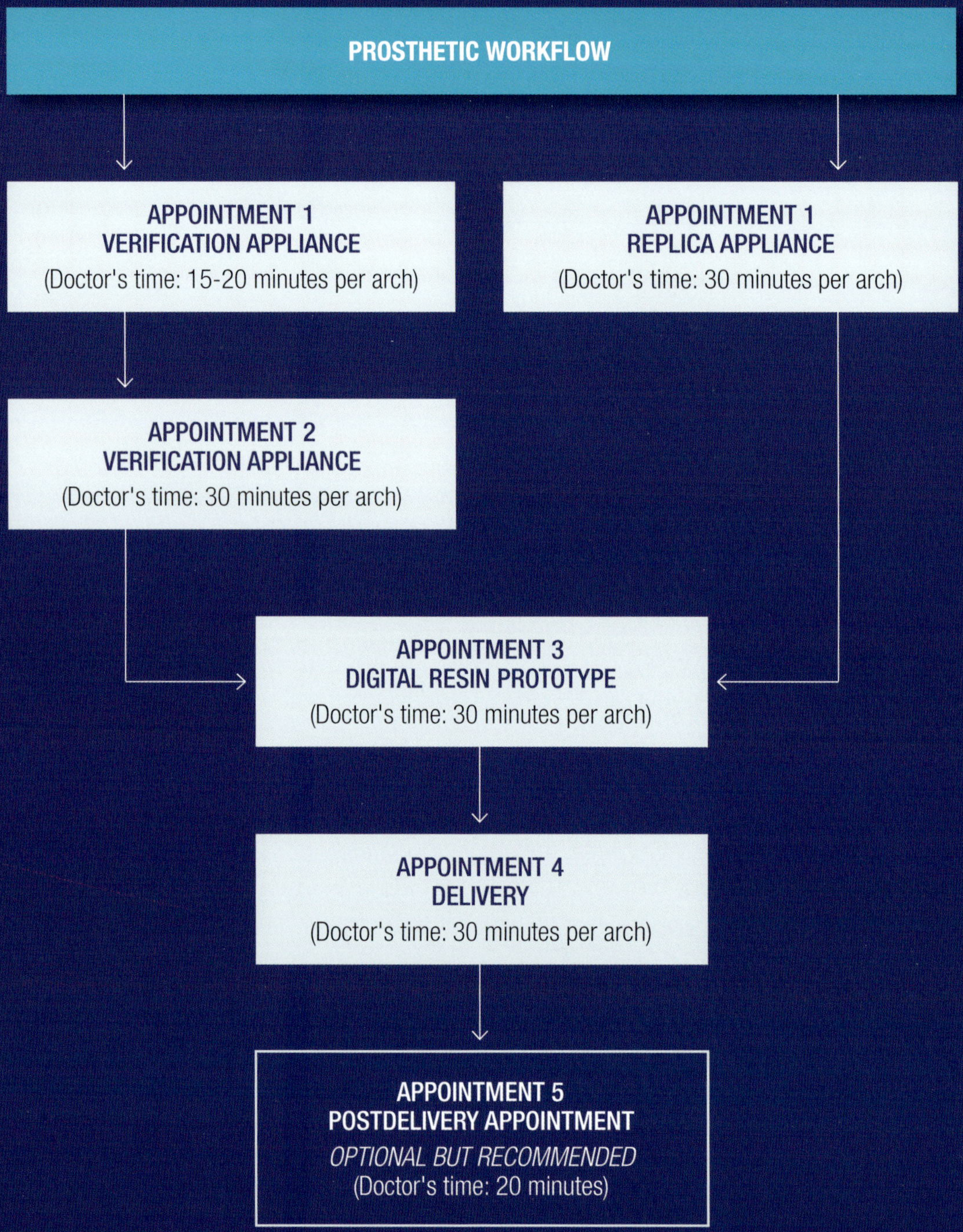
PROSTHETIC WORKFLOW
APPOINTMENT 1
VERIFICATION APPLIANCE
(Doctor's time: 15-20 minutes per arch)
APPOINTMENT 1
REPLICA APPLIANCE
(Doctor's time: 30 minutes per arch)
APPOINTMENT 2
VERIFICATION APPLIANCE
(Doctor's time: 30 minutes per arch)
APPOINTMENT 3
DIGITAL RESIN PROTOTYPE
(Doctor's time: 30 minutes per arch)
APPOINTMENT 4
DELIVERY
(Doctor's time: 30 minutes per arch)
APPOINTMENT 5
POSTDELIVERY APPOINTMENT
OPTIONAL BUT RECOMMENDED
(Doctor's time: 20 minutes)

STEP-BY-STEP PROSTHETIC WORKFLOW

CHAPTER **9**

Commitment: Stay active, exercise, eat clean.
A healthy body and mind are important to longevity and fulfilling your purpose. You are your best investment. Take the time to make healthy decisions.

As discussed in Chapter 8, the prosthetic workflow for fixed full-arch implant prostheses is completed in three to five appointments, depending on whether a replica appliance pick-up was performed after the interim prosthesis pick-up procedure during the surgical phase. The replica appliance technique provides the fastest and most efficient pathway to completing the prosthetic workflow, but it is not an option in every case. For cases in which *(a)* the surgeon does not pick up a replica appliance or *(b)* a new patient presents for the first time already wearing a fixed full-arch implant prosthesis, a verification appliance technique can be used. Both workflows are similar in the final two appointments (see flowchart).

This chapter begins with the first two appointments of the verification appliance technique; after that, the first appointment of the replica appliance technique is presented. As the flowchart shows, the workflow then follows a single pathway ending with delivery of the definitive prosthesis (and an optional postdelivery appointment). I encourage you to read through the entire chapter at least once. After that, you can skip the verification appliance technique if you have a patient with a replica appliance (and vice versa) when you want to review the process.

VERIFICATION APPLIANCE TECHNIQUE: APPOINTMENT 1

Although the verification appliance technique is not the most efficient pathway to the definitive prosthesis, it can be employed in place of the replica appliance technique when a replica appliance from the patient's surgery was not made or is not available—for example, when a patient already in a fixed full-arch prosthesis shows up in your practice needing a replacement. If you are working with such a patient, you can follow the same steps you would for a patient who is ready to move forward from an interim prosthesis to a definitive prosthesis 3 to 4 months after surgery but for whom a replica appliance was not made.

Operatory setup. In addition to a basic chairside exam kit, the following items will be helpful:

- Intraoral scanner
- Dental implant prosthetic setup with drivers and torque wrench
- Dental implant scan analogs for multiunit abutments (MUAs) (usually implant-specific)
- Dental handpiece and bur kit for intraoral adjustments
- Polyvinyl siloxane (PVS) impression material
- Articulating paper and digital jaw relation device
- Cheek and lip retractors, such as OptraGate® (Ivoclar Vivadent)
- Periotest M® (Medizintechnik Gulden) or similar osseointegration testing device (optional but recommended)

A. Verify the vertical dimension of occlusion and maxillomandibular relationship

Check the status of the patient's vertical dimension of occlusion (VDO) and maxillomandibular relationship (Fig. 9.1a). These indices should be fairly accurate by now as they have most likely been adjusted during the preceding postoperative visits. At this point, the patient is probably functioning comfortably at their current VDO and occlusion. If you have a patient whom you did not see for postoperative visits (for whatever reason) and the VDO is not where it should be, do not spend too much time addressing it unless it is significantly off. Once you have the verification appliance in its final form, you will be able to adjust the VDO easily.

To check the occlusion, you should inspect it visually and with the use of articulating paper (Fig. 9.1b). Ask for feedback from the patient about where the contact is felt. Your goal should not be to get the occlusion perfect at this time, but to have sufficient contact bilaterally to allow the lab to mount the case predictably. Make any necessary adjustments to the occlusion with a high-speed handpiece and a bur. I prefer a football-shaped bur that allows for efficient removal of the polymethylmethacrylate (PMMA) or acrylic material your interim prosthesis is made of (Fig. 9.2).

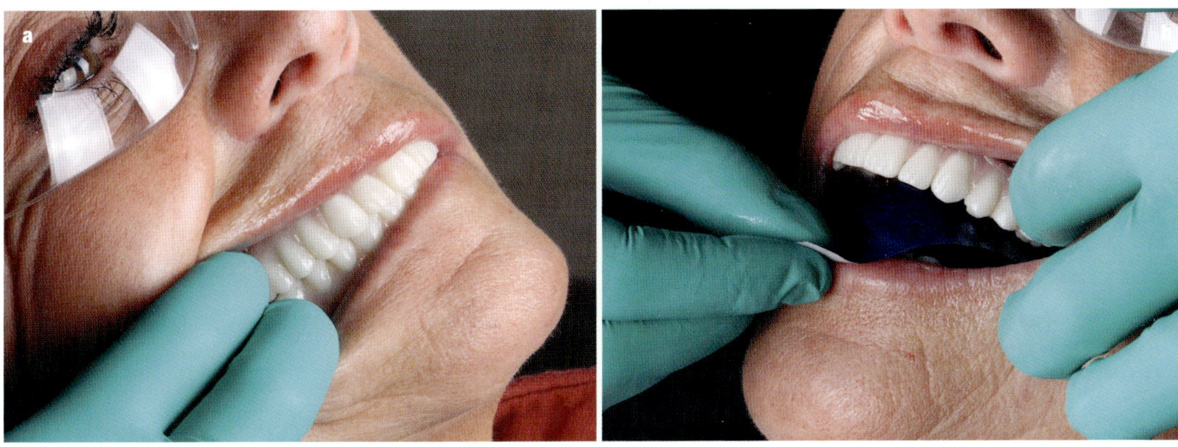

Figure 9.1 (a) Visual examination of patient's occlusion and maxillomandibular relationship; (b) Use of horseshoe-shaped articulating paper to check the occlusion in the arch.

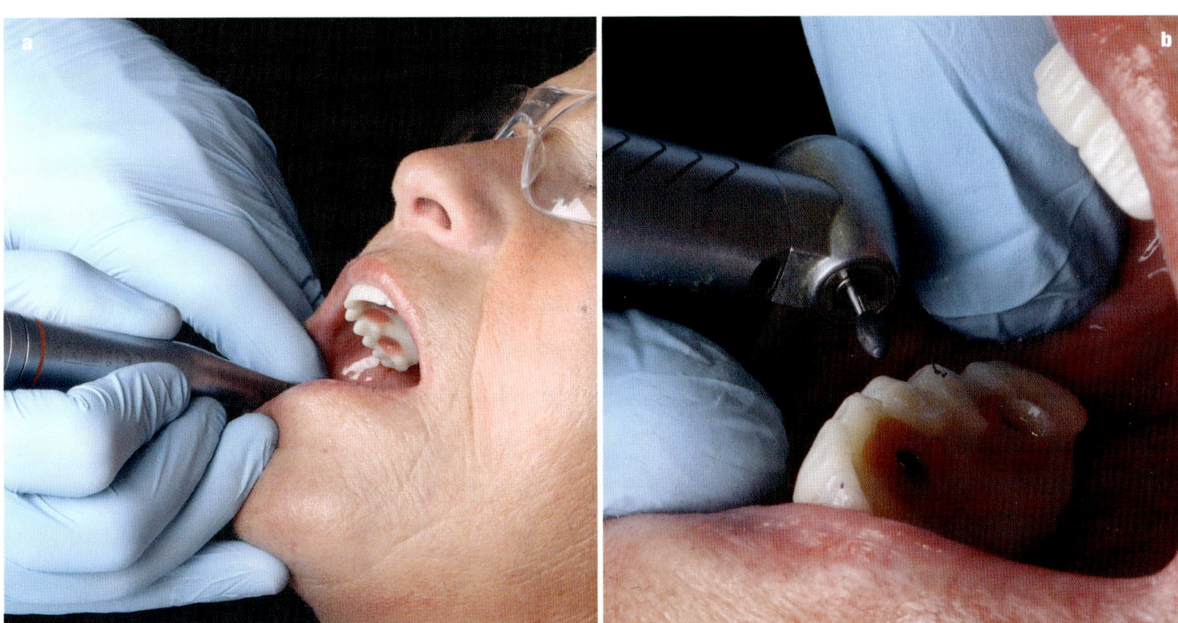

Figure 9.2 (a, b) Adjusting the occlusion of the interim prosthesis intraorally.

B. Remove the interim (or current) prosthesis

At the first appointment of the prosthetic workflow, the patient usually has an interim prosthesis in place. If the patient is new to your practice or it is the first time you (or your team) have removed the prosthesis, I suggest that the dentist be the one to take it out. To make the process easier and more efficient, use a cheek retraction device for better visualization of the access channels and movement around the arch (Fig. 9.3). I prefer the latex-free OptraGate (Ivoclar Vivadent) because it is easy for auxiliaries to manipulate, disposable, and very comfortable for the patient.

Most fixed full-arch prostheses have screw channels that exit either through the occlusal table or on the lingual surface. Identify where these screw access channels are located using an intraoral mirror. The material covering the screw channel or temporary cylinder will need to be removed first. In my surgical cases, I prefer to use a heavy- or medium-body PVS in the temporary cylinders because it is easy to see and remove.

A dental explorer generally works well for picking out the PVS material (Figs. 9.4a, 9.4b). (When a definitive prosthesis is removed, the screw access channels have a more durable restorative material such as composite or resin, which requires the use of a dental handpiece and bur.) Once the filling materials have been removed from each screw channel, you should have access to the prosthetic screws that attach the prosthesis to the MUAs (Fig. 9.4c).

PRO TIP: Placing and removing appliances

During the prosthetic workflow, the different appliances are removed and replaced several times. This process can be time consuming in the beginning, but with enough practice, a dental auxiliary or assistant can perform it very efficiently. Most often, delegating this task to the dental auxiliary or assistant will free up valuable time for the dentist to do other more productive activities.

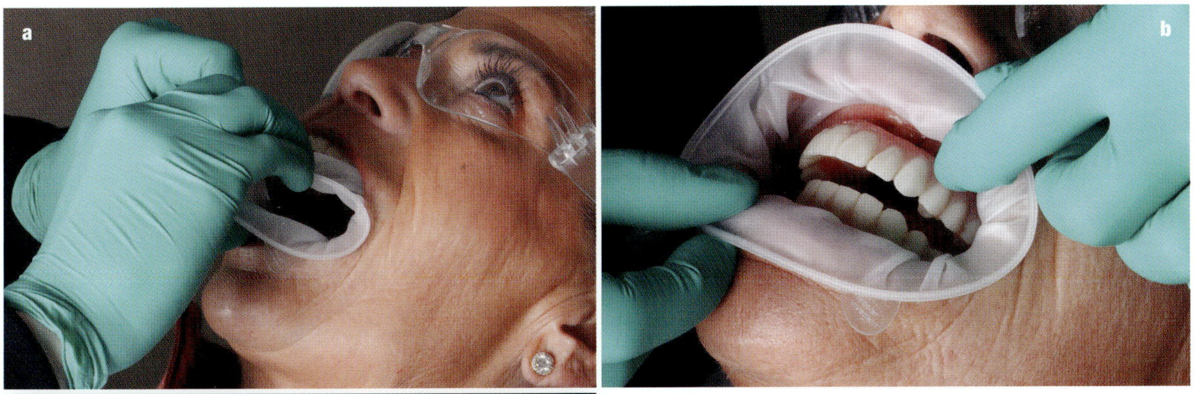

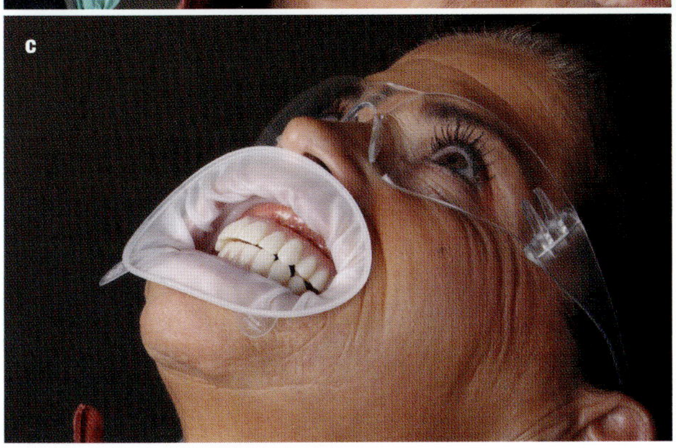

Figure 9.3 (a) Placing an OptraGate cheek retractor (Ivoclar Vivadent); (b) Positioning the retractor comfortably under the patient's lips; (c) Retracted cheeks and lips allow for optimal visualization and patient comfort.

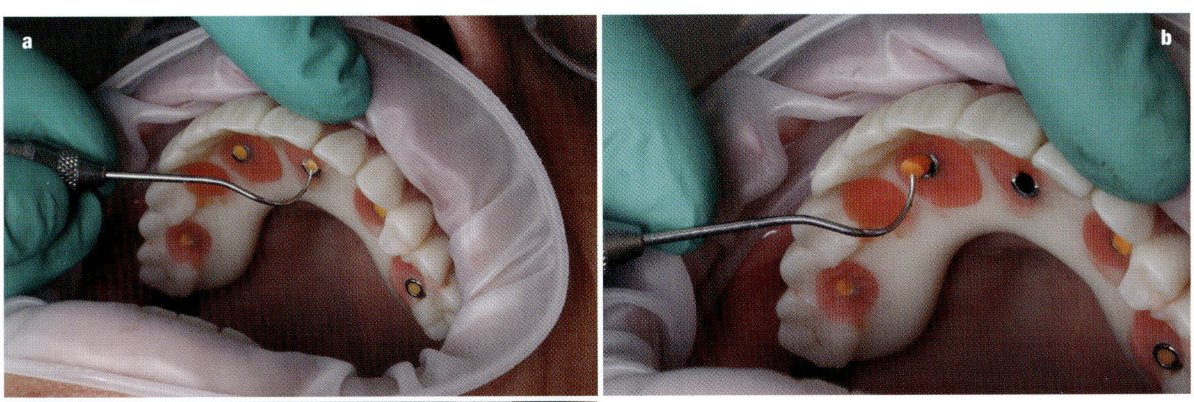

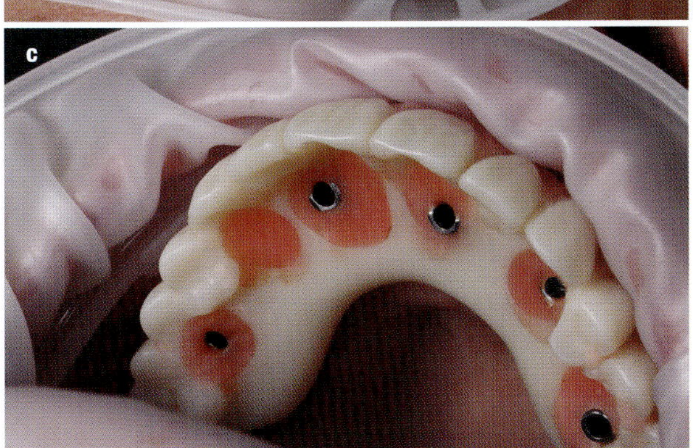

Figure 9.4 (a, b) Using a dental explorer to remove polyvinyl siloxane (PVS) plugs from the temporary cylinders in the interim prosthesis; (c) Appearance of the prosthetic screw access channels after the PVS plugs are removed.

Removing the prosthetic screws from the temporary cylinders or screw-access channels requires the appropriate driver and torque wrench. Once you have identified the implant system and the correct driver, place it into each screw and turn it counterclockwise to remove them (Figs. 9.5a, 9.5b). Place the screws in a dappen dish to avoid losing them and to help you keep count of them (Fig. 9.5c). Once all the screws have been removed, the prosthesis should detach easily from the MUAs (Fig. 9.5d).

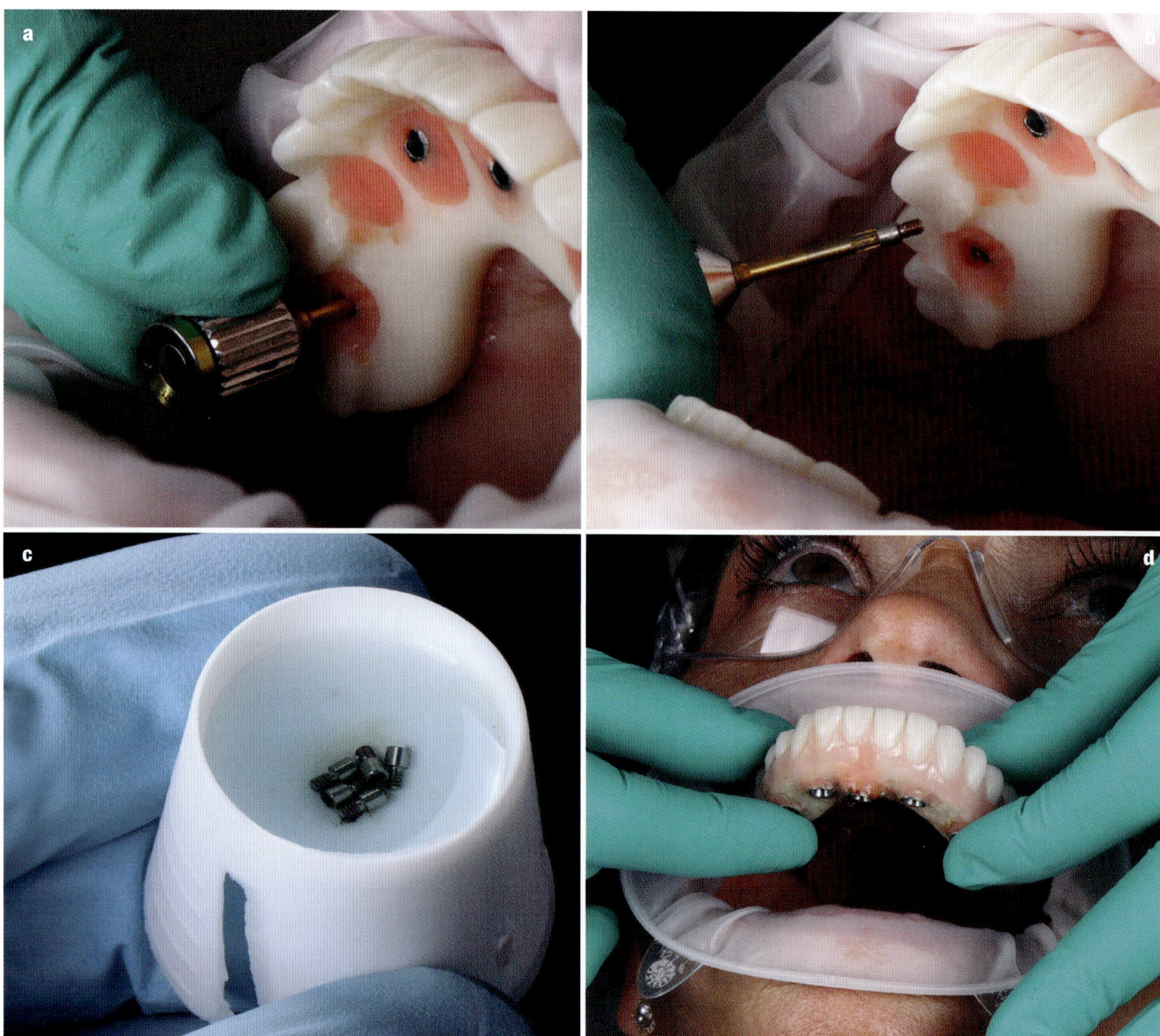

Figure 9.5 (a, b) Use of an implant driver to remove the prosthetic screws from the screw access channels; (c) Prosthetic screws soaking in a small dappen dish filled with OraCare rinse; (d) Removal of a mandibular interim prosthesis from the MUAs.

Beware of the second screw phenomenon

If you loosen the screws from the prosthesis and it will not budge, do not panic. It is likely that one of the access channels has an extra screw on top of a screw that is still torqued into the MUA. I refer to this in my office as the "second screw phenomenon." Sometimes a clinician or auxiliary will inadvertently place more than one prosthetic screw into a screw channel or temporary cylinder. This can happen during initial placement, at a subsequent visit, or at a hygiene appointment. One clue that this has happened is that, during placement, a screw will not torque, or it will spin because it is hitting the head of the screw below it. Either remove the extra screw at that point or make a note about the additional screw to avoid confusion and frustration for the assistant or dentist who will be removing the prosthesis at the next visit.

Loosening screws from a prosthesis is straightforward, but it is not always easy to remove them from the screw access channels, and it is not always necessary. However, if you encounter the second screw phenomenon, you will need to remove all the screws from the prosthesis in order to determine which access channel is hiding the second screw. In some implant systems, the driver fits very intimately with the prosthetic screws, and removing them is relatively easy. In other implant systems, the fit is less intimate and screws are not as easily removed.

PRO TIP: Avoiding the second screw phenomenon

To avoid the second screw phenomenon, use dappen dishes or other small containers to keep track of all the screws as you remove them from appliances. One of the most common causes of the second screw phenomenon is when screws are not entirely removed from prosthetics and another screw is inadvertently placed on top of an existing one. Therefore, removing all screws from appliances can help you avoid this problem. If you encounter a screw that is particularly difficult to remove, especially from a definitive prosthesis, the fastest method I have found to remove it is to use a reverse-thread implant screw removal tool. Make sure the tool is designed to work with your implant system, and do not reuse a prosthetic screw after it has been removed with it.

To remove a stubborn prosthetic screw from an access channel, apply one or more of the techniques that have worked for me in the past:

- Use a reverse-thread screw removal tool from your implant manufacturer. This is the technique I use first because it is the quickest, but the screw will not be reusable once it is removed.
- Use an ultrasonic scaler such as a Cavitron unit (Dentsply Sirona) with an old tip to vibrate the screw out of the channel.
- Use a low-speed handpiece very carefully *in reverse* with a round bur sized appropriately for the access channel. Apply light pressure with the bur on top of the screw head to vibrate and reverse out the screw.
- If the access channel is shallow, you may be able to pick the screw out with a periodontal probe or endodontic explorer.
- Use an air-water syringe to dry out the screw access channel, then place a very small amount of super glue on the tip of the driver. Place the driver into the screw access channel and then down into the screw head. Wait about 60 seconds and pull it out. Be sure to clean your driver well and discard the screw.

Right after you remove the interim prosthesis is the optimal time to examine its integrity and look for any areas of failure, including fractures, delamination, loose temporary cylinders, excessive wear, and so forth (Fig. 9.6a). If the interim prosthesis exhibits any problems that might affect its integrity over the next few months, consider repairing them in your onsite laboratory or having them repaired by your dental lab. Owning the armamentarium to make small repairs within your office and by your team is very helpful in keeping the workflow as efficient as possible. A well-trained dental assistant can perform many of the duties of a lab technician and will save time for the doctor and the patient. After inspecting the patient's prosthesis, have a dental assistant or auxiliary remove any debris found on it and place it in a cleaning/tartar removal solution within a resealable zipper-closure bag (Figs. 9.6b, 9.6c) and then into the office ultrasonic cleaner/shaker.

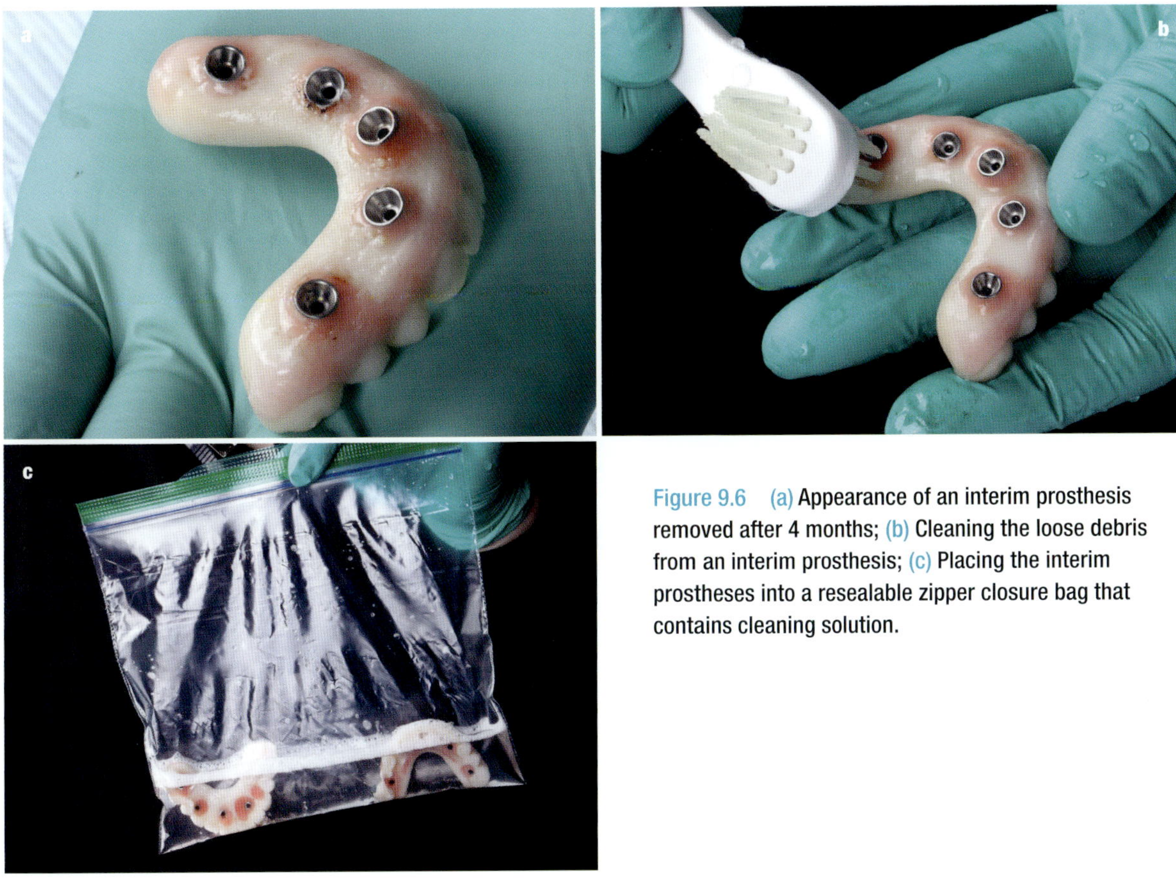

Figure 9.6 (a) Appearance of an interim prosthesis removed after 4 months; (b) Cleaning the loose debris from an interim prosthesis; (c) Placing the interim prostheses into a resealable zipper closure bag that contains cleaning solution.

C. Check the stability of the MUAs

Once the interim prosthesis has been removed and inspected, it is time to survey the implant and tissue landscape. As discussed in Chapter 8, it is important to examine the soft tissues and check the stability of the MUAs and implants (Fig. 9.7a). After you examine the soft tissue, carefully tap or gently press on each MUA with the end of a metal instrument such as a mouth mirror, checking for any loose abutments or movement (Fig. 9.7b). Your objective is to make sure each MUA is still torqued properly into its corresponding implant. You may also want to take the driver and make sure each MUA is at least hand-tight (Figs. 9.7c, 9.7d). If any of the abutments have become loose, as you tighten them be sure you do not lose the original direction or indexing on the MUA.

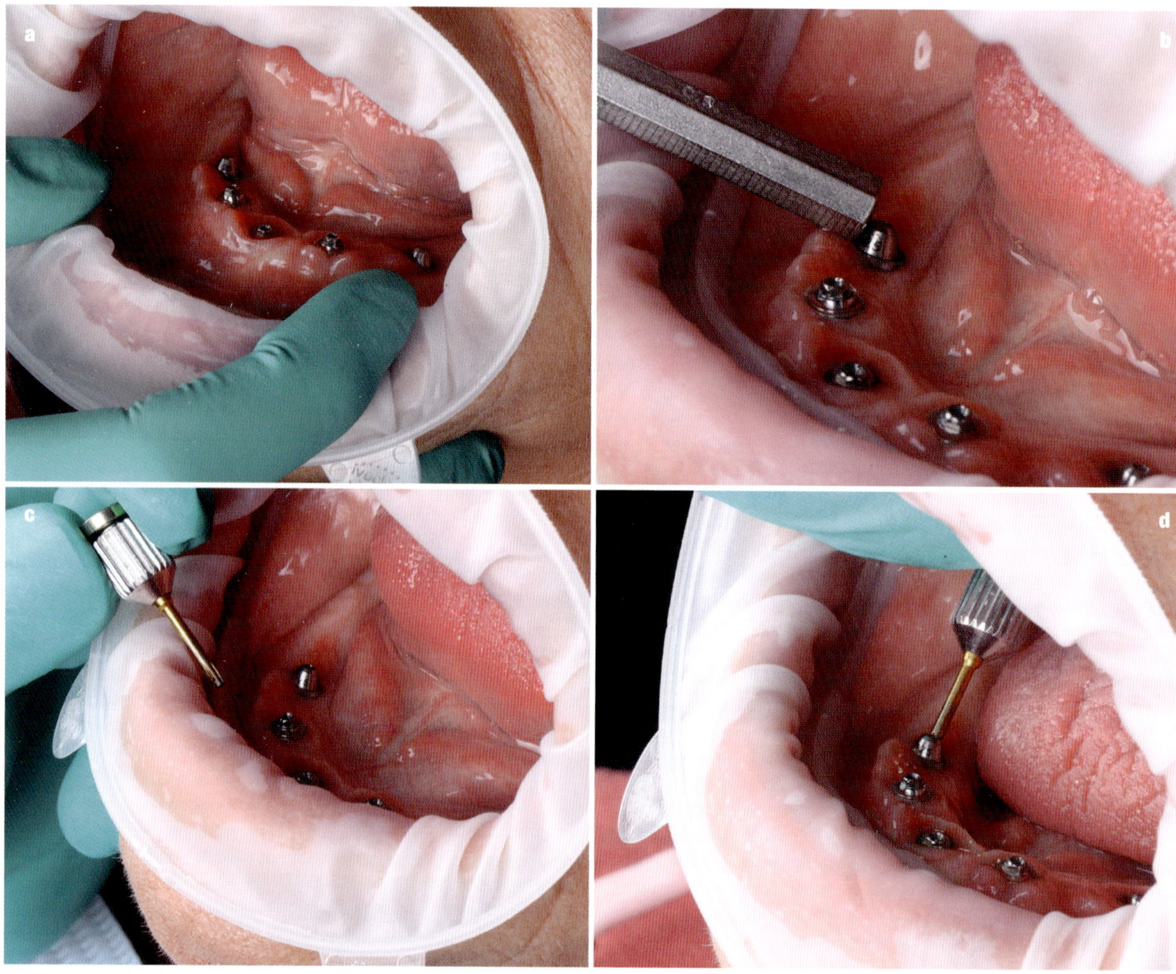

Figure 9.7 (a) Examination of the soft tissues around the MUAs and in the edentulous areas; (b) Tapping on the MUAs with an intraoral mirror handle to check their stability; (c, d) Using an implant driver to hand tighten any loose MUAs.

D. Test the implants for osseointegration

In our practice, we check each dental implant for stability using an osseointegration device and record each reading by implant number. With the device we use (Periotest M,® Medezintechnik Gulden), the lower the reading, the higher the stability of the implant. Thus, a reading of -2 or lower indicates that an implant is stable and integrating, and a reading of -6.2 suggests even more stability and complete integration (Fig. 9.8). There are several other devices available that measure implant stability using either implant stability quotient (ISQ) or implant stability test (IST) readings.

If you use an osseointegration device and do not get an acceptable reading, consider doing the following:

- Retighten the MUA(s) on the implant(s) in question.
- Recheck the reading by testing the abutment from a different angle.
- Take a periapical radiograph to verify correct seating of the MUA within the implant. Also verify that the diameter of the MUA and implant are correctly matched.
- Wait an additional 4 to 6 weeks and retest.

After you have retightened the MUA (and verified that it is the correct size), your reading should improve. If it does not, you may want to take some radiographs or an additional CBCT. After 4 months of healing, it is not necessary to retake radiographs or a CBCT unless integration of the implant is in question. We generally try to take only as many films as necessary to avoid overexposing our patients to dental radiation. However, additional films may be needed to investigate whether an implant is failing, as it is best to identify and address this early on in the workflow. That may mean an implant(s) needs to be removed and replaced or, in a worst-case scenario, that the arch needs to be replanned, re-engineered, and re-operated.

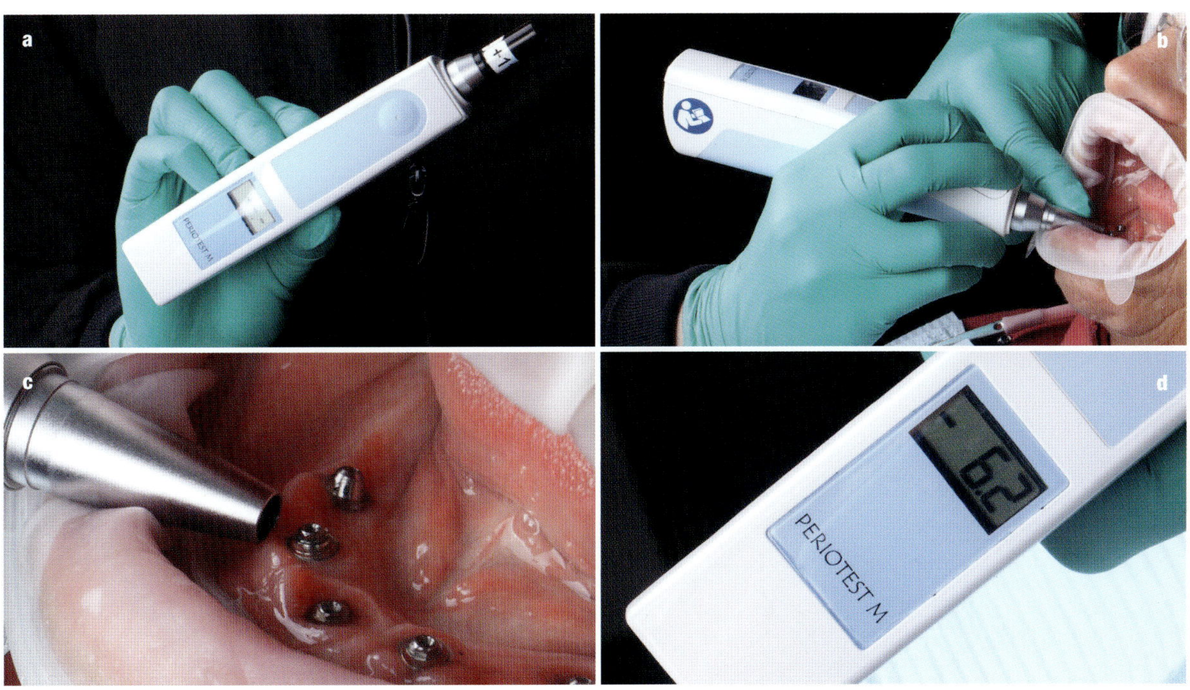

Figure 9.8 (a) Periotest M® device (Medezintechnik Gulden); (b) Holding the Periotest M in place as it taps on an MUA and then displays a value; (c) Demonstration of the proper distance and angulation of the Periotest M in relation to an MUA to obtain an accurate reading; (d) A Periotest M device displaying an ideal reading that suggests excellent osseointegration.

Assuming that your implants are stable and integrating, verify the torque values of your straight and angled MUAs. Using your torque driver, apply the manufacturer's recommended torque to each MUA in order (Fig. 9.9). Be aware that in many implant systems, straight MUAs have a different torque value assigned to them than angled MUAs. Once the MUAs are torqued properly, it is time to begin collecting the data that will help the laboratory build your verification appliance.

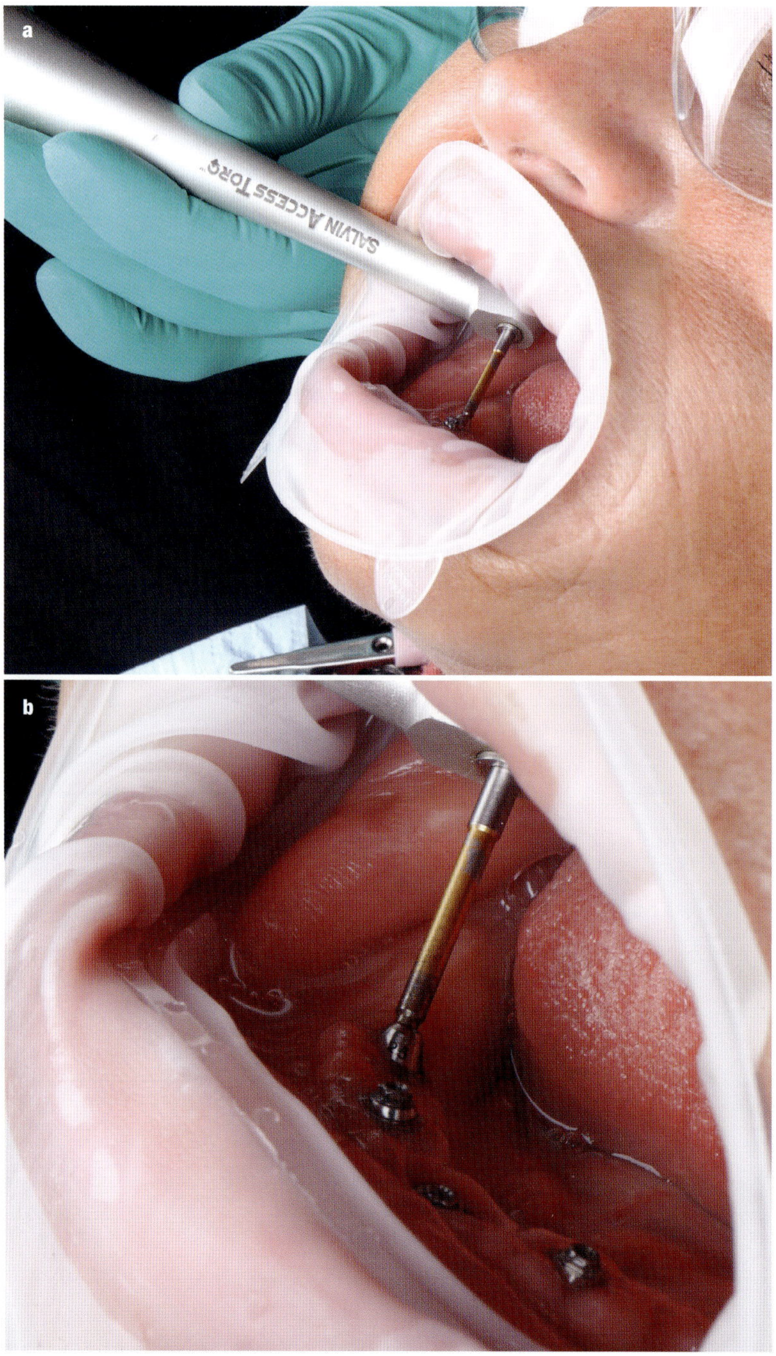

Figure 9.9 (a, b) Use of a torque driver to apply the manufacturer's recommended torque on each MUA.

E. Obtain a digital scan of the interim prosthesis

The following steps are easily delegated to a team member/auxiliary. Retrieve the interim prosthesis from the cleaning solution where it was placed earlier. If the integrity of the prosthesis is acceptable, attach MUA lab analogs to the undersides of the temporary cylinders (or titanium bases if this was a long-term prosthesis). Use the same screws that you removed from the prosthesis to stabilize the MUA analogs in place, and hand tighten only (Fig. 9.10). Make sure each analog is flush with the underside of each temporary cylinder and/or titanium base.

Depending on the type of scanner you have, you may need to make modifications to the prosthesis itself. With some older models, scan sprays were helpful for picking up all the details of the appliance and the analogs. The software in the latest generation of intraoral and laboratory scanners has improved dramatically, and these prostheses require far less preparation to achieve a successful scan. Follow your manufacturer's recommended scanning technique to obtain a 3D digital model of the prosthesis with the analogs in it (Fig. 9.11). When scanning two prostheses for a dual-arch case, repeat the entire process for the opposing arch.

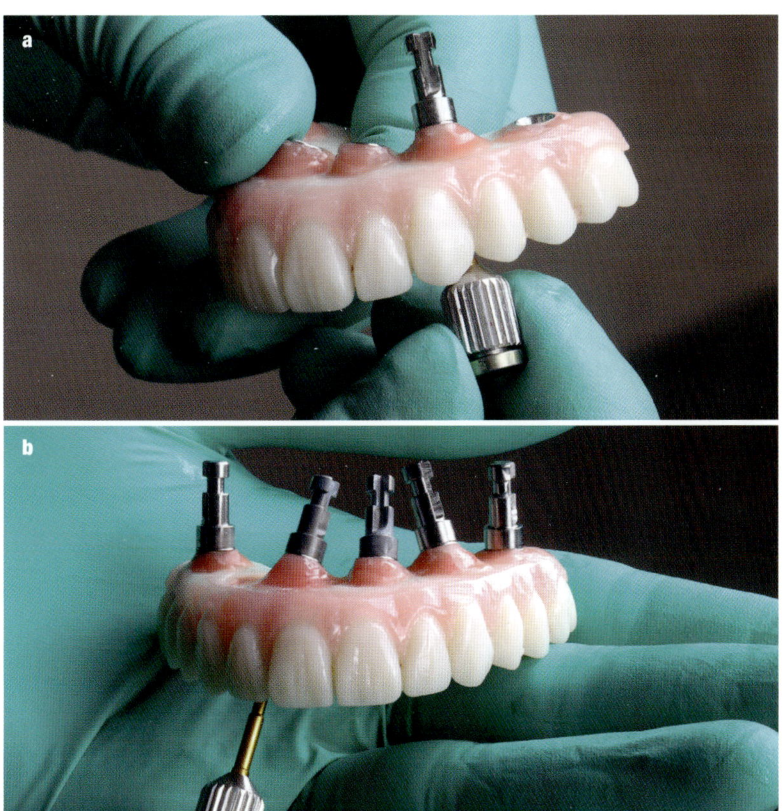

Figure 9.10 (a, b) Tightening the MUA scan analogs in place using a torque driver.

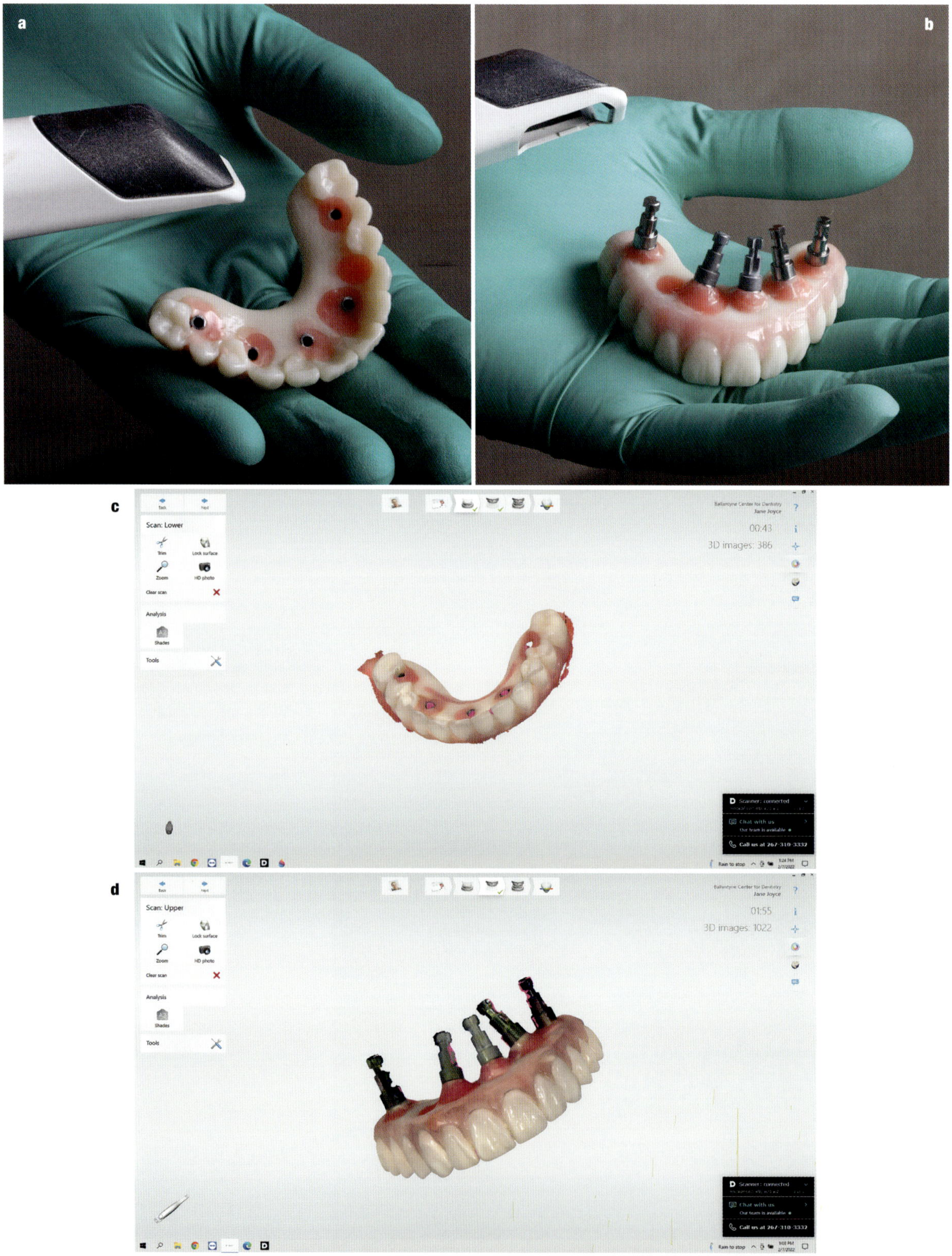

Figure 9.11 Scanning the (a) occlusal and (b) intaglio surface, with scan analogs, of the interim prosthesis; (c, d) Digital model displaying the same surfaces, respectively.

F. Replace the interim prosthesis

After you have obtained a 3D scan of the interim prosthesis, remove the screws from the implant analogs using the implant driver and set them aside. Again, keep careful track of the screws as you put them in and take them out of the prosthesis, and use a dappen dish or small bowl to keep them organized. Replace the interim prosthesis back in the patient's mouth over the MUAs and torque the screws to the appropriate value. Rinse and dry the access channels and backfill them with heavy-body PVS impression material (Fig. 9.12).

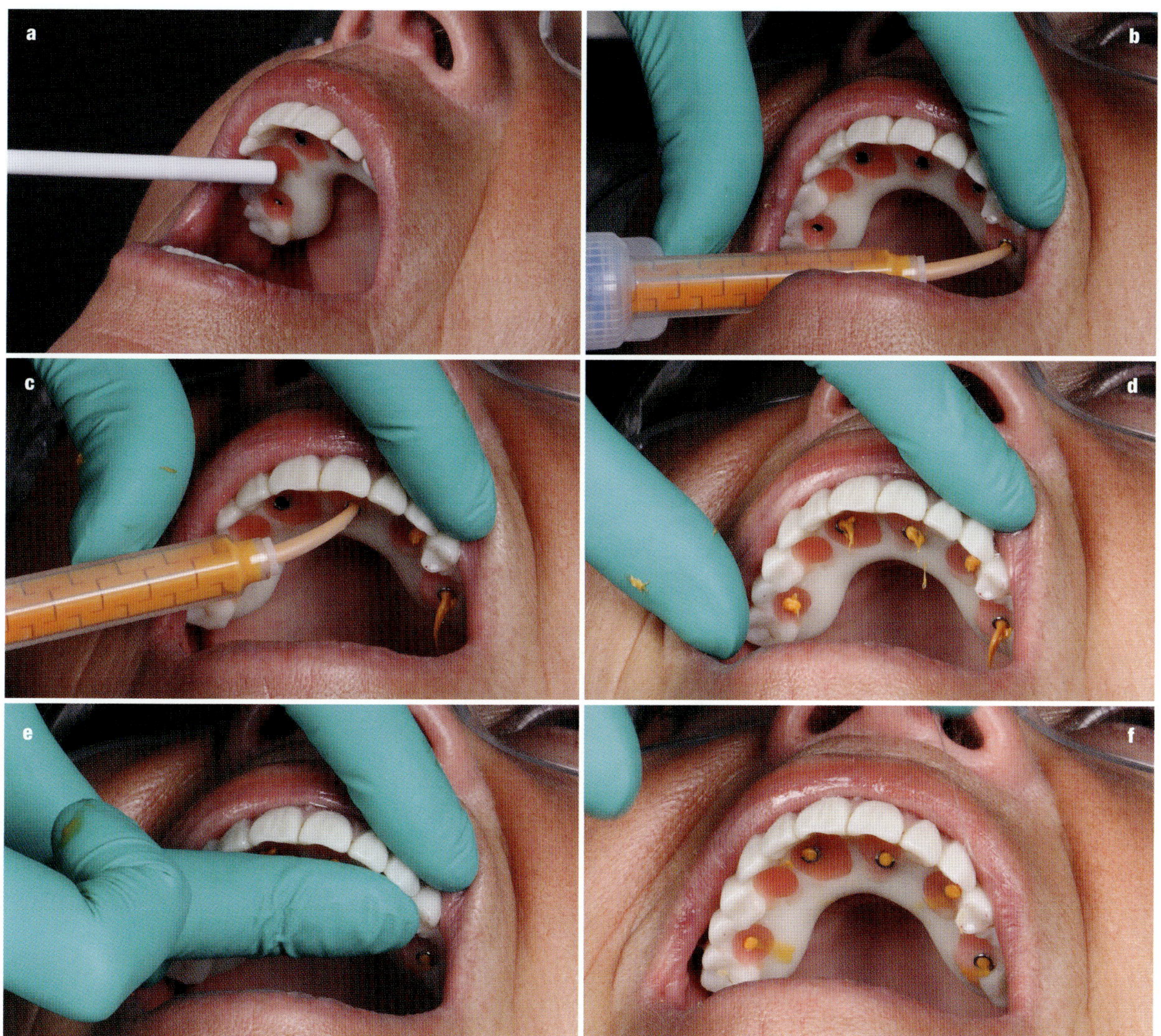

Figure 9.12 Filling the access channels of the interim prosthesis with PVS impression material. (a) Rinse and dry the access channels; (b, c) Place heavy-body PVS in the access channels; (d, e) Wipe off any excess PVS material; (f) Appearance of the interim prosthesis access channels filled with heavy-body PVS material.

G. Scan the opposing arch and obtain the maxillomandibular relationship record

To enable the laboratory to provide the most accurate verification appliance, you will need to obtain an intraoral scan of the opposing arch (Fig. 9.13a). In a dual-arch case, you will have already obtained this record, but you should scan the opposing arch using the intraoral scanner when you have an opposing arch that you are not making a verification appliance for. You will also record the patient's maxillomandibular relationship, either digitally with your scanner or with an analog bite registration. My preference is the former if you are already working within a digital workflow, not only because it helps maintain consistency and avoid confusion, but it also provides the most accurate records in most cases (Figs. 9.13b, 9.13c).

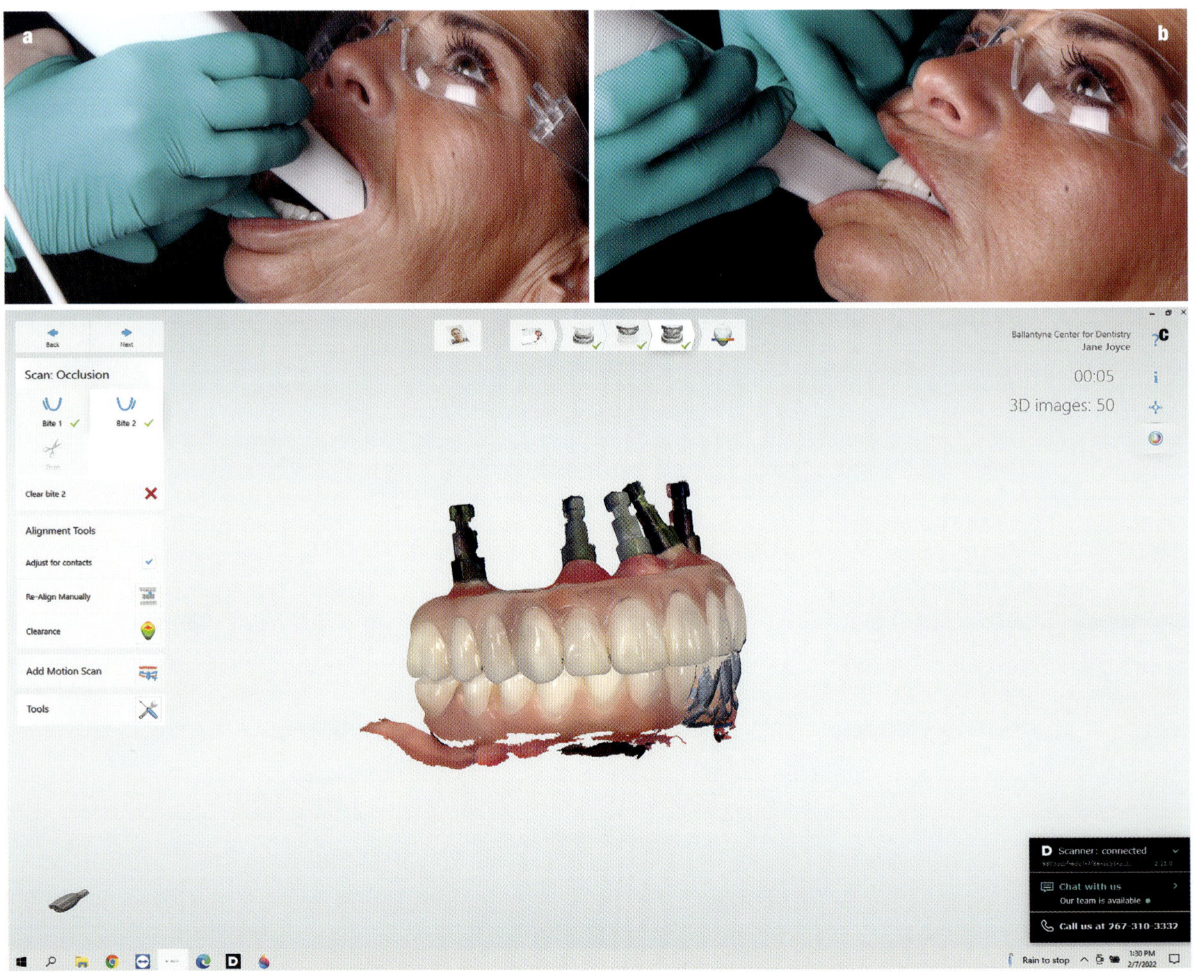

Figure 9.13 (a) Intraoral digital scanning of the opposing arch; (b) Intraoral digital recording of the patient's maxillomandibular relationship; (c) Resulting digital models of the interim prosthesis with the opposing arch and maxillomandibular relationship.

H. Dismiss the patient and communicate with the laboratory

Advise your patient that they have successfully completed their first prosthetic appointment and that you will be sending the records to your laboratory. Generally, the major share of this appointment can be delegated to a well-trained dental assistant. If you collected all your data digitally, you should have one of your assistants upload it from your intraoral scanner to the laboratory and explain in prescription form what you need from them.

You may also want to take photos at this visit, especially if the patient is already wearing a definitive prosthesis that you are planning to replace with a new (and significantly modified) prosthesis (Fig. 9.14).

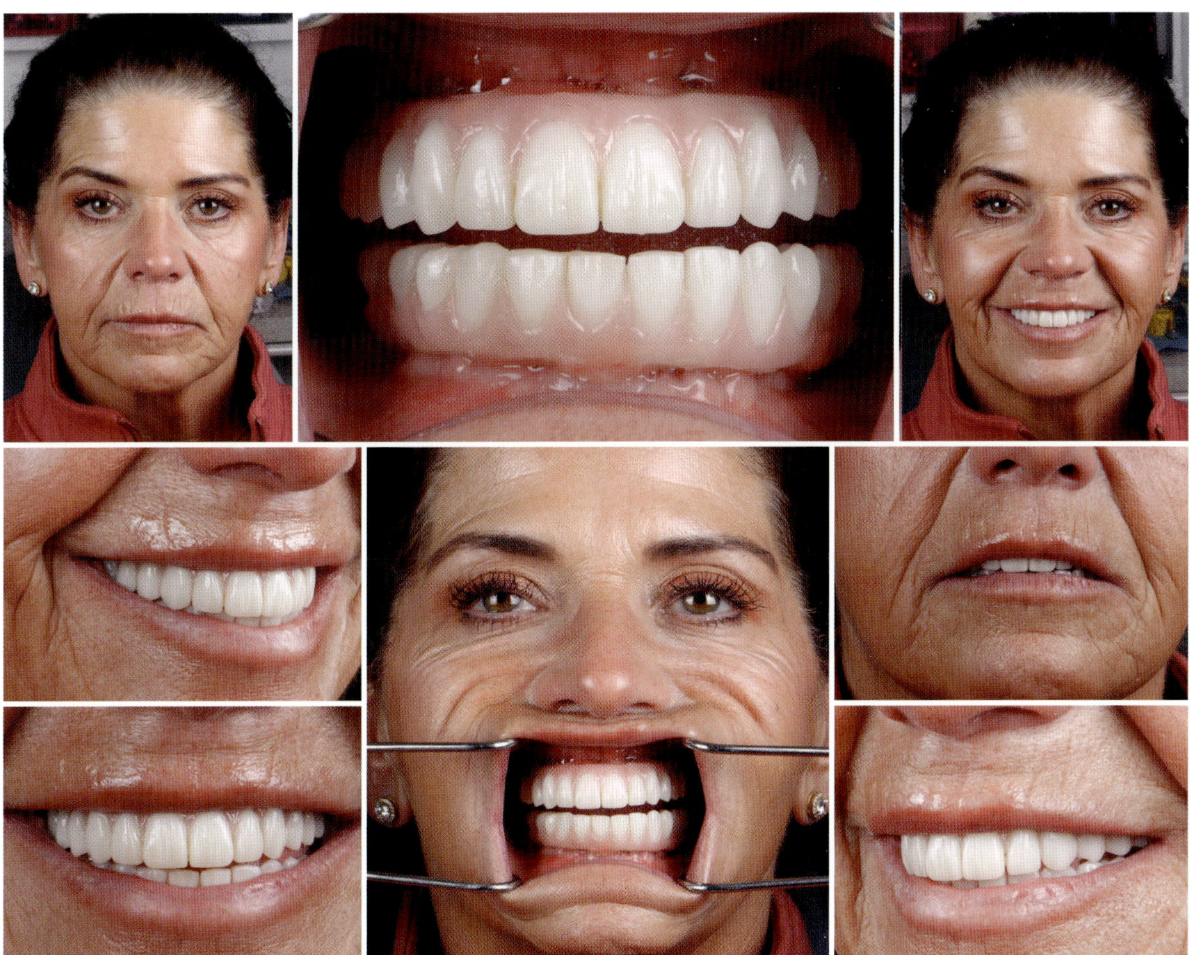

Figure 9.14 Sample photo series of the interim prosthesis used for lab communication.

Throughout the prosthetic workflow, you will be sending appliances, maxillomandibular relationship records, photographs, and possibly other nondigital components to your dental lab. Some labs prefer to have a hard copy laboratory prescription from the very beginning of the process in addition to any digital files you may send. Having an easy-to-follow laboratory communication tool can be helpful for you and your team. An easy to understand lab prescription for fixed full-arch implant prosthetics was developed by Drs. Nate Farley and Kent Howell, the founders of Renew Digital Design Lab (Fig. 9.15). You may find this form useful for keeping track of where you are in the workflow process and to let your lab know the details of your cases.

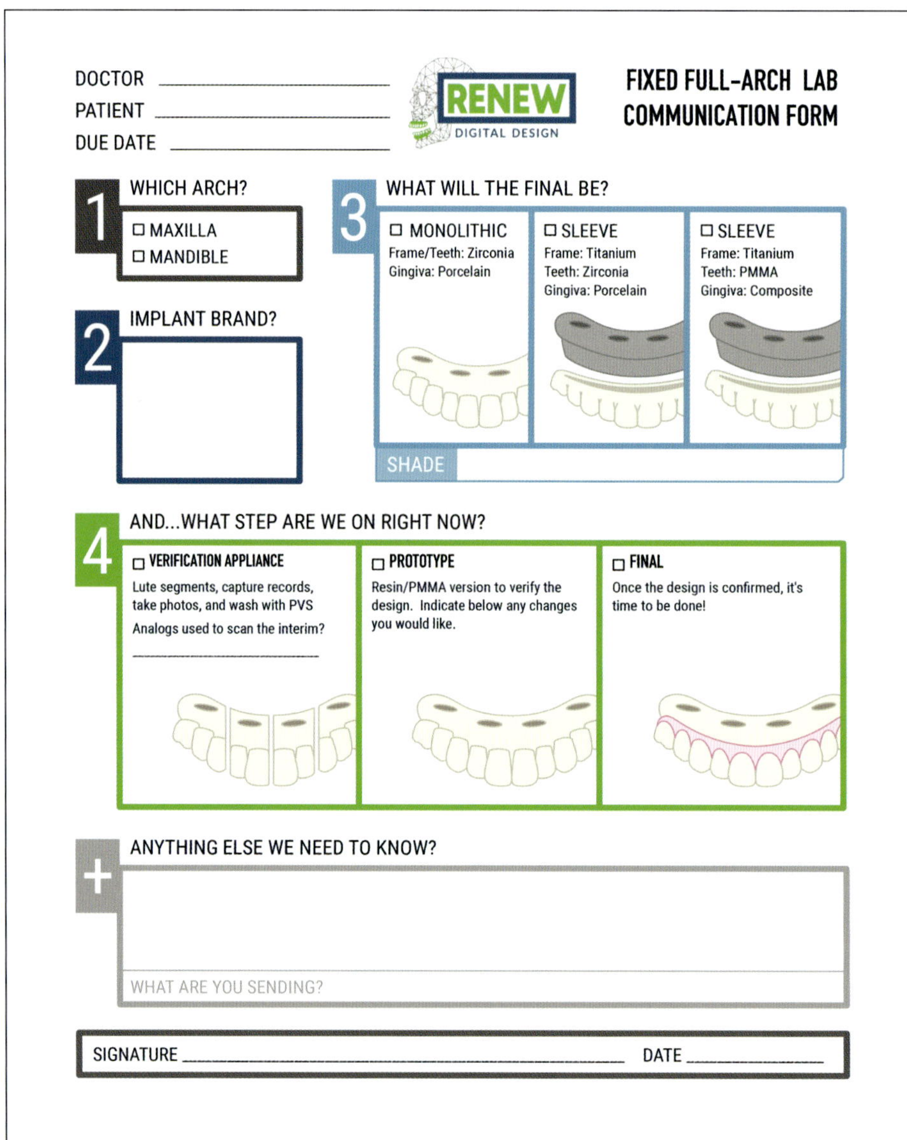

DOCTOR ______________
PATIENT ______________
DUE DATE ______________

RENEW DIGITAL DESIGN

FIXED FULL-ARCH LAB COMMUNICATION FORM

1 WHICH ARCH?
☐ MAXILLA
☐ MANDIBLE

2 IMPLANT BRAND?

3 WHAT WILL THE FINAL BE?

☐ MONOLITHIC
Frame/Teeth: Zirconia
Gingiva: Porcelain

☐ SLEEVE
Frame: Titanium
Teeth: Zirconia
Gingiva: Porcelain

☐ SLEEVE
Frame: Titanium
Teeth: PMMA
Gingiva: Composite

SHADE

4 AND...WHAT STEP ARE WE ON RIGHT NOW?

☐ VERIFICATION APPLIANCE
Lute segments, capture records, take photos, and wash with PVS
Analogs used to scan the interim?
____

☐ PROTOTYPE
Resin/PMMA version to verify the design. Indicate below any changes you would like.

☐ FINAL
Once the design is confirmed, it's time to be done!

+ ANYTHING ELSE WE NEED TO KNOW?

WHAT ARE YOU SENDING?

SIGNATURE ______________ DATE ______________

Figure 9.15 **Prosthetic workflow laboratory communication form developed by Drs. Nate Farley and Kent Howell of Renew Digital Design Lab.** ***(Reprinted with permission.)***

VERIFICATION APPLIANCE TECHNIQUE: APPOINTMENT 2

Before beginning the second appointment, it is helpful to make sure that the verification appliance returned by your laboratory is ready to go.

Operatory setup. In addition to a basic chairside exam kit, the following items will be helpful:

- Dental implant prosthetic setup with drivers
- Cheek and lip retraction device
- Luting material, such as Stellar DC® (Taub Products)
- Handpiece and bur kits (both chairside and lab)
- PVS tray adhesive
- PVS impression material
- Occlusal registration material
- Articulating paper
- Digital occlusal analysis device (optional)
- Camera

A properly designed verification appliance should be shorter in height than the patient's interim prosthesis in order to accommodate the PVS impression material. It should have a flat platform with a flange that protrudes slightly to hold the PVS impression material, which will be used to capture the intaglio surface (Fig. 9.16). In order for the PVS impression material to accurately pick up an impression of the soft tissues around the MUAs, the intaglio surface of the appliance must be coated with PVS adhesive. Use the adhesive that is designed to work with the impression material you are using (Fig. 9.17). It is also helpful to paint the adhesive just over any flanges or onto the buccal aspect of the appliance, just short of the teeth. This will make the PVS material less likely to peel away from the appliance.

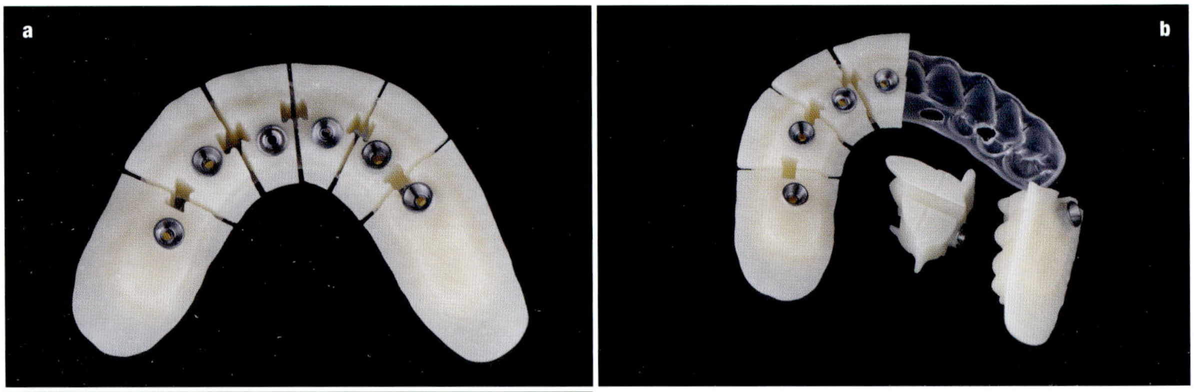

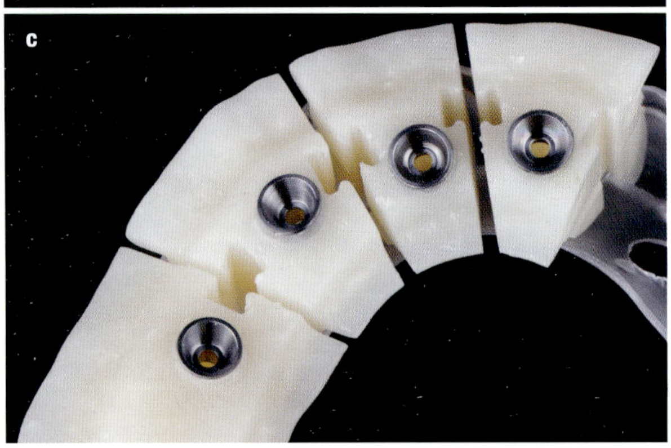

Figure 9.16 Verification appliance. (a) Platform and interlocking spaces; (b) Individual sections with titanium bases; (c) Close-up view of the space between the sections to allow for PVS material.

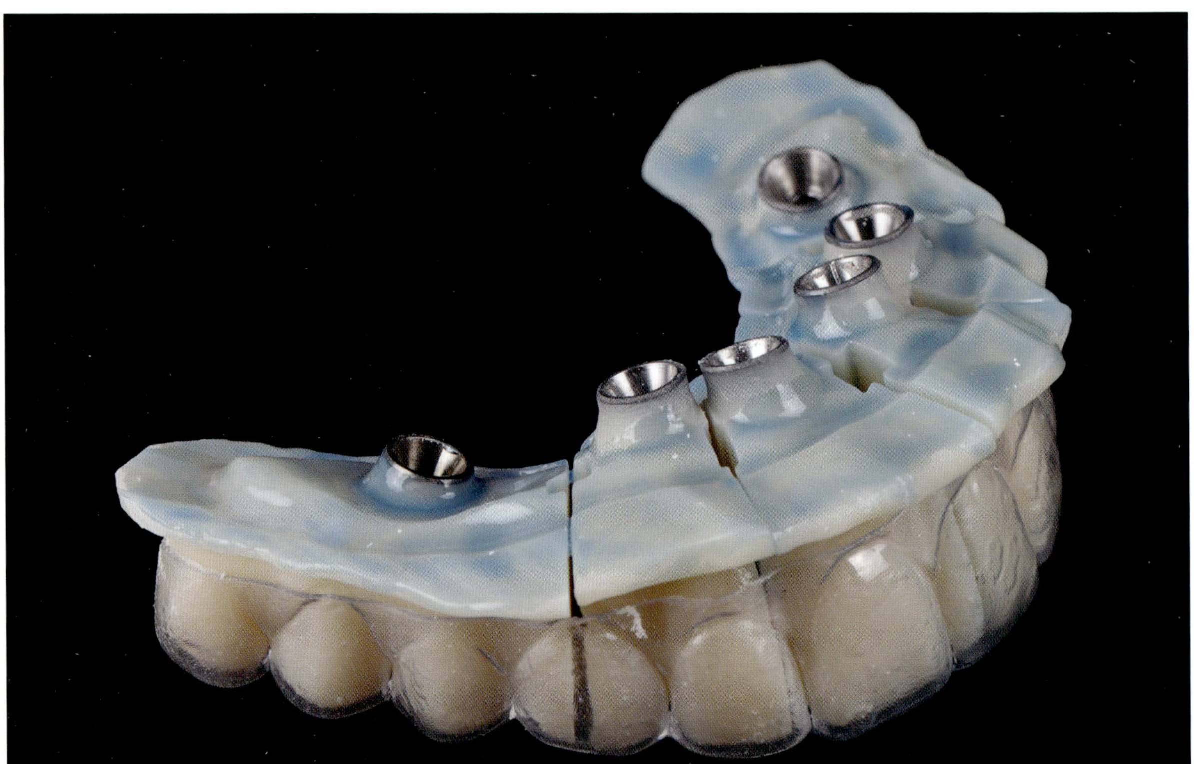

Figure 9.17 PVS adhesive applied to the intaglio surface of the verification appliance.

A. Remove the interim prosthesis

The task of removing the patient's interim prosthesis (or prostheses) can be delegated to your dental auxiliary. As before, start by removing the PVS plugs in the screw access channels, then use the implant driver to loosen the MUA screws and remove the prosthesis from the MUAs (Fig. 9.18a). Be sure to place the prosthetic screws into a dappen dish or small bowl. I emphasize this because losing screws can become expensive over time, and it is easy to do if you are not organized. At the prior appointment, you checked over the prosthesis, examined the soft tissues, tested for osseointegration of the implants, and re-torqued the MUAs, and these steps do not need to be repeated at this appointment. Retraction of the lips and cheeks using the OptraGate can be very helpful during the luting process. As noted earlier, this device also allows for better visualization and movement around the arch (Figs. 9.18b, 9.18c).

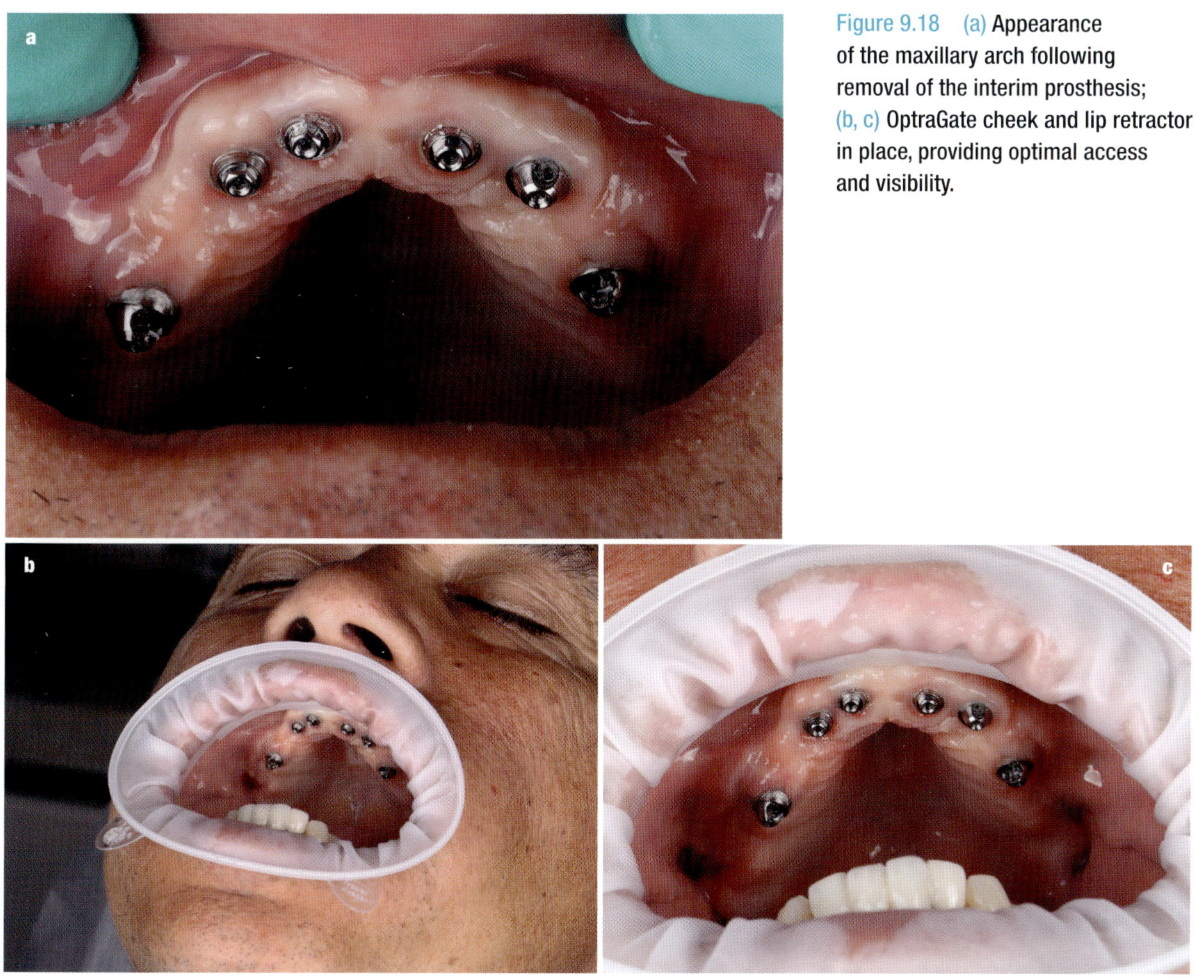

Figure 9.18 (a) Appearance of the maxillary arch following removal of the interim prosthesis; (b, c) OptraGate cheek and lip retractor in place, providing optimal access and visibility.

B. Place the verification appliance sections

Once the interim prosthesis (or prostheses) is removed, you can attach the sections of the verification appliance to the MUAs. I generally recommend that the dentist be responsible for completing this procedure, as it can be challenging: If you discover that one of the sections was seated improperly after all the sections have been luted together, it can have a negative effect on the efficiency of future visits and potentially result in a definitive prosthesis that does not fit well.

Some labs use a plastic retainer-like tray to hold the sections of the verification appliance together (Fig. 9.19a). The idea is to place the entire tray with the sections over the MUAs and then use the driver to place the screws through the access channels and tighten all the parts down (Fig. 9.19b). I have found that this works only if the tray is somewhat flexible, the scan was very accurate, and the lab lined everything up well in the software; otherwise, it is easier to place each section of the verification appliance separately. My suggestion is to do what takes the least amount of time and creates the least amount of frustration for you and your patient.

The sections of the verification appliance should be placed consecutively, following the curve of the arch. Once all the sections have been screwed into the MUAs, make sure they are hand-tight or even torqued to approximately 10 Ncm (Figs. 9.19c, 9.19d). What is important is that each section of the verification appliance is seated securely and in alignment over each MUA. If any of the sections are spinning or not tightening the way they should, remove that section and inspect it for a loose temporary cylinder or titanium base. In some cases you will have sections of the verification appliance that are not in perfect alignment with adjoining sections. This is acceptable if the titanium bases are seated completely on the MUAs. If there are spaces between the sections for the luting material, further adjustments can be made with a handpiece and a bur to correct for most of the misalignments.

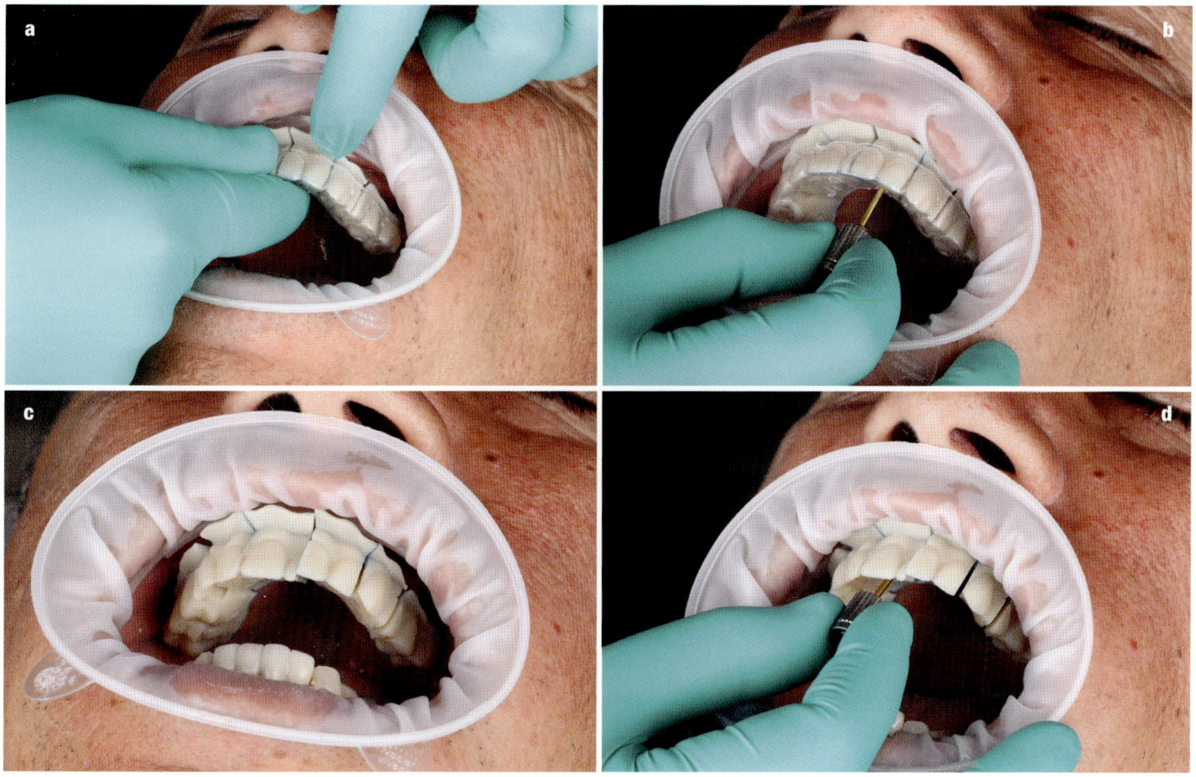

Figure 9.19 **Placement of the verification appliance.** (a) **Place all sections of the appliance at once using the plastic tray matrix (if provided), or please one section at a time consecutively following the curvature of the arch;** (b) **Use the driver to screw the verification appliance in place over the MUAs;** (c) **Close-up view of the verification appliance in place. Note that the individual sections of the appliance are not perfectly aligned;** (d) **Hand-tighten the individual sections of the verification appliance after removing the plastic tray matrix (if provided).**

C. Lute the verification appliance

When all the sections of the verification appliance are in place and have been hand tightened, use an air-water syringe to rinse it off and remove any moisture or saliva that is on it, then lute the sections together. This is another procedure that I recommend the dentist perform or directly oversee.

Luting the sections of the verification appliance does not have to be a complicated or messy job. In the past, dentists have relied on self-curing acrylics that required time-consuming mixing techniques and were not always easy to manipulate. Stellar DC by Taub Products solves this problem. This material is a dual-cure acrylic resin that comes in a familiar syringe dispenser. The tip delivery system makes it easy to inject the material into the spaces between the verification appliance sections, and it can be tack-cured with a curing light in a few seconds (Fig. 9.20). As noted in the surgical workflow (Chapter 7), I also use Stellar DC in the pick-up of the temporary cylinders during surgery as well as for small repairs to the interim prosthesis. Having one material for multiple uses within the complete full-arch implant workflow is just another way to simplify the process.

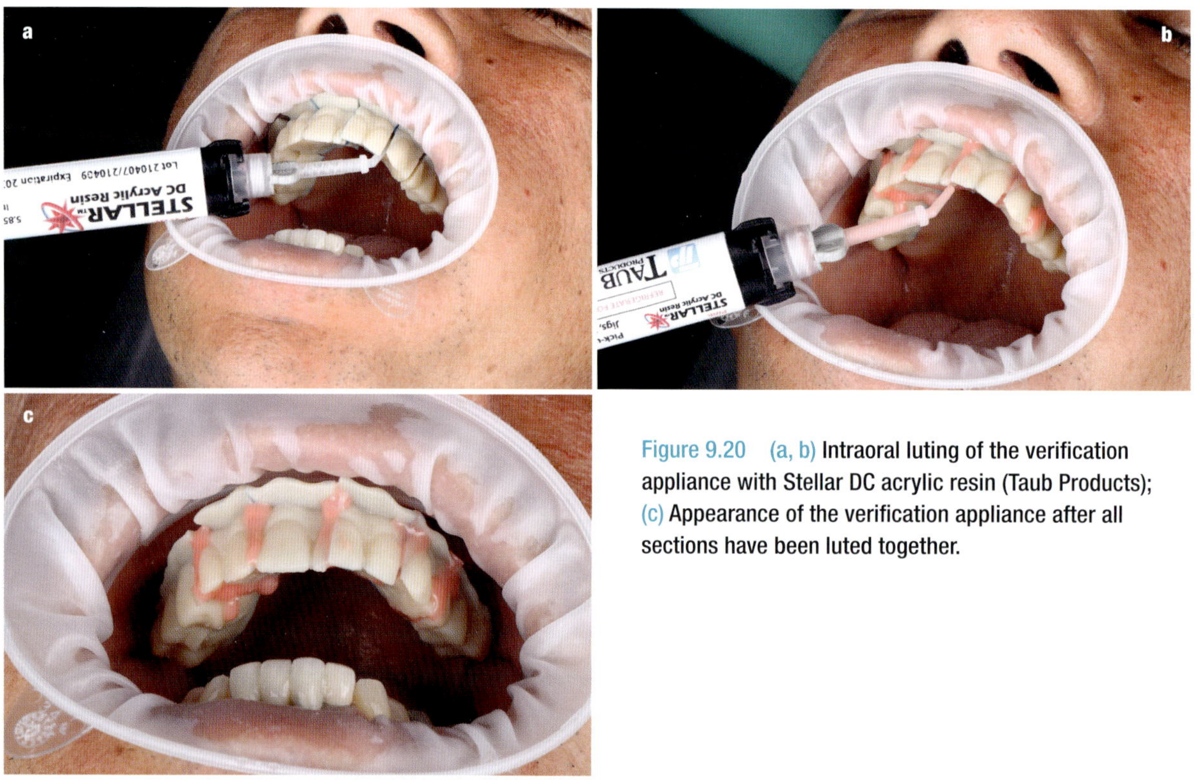

Figure 9.20 (a, b) Intraoral luting of the verification appliance with Stellar DC acrylic resin (Taub Products); (c) Appearance of the verification appliance after all sections have been luted together.

D. Remove the luted verification appliance and check it for stability

Once the sections are luted together, the verification appliance can be removed and inspected. It is important for all the sections of the appliance to be secured together well. In some cases, you may find that the luting materials did not completely seal the sections of the appliance as well as you may have thought. This is the time to make certain that your verification appliance is stable. If it is not, place the verification appliance back on the MUAs in the patient's mouth and use the Stellar DC to reinforce those areas. I recommend adding luting material for additional strength even if the appliance is secure and the sections are not moving independently (Fig. 9.21). Once it has passed inspection, place the verification appliance back into the patient's mouth and use the implant driver to hand tighten the screws through the access channels into the MUAs (Fig. 9.22).

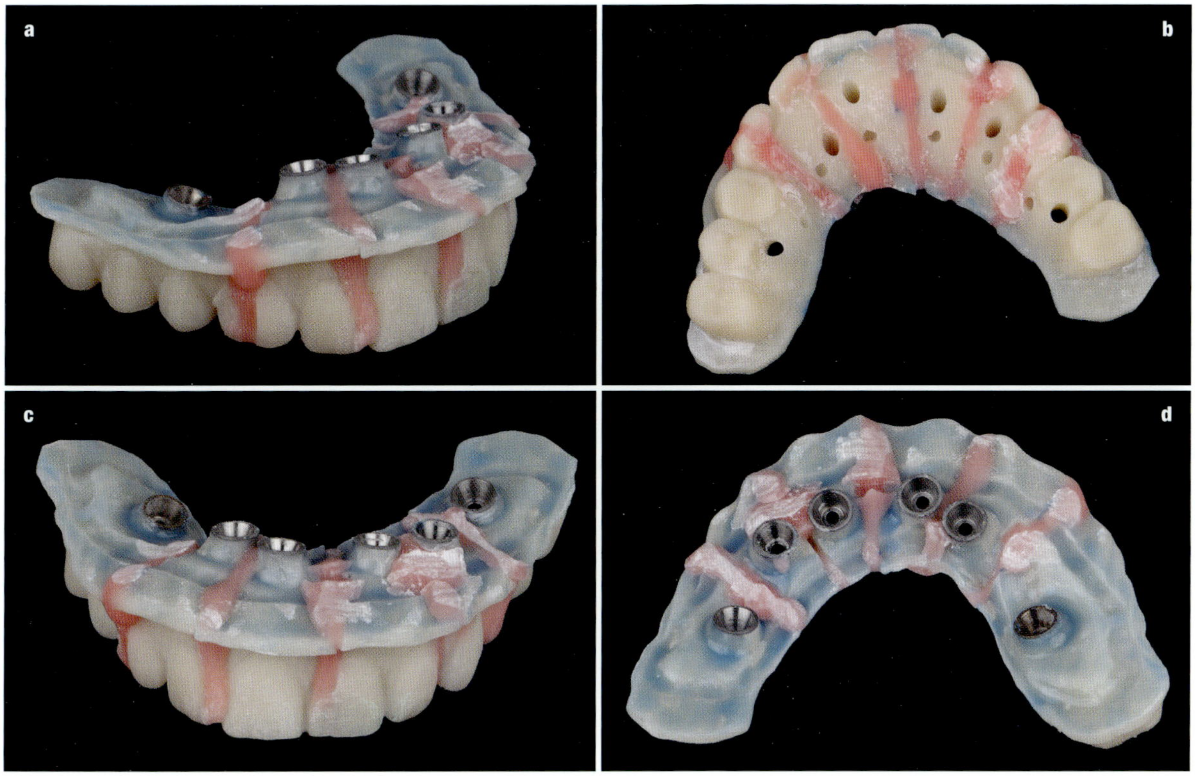

Figure 9.21 (a-d) Extraoral view of the verification appliance after additional luting material was added for strength.

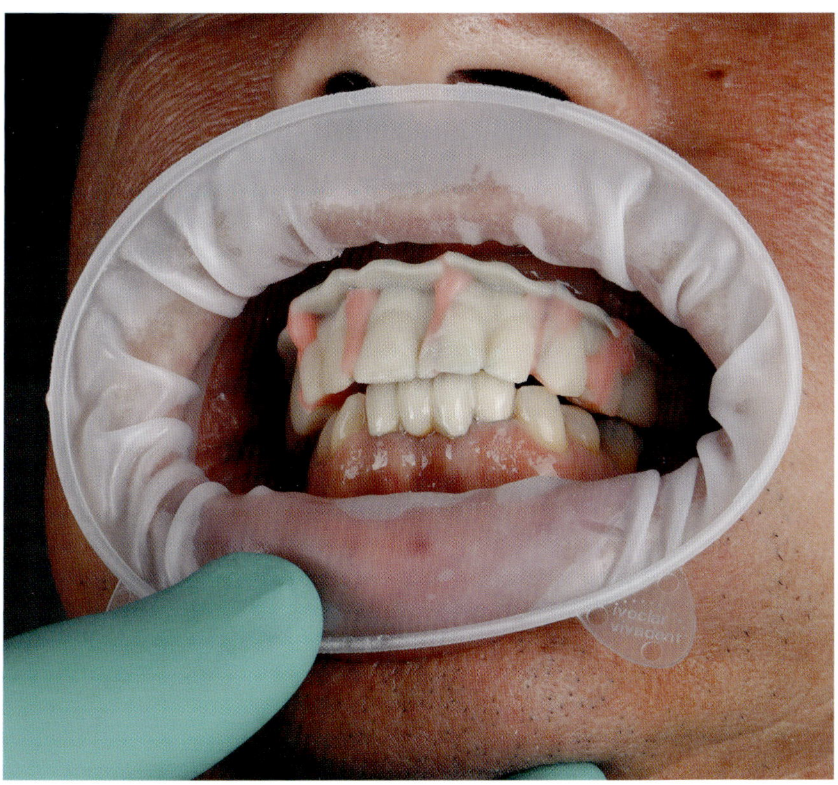

Figure 9.22 Luted verification appliance reseated and secured with screws on the MUAs.

E. Verify the horizontal plane, midline, and VDO

With the verification appliance in the patient's mouth, evaluate three reference indicators. Depending on the accuracy of the scans and data collected at the first visit, you might have some work ahead of you. Fortunately, the process is simple if you follow the three steps detailed below. These steps affect the maxillary prosthesis more than the mandibular prosthesis, but it is wise to check both. They should be completed by the dentist, not a dental assistant or auxiliary.

Step 1. Determine whether the appliance is canted in the mouth and make any necessary adjustments.

Place the patient in a sitting position and look at them straight on. For the maxillary appliance, I have found it easiest to ask the patient to smile and then observe how the incisal edges of the anterior teeth follow the patient's lower lip and where the posterior buccal cusps align with the oral commissures. You can also look at the highest point of each tooth and the gingival border to evaluate the curve along the upper lip (Fig. 9.23a). In the mandible, have the patient open and then inspect how well the incisal edges of the lower teeth align with the lower lip and how much incisal edge is showing. When adjusting the appliances to correct the cant, at this point you only really need to focus on getting the edges of the six anterior teeth approximately where you want them. You may want to do this even if the smile is not canted, just to help the lab know about where you want the incisal edges to be. These adjustments can be made intraorally with a handpiece and bur (Fig. 9.23b).

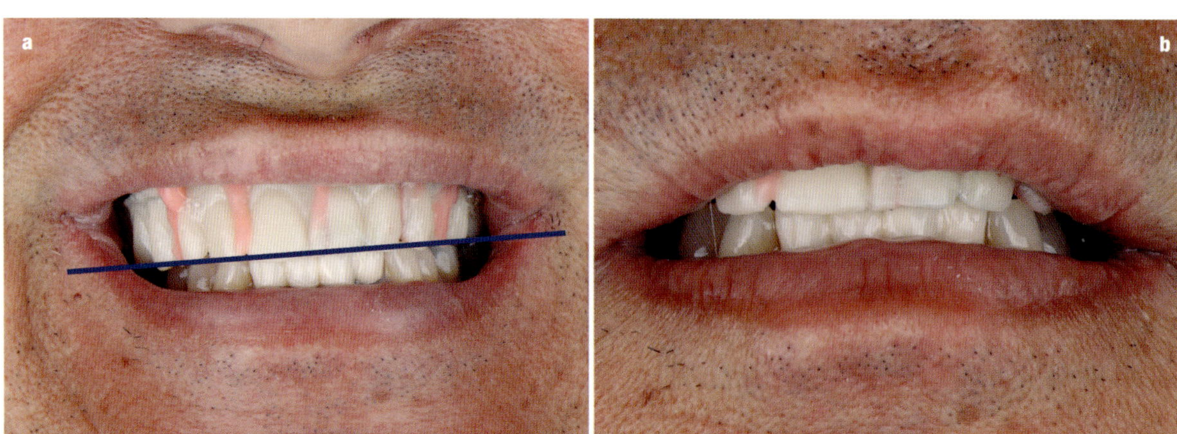

Figure 9.23 (a) Black horizontal line showing that the horizontal plane of the appliance is canted to the patient's right. Note the position of the teeth in relation to the incisal edges, oral commissures, and gingival line; (b) Appearance of the same patient after adjustments were made. Note the incisal edge position.

Step 2. Evaluate the facial midline.

Based on the patient's facial landmarks—including the forehead, eyes, nose, mouth, lips, and chin—determine where the facial midline should be. If the midline of the appliance is off, use a sharp pencil to mark where it should be (Fig. 9.24). Determining where the midline should be is more of an art than a science, and the laboratory can help you decide where the midline will be in the definitive prosthesis. After a few more steps you will be taking photos, which will allow you to make a better evaluation. At that time, you can always remove the pencil mark and change it.

Step 3. Determine whether the VDO is in the right position.

If you have planned well and made appropriate adjustments to the interim prosthesis throughout the healing period, you may not have much work to do here. However, if the patient is one you have inherited or did not see postoperatively, this step may require more time. If, after going through the process, you decide that the VDO needs to be increased, the easiest way to do so is by adding resin to the occlusal surfaces of the appliance in the posterior, a small amount at a time. First, dry the appliance while it is seated in the patient's mouth, then apply some composite bond and cure small amounts of flowable composite until you are happy with the patient's new position. If the occlusion needs to be closed and the verification appliance is too "tall," start by reducing the occlusion gradually in the posterior areas.

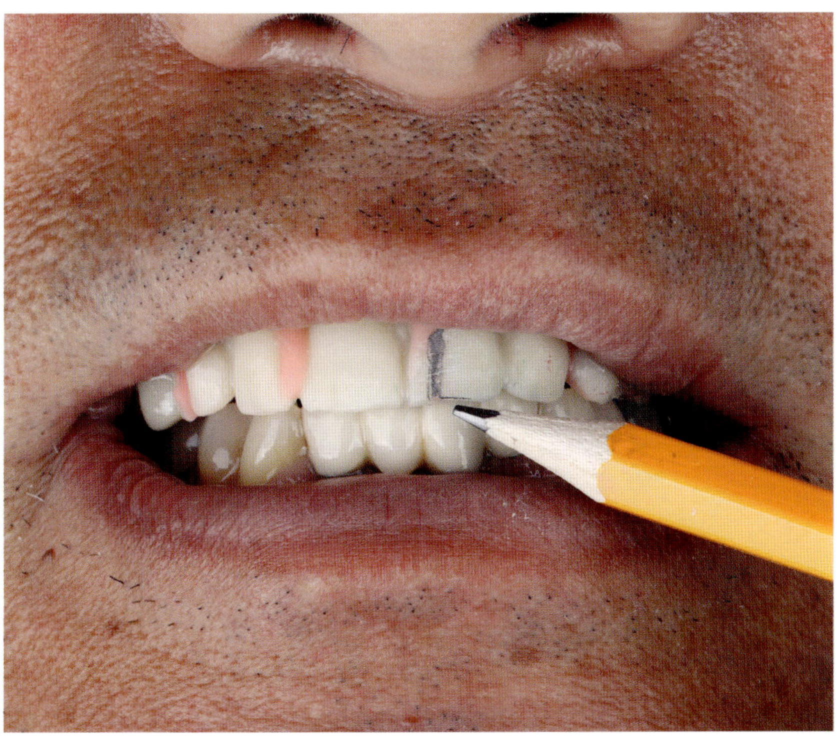

Figure 9.24 **Using a pencil to mark the patient's midline on the verification appliance.**

F. Verify/adjust the occlusion and capture the maxillomandibular relationship

With the luted verification appliance seated, it is okay if the occlusion is not exactly where you want it. However, you should obtain at least a few points of contact balanced around the arch. The lab will help you perfect the occlusion when the resin prototype is fabricated from the verification appliance. What is important is that you get at least three balance points—more like occlusal stops—around the arch.

Use articulating paper to check for contacts (Figs. 9.25a, 9.25b). To make adjustments, use an intraoral handpiece and football-shaped diamond or carbide bur and remove material that is holding up contacts (Figs. 9.25c, 9.25d). Bear in mind that doing this will reduce the patient's vertical dimension. If you are trying to maintain the current VDO, you may need to add composite resin (as noted in Step 3, on the previous page), then create three or four points of balance, keeping the VDO where it is. When you are finished, use your preferred registration material to index and record the maxillomandibular relationship. I recommend obtaining a maxillomandibular relationship record in the centric relation (CR) position (Figs. 9.25e, 9.25f).

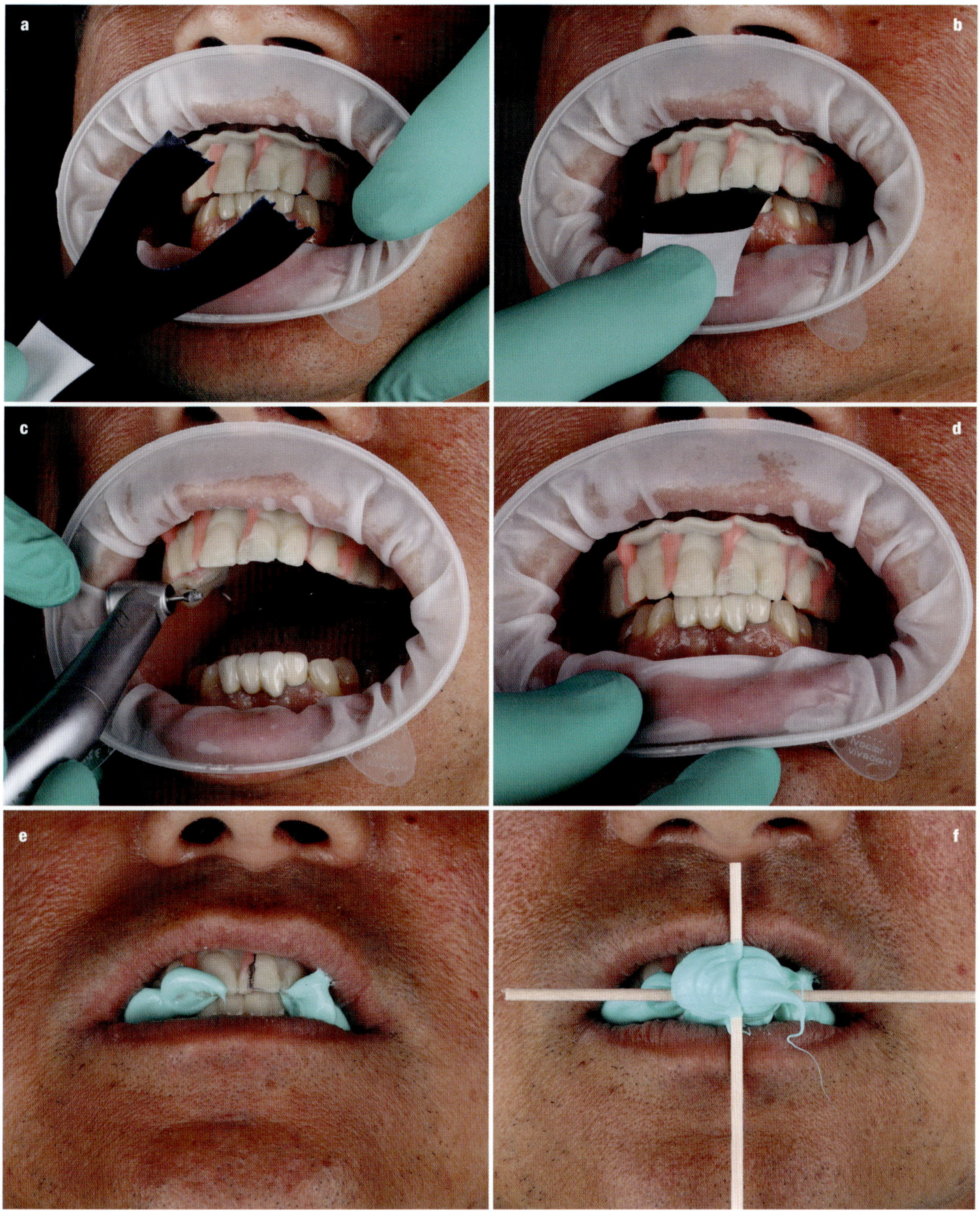

Figure 9.25 Verification and adjustment of the occlusion in the verification appliance. (a, b) Check the contacts in the verification appliance with articulating paper; (c) Adjust the contacts using a high-speed handpiece and football-shaped carbide (or diamond) bur; (d) Appearance of the adjusted occlusion with the patient in centric relation (CR) position; (e) Use registration material to record the patient's maxillomandibular relationship; (f) Use applicator sticks to communicate the midline and horizontal plane to the lab (also referred to as the "poor man's facebow").

G. Take photos to use for laboratory communication

If you are satisfied with the position of the appliance in the patient's smile, take photos for the laboratory. Several pictures will be helpful, but the entire series is probably not needed. I find that the lab can do a very nice job of developing a resin prototype from the verification appliance with the following photographs (Fig. 9.26):

- Retracted portrait
- Close-up smile
- Close-up repose

These three photos give the laboratory most of the information they will need. In our practice, we almost always take photographs at this step in the workflow because the next steps can get a little messy and create distractions in your photographs.

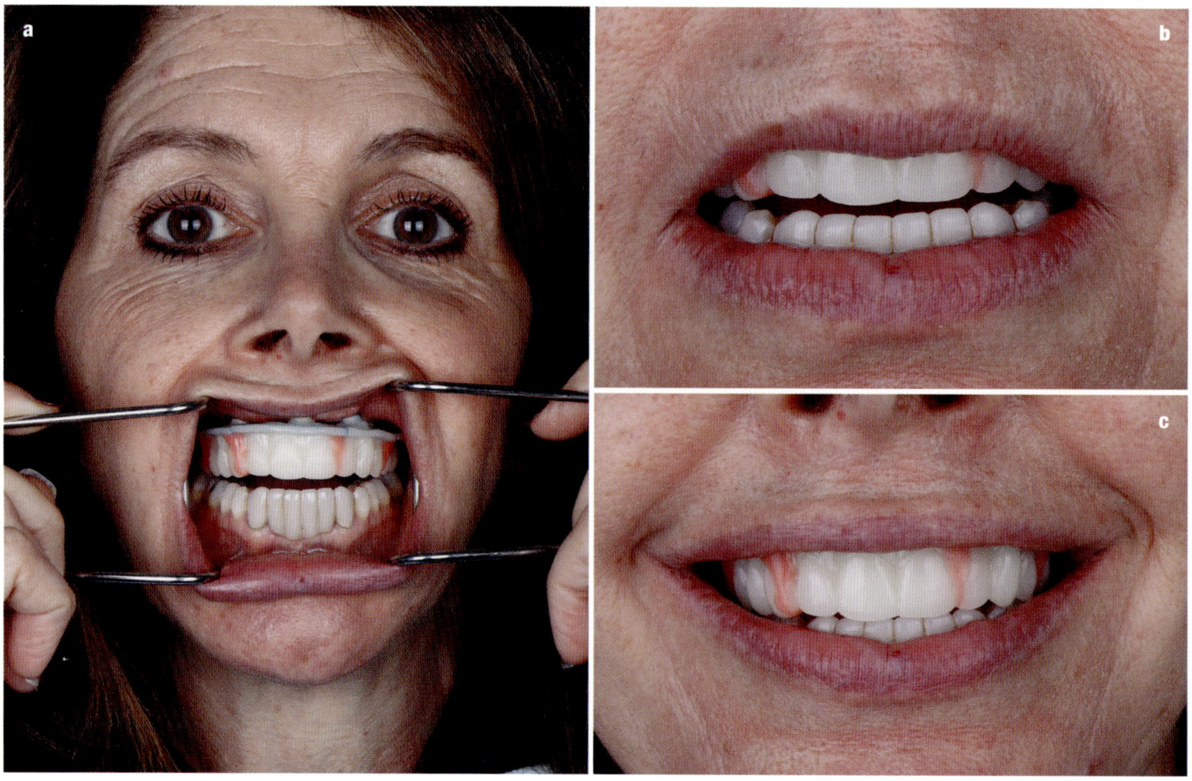

Figure 9.26 **Photos taken to communicate the position of the verification appliance to the lab: (a) Retracted portrait; (b) Close-up repose; (c) Close-up smile.**

H. Take an analog impression of the soft tissues

The workflow I use is almost entirely computer- and software-assisted, with the exception of this step. As of the publishing of this book, I have not found a fast, efficient way to provide the laboratory with a more accurate record of the intaglio surface for the definitive prosthesis than by taking an analog impression. The limited ability of intraoral scanners to pick up this information accurately is partly responsible, although that is about to change. The good news is that this analog step is a simple process and takes only a few minutes.

Begin by preparing a medium-body PVS impression material in an impression syringe with a tip that is small enough to inject into the spaces beneath the verification appliance. I prefer a medium-body impression material because it flows better than heavy-body and has sufficient weight, unlike a light-body wash. Also, choose a PVS material with a longer setting time as this has proven to be helpful compared with some of the more popular fast-set materials.

Use the OptraGate retractor to retract the lips and cheeks from around the appliance(s), then dry the tissues and the verification appliance with an air-water syringe and make sure the patient is comfortable. Start your impression under the appliance on the buccal aspect, either from left to right or right to left. Once you have completed the buccal/facial aspect, repeat the process on the lingual/palatal aspect of the appliance (Fig. 9.27). Make sure the impression material comes over the edges of the appliance onto the buccal and lingual surfaces but does not cover the teeth. (If you do inadvertently place more impression material than is necessary and it flows over the teeth, do not panic; you can remove it once the material is set.) Make sure you have captured the entire arch into the vestibule and around the lingual or palatal, and go far enough distally that you capture any tissue that will be covered in a cantilever within your definitive prosthesis.

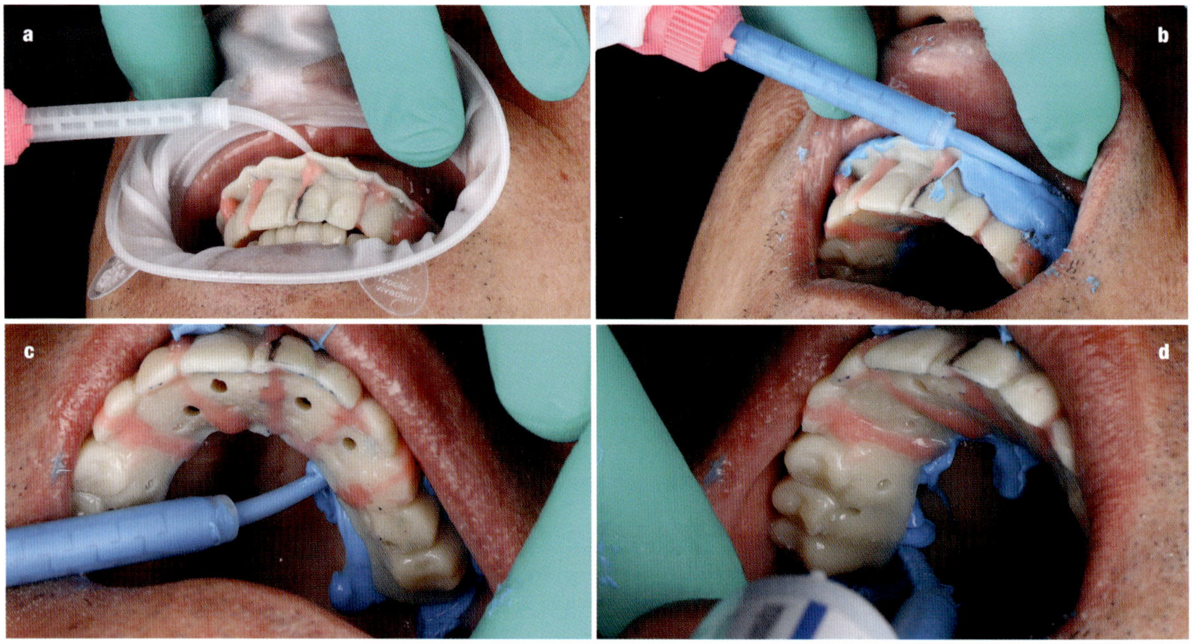

Figure 9.27 Taking an analog impression of the soft tissues. (a) Retract the lips to allow PVS materials to flow under the verification appliance; (b) Capture the buccal vestibule and edentulous areas; (c) Capture the palatal aspects of the tissue under the verification appliance; (d) Complete the impression of the intaglio surface of the verification appliance.

I. Remove the verification appliance and re-seat the interim prosthesis

Once the PVS material has set, you can carefully remove the verification appliance(s) by using the implant driver to remove the screws from the temporary cylinder access channels (Figs. 9.28a, 9.28b). As soon as the appliance is out of the mouth, inspect the intaglio surface for uniformity of the PVS material. If you are satisfied with the way it looks, proceed with placing the patient's interim prosthesis back in the patient's mouth. Torque the screws to the appropriate tightness and fill the access channels with heavy-body PVS material. You will send the verification appliance and maxillomandibular relationship record to the laboratory (Figs. 9.28c, 9.28d). It is important to note here that if the case is a single arch, make sure you have an analog or a digital impression of the opposing arch to send to the lab (Fig. 9.28e). If it is a dual-arch case, the point is moot because you will have repeated the processing of the verification appliance in both arches.

You now have an accurate impression of the patient's arch as well as a way for the lab to determine the appropriate VDO and maxillomandibular relationship. The shape of the teeth, the horizontal plane, and the midline are also marked on the verification appliance. All this information was able to be collected in two short appointments.

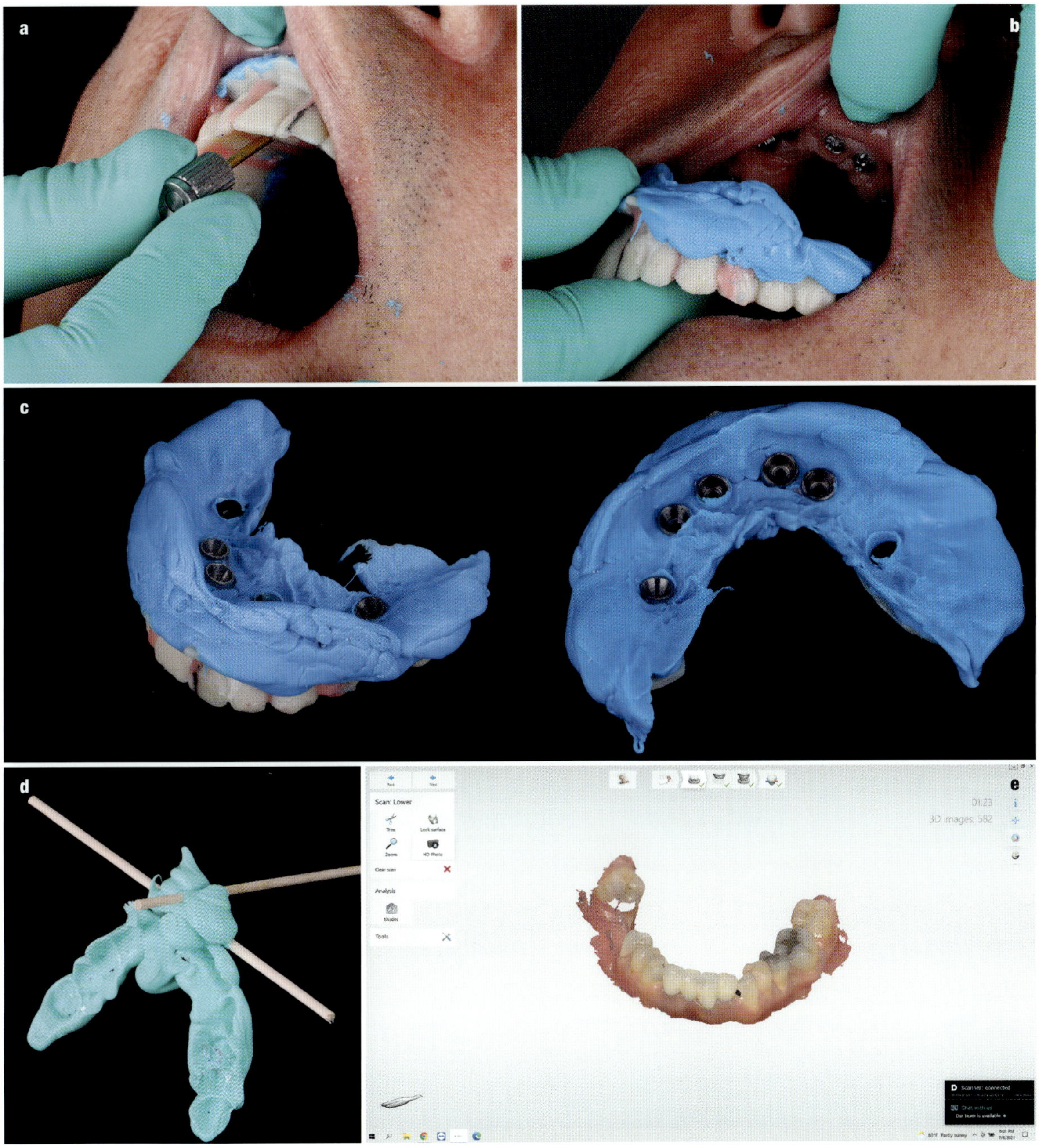

Figure 9.28 Removing the verification appliance from the patient's mouth. (a) Use a driver to remove the prosthetic screws from the temporary cylinder access channels after the PVS impression material is set; (b) Remove the verification appliance from the mouth; (c) Appearance of the PVS impression of the intaglio surface of the verification appliance; (d) Send the record of the maxillomandibular relationship, horizontal plane, and midline to the lab; (e) Intraoral digital impression of an opposing arch.

PRO TIP: Verifying complete seating of an appliance

If you see PVS impression material on the underside of the temporary cylinders or titanium bases, it means that either the verification appliance was not seated completely during the impression or the original luting procedure. Troubleshoot this problem now to avoid inaccuracy in the resin prototype appliance. Individual radiographs can be taken of the MUAs once the verification appliance is screwed back into place and hand tightened. Often a radiograph taken perpendicular to the MUA will show if a temporary cylinder is not seated completely. The one-screw test or Sheffield test (see page 370) is another good method to use when trying in the digital resin prototype at the next visit.

J. Dismiss the patient and communicate with the laboratory

Once you have re-seated the interim prosthesis and scheduled the next appointment to try in the resin prototype, the patient can be dismissed. Create a lab prescription for the case and attach or digitally send any photographs you have taken. If you are following the verification appliance technique workflow, you can skip the next section covering the replica appliance technique. Regardless of which technique you follow in the prosthetic workflow, the outcome is the same: an appliance that your dental laboratory can use to develop a resin prototype.

REPLICA APPLIANCE TECHNIQUE: APPOINTMENT 1

The replica appliance technique is more efficient, requiring only one visit in lieu of the two needed for the verification appliance technique, and thus is my preferred technique. However, it is an option only if a second prosthetic pick-up impression was completed during the patient's surgical visit.

Many of the steps involved in creating the replica appliance are identical to those just described in appointments 1 and 2 of the verification appliance technique. Therefore, to avoid repetition, most of the steps in this section are presented in outline form accompanied by photos. The details of each step can be found in the previous section.

Operatory setup. In addition to a basic chairside exam kit, the following items will be helpful:

- Dental implant prosthetic setup with drivers
- Cheek retraction device
- Handpiece and bur kit (both chairside and lab)
- PVS tray adhesive
- PVS impression material
- Occlusal registration material
- Articulating paper
- Digital occlusal analysis device (optional)
- Camera

A. Verify the patient's VDO and maxillomandibular relationship (Fig. 9.29)

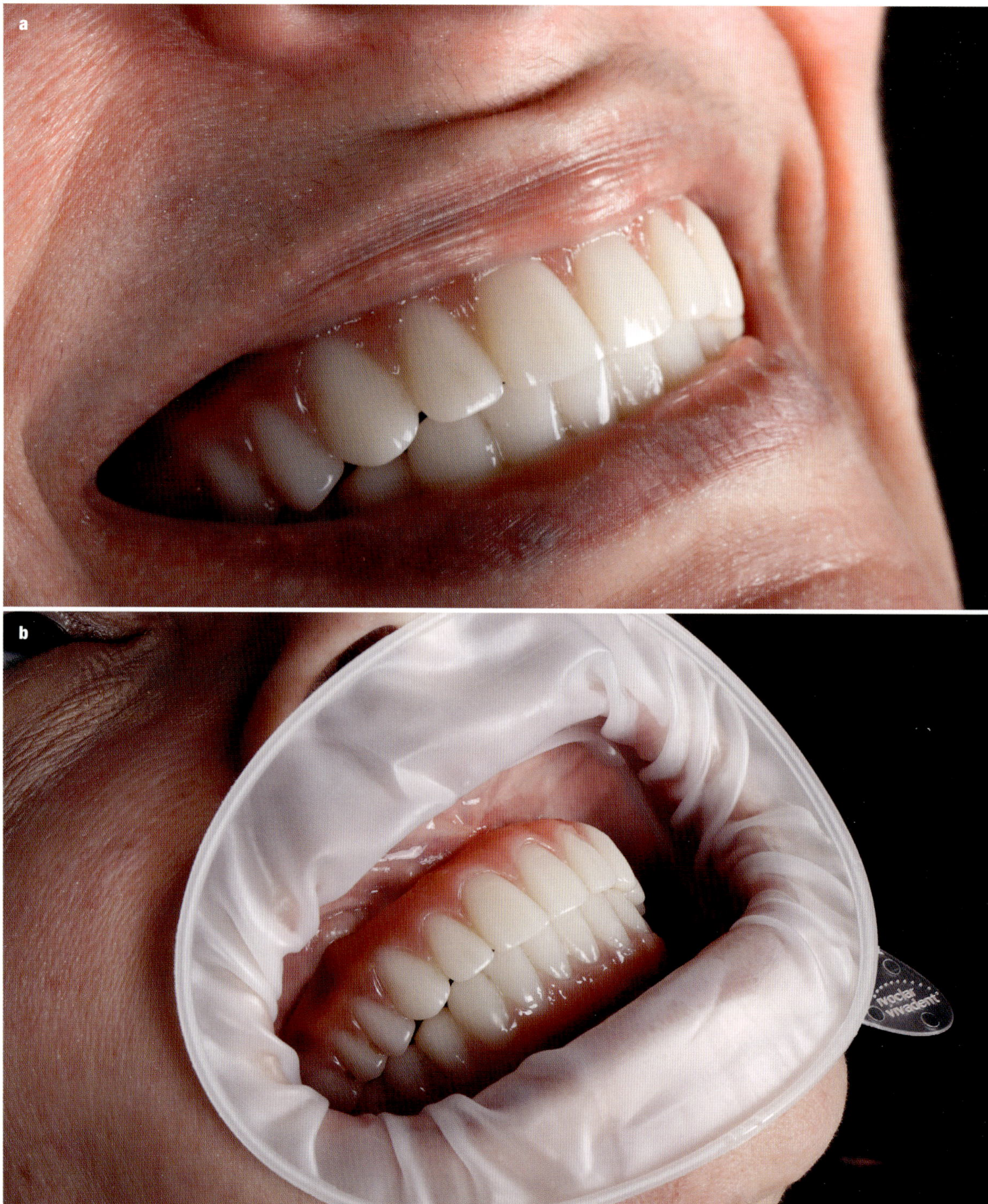

Figure 9.29 (a) Display of the maxillomandibular relationship; (b) Placement of the cheek and lip retraction device (OptraGate) for optimum visibility.

B. Remove the interim (or current) prosthesis (Fig. 9.30)

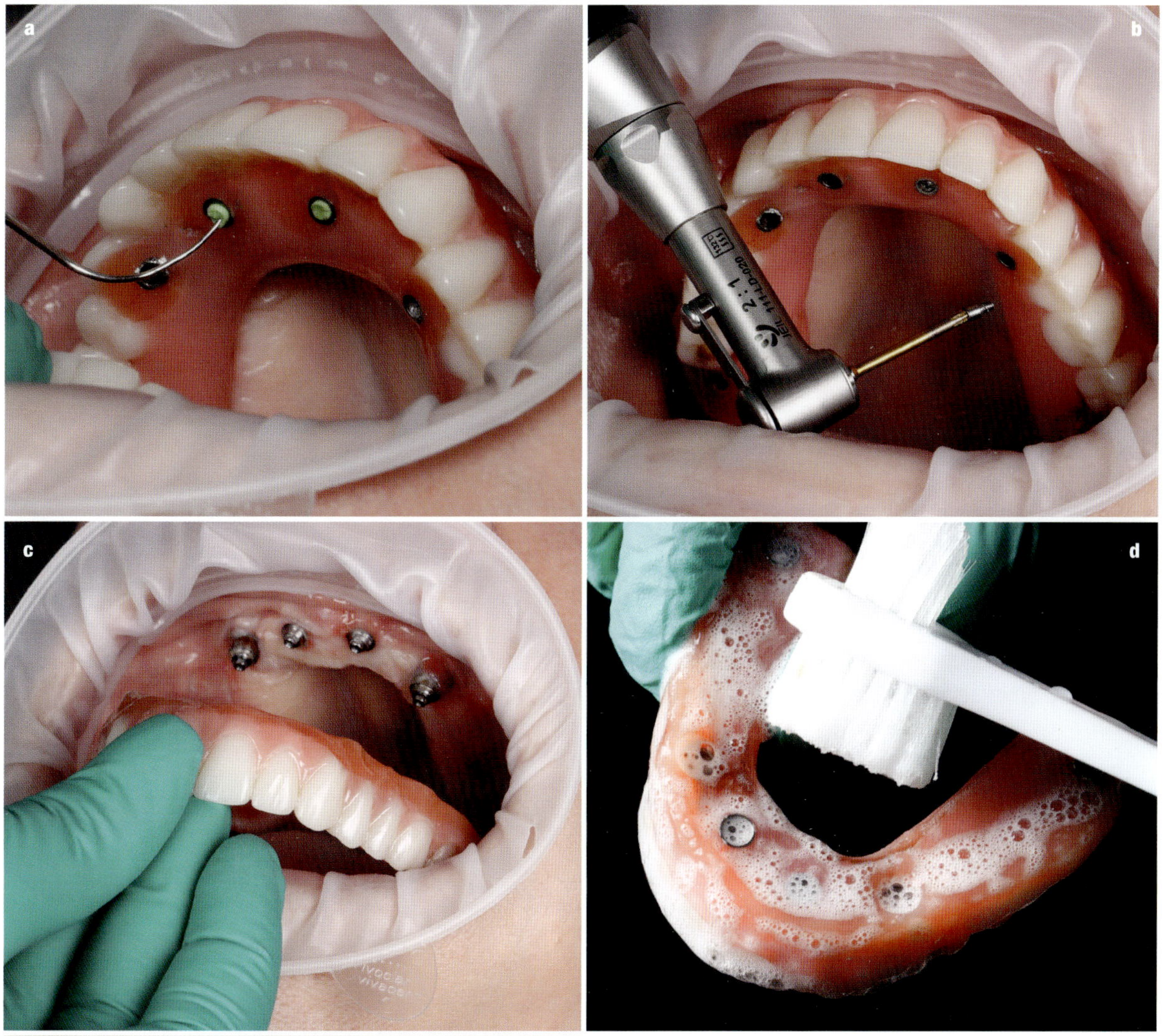

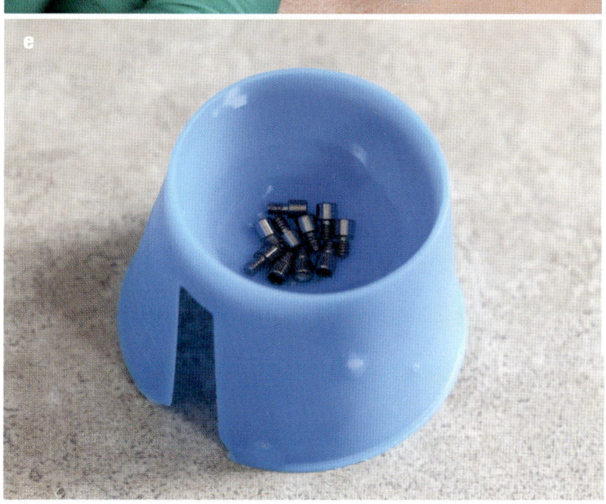

Figure 9.30 Removing the patient's maxillary interim prosthesis. (a) Use a dental explorer to extract the PVS plugs from the screw access channels; (b) Use a torque driver to remove the prosthetic screws from the MUAs; (c) Manually remove the prosthesis from the mouth; (d) Clean the interim prosthesis with a denture brush and soap; (e) Place the prosthetic screws in a dappen dish with OraCare solution to disinfect them.

C. Check the stability of the MUAs (Fig. 9.31)

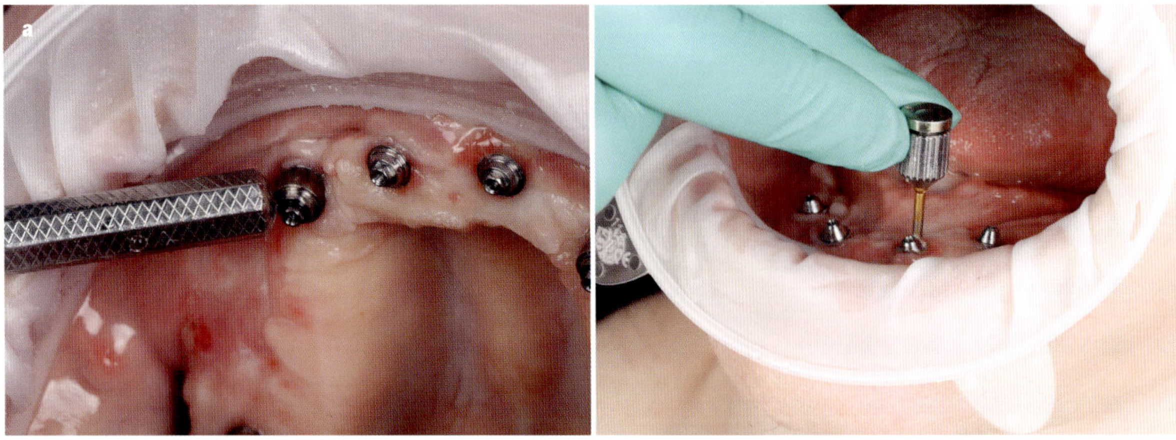

Figure 9.31 (a) Tapping the MUAs in the maxillary arch with the handle of an intraoral mirror for auditory feedback of stability; (b) Hand tightening the mandibular MUAs with an implant driver.

D. Test the implants for osseointegration (Fig. 9.32)

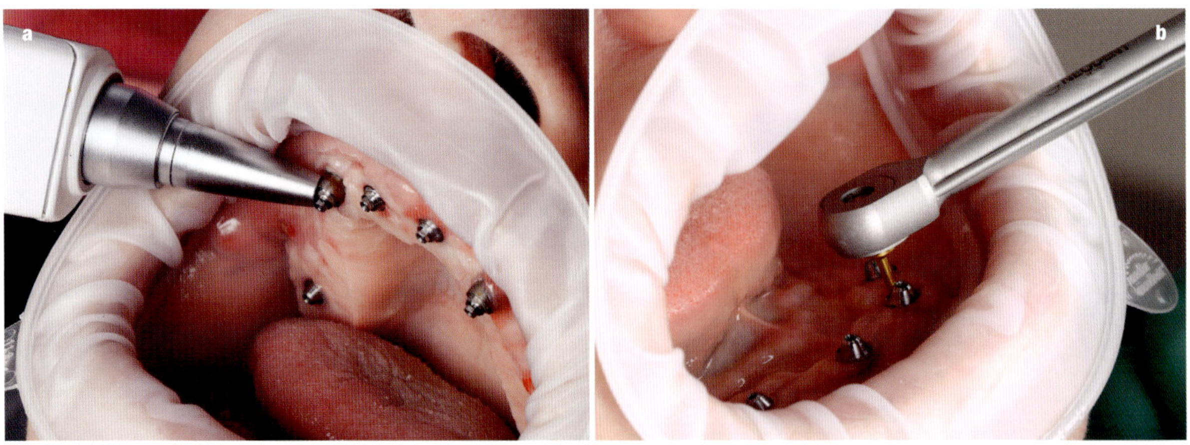

Figure 9.32 (a) Using a Periotest M device to verify osseointegration of implants in the maxillary arch; (b) Retorquing the MUAs in the mandibular arch.

E. Prepare the replica appliance

Having assessed the dental implants and tissue and verified that you have a stable foundation, it is time to prepare the replica appliance. The first step is to determine whether you need to reduce the intaglio surface of the appliance to make room for a pick-up impression. In some cases the tissue will have receded in many places, and you may only need to make minor adjustments to allow for the flow of PVS around the temporary cylinders and over the tissue. Reduce the replica appliance only enough to allow for about 2 to 3 mm of PVS impression material to flow under it. Next, to pick up an accurate impression of the soft tissues, you will need to coat the intaglio surface with PVS adhesive. Use the adhesive that was designed to work with the impression material you are using. If you paint the adhesive over the buccal of the appliance just short of where the teeth are, the impression material will be less likely to separate from the appliance (Fig. 9.33).

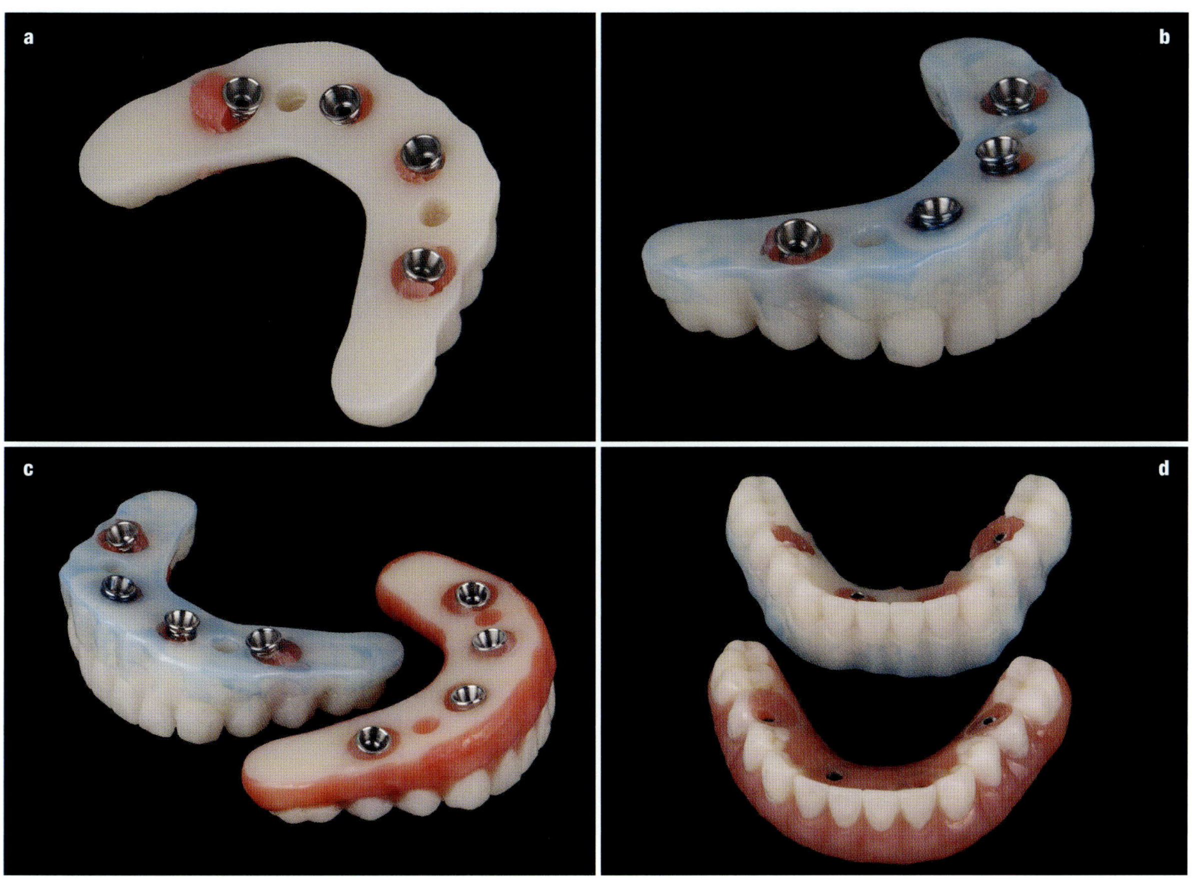

Figure 9.33 (a) Intaglio surface of a mandibular replica appliance; (b) Appearance of the same appliance after impression adhesive has been applied; (c) Side-by-side appearance of the intaglio surfaces of the mandibular replica appliance and the same patient's interim prosthesis; (d) Occlusal surfaces of the same appliance and prosthesis.

F. Verify the fit and alignment of the replica appliance

Place the replica appliance painted with adhesive back into the patient's mouth and use the implant driver to hand tighten the screws through the access channels into the MUAs (Figs. 9.34a, 9.34b). If your replica appliance pick-up was accurate, you should be able to tighten all the screws easily and passively. Check the appliance for mobility and make sure that it is stable (Fig. 9.34c).

If you have any concerns about the fit or see signs that the replica appliance is not seating completely, I recommend that you perform a "one-screw" test as described on page 370. It is relatively easy to section the replica appliance if necessary in order to achieve an intimate fit of the temporary cylinders with the MUAs. (Before doing this, review appointment 2 of the verification appliance technique, page 339)

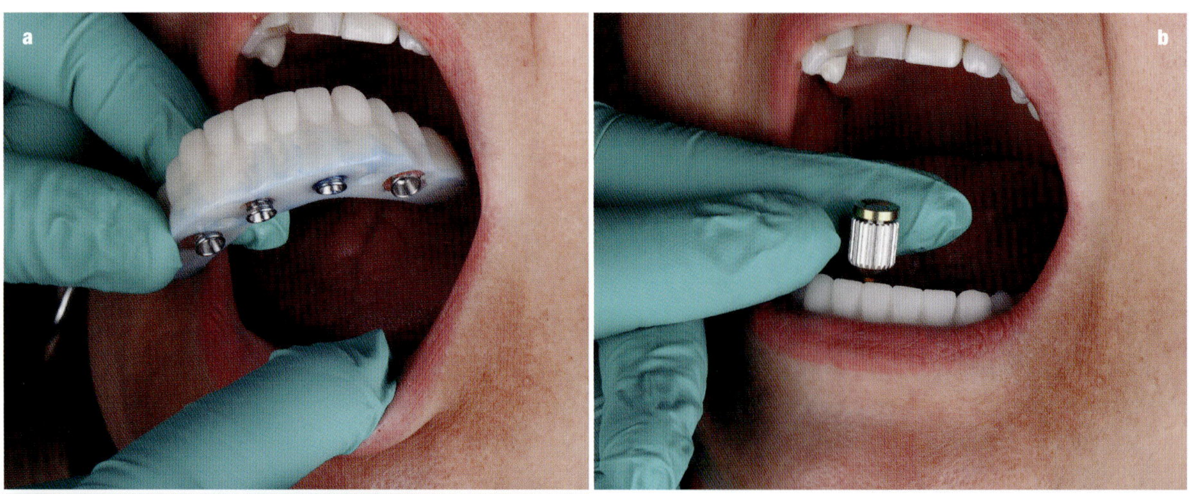

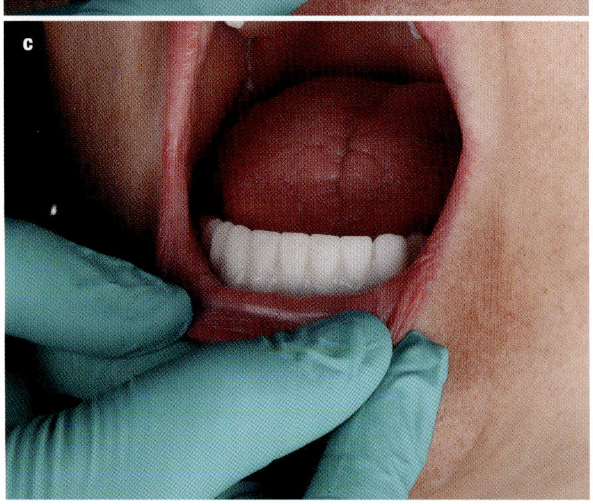

Figure 9.34 **Verifying the fit of the replica appliance.** (a) **Place the replica appliance in the mouth;** (b) **Use an implant driver to hand tighten the prosthetic screws in the replica appliance;** (c) **Once the appliance is fully seated and screwed into the MUAs, check for mobility and overall stability.**

G. Verify the horizontal plane, midline, and VDO

Step 1. Determine whether the appliance is canted in the mouth (Fig. 9.35)

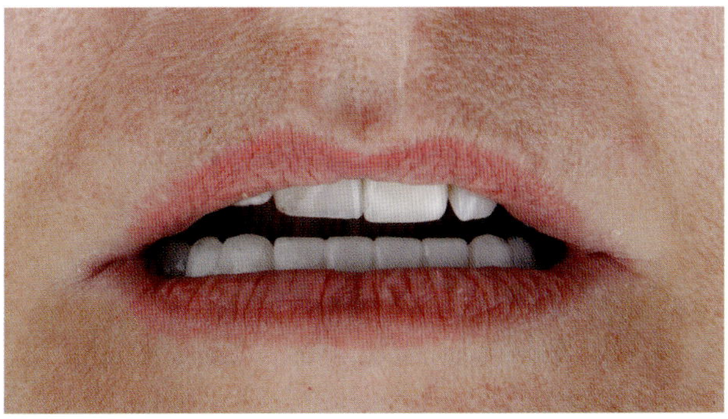

Figure 9.35 Evaluate the horizontal plane with the patient in repose. Note the slight cant in the horizontal plane of this mandibular replica appliance.

Step 2. Evaluate the midline (Fig. 9.36)

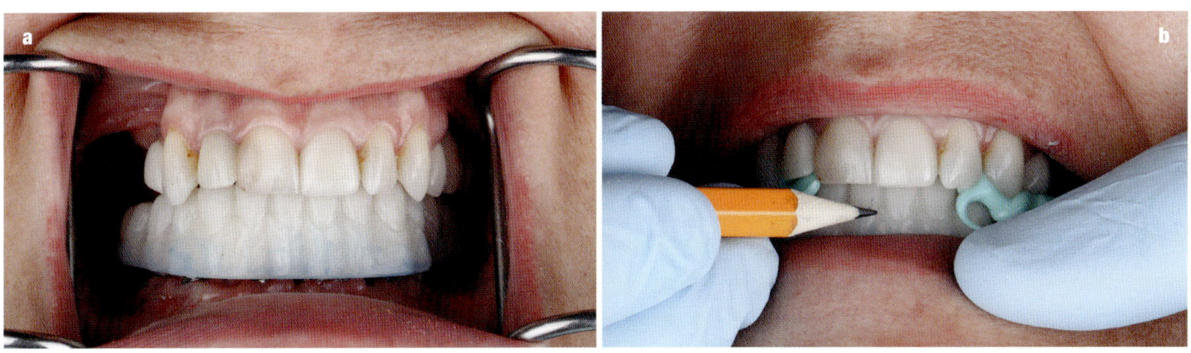

Figure 9.36 Evaluating the midline of the mandibular replica appliance. (a) Retract the lips and soft tissues; (b) Use a pencil to mark the midline on the appliance.

Step 3. Determine whether the VDO is in the right position (Fig. 9.37)

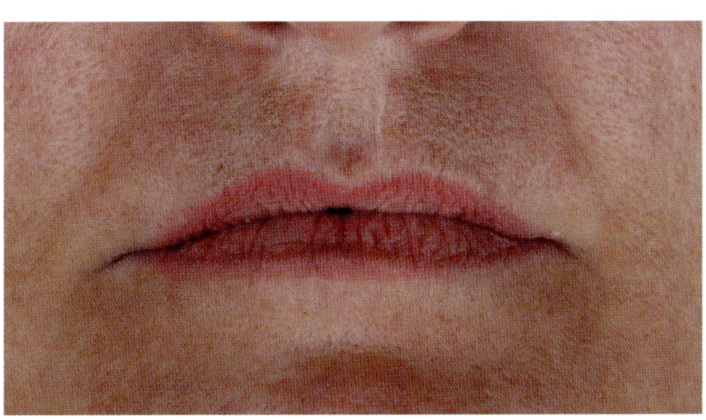

Figure 9.37 An appropriate VDO allows the patient to close in rest position without straining the mentalis muscles.

H. Verify/adjust the occlusion and capture the maxillomandibular relationship (Figs. 9.38, 9.39)

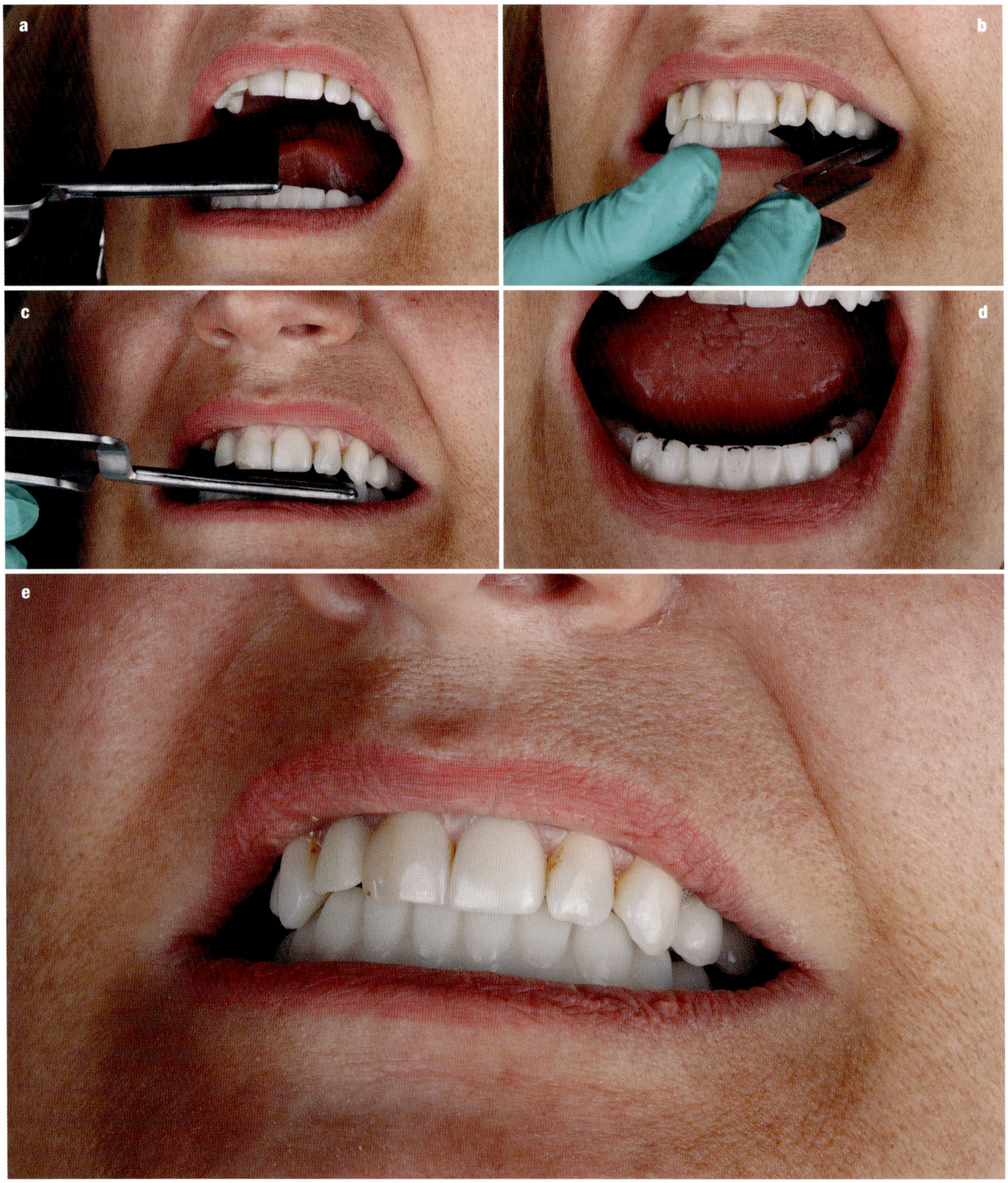

Figure 9.38 (a-d) Using articulating film to mark the contacts on a mandibular replica appliance; (e) Balanced bite in CR confirmed after adjustments.

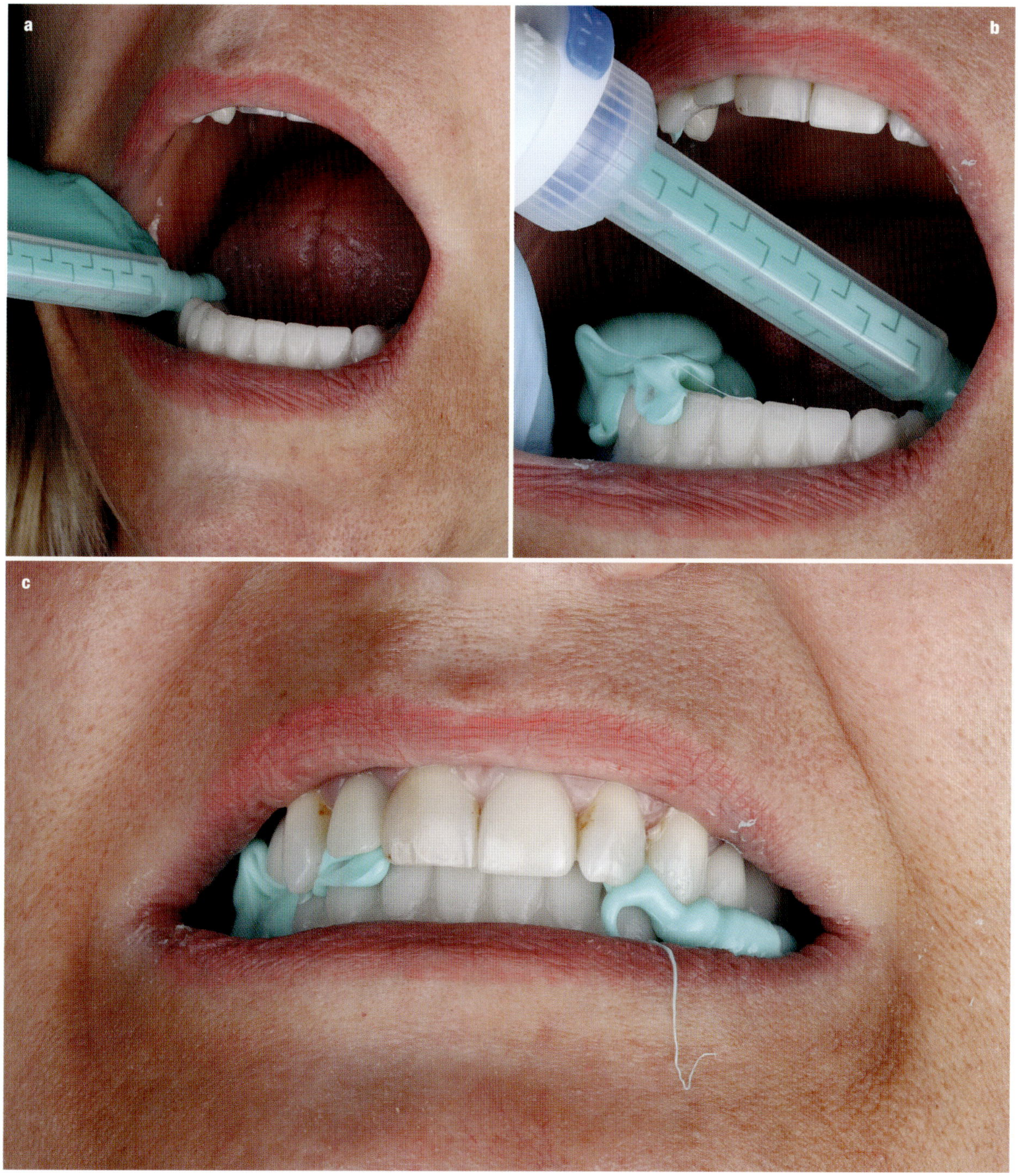

Figure 9.39 Recording the maxillomandibular relationship. (a, b) Place bite registration material in the posterior areas of the mandibular replica appliance; (c) Ask the patient to close and bite down.

I. Take photos for laboratory communication (Figs. 9.40, 9.41)

- Retracted portrait
- Close-up smile
- Close-up repose

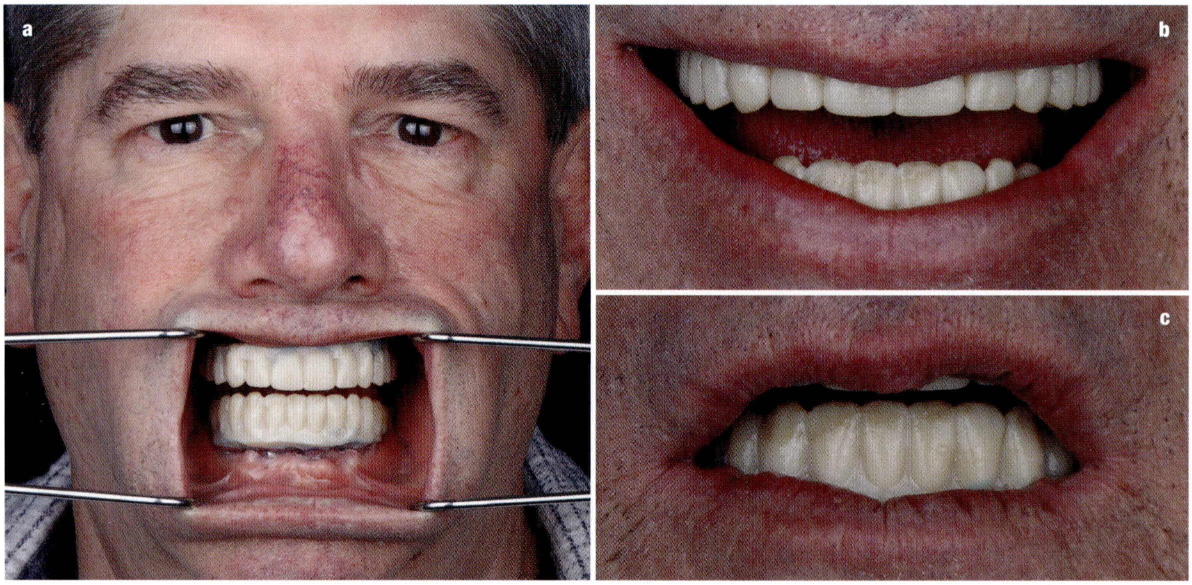

Figure 9.40 The three views used most commonly by the author for lab communication at the replica appliance stage: (a) Retracted portrait; (b) Close-up smile; (c) Close-up repose.

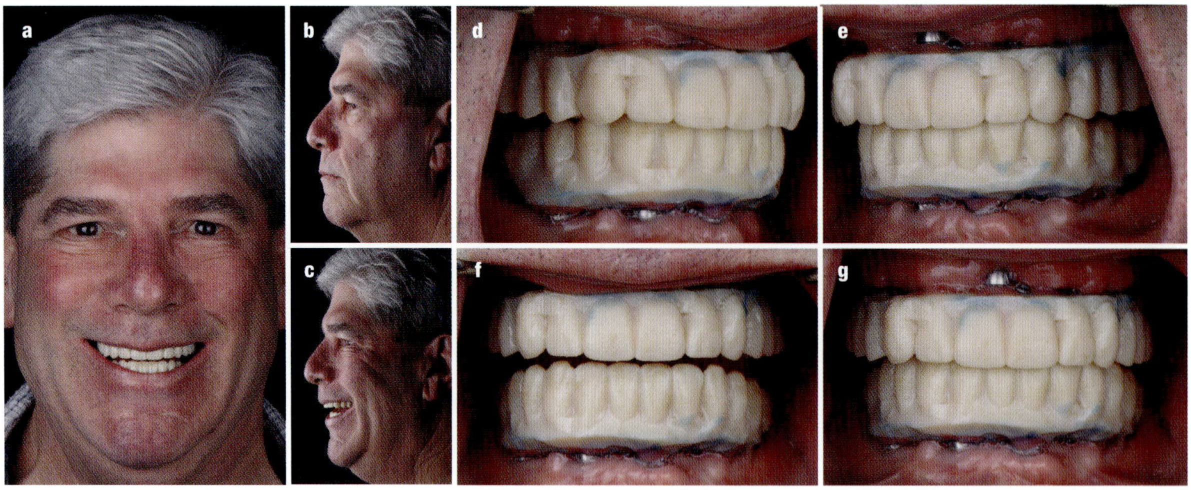

Figure 9.41 Examples of additional views of the replica appliance that may be taken for lab communication: (a) Portrait smile; (b) Profile portrait no smile and (c) smile; (d) Retracted close-up right and (e) left in maximal intercuspal position (MIP); (f) Retracted close-up frontal in open position; (g) Retracted close-up frontal in MIP.

J. Make an analog impression of the soft tissues (Fig. 9.42)

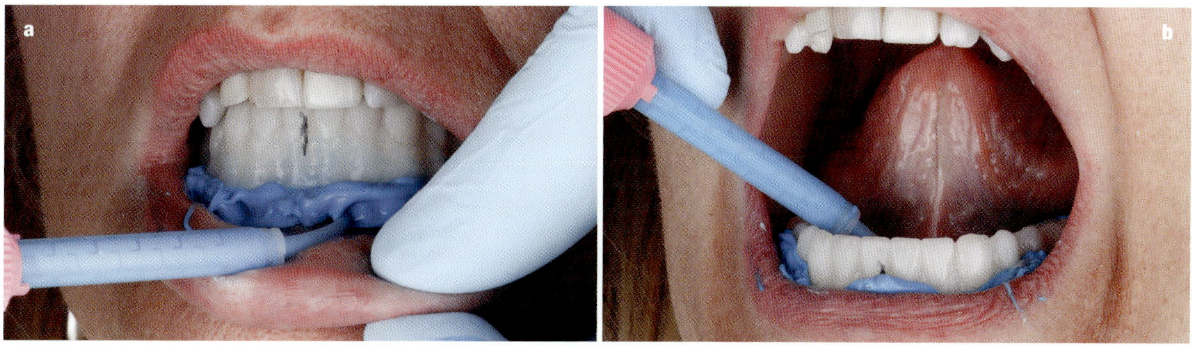

Figure 9.42 Injection of medium-body impression material to capture the tissues (a) under and around the buccal surface and (b) under and around the lingual aspect and intaglio surface of the mandibular replica appliance.

K. Remove the replica appliance and replace the interim prosthesis (Figs. 9.43, 9.44)

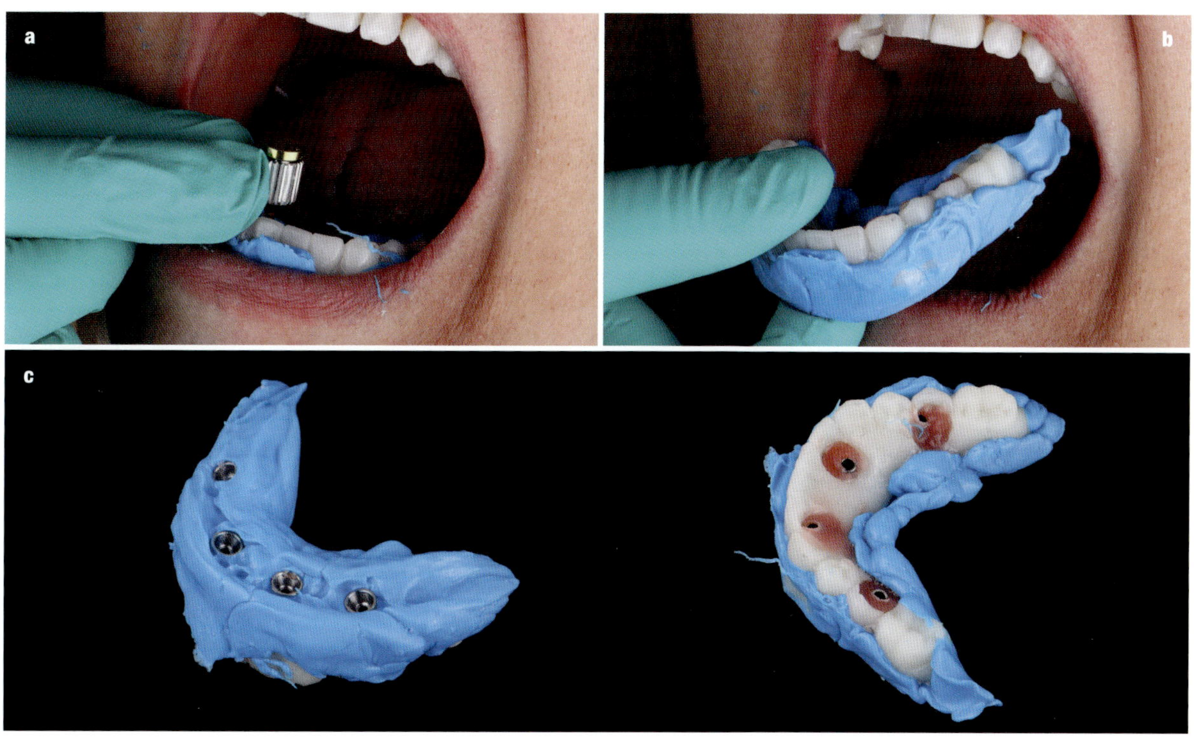

Figure 9.43 Removing the replica appliance from the patient's mouth. (a) Use an implant driver to remove the prosthetic screws; (b) Remove the replica appliance from the patient's mouth; (c) Appearance of the mandibular replica appliance after an impression of the intaglio surface was taken using a medium-body PVS material.

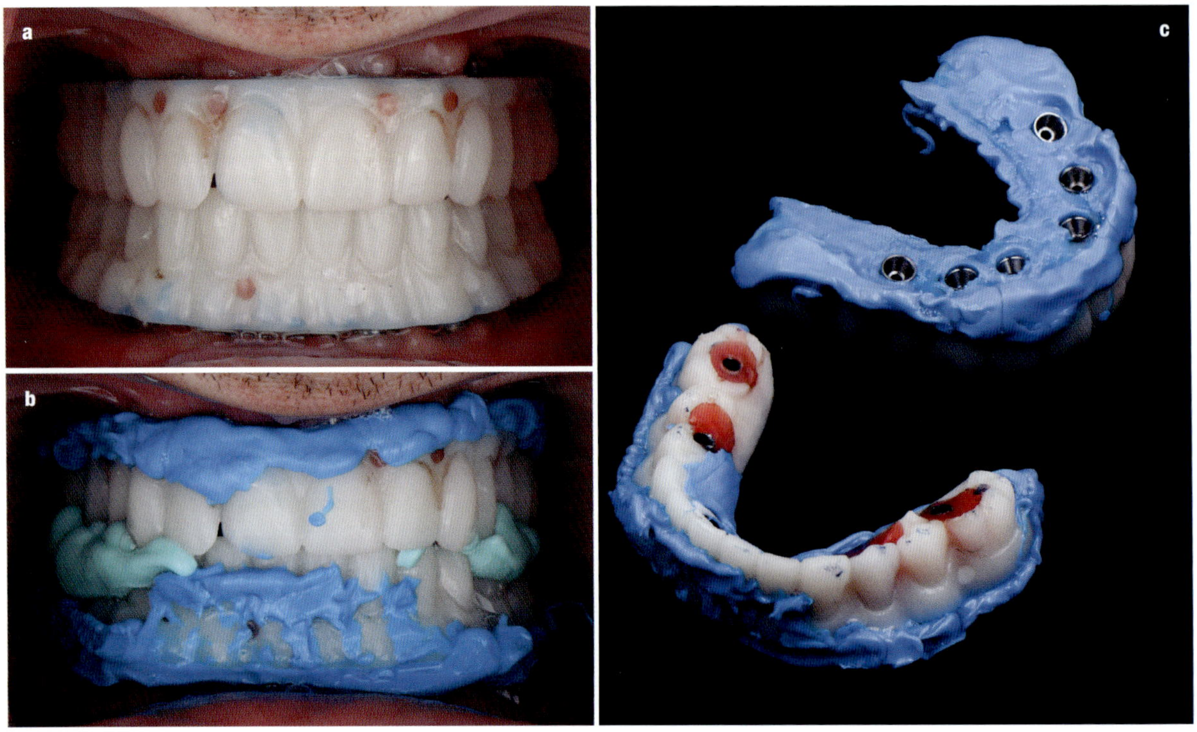

Figure 9.44 Appearance of the replica appliances (a) before and (b, c) after analog impressions were taken of maxillary and mandibular intaglio surfaces.

L. Dismiss the patient and communicate with the laboratory

Send the completed replica appliance(s) and the maxillomandibular relationship record to the dental lab and schedule your patient for the resin prototype appointment.

RESIN PROTOTYPE: APPOINTMENT 3

This is the third appointment in the prosthetic workflow for patients who needed a verification appliance and the second appointment for patients who had a replica appliance. The purpose of this visit is to evaluate the resin prototype appliance and complete a checklist with the patient that will prepare them for the definitive prosthesis. It can be an efficient process and should require minimal doctor time.

Operatory setup. In addition to a basic exam kit, the following items will be helpful:

- Dental implant prosthetic setup with drivers
- Handpiece and bur kit (both chairside and lab)
- Articulating paper
- Digital occlusal analysis device (optional)
- Occlusal registration material (not always necessary)
- Bonding agent and flowable or packable composite and restorative kit
- Pencil or Sharpie marker
- Camera and retractors
- Shade guide
- The Esthetic and Functional Checklist (provided below)

A. Remove the interim prosthesis

Remove the PVS material from the screw access channels and use the implant driver to loosen the MUA prosthetic screws. Once the interim prosthesis is loose and removable, take it out of the patient's mouth and inspect it. If it appears to be in good working condition, with no fractures, loose temporary cylinders, or any other issues, set it aside.

PRO TIP: Master cast test

Over the years, in my efforts to make the prototype appliance appointment as efficient as possible, I discovered a technique that my team could perform to rule out poor fit of the resin prototype appliance before I ever entered the operatory. After the interim prosthesis has been removed and cleaned, it is placed on the master cast provided by the lab when they sent the prototype appliance. If the position of the implants was communicated accurately, the interim prosthesis will fit intimately on the cast without resistance. If it has a passive fit, seats completely, and can be screwed into the cast, then the resin prototype appliance should fit on the MUAs in the mouth. This means the team can proceed with placing and fitting the resin prototype intraorally.

B. Place the resin prototype in the mouth and verify or adjust the fit if necessary

I recommend that the dentist perform or directly oversee this part of the workflow, as one mishap can create problems with the definitive prosthesis. Place the resin prototype(s) in the patient's mouth and check whether the titanium bases used by the lab align with the MUAs (Fig. 9.45). Fit the resin prototype over the MUAs and check for stability (Fig. 9.46). The appliance should not rock or feel imbalanced and should fit intimately over the MUAs. Even if you are satisfied with the fit of the appliance, you may want to confirm it visually and using the one-screw test, as described below.

If the resin prototype appliance is not stable and rocks in the mouth, you will need to identify the cause of the instability. Check whether the appliance is being held up by soft tissue on the edentulous ridge. Commonly, the intaglio surface of the prototype creates pressure on the ridge and simply needs to be adjusted with a laboratory bur. Remove the resin prototype and make the appropriate adjustments until the resin prototype fits securely over the MUAs. If the appliance is not impinging on the soft tissues, there may be some inaccuracy within the prototype itself. Find the area(s) where the prototype is not fitting well and then remove the appliance from the mouth. Using your laboratory handpiece, section the resin prototype in the area between the MUAs where the instability is occurring. You may have to section it in multiple areas to get it to fit perfectly. Be sure to create enough space between the sections to allow the flow of the Stellar DC or other acrylic material. Once you have achieved a good fit of your sectioned resin prototype over the MUAs, use the Stellar DC acrylic material to lute the pieces together, as described in the verification appliance workflow, and proceed with the next step.

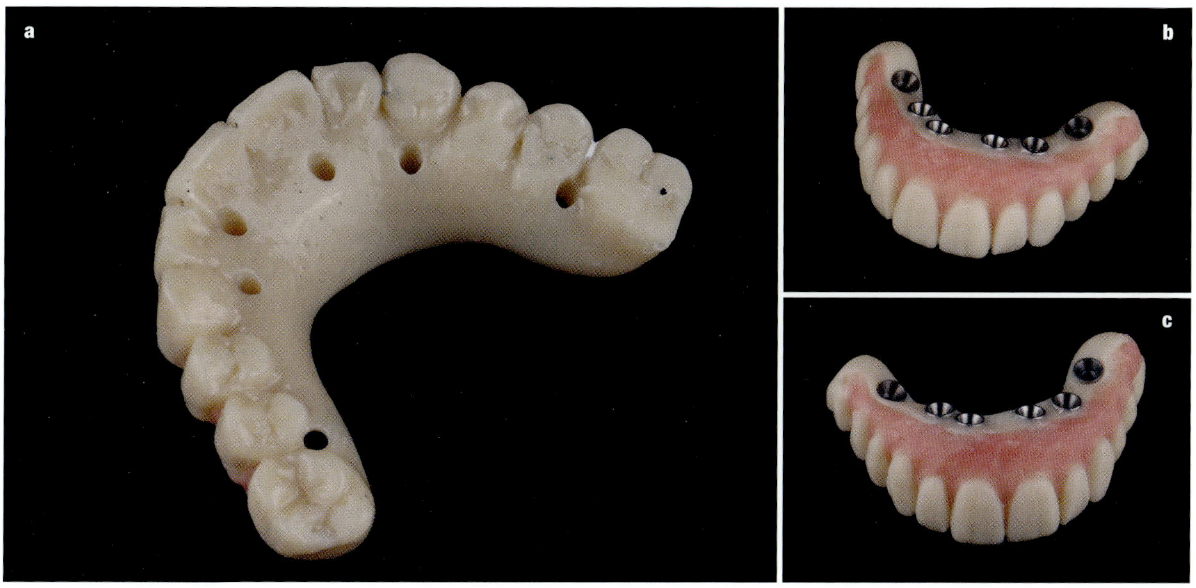

Figure 9.45 (a) Occlusal surface of a maxillary resin prototype appliance; (b, c) Intaglio surface with titanium bases.

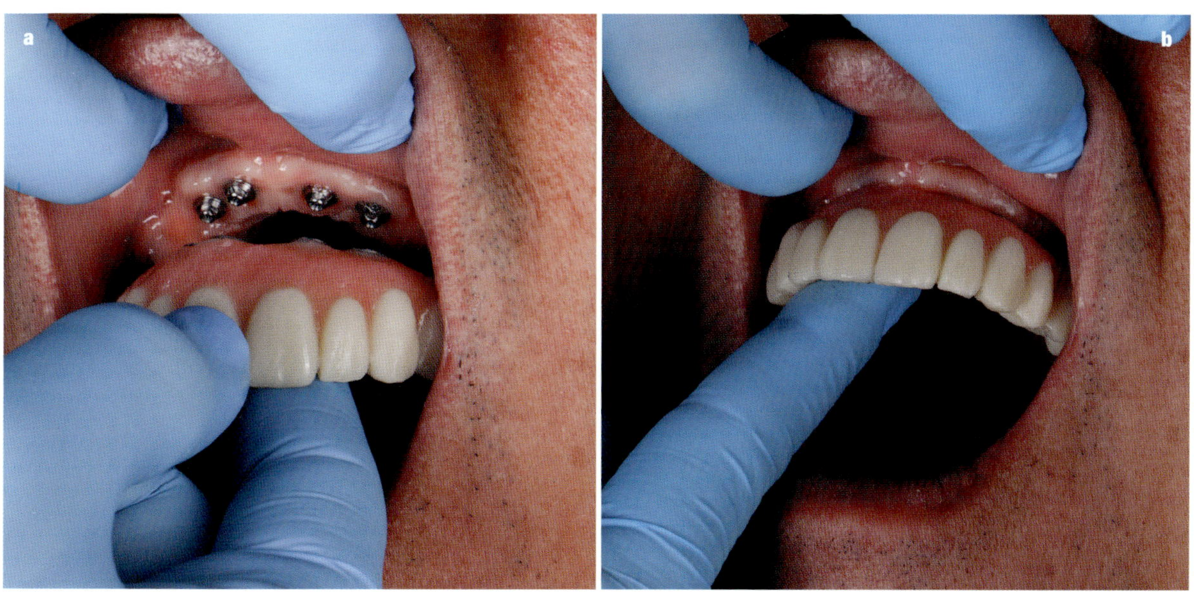

Figure 9.46 (a) Placement of a maxillary resin prototype appliance over the MUAs; (b) Checking the stability of the resin prototype appliance.

Sheffield or "one-screw" test

The one-screw test is a traditional technique that is employed to verify the passive fit of a fixed full-arch implant prosthesis. A passive fit reduces stress along the implants and surrounding bone and is fundamental to the success of the prosthesis. The one-screw test can be applied throughout the prosthetic workflow to test the fit of the verification appliance, replica appliance, resin prototype, and definitive prosthesis.

To perform the one-screw test, use your driver to place a single screw into one of the terminal implant abutments until it is hand-tight (Fig. 9.47a). Next, take a radiograph of the terminal abutment on the side contralateral to where the screw was placed, as parallel to the abutment as possible (Fig. 9.47b). If the prosthesis rises or you detect a space between the MUA and titanium base connection, there may be a misfit.

The one-screw test can be used in conjunction with direct vision and tactile inspection with an explorer or other fine instrument. Misfits in your definitive prosthesis can cause a multitude of issues including the alteration of biomechanical function, increased stress on the entire implant system, and mechanical failure of the definitive prosthesis framework. If the inaccuracies that may exist in the resin prototype are not corrected, your definitive prosthesis will not fit properly and may have to be completely remade. I have experienced this more than once when I first started providing fixed full-arch treatment and paid the consequences, quite literally.

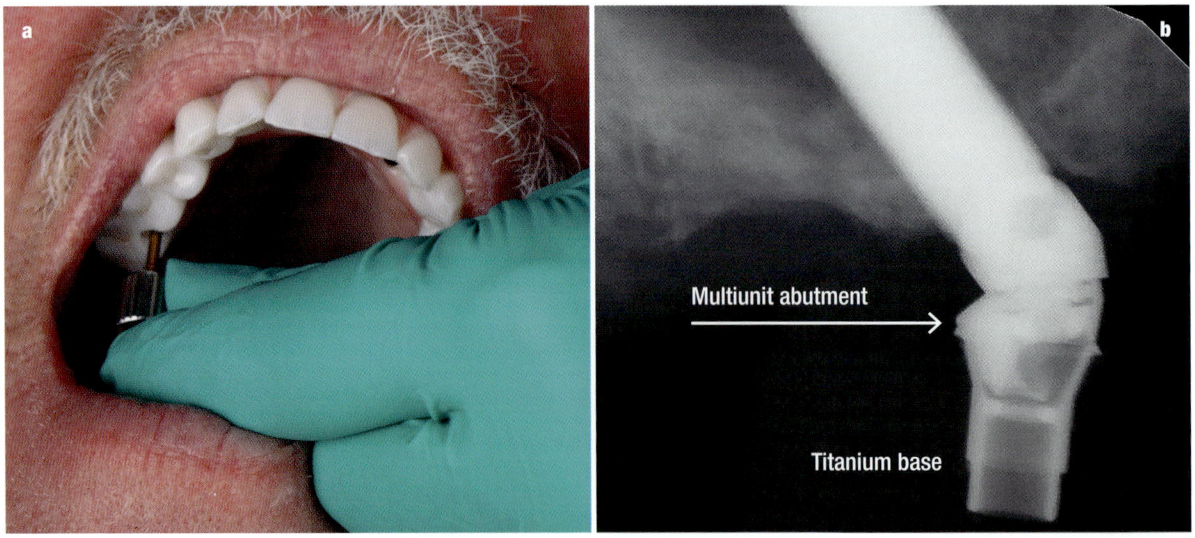

Figure 9.47 (a) Placing and tightening a screw in a terminal access screw channel of a fixed full-arch implant prosthesis; (b) Radiograph of the connection between the MUA and titanium base on the opposite side of the arch. Note the intimate fit of the connection, with no gap between the two components.

C. Evaluate the esthetics and function of the resin prototype appliance and make adjustments

Once you have a stable and verified resin prototype that is securely fixed in the mouth, it is time to evaluate it esthetically and functionally and make any final changes that are needed (Fig. 9.48). This step will bring you as close as possible to finalizing the definitive prosthesis. Any changes you asked the lab to make in the verification or replica appliance should be apparent (Fig. 9.49). Resin prototype appliances sometimes come from the lab without gingival coloring (Fig. 9.50); however, I have found that gingival coloring makes it easier for patients to visualize and agree to move forward with the definitive prosthesis (Fig. 9.51).

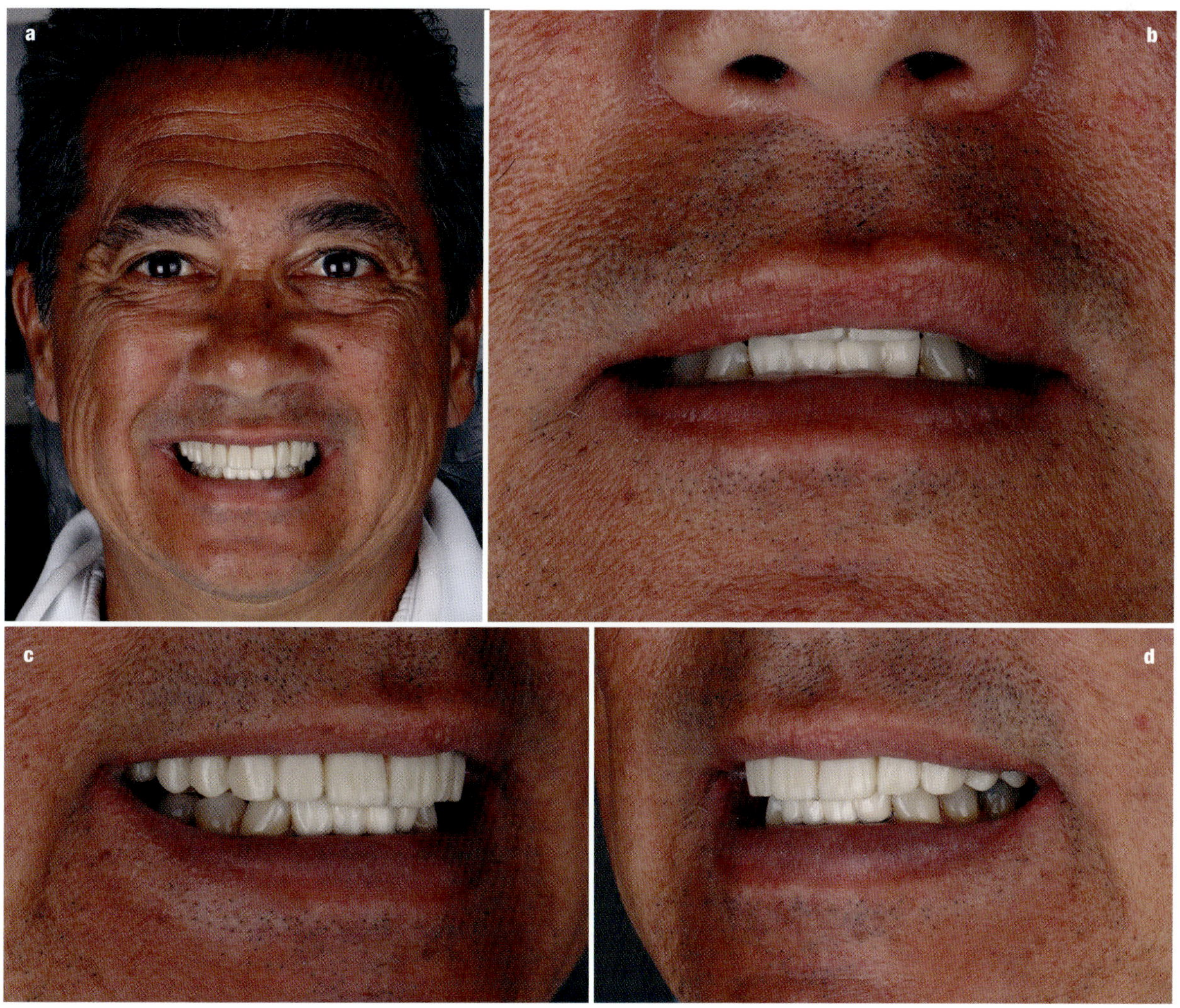

Figure 9.48 Photos taken with the maxillary resin prototype in place: (a) Portrait smile; (b) Close-up repose; (c, d) Left and right close-up in MIP.

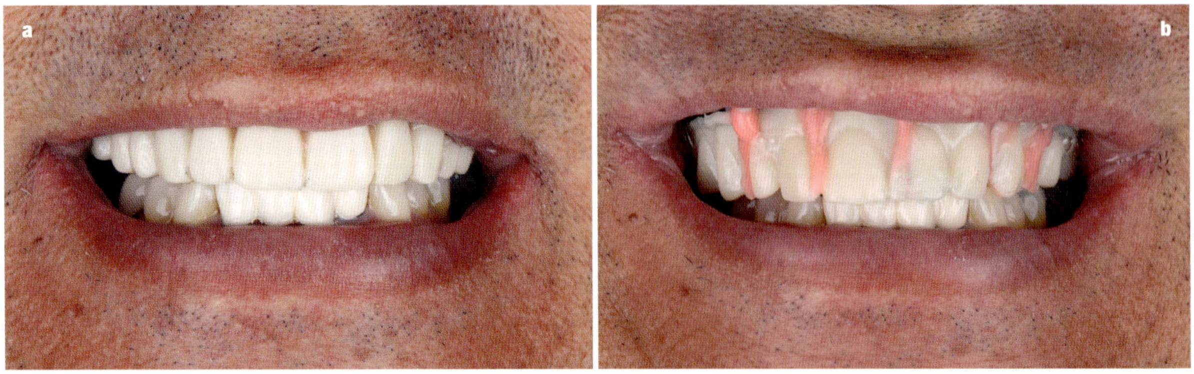

Figure 9.49 Side-by-side comparison of (a) the maxillary resin prototype appliance and (b) the verification appliance in the same patient. Note the adjustments that were made in the position of the verification appliance, which corrected the horizontal plane, midline, and midline cant, as well as the height of the prosthesis.

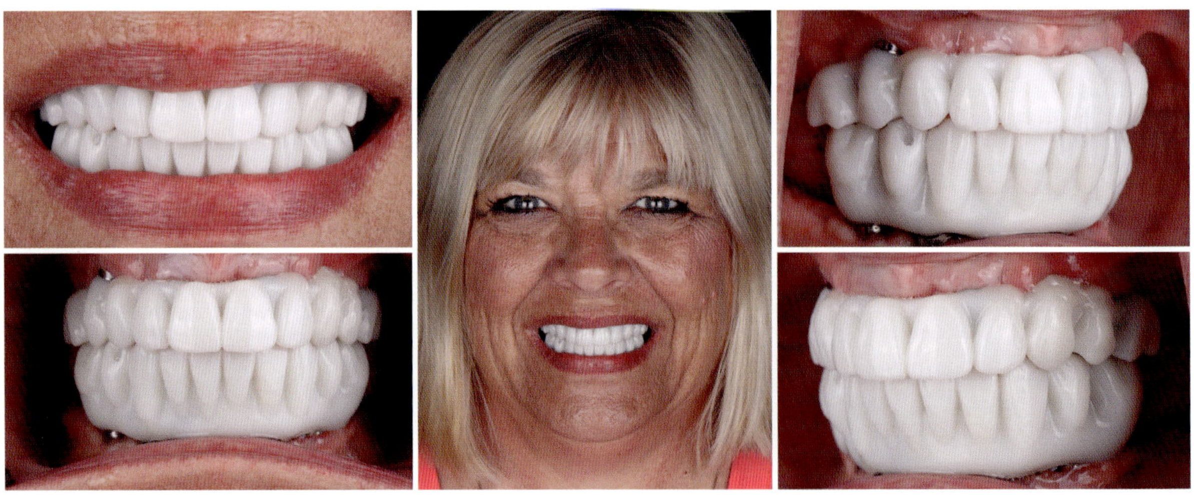

Figure 9.50 Dual-arch resin prototype appliances without gingival coloring.

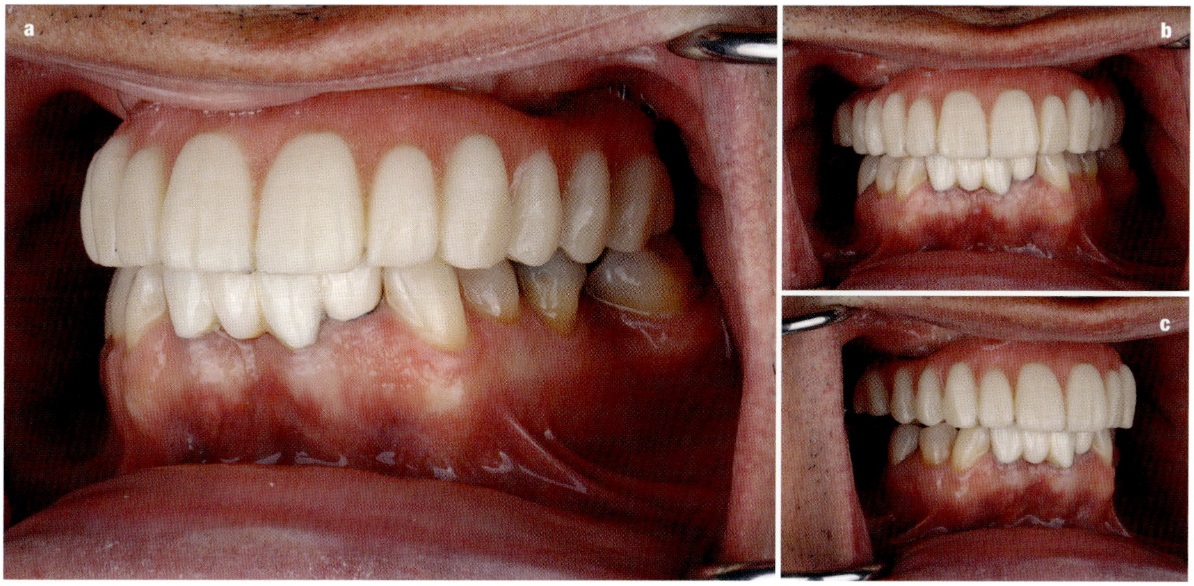

Figure 9.51 (a-c) **Maxillary resin prototype appliance with gingival coloring.**

For consistency of process and to help you educate your team, I developed an Esthetic and Functional Prosthetic Checklist in conjunction with Absolute Dental Services (Fig. 9.52). This is another part of the appointment that I suggest the dentist take the lead in. It is important to most patients that their dentist participate in decisions about how their definitive prosthesis will look and function. Having an assistant with a good eye for esthetics, who can catch little nuances that dentists sometimes miss, is also helpful. Some of the items on the checklist may have been reviewed or identified at earlier appointments. I like to focus on the finer points of the patient's esthetics, occlusion, and phonetics at this appointment. Critically evaluating and adjusting the resin prototype will make the delivery appointment more efficient and less complicated. Use the Esthetic and Functional Prosthetic Checklist to make this appointment easy and more efficient.

To begin, have the patient seated in an upright position; trying to evaluate a patient's esthetics and function while the patient is supine is difficult. Go through each section of the checklist in order and have your assistant take notes. You can either fill out the form first and then go back and make corrections or make corrections as you go through the list. You will find that many of the changes you need to make are straightforward and easy to do chairside. Note which changes you are going to make and which changes your laboratory will make. Share this checklist with your laboratory and save it in the patient's chart.

ESTHETIC & FUNCTIONAL PROSTHETIC CHECKLIST

Can be used throughout steps of the prosthetic workflow

ESTHETICS

Esthetic VDO
- ☐ Appropriate ☐ Needs to be Increased ☐ Needs to be Decreased

Lip Support
- ☐ Lips Supported Properly
- ☐ Lip Support Inadequate ______
- ☐ Lip Support Exaggerated ______

Skeletal & Teeth Classification
- ☐ Class I ☐ Class II ☐ Class III
- Changes? ______

Smile/ Transition Line
- ☐ Appropriate
- ☐ Needs Changes ______

Anterior Tooth Display

Upper
- ☐ Appropriate
- ☐ Shows too much - Shorten by ______ mm
- ☐ Shows too little - Lengthen by ______ mm

Lower
- ☐ Appropriate
- ☐ Shows too much - Shorten by ______ mm
- ☐ Shows too little - Lengthen by ______ mm

Midline
- ☐ Midline is Appropriate
- ☐ Midline needs to be moved to Left/Right ______ mm
- ☐ Vertical Angle of Midline is appropriate
- ☐ Vertical Angle of Midline needs to angle to Left/Right ______ mm

Diastemas?
- ☐ Yes Locations ______ Size ______ ☐ No

Tooth Size & Shape
- ☐ Match teeth design in Interim prosthesis
- ☐ Change design of teeth
  - Describe: ______
- ☐ Characterization

Tooth Characterization

Facial Anatomy
- ☐ Heavy ☐ Medium ☐ Light

Teeth Rotation
- ☐ Moderate ☐ Slight ☐ None

Figure 9.52 Esthetic and Functional Prosthetic Checklist (*cont'd*).

ESTHETIC & FUNCTIONAL PROSTHETIC CHECKLIST

Can be used throughout steps of the prosthetic workflow

Incisal Edge Design

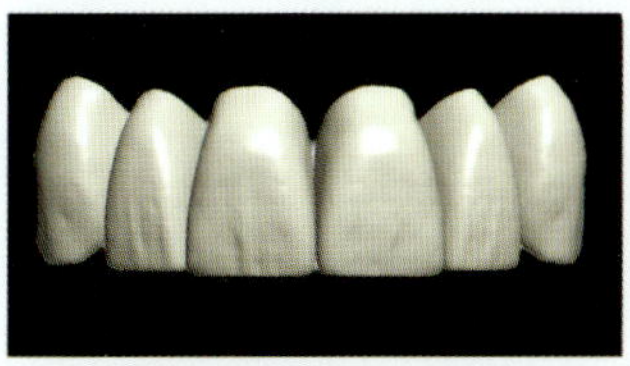

MATURE

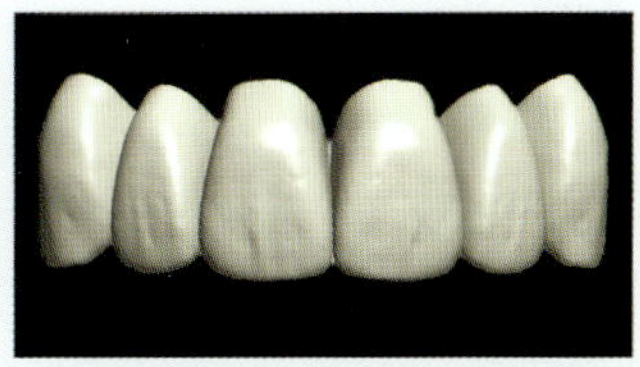

YOUTHFUL

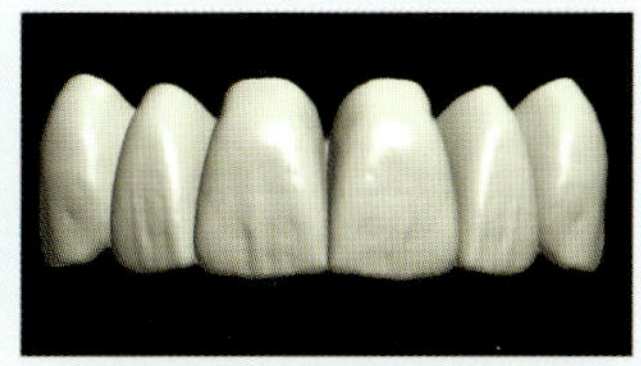

NATURAL

Horizontal Plane of Teeth
- ☐ Level
- ☐ Canted   Keep or Change ______________

Arch Width/ Buccal Corridor
- ☐ Appropriate
- ☐ Needs to be Changed ______________

Tooth Shade ______________

Material of Definitive Prosthesis ______________

OCCLUSION

Occlusal Scheme
- ☐ Bilateral Balanced
- ☐ Group Function
- ☐ Mutually Protected

CR/CO Shift? ☐ Yes ☐ No

____

____

____

Planes of Occlusion
- Curve of Spee ☐ Appropriate ☐ Needs to be Changed ______________
- Curve of Wilson ☐ Appropriate ☐ Needs to be Changed ______________

Figure 9.52 (*cont'd*) Esthetic and Functional Prosthetic Checklist.

ESTHETIC & FUNCTIONAL PROSTHETIC CHECKLIST

Can be used throughout steps of the prosthetic workflow

OCCLUSION

Opposing Arch

- ☐ To be restored in the future?
- ☐ New prosthesis to follow existing opposing occlusion
- ☐ New prosthesis to be idealized and opposing
- ☐ Not applicable

PHONETICS

D, N, T - Have the patient say "donut"	☐ Acceptable	☐ Needs to be Changed ____________
L, TH, SH/CH - Have the patient say "thirty-three" & "shoeshine"	☐ Acceptable	☐ Needs to be Changed ____________
S, Z - Have the patient say "sixty-six"	☐ Acceptable	☐ Needs to be Changed ____________
F, V - Have the patient say "fifty-five"	☐ Acceptable	☐ Needs to be Changed ____________
B, M, P - Have the patient say "bump"	☐ Acceptable	☐ Needs to be Changed ____________

PHOTOS

☐ Taken ☐ Not necessary

I, ____________________ approve and understand the design for my **Implant Prosthesis** discussed and presented on ____________.
The esthetics, functional design, and phonetics (speech) in the prototype appliance are acceptable to me, except for any changes discussed and noted on this checklist. Any changes to the definitive prosthesis after this approval will be at my expense.

Doctor Signature ____________________

Assistant Signature ____________________

Patient Signature ____________________

Date ____________

Figure 9.52 **Esthetic and Functional Prosthetic Checklist.**

Esthetics: Face

Vertical dimension of occlusion (VDO) Step back and observe how the patient's face looks once the resin prototype has been placed, beginning with the face in repose. Does the patient look relaxed? Are the muscles of the face strained? Does the appliance look too large for the patient's mouth? Is there muscle strain around the lips or at the chin? All of these can be signs that the VDO is not where it should be. To evaluate this, ask the patient to bite down in maximal intercuspal position (MIP) with their lips closed. (Although the VDO appears in the esthetics section of the checklist, it should also be evaluated as a functional process.)

If the VDO is appropriate and there is adequate freeway space, you will have less to worry about when evaluating phonetics and occlusion. Because the VDO was evaluated at the previous appointment, there may be very little adjustment necessary. However, if the VDO is excessive, you will probably want to reduce the occlusion on the resin prototype. When doing so, remember that 1 mm of adjustment in the posterior area can create about 2 to 3 mm of change in the anterior. If the appliance looks sloppy after you have made the adjustments, you might have to send it back to the lab with the new VDO recorded (along with a maxillomandibular relationship record) and ask them to create another resin prototype for you.

Lip support/labial position In most patients, the labial position can be assessed by looking at their profile and visualizing an imaginary line drawn perpendicular to the Frankfort plane through nasion and the tip of the chin. The upper lip should be about 1 to 2 mm in front of this line. Keep in mind that soft tissue and skeletal norms vary by race, so this simple measurement will not apply in all cases, and you and the patient may have to use your best judgment about labial position. If lip support is lacking, I bond resin to the anterior teeth to bring the position more anterior. If there is too much lip support, I generally just let the lab know and take pictures for them to evaluate. If these landmarks are way off, take measurements and ask the lab to make changes digitally and provide another resin prototype for try-in.

Skeletal and teeth classification Mention skeletal and teeth classification, and most of us think of orthodontics and occlusion. However, here I want you to consider these concepts in terms of how they affect the patient's esthetics. In the checklist, I have purposely avoided referring to different types of crowding, spacing, divisions, etc. Following are the guidelines I use when documenting a patient's skeletal and teeth classification for fixed full-arch implant prostheses.

- **Class I:** This is what I will refer to as "normal" tooth relation and a balance to the face when it comes to the positions of the maxilla and the mandible.

- **Class II:** This is when the maxillary anterior teeth protrude considerably over the mandibular anterior incisors. Patients with this occlusion may describe it as having "buck teeth." From the skeletal aspect, such patients may have a smaller than normal mandible that is retruded. I have observed many patients, especially males, that posture their mandible forward to compensate for a Class II appearance. Sometimes their muscles have adapted to this new position, and this leads to differences in where their MIP ends up.
- **Class III:** This is when the mandibular anterior teeth are anterior or facial to the maxillary incisors. This so-called crossbite can create functional issues in a prosthesis, and therefore it is best to try to modify the occlusion so that the central and lateral incisors are at least edge to edge. The face of the patient with a Class III skeletal occlusion has been referred to as having a bulldog-like appearance. This occlusion is harder for an individual to mask using facial posturing.

Describing to a patient the limitations of where their teeth will end up and what their face will look like because of space considerations and the location of their jaws can be challenging at times. I tell patients early in the process, during data collection, that without expensive and invasive surgery, we often must place the teeth within specific boundaries. I use analogies such as the size of a parking lot and the number of cars we can put in it: "If I have a very large parking lot (jaw), we might be able to fit a lot of cars (teeth) in it. Smaller parking lots restrict that to some degree." Patients who present in a Class I skeletal position are usually okay maintaining it. Patients with Class II or Class III skeletal positions are not always pleased with their facial profile or appearance, and we often cannot change that (with some exceptions).

PRO TIP: Occlusion, part 1

You may find that some patients have two positions to their jaw: a retruded position and a more anterior position. I commonly encounter this in patients who are significantly skeletal Class II and for years have postured forward to mask a retruded appearance of their jaw. Their muscles seem to have adapted to this new position. Be prepared to identify the most comfortable position for this patient to function but also to be in rest position. Your lab can help you avoid potential hazardous interferences and complications if you can accurately communicate the positions of the jaw to them.

Esthetics: Mouth

Smile/transition line As I noted earlier, the smile or transition line is an area that can be fraught with challenges when it comes to fixed full-arch implant rehabilitation. If a patient shows their actual gingiva as well as the pink gingiva of the appliance, the esthetic appearance of the smile will be less than ideal. Fortunately, you determined what the appropriate amount of bone reduction would be during the planning stages, and the lab used that measurement when they designed the implant guide and placement. Now you are simply confirming that the transition line is acceptable.

If, despite all your planning, you now find that the transition line is unesthetic, you will need to have a discussion with the patient about options for reducing lip movement, such as botulinum toxin (Botox) injections and/or a surgical procedure that can restrict the height of the smile. Take photographs for the lab and measure the distance in millimeters from the edge of the lip to the transition line. In some circumstances, minor transition line issues can be hidden, but do not compromise the convexity and hygienic design of the definitive prosthesis or put a flange on the prosthesis to hide it.

Anterior tooth display Evaluate the anterior tooth display with the patient smiling as well as in repose. Generally, if the incisal edge of the appliance hits the lower lip while the patient is smiling comfortably, you will need to shorten them using your handpiece and bur. If the patient does not show enough tooth display when smiling or in repose, you may want to add to the incisal edges (unless the patient has a very long upper lip and/or has phonetic difficulties with longer teeth). The easiest way to add length is to bond composite resin to the edge of the teeth. Deciding on the length of the incisal edges can be more of an art than a science. I have found that women tend to want to show more incisal edge because it can make them look younger, whereas men generally seem less concerned about the way it makes them look and focus more on phonetics, comfort, and function.

Midline With the patient smiling, take a step back and confirm the facial midline based on their facial features, just as you did at the last appointment in the verification or replica appliance technique. Usually it is easy to determine whether the midline is accurate or not. If it is off, you will need to make an adjustment again by using a pencil or Sharpie and marking on the appliance itself. Decide not only whether the horizontal position of the midline needs to be changed but also whether any vertical angulation changes need to be made.

Diastema On occasion, a patient who presents with a diastema will ask me if we can keep the space between their teeth. Some people consider their diastema part of their character and would not see themselves the same without it. A diastema is not difficult to add to a fixed full-arch prosthesis, whether between the central incisors or just about anywhere in the arch. It also will not impact the function or longevity of the prosthesis. So if your patient has or wants a diastema, use your hand piece and a bur to create one if you have not already asked the lab to do it for you.

Tooth size, shape, characterization, and incisal edge design

The size and shape of the teeth can significantly affect the esthetics of the prosthesis, so this is another category that patients like to take part in evaluating. Many people request specific sizes and shapes based on what their teeth looked like years before or what resonates with them when they peruse the pages of a fashion magazine. Characterization of the teeth—which refers to facial anatomy in general and/or their rotational position in the arch—is a design area you and your patient may want to consider as well. By creating characterization, the teeth can look more natural. The incisal edge design also plays a part in how the teeth look and can be very patient-specific.

We usually help patients through this process by considering what might work best based on their age, gender, desires, etc. In most cases, a creative laboratory technician who is well-versed in smile design can do a great job of setting up the resin prototype with a size and shape that is complimentary to your patient's smile.

Horizontal plane of the teeth

The horizontal plane, or "cant" of the teeth, was evaluated and adjusted (if necessary) in the verification or replica appliance, so there should not be too much to adjust. However, do not overlook it. If the horizontal plane is not even with the lips, the patient will generally notice that something is off. Use the frame of the mouth, especially the lower lip and oral commissures, as a reference point for evaluating the cant. The features of the face can also provide reference; however, many people have asymmetry in their faces, so using only facial features as a guide is less predictable. If the horizontal plane is acceptable, you can move on to the next step. If it still needs work, you can mark the horizontal plane on your appliance with a pencil or Sharpie and take photographs with measurements, as you did in the verification or replica appliance. You may also want to consider using a traditional facebow and articulator or one of the many digital facebows available. If a significant change is made in the horizontal plane at this stage, I would recommend having a new resin prototype appliance fabricated.

PRO TIP: "Poor man's facebow" technique

I have used a technique that I call the "poor man's facebow" to communicate the midline and horizontal plane to the lab. Although it is not nearly as accurate as using an actual facebow, I recommend it for situations where the midline and/or horizontal plane need to be modified by the lab (and you do not own a facebow). To use this technique, take a new analog maxillomandibular relationship record in the anterior incisor region and place two intersecting cotton swab applicators into the material to indicate the patient's facial midline (vertical stick) and the corrected horizontal plane position (horizontal stick) (see Fig. 9.25).

Arch width and buccal corridor

Determining where the teeth will fit in the patient's mouth requires consideration of the width of the arch. Most patients want a wider smile because that is more esthetically pleasing. Patients with narrow arches often have prominent buccal corridors when smiling, which makes it look like they are missing their posterior teeth.

Although the location of the edentulous ridges of both arches and the position of the dental implants limit what we can do, it is sometimes possible to camouflage the arch and make the buccal corridors less dark in a patient with a narrow arch and a relatively large mouth. This usually involves making the prosthesis a bit wider in the mid to posterior areas. Your lab technician can often design just enough difference in the prosthesis to change the look dramatically. You can make changes by bonding some composite to the resin prototype on the facial surface where you want to expand it. If you add too much, simply remove or reshape it with your handpiece. Be careful not to create a ledge or buccal step in the appliance, as this can lead to food impaction or make it difficult to maintain proper hygiene. Also note that expanding into the buccal corridor too much may cause parafunctional activity. You can test this by having a patient wear the prototype home for a period before sending it to the lab.

Tooth shade

The tooth shade of the definitive prosthesis is one of the most important factors to consider with your patient. Unless you instruct your lab otherwise, the resin prototype appliance will likely be a monolithic A2 or some other shade that is unappealing. Because of this, the patient may not be able to accurately perceive what their final shade will be. Over the years, I have found that almost all of my patients want to have whiter teeth and usually choose a color that falls within a very narrow range, which honestly has been a little disappointing to me. As a dentist, I want the patient to have a natural-looking and age-appropriate smile, but patients usually tell me that they paid so much for their new teeth, they want them to be white!

Shade can be very difficult to change once the definitive prosthesis has been fabricated, so take several factors into consideration when choosing it. If you have a single-arch prosthesis, look at the color of the opposing dentition and give the patient options available to them if they want to change the color of their natural teeth. If both arches are being restored with prostheses made of different materials (such as an acrylic denture opposing a zirconia prosthesis), consider the different opacity levels and shades of these materials and the contrast between them. In some cases, I have used a shade tab guide that is made from the material I will use for the patient's definitive prosthesis. Your lab can make you one of these inexpensively. In the end, you want the patient to get the color they will be most satisfied with. Have the patient pick the final shade and tell them you will note that in their chart as well as on the checklist. The patient must understand that once the color is chosen, it cannot be changed without significant cost and effort. It is helpful to have your patient sign the Esthetic and Functional Prosthetic Checklist form so they take this seriously and know that once they approve it, any esthetic changes to the definitive prosthesis may be costly.

Occlusion

General principles related to fixed full-arch implant occlusion The fixed full-arch implant prosthesis literature is somewhat lacking in controlled studies on occlusion, whereas entire books have been written and entire dental academies have been established around the role of occlusion in natural teeth. As you read this section, remember that teeth and implants respond differently to forces placed on them. Consider that in dentistry, much of what we apply to dental implant occlusion has been taken from years of studying the occlusion of the natural dentition as well as removable prosthetics. I will only be sharing my personal philosophy and the types of occlusions I subscribe to in my designs for fixed full-arch prostheses. Much of this knowledge I obtained from the concepts developed and discussed by Dr. Carl Misch and his concepts for implant-protected occlusion (IPO) as well as the book *Fundamentals of Implant Dentistry* by Beumer et al.[1,2]

Based on their skeletal classification, some patients may be outliers to the following discussion on occlusion, which cannot account for all potential variables. I encourage you to use it as a reference as you begin your journey into fixed full-arch dentistry and be aware that dental research and science may become clearer on this subject as time goes on.

The variables I consider when designing and engineering the occlusion for fixed full-arch prostheses are:

- The number of dental implants present
- The position of the implants in the arch
- The surface area of the implants
- The opposing dentition
- Parafunctional habits the patient may have
- Muscle and temporomandibular joint (TMJ) issues the patient may have
- The presence of cantilevers in the arch

Occlusal schemes The three types of occlusal schemes I use in fixed full-arch implant dentistry are:

1. Bilateral balanced occlusion (BBO). In this occlusal scheme, the anterior and posterior teeth are in contact in centric and eccentric positions. When the patient moves their jaw, the teeth are "balanced" all around—as if the teeth were skating on an ice rink. This type of occlusion is commonly designed for removable dentures. BBO is an occlusal design I might consider when:
   - The prosthesis opposes a conventional removable denture
   - The prosthesis opposes a removable overdenture that is implant-retained but not implant-supported.
2. Group function (GF). This occlusal scheme is similar to bilateral balanced occlusion in that the teeth are balancing together but only unilaterally. During excursive movements of the mandible, the teeth on the working side are contacting and balanced and the teeth on the opposing or nonworking side are not contacting. In other words, when a patient moves their teeth to the left, the teeth on the left side are contacting and the teeth on the right are not, and vice versa. GF is an occlusal design I might consider when:
   - It is the occlusal scheme the patient had in their previous dentition
   - The prosthesis opposes natural dentition
   - The canines of the opposing arch are worn and will not be restored (for whatever reason)
3. Mutually protected occlusion (MPO). This occlusal scheme, often referred to as *canine-protected* or *canine rise*, is commonly used in everyday restorative dentistry. In this design,

the anterior teeth are in contact during protrusive or forward movements of the mandible and the posterior teeth are in disocclusion. During lateral movements of the jaw, the canines are the only teeth that contact, keeping the anterior and posterior teeth out of contact. In centric occlusion, the teeth are in balanced contact throughout the arch, although in some Class divisions of the design, they may only be in contact on the posterior teeth. MPO is an occlusal design I might consider when:

- The prosthesis opposes healthy natural dentition
- The prosthesis opposes another fixed or implant-supported prosthesis
- The prosthesis opposes a removable implant-supported overdenture

When communicating the type of occlusion you want to develop for your patient, it may be useful to discuss it with an experienced laboratory technician. Such individuals can be very helpful when you are just starting to restore fixed full-arch implant cases. Some other concepts to consider planning into the occlusion of your definitive prosthesis are:

- Stability bilaterally when the patient is in a reproducible centric occlusion
- Wide freedom of movement in centric occlusion
- A narrow occlusal table with minimal cusp heights
- Contacts that are evenly distributed throughout the arch
- Reducing any interferences that exist between the patient's retruded position (commonly referred to as *centric relation*), if it exists, and their MIP
- Smooth and even lateral excursive movements that do not create working and nonworking interferences
- Shallow anterior guidance

PRO TIP: Occlusion, part 2

If a patient cannot touch their maxillary central incisors with balanced contact against their mandibular anterior incisors when they move their mandible forward, they will complain that they are not able to bite or tear with their front teeth. Make sure you remove any posterior interferences when the patient is in this position.

The Esthetic and Functional Prosthetic Checklist includes several other collectible data points pertaining to occlusion.

Planes of occlusion The *curve of Spee* is the anteroposterior curve of the teeth in the arch, or the amount of curve the teeth have from back to front. This curve varies depending on the type of occlusion you create for your patient. The *curve of Wilson* is the curve created by the teeth across the arch laterally. Do not confuse this curve with the horizontal plane of occlusion; it is less about the cant of the teeth and more about the actual curve itself.

When documenting or communicating these curves to the lab, the idea is to note any abnormalities or exaggerations. In dual-arch cases, you will probably not have much to note as the technician who designed the interim prosthesis probably built very little curvature into it. It may become more important when you have a prosthesis opposing natural dentition, where these curves can vary.

Opposing arch Rather than documenting what is present in the opposing arch, this section of the checklist allows you to communicate your plans to the lab. It should also remind you to have a discussion with your patient when they have a compromised opposing arch. In my practice, I start by asking the patient, when their prosthesis is finished, what their timetable is to address any issues that remain untreated in the opposing arch. Ideally, you will have had at least some discussion about this earlier in the process, but your patient may not have been ready to make any concrete decisions at that time. There may be circumstances in which you will restore a single arch and have a less-than-ideal situation opposing it. If your patient understands the limitations that this creates, you will have a much better outcome as well as a patient with the appropriate expectations.

Phonetics

How the patient will pronounce their words and certain letter sounds is important to evaluate, not only preoperatively but also postoperatively in the interim prosthesis and before the patient's definitive prosthesis is created. Speech problems can cause emotional issues for patients who are struggling to pronounce their words. Patients' speech is commonly affected by the length of the teeth, the VDO, freeway space, and the width of the maxillary arch in the posterior region. Common complaints from patients are slurred speech, hissing, lisping, spitting while talking, and the pronunciation of certain words. Managing a patient's phonetics chairside before fabricating the definitive prosthesis will save you time, money, and frustration. I have used the following speech sounds to evaluate my patients' phonetics and document them on the Esthetic and Functional Prosthetic Checklist.

Sound groups

- Tongue to hard palate sounds: *D, N, T*

When these letters are formed, the tip of the tongue reaches out to the area where the incisive papilla would be located. That is why it was important to consider the angle of trajectory of the screw access channel during the planning stages of the case. If the appliance is too thick and covers too much of the area around the incisive papilla, a patient may struggle with the *D*, *N*, and *T* sounds. If you need to make corrections, you can thin the patient's resin prototype appliance on the lingual in this area, but be careful not to weaken it too much. The definitive prosthesis will need at least 3 mm of thickness around the screw access channel. Also, you may consider replacing any abutments in the area that have the screw access channel trajectory toward the lingual and reposition them to be more buccal. Of course, this will require you to pick up new temporary cylinders in the patient's interim prosthesis and the resin prototype, so consider this only as the final option.

- Tongue to teeth sounds: *L, Th, Sh/Ch*

The letter *L* is formed when the tip of the tongue just touches the cingulum of the maxillary anterior teeth. If these teeth are positioned too far buccal or too lingual, it will be difficult for patients to pronounce *L*. You can adjust this position by either adding flowable composite resin to the resin prototype appliance on the lingual or by adding resin to the facial of the anterior teeth and removing material from the lingual. Remember, with the resin prototype appliance the laboratory can digitally modify any adjustments you make, so do not be afraid to whittle away on it a bit. The worst that can happen is that you will need to ask them to make an additional resin prototype appliance for you to test.

The *Th* sound is formed when the tip of the tongue passes through the anterior teeth, just lightly touching the edges of the maxillary central incisors. When a patient has trouble pronouncing this sound, it has to do with the VDO and freeway space. Make sure the patient has 2 to 3 mm of distance between the maxillary and mandibular central incisors in the rest or repose position. If they do not, adjust the VDO by giving them more space, or shorten the length of the anterior teeth. Just be sure to consider the esthetic consequences of shortening the teeth—how it will affect the anterior tooth display, for example.

Sh and *Ch* sounds are created when the tongue moves up toward the palate and is in contact with the lingual aspect of the posterior teeth. Posterior arch width is responsible for changes in these sounds. If the tongue is large and the arch width is narrower than it should be because the appliance is too bulky, issues like slurred speech can result. You can correct this by reducing the material on the prototype appliance in the posterior lingual areas.

- Teeth to teeth sounds: *S, Z*

Most patients make the *S* and *Z* sounds by putting the front teeth together; however, some Class II and Class III patients make these sounds without the teeth contacting (see Tongue to teeth sounds on the previous page). If a patient is having difficulty pronouncing their *S* and *Z* sounds, there may be too much contact with the incisal edges, creating a lisping noise. You can correct this by making the edges of the front teeth shorter or longer. In addition to teeth corrections, you may also want to check whether the prototype appliance has too much space between the intaglio surface and the ridge in the anterior. A wide gap that allows air to pass through too easily will create a hissing noise that patients are not fond of. Closing this space with some composite or placing some impression material in the area can be helpful to give the lab a more accurate idea of where the ridge is when they make the definitive prosthesis.

- Teeth to lip sounds: *F, V*

These sounds are made when the incisal edges of the maxillary teeth contact the vermilion border of the lower lip. You may notice a patient "reaching" with the lower lip to create these sounds if the VDO is too great. If the teeth are too long, the patient will feel as if there is too much pressure on the lower lip when pronouncing words beginning with *F* and *V*. To correct any of these issues, simply make the maxillary anterior teeth longer or shorter, or consider changing the patient's VDO.

- Lip to lip sounds: *B, M, P*

To make these sounds, the lips need to be in contact. If a patient cannot get their lips together for whatever reason, it will be difficult for them to pronounce these letters. You will observe this in patients whose VDO is too great or if their teeth are flared too far forward, not allowing the lips to close. This, again, can be adjusted by shortening the anterior teeth or closing the VDO.

Final occlusal adjustments and maxillomandibular relationship record

After you complete the Esthetic and Functional Prosthetic Checklist, make any final adjustments to the patient's occlusion. Be sure to do this while the patient is wearing the resin prototype appliance and comfortably seated in an upright position. Start by using articulating paper to identify the points of contact and then fine tune the occlusion using an OccluSense® (Bausch) or a T-Scan Novus® (Tekscan) device **(Figs. 9.53-9.55)**. I find that getting the occlusion as close as possible to where I want my definitive prosthesis makes the delivery appointment much more efficient. Also, by fine-tuning the accuracy of the occlusion at this visit, you can avoid issues that can arise while making unnecessary adjustments to the definitive prosthesis. When you are finished, take a final analog or digital maxillomandibular relationship record for the laboratory (Fig. 9.56).

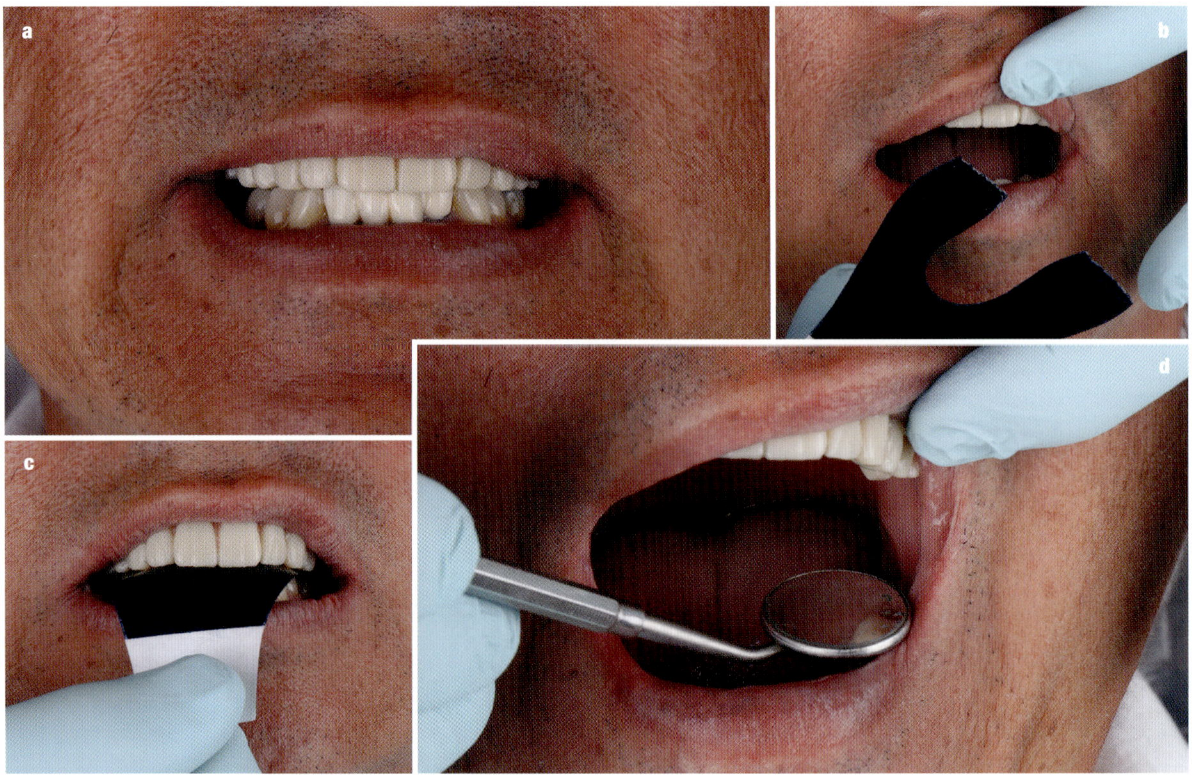

Figure 9.53 (a-d) Checking the contacts on the prototype appliance with articulating paper.

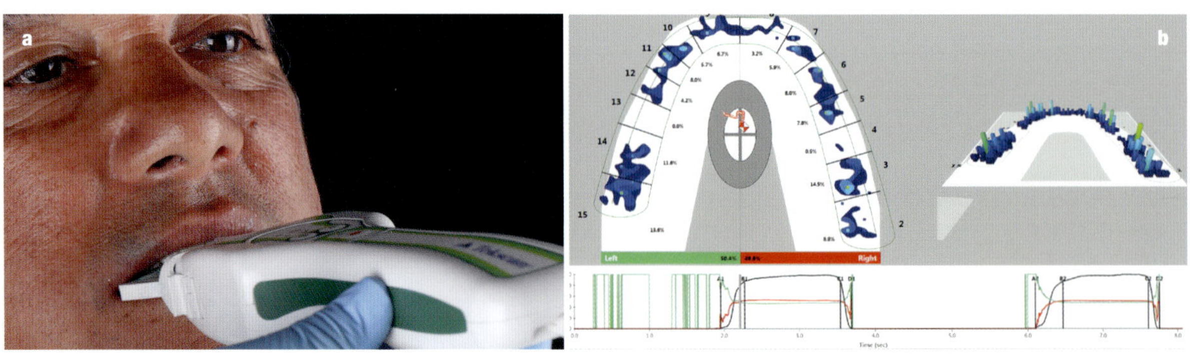

Figure 9.54 (a) Using a Tekscan device to measure the patient's occlusion; (b) Screenshot of T-Scan software readout taken while the patient is occluding.

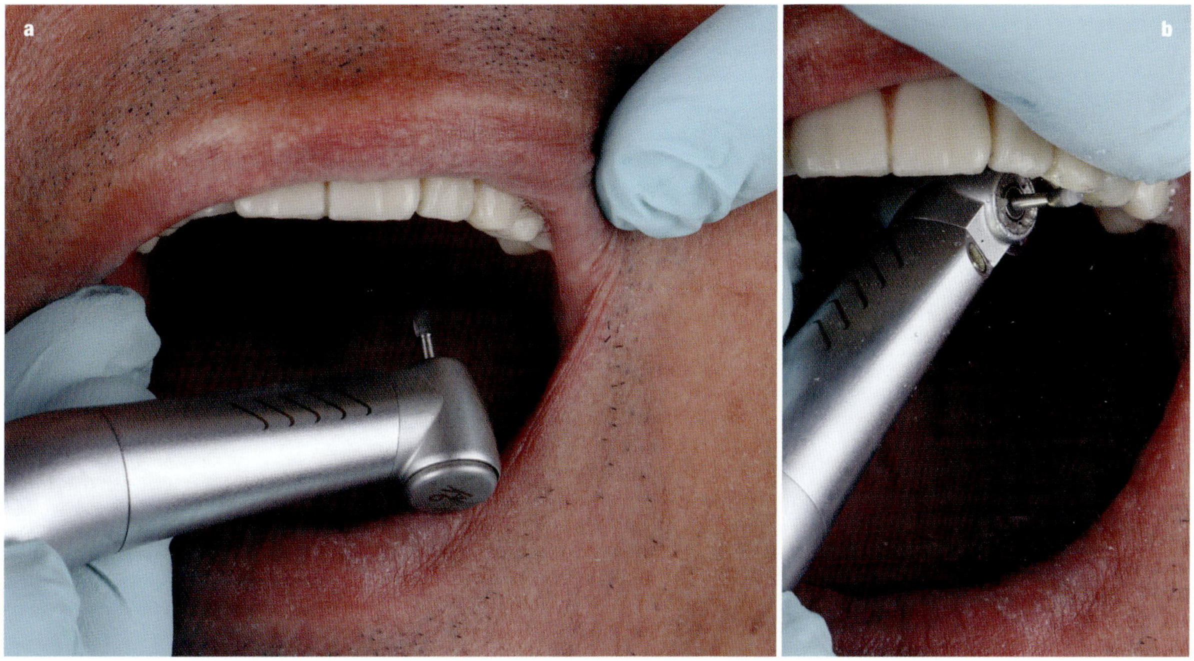

Figure 9.55 (a, b) Making final adjustments to the occlusion on the resin prototype appliance with a dental handpiece.

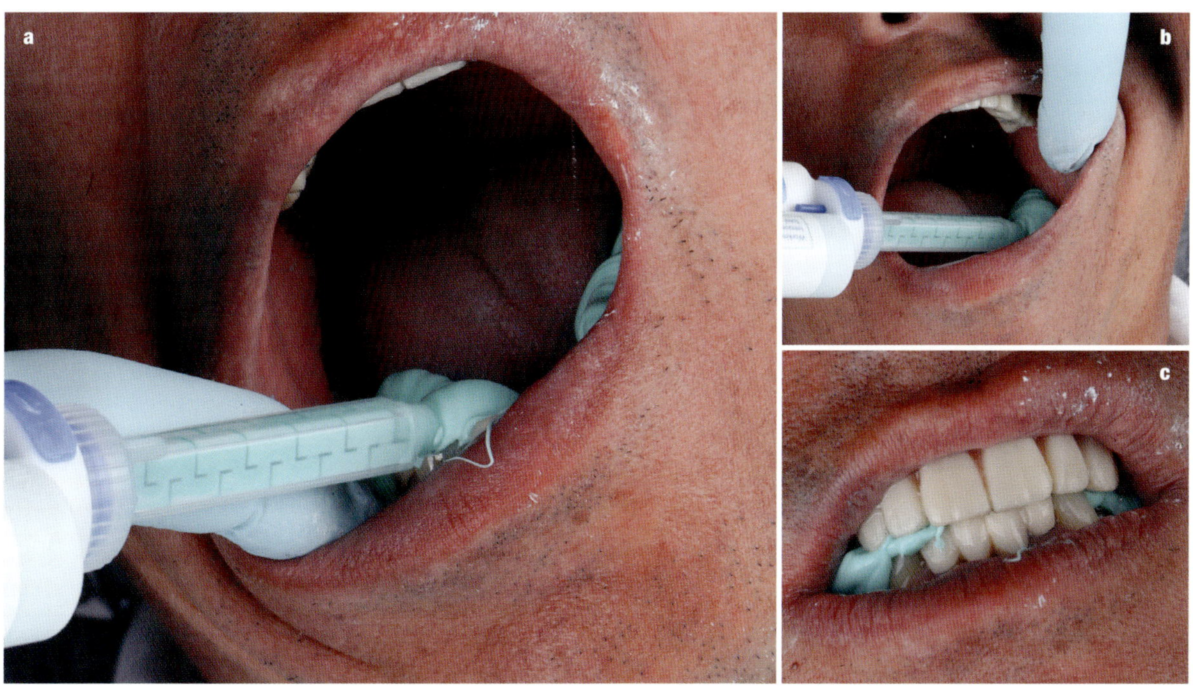

Figure 9.56 (a-c) Obtaining an analog maxillomandibular relationship record of the resin prototype opposing natural dentition.

D. Select the material and design of the definitive prosthesis

Materials

There are several materials on the market that can be used in a definitive fixed full-arch implant prosthesis. I hesitate to list all of them because more will be available by the time you read this book, and some of the materials we are now using may be taken off the market. I have worked with several dental labs and multiple materials in the last several years. Based on that experience, my advice about materials is: Choose one that is tried and true and avoid the latest fad or untested material your lab or a dental materials company might introduce to you. This choice can literally make or break your ability to be profitable. One materials manufacturer has been aggressively marketing their nanoceramic product for several years. I used it in at least a dozen fixed full-arch implant cases but discontinued immediately after I had a few complications. Every prosthesis I fabricated from this material has catastrophically failed. Leading experts in the field are now recognizing that the material does not hold up to its claims. A highly reputable lab I work with reported that 100% of their cases failed within 2 years of being in service. The moral of this story is that you should use a material that has at least a 2- to 3-year predictable track record and let others ride the bleeding edge.

In my practice, I currently use zirconia almost exclusively. Zirconia is not perfect, but it tends to be predictable over time, and I have had significantly fewer prosthetic failures with it than with any other material I have used. In my experience, fixed full-arch implant dentistry is somewhat muddled with misinformation and varied opinions about the best materials for fabricating a definitive prosthesis. My suggestion is to work with a high-quality laboratory that has a successful track record with these cases and guarantees their work. I rely on one of the world's leading zirconia experts—Mr. Jack Marrano, CDT, director of prosthetics at Absolute Dental Services—for advice on materials that are currently available as well as those just being introduced into fixed full-arch implant dentistry. Use a trusted resource to help you choose the right material for your patients and discuss with them all the variables that might come into play.

Design

Most of the factors related to definitive prosthesis design are covered in the Esthetic and Functional Prosthetic Checklist, with one exception: the intaglio surface. Make sure the intaglio surface is convex, as this is essential to its cleansability and the long-term health of the implant foundation. It was not so long ago that dental laboratories and clinicians seemed naive to this fact. Many cases I have inherited in the past few years overlooked this area, and the prostheses have small flanges and a concave intaglio surface. In Chapter 10 I share one of my cases from many years ago, before I really understood the importance of this design concept.

E. Obtain patient permission and approval

Once you have completed the Esthetic and Functional Prosthetic Checklist with your patient and discussed the materials and design of the definitive prosthesis, your patient should be ready to sign off on the Checklist. For documentation purposes and accountability, you and your assistant should also sign the Checklist. Tell your patient that in signing the checklist, they give you permission to move to the definitive prosthesis and are happy with the changes you have made or are making. Most patients will notice the time you took to walk them through their options as well as your attention to detail. My patients generally appreciate the opportunity to participate in the process, and this will set you apart from other practices and facilities that provide this service.

F. Take photos (if necessary)

If you will be asking your laboratory to make any changes after completing the Esthetic and Functional Prosthetic Checklist, take photographs or video to document the changes you want to communicate (Fig. 9.57). Follow the same guidelines for photos outlined in other parts of the workflow. If you made only minor adjustments to the patient's resin prototype appliance that will not significantly affect its esthetics or function, or if it did not require any adjustments, photos may not be necessary at this point.

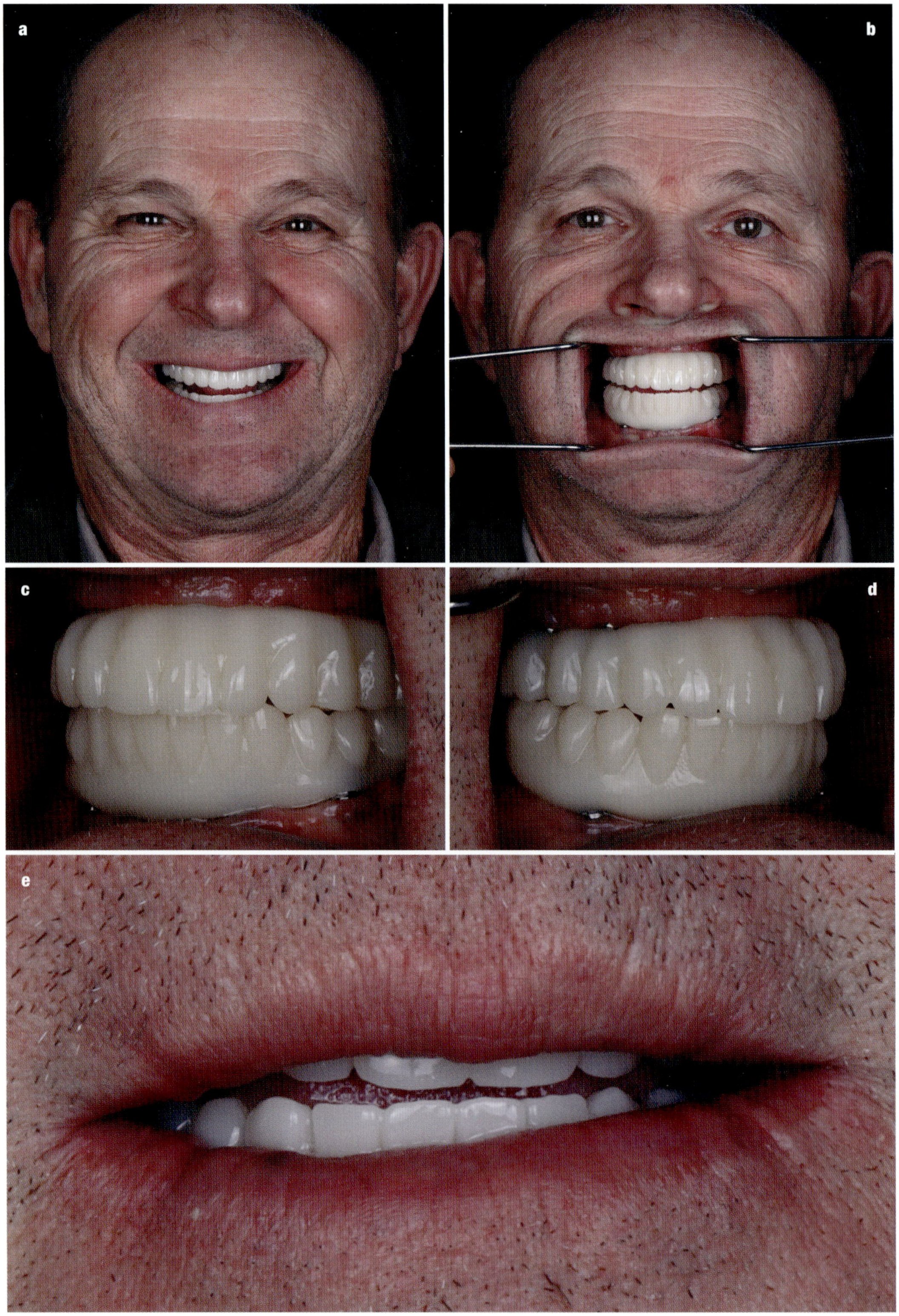

Figure 9.57 Examples of photos taken for lab communication of a patient with maxillary and mandibular resin prototype appliances: (a, b) Portrait smiling and retracted portrait; (c, d) Retracted close-up left and right in MIP; (e) Close-up repose. It may not be necessary to take photos of the views needed in earlier stages of the process.

G. Remove the resin prototype appliance and reseat the interim prosthesis—Or, consider your other options

Depending on the complexity of the case, the needs of the patient, and any concerns you have, there are a couple of options at this juncture. If you are comfortable with all the changes and the patient is ready to move forward with the next step—that is, fabrication of their definitive prosthesis—you can remove the resin prototype appliance and replace it with the interim prosthesis. If, for any reason, you feel that going to the definitive prosthesis is not the best idea just yet, I recommend doing one of the following:

- Consider letting the patient wear their resin prototype home for evaluation over a few days. This gives the patient a chance to share their new smile with friends and family and inspect it more carefully themselves, without the pressure they may feel in your office. This is also helpful if there are phonetic issues the patient wants to try to accommodate to. If you do this, it is important to tell the patient that they can only eat very soft foods and keep chewing to a minimum. Occasionally I ask my lab to fabricate the resin prototype appliance from material that has been approved for intraoral use and is more durable than some of the cheaper printed materials on the market. I may also ask my lab to send me a resin prototype appliance that has simulated gingival tissue instead of all one color, which makes it easier for patients to imagine what their definitive prosthesis will look like.
- If you do not have a resin prototype appliance that can be worn home by the patient, remove the prototype, replace the patient's interim prosthesis, and then ask your lab to send you a provisional prosthesis that the patient can wear for a time. This option makes sense when dramatic esthetic changes need to be made to a resin prototype, the patient's occlusion is difficult to establish, or the patient is having difficulty committing to the final design. Although these options increase the workflow timeline and (potentially) the lab expenses, they far outweigh having to send back and remake an expensive zirconia prosthesis.

H. Dismiss the patient and communicate with the laboratory

When the patient has left, you are ready to order the definitive prosthesis and begin the process of gathering all the materials you will need to send to the lab. Fill in the details of the lab prescription, send the information in the Esthetic and Functional Prosthetic Checklist, and attach any photos you have taken. I often call my lab to discuss the final touches that will be made, knowing that this is the last chance I have to do so before a very expensive prosthesis is fabricated. If you have any concerns that are difficult to articulate, ask your lab to let you view the case design before it goes into production. I frequently have the lab send me photos of the digital proposal or get on a video conferencing call so that I can see how the changes look (Fig. 9.58).

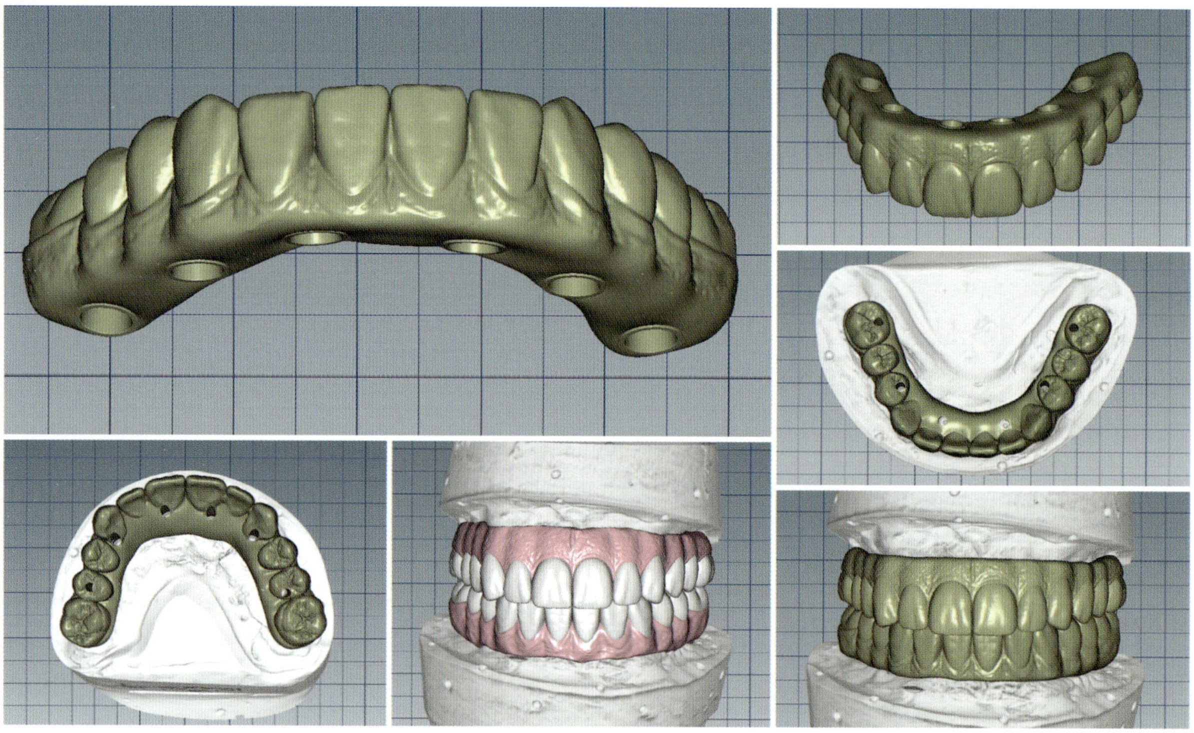

Figure 9.58 **A design proposal prepared by the lab for previewing changes being made before production of the definitive prostheses.**

DELIVERY: APPOINTMENT 4

The delivery appointment is probably my favorite visit of the prosthetic workflow. We usually tell our patients to come to this appointment ready to have portrait pictures taken. This can be a fun appointment for your team to be creative with some patients. For example, one of our patients told us she just wanted to be able to bite into an apple again without worrying about breaking off her teeth. After her definitive prosthesis was delivered, we surprised her with a large apple, and she finally had the opportunity to make her wish a reality. Gift certificates for steak dinners, oversized candy bars, and a jar of peanuts have also been real winners with patients. I encourage you to spend a little time making this appointment a big deal and roll out the red carpet. A positive patient experience at the end of their journey can create a boost in office culture, marketing opportunities, and future referral of friends and family, plus it is just a nice thing to do that distinguishes your practice from everyone else.

Operatory setup. In addition to a basic exam kit, the following items will be helpful:

- Dental implant prosthetic setup with drivers
- Chairside handpiece and bur kit
- Articulating paper
- Digital occlusal analysis device
- Teflon tape and flowable temporary resin material
- Camera

A. Remove the interim prosthesis

With the patient seated comfortably, remove the PVS plugs from the interim prosthesis, then remove the prosthetic screws, and take out the interim prosthesis (Fig. 9.59). Make sure you place all the screws in a small dish after completely removing them from the prosthesis. Check the integrity of the prosthesis, looking for any cracks, breaks, or other problems. If you find any issue that affects the integrity of the interim prosthesis, consider repairing it yourself or send it to the laboratory for refurbishing. Clean the prosthesis thoroughly, removing plaque, tartar, and other debris. You will want to set the prosthesis aside with the other components of the patient's case and eventually package it all together for the patient to take home (Fig. 9.60).

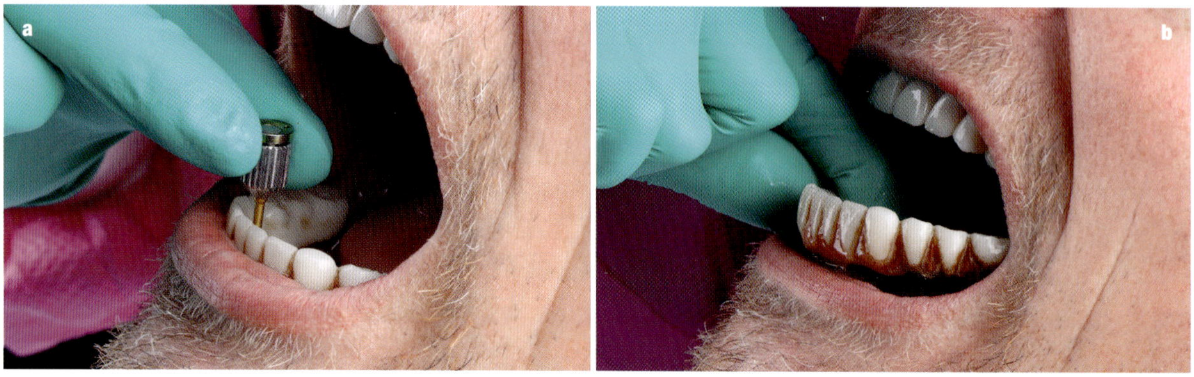

Figure 9.59 (a, b) Removal of the patient's mandibular interim prosthesis.

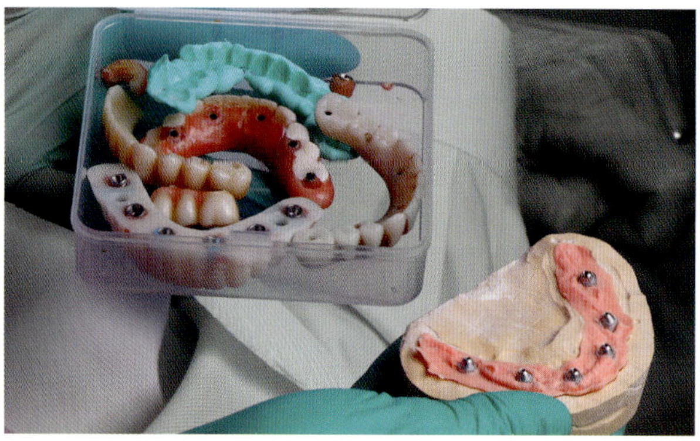

Figure 9.60 Collecting the patient's interim prosthesis, master cast, maxillomandibular relationship record, replica appliance, and other components to send home with the patient.

PRO TIP: Delivery of the definitive prosthesis, part 1

When you finish a fixed full-arch implant case, give the patient all the components of it, including master casts with the implant analogs, appliances, maxillomandibular relationship records, opposing casts, laboratory and implant details, spare dentures, and so forth. If you try to store all your patients' cases in the office, over time you may run out of space. Also, having the patient keep these components makes sense: If something happens to the definitive prosthesis, the patient has possession of their interim prosthesis and other components of the case. Definitive prostheses can break or become damaged on rare occasions, and it can be stressful for you to have to search for the back-up in an emergency. When the patient has everything at home in a safe place, it is much easier to deal with unforeseen circumstances that may arise.

B. Inspect the prosthesis (or prostheses), MUAs, and soft tissues

As before, carefully inspect the patient's ridges, looking for anything unusual (Fig. 9.61). Examine the MUAs and clean away any plaque, tartar, or other debris. This may be a good time for you to introduce your hygienist to the patient and offer some advice about at-home hygiene. For patients whose hygiene has been less than acceptable during the course of treatment, I recommend they visit hygiene the day of delivery. Eventually, the patient should be seen regularly in hygiene, and the delivery visit is a good time to reinforce that. Make note of any areas around the MUAs that lack adequate keratinized tissue and take intraoral occlusal photographs of the tissue at delivery as a baseline for future visits. Retorque the MUAs with the appropriate driver and torque wrench.

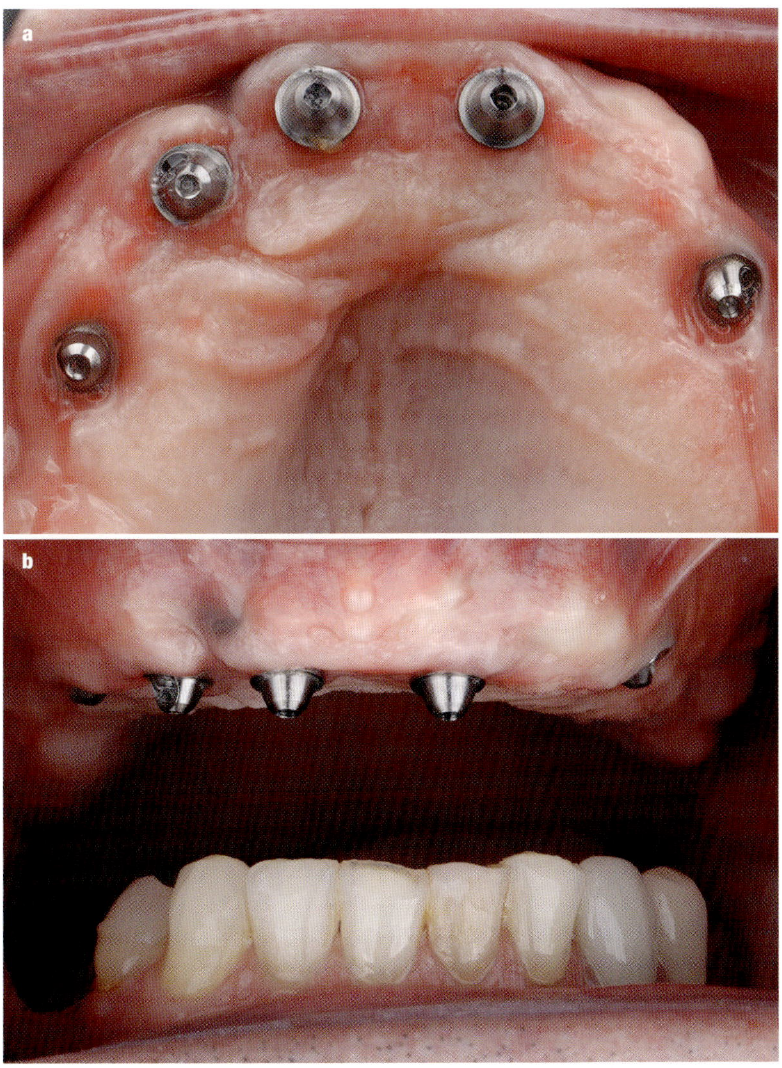

Figure 9.61 (a) Occlusal and (b) facial views of a maxillary arch immediately after removal of the interim prosthesis.

C. Seat the definitive prosthesis in the patient's mouth

Before placing the definitive prosthesis, examine it extraorally. If it has titanium bases, verify that they are firmly in place and check for any fractures or discrepancies from what you ordered. Make sure the intaglio surface of the prosthesis is convex and highly polished. Any qualified laboratory understands how to design full-arch prostheses, and in most cases you should have little to worry about (Fig. 9.62).

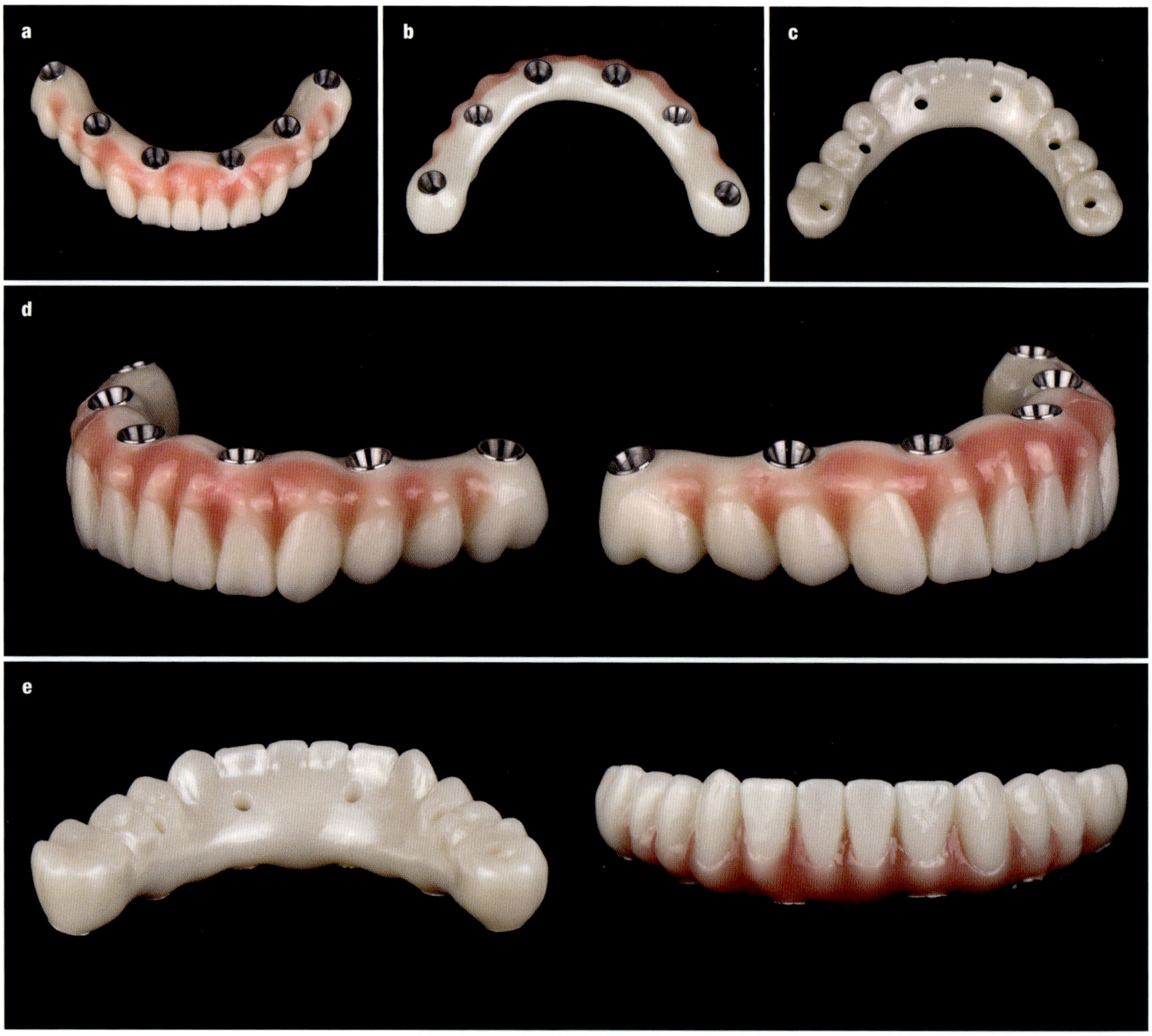

Figure 9.62 (a-e) A definitive dual-arch monolithic zirconia prosthesis with titanium bases as seen from different perspectives.

Place the definitive prosthesis over the MUAs, then insert new prosthetic screws into the access channels in the prosthesis and hand tighten. Be sure to use new titanium prosthetic screws that have not been torqued before, and put the used screws you set aside earlier with the patient's case to take home. The new screws should all go in passively, with little or no resistance. If you are unable to screw the prosthesis in place, review the earlier section on placing and fitting the resin prototype appliance, including the one-screw test, and go through the same thought patterns and exercises to identify the source of the problem. As you are screwing the prosthesis in place, do not be surprised if your patient feels some tightness or pressure, or possibly a pinching feeling, as the fit of the definitive prosthesis is much more precise than the other appliances and prostheses. Take your time, just as you would with a single-unit implant abutment that slightly constricts the tissue, and give the patient small breaks to allow the tissue to expand. If the tissue compression is not excessive or unreasonable, the patient will feel relief and you can continue. Finally, torque all the prosthetic screws into place following the implant manufacturer's guidelines (Figs. 9.63, 9.64).

PRO TIP: Delivery of the definitive prosthesis, part 2

If your patient experiences pain during the delivery of the definitive prosthesis that does not subside after a short period, the prosthesis may be compressing the tissue more than it should. In my experience, such compression most commonly occurs between two MUAs or at the cantilever area of the prosthesis. Identify the area with the patient's help and then consider removing the soft tissue that is being compressed or reducing the prosthesis. Reducing the prosthesis is often the easiest solution, but make sure that once the section is adjusted, you finish and polish it. It may be helpful to take a radiograph of the area in the patient's mouth as well to rule out the presence of pathology.

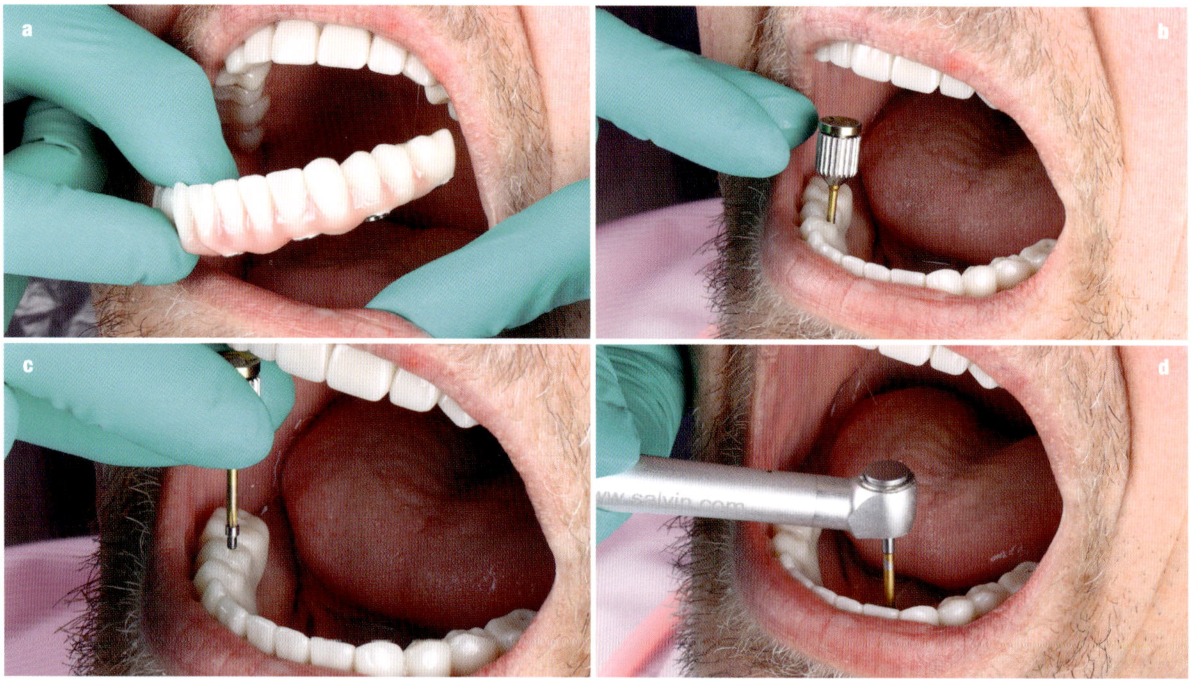

Figure 9.63 (a-d) Delivery of a definitive mandibular monolithic zirconia prosthesis.

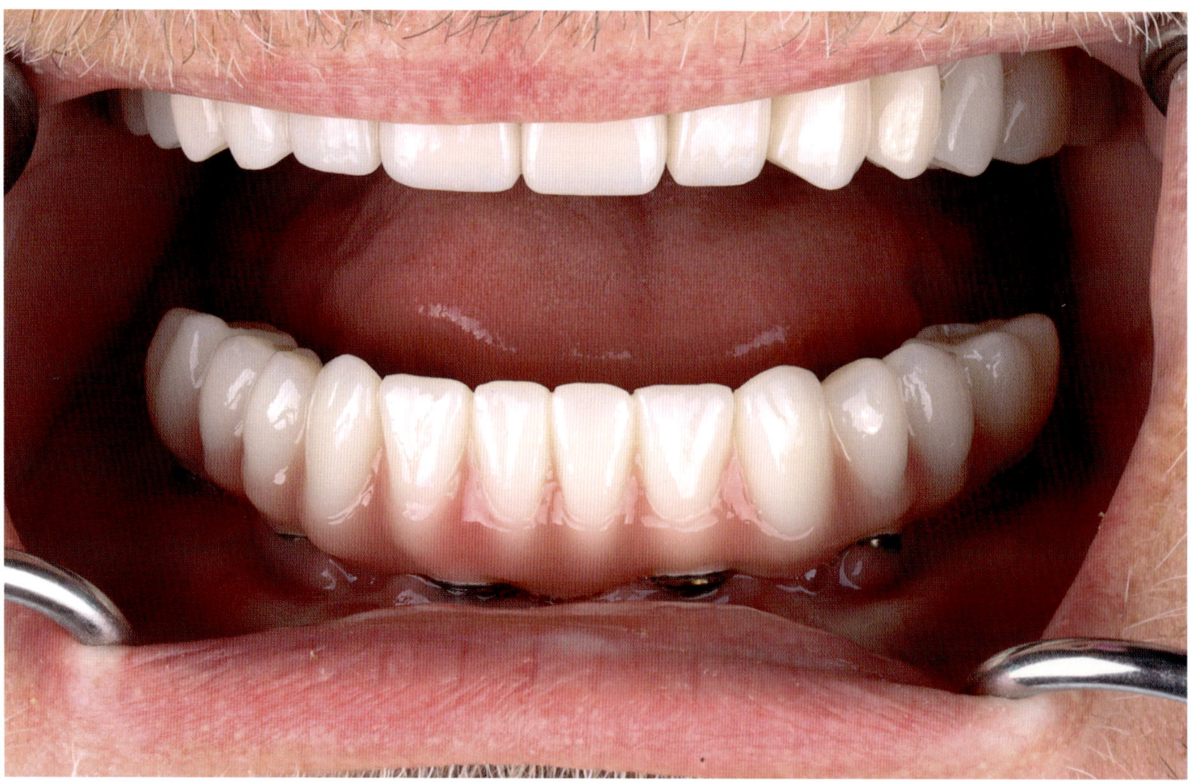

Figure 9.64 Definitive mandibular zirconia fixed full-arch implant prosthesis in place after torquing of the prosthetic screws.

D. Evaluate the definitive prosthesis

When the prosthesis is torqued and in position, go through the Esthetic and Functional Prosthetic Checklist once again with your patient and assistant. Verify that the esthetics, phonetics, and occlusion are precisely correct. This process should take little time because of all the adjustments made and planning performed at the resin prototype appointment. Patients will often comment that their definitive prosthesis feels so much smoother and less bulky than their interim prosthesis and that their speech is less labored. Regarding occlusion, I almost always have a digital occlusion device set up to verify that the contacts are balanced, excursion patterns are void of interferences, and pathways of chewing are correct. Adjust and polish as needed with a high-speed handpiece and a bur that is appropriate for the prosthesis material (Fig. 9.65). The esthetics of the new prosthesis are almost always the highlight of this visit.

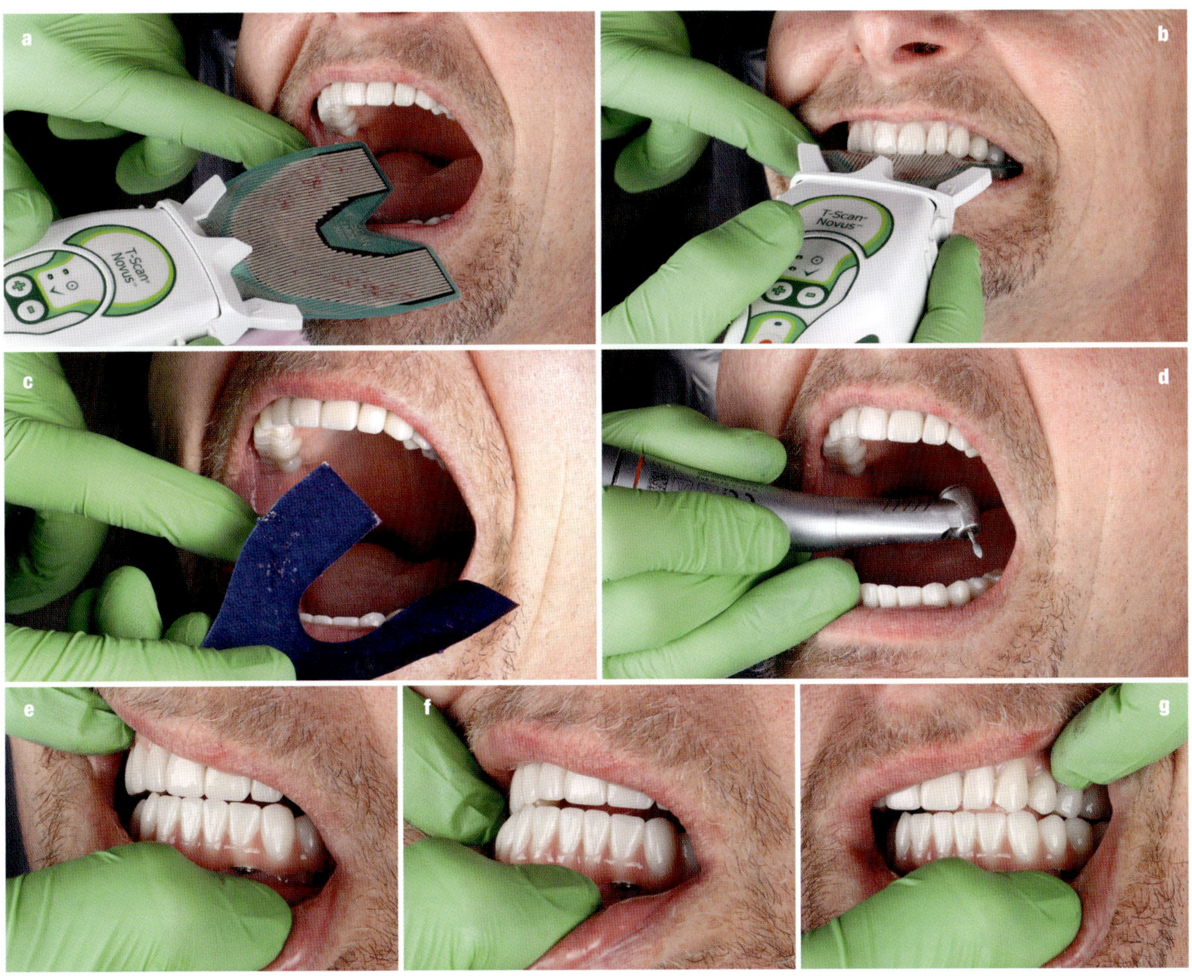

Figure 9.65 (a-g) Checking the occlusion, excursions, and chewing pathways of the definitive prosthesis.

E. Finalize delivery

Finalize the case by filling in the screw access channels (Figs. 9.66a-9.66c). The question of what to put in the access channels has been a subject of debate for several years. Some dentists use PVS because of its retrievability and ease of removal, but it has the disadvantages of being unstable and the color generally does not match the prosthesis, which can be off-putting to the patient. Other dentists have opted for some form of block-out material such as Teflon tape, along with resin composite to obturate the screw access channels. This method fills the channels effectively but makes retrieval, especially in the hygiene department, a time-consuming and inefficient process. Over the past few years, I have tried multiple materials and methods for filling the screw access channels. Currently, we are using Teflon tape and temporary flowable resin (Clip Flow, VOCO Dental), which can be placed by an auxiliary or dental hygienist and removed without a high-speed handpiece at maintenance visits (Figs. 9.66d-9.66g).

After the screw access channels are filled, I like to take final photos of the patient and ask for their feedback and a testimonial. However, not all patients are ready to do this without the proper "test drive," so to speak. If your patient is ready, go ahead and complete these tasks. If your patient would be more relaxed and amenable to giving a testimonial and positive feedback later, as well as sitting for final photographs, save these tasks for the postdelivery appointment.

For most of my cases, I order a resin occlusal guard from the lab for the patient to wear at night, and it is often delivered at this appointment. However, some labs we have worked with ask us to take digital impressions for the occlusal guard at the delivery appointment. Recently we have begun 3D printing nightguards and other orthotic devices in our office. We either have the lab create the design or we use AI software to do this. If you decide to make this part of your workflow, one of your dental auxiliaries can easily obtain a digital impression of the patient's arches along with the maxillomandibular relationship record and then print an occlusal guard or orthotic device and deliver it at the postdelivery appointment.

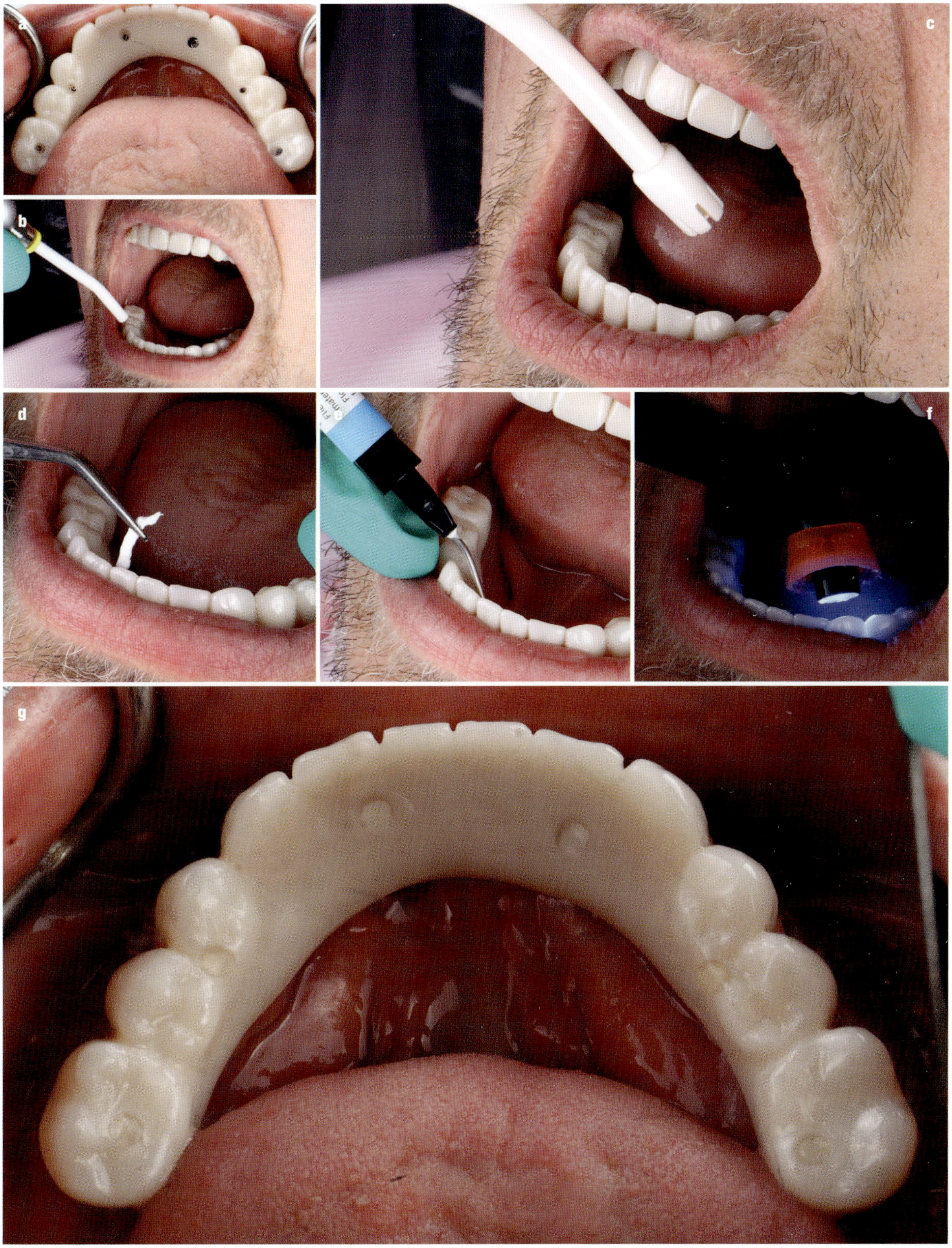

Figure 9.66 Finalizing delivery of the mandibular prosthesis. (a-c) Rinse and dry the screw access channels; (d) Place a small amount of Teflon tape over each access channel; (e, f) Apply Clip Flow temporary flowable resin (VOCO Dental) over the Teflon tape and light-cure; (g) Lingual view after the definitive zirconia prosthesis access channels have been filled.

POSTDELIVERY: APPOINTMENT 5

(OPTIONAL BUT RECOMMENDED)

Although this appointment is optional, I frequently ask my team to schedule it for patients who have gone through the prosthetic workflow. If we took final photos and requested a testimonial and feedback at the delivery appointment, this visit will be short and sweet.

This appointment usually takes place 2 to 4 weeks after delivery of the definitive prosthesis and takes about 20 minutes. The first few minutes should be spent listening to any concerns your patient may have, answering questions, and being supportive. Typically, we will again verify the VDO and maxillomandibular relationship. In some cases, a patient's muscles will adapt differently than expected based on what was observed at the delivery appointment. Locating any interferences or strong contacts and making adjustments to eliminate them can greatly improve the patient's comfort and increase the longevity of the prosthesis and opposing dentition. We also deliver the patient's protective occlusal appliance or guard for those who did not receive it at the delivery appointment. I recommend a nightguard appliance to almost all my patients, and after a few weeks of wearing their new prosthesis, most patients agree with me. Occlusal guard designs vary, but in my practice the objective is just to protect the patient's prosthesis/prostheses and provide a buffer between the opposing arches.

Repeating the discussion on home hygiene and reminding the patient about our maintenance program/contract is valuable to do at this visit. We strongly advise our patients to maintain the investment they have made in their oral health and appearance by having consistent and regular visits in our hygiene department. Finally, if you have not done so already, be sure to give the patient their completed case in a sealed box or package and encourage them to keep it in a safe, dry place where it will not be damaged.

If you have not formally asked your patient to provide a written testimonial or taken the final post-treatment photos, do so during this appointment (Figs. 9.67-9.71). Building the relationship, not just fixing our patient's teeth, is top priority, and the entire team can be part of this process. Getting feedback and taking the photographs is a great opportunity not only to celebrate with your patient but also to document the case and begin building a portfolio to show other potential patients. Get creative and have fun with this. Your patient and everyone on the team will appreciate making this memory.

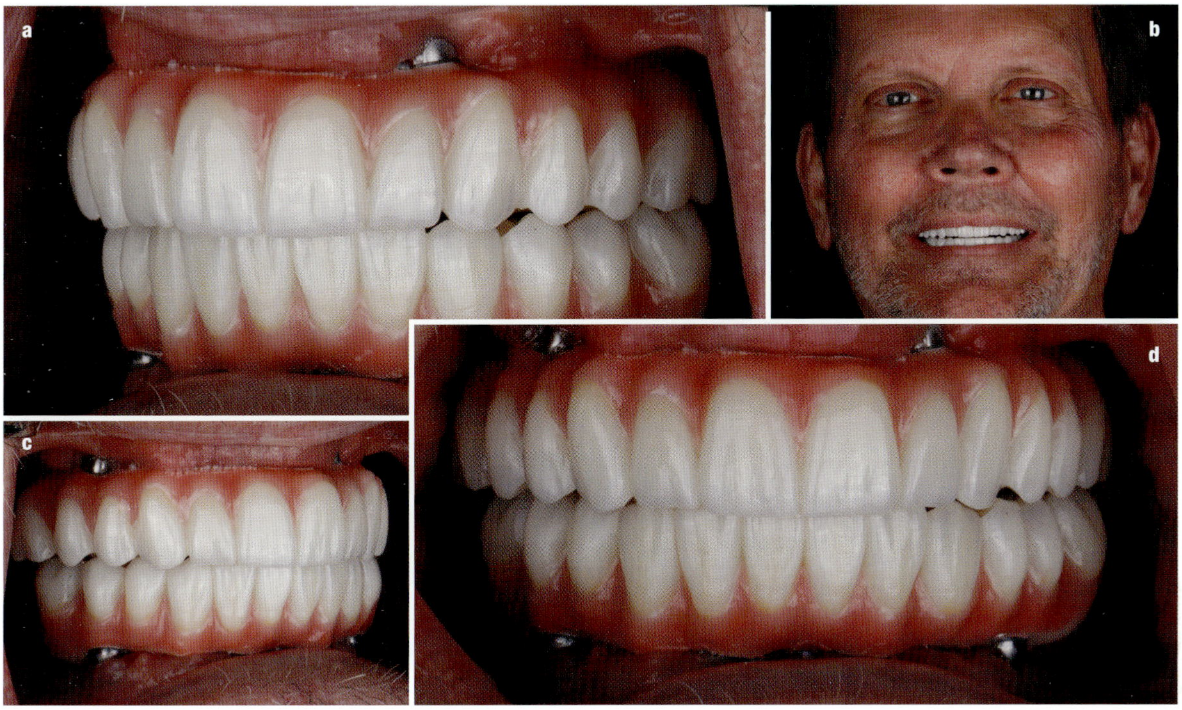

Figure 9.67 (a-d) Postdelivery photographs of a portrait smile and retracted views.

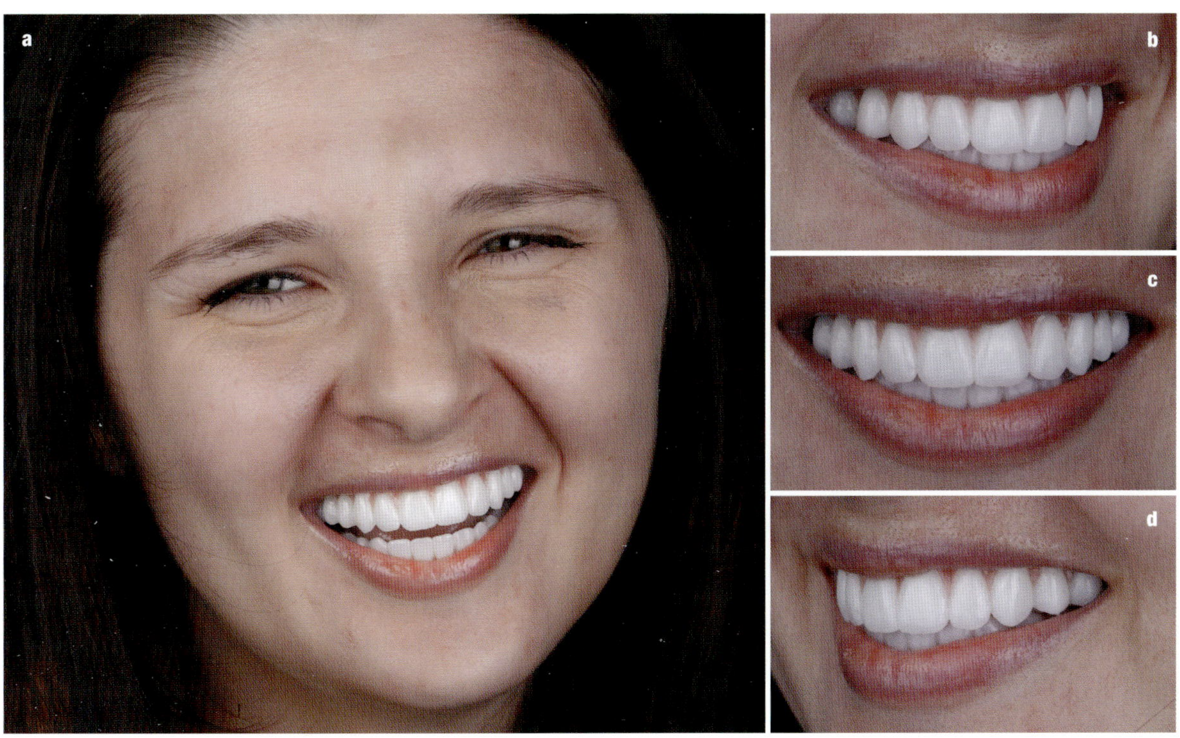

Figure 9.68 (a-d) Postdelivery photographs of a portrait smile and close-up smile views.

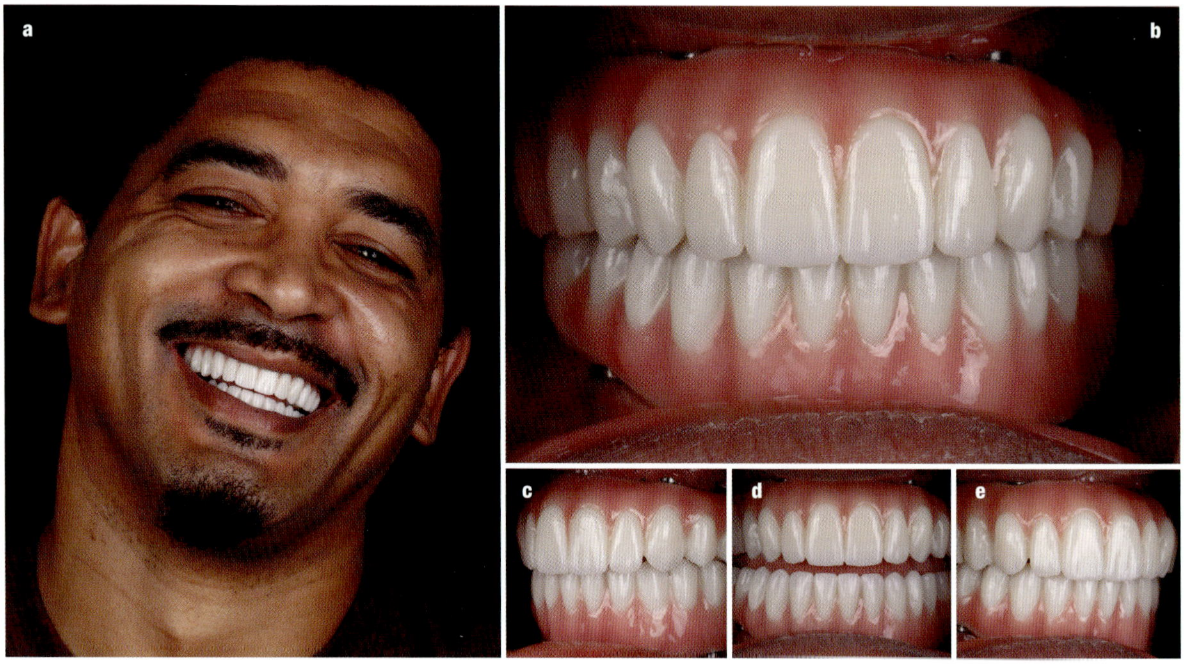

Figure 9.69 (a-e) Postdelivery photographs of a portrait smile and retracted views.

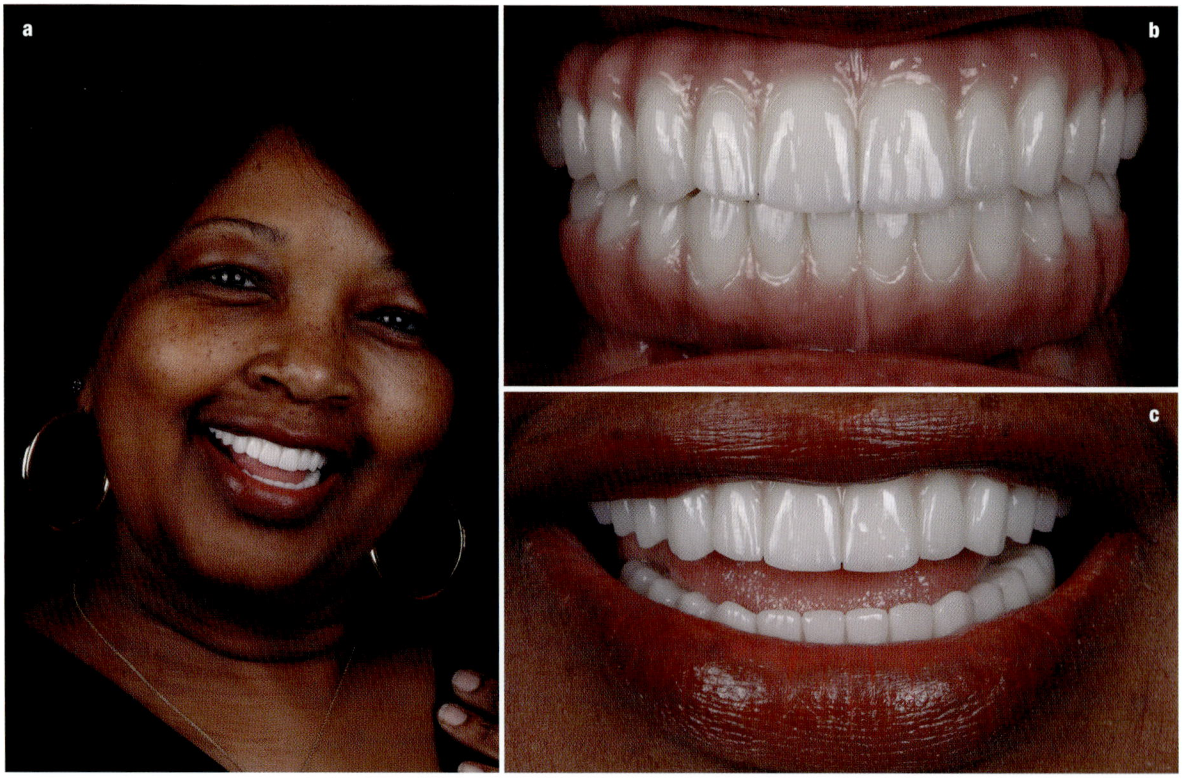

Figure 9.70 (a-c) Postdelivery photographs of a portrait smile and retracted and close-up smile views.

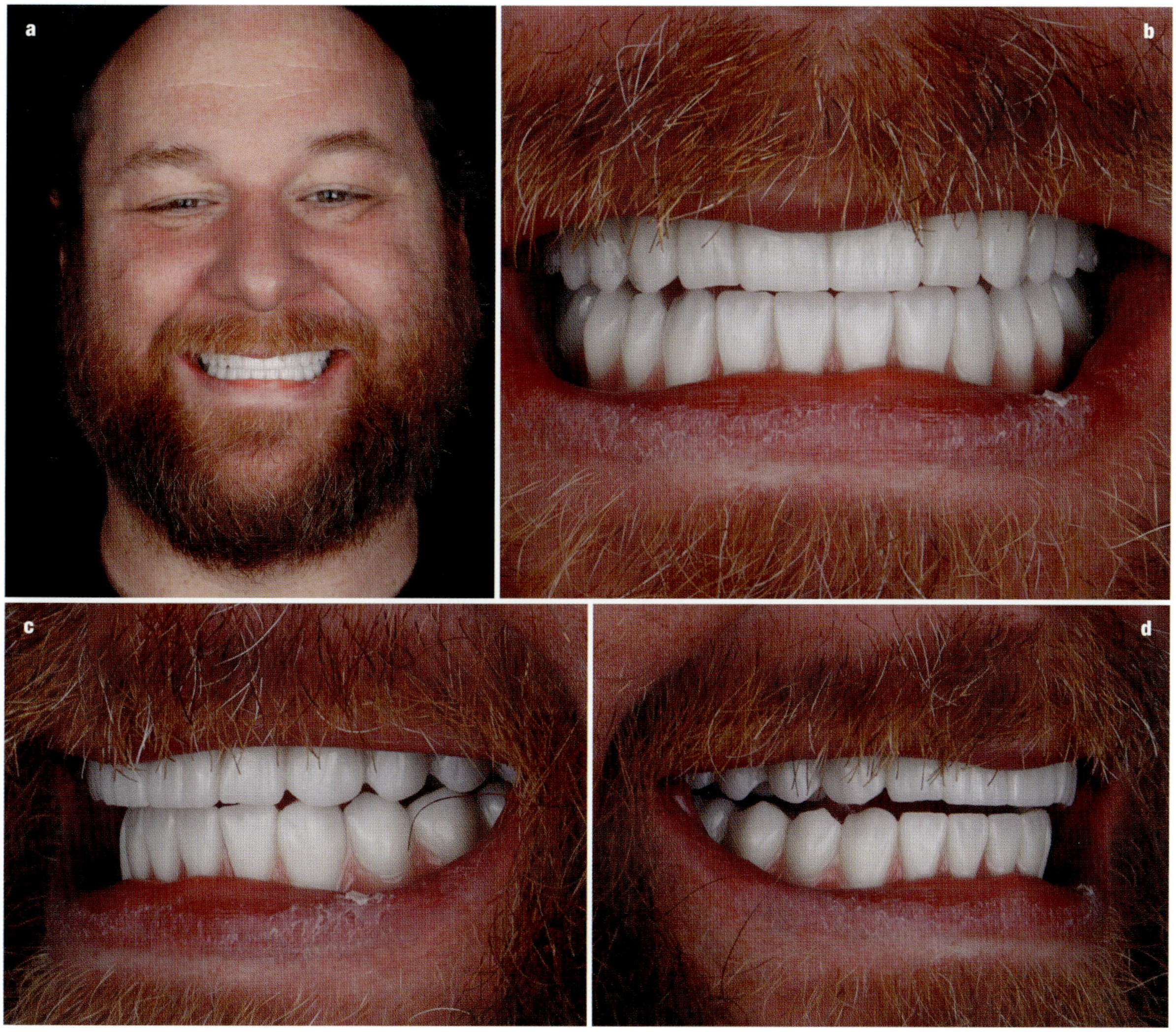

Figure 9.71 (a-d) Postdelivery photographs of a portrait smile and close-up smile views.

THE FUTURE OF THE PROSTHETIC WORKFLOW

While writing this text, I have been introduced to new processes and technology that have begun to impact my prosthetic workflow. I anticipate that these new techniques and technologies will significantly affect how we deliver care to our patients and will further simplify the process.

One recent technology that could revolutionize how we attach and stabilize full-arch and single-unit implant restorations to abutments and MUAs is Smileloc® (RODO Medical). Smileloc is a screwless, cementless system that allows retrieval of an appliance from abutments using a device that creates induction energy to unlock sleeves made of nitinol, a nickel and titanium alloy known for its superelasticity and shape memory. This solution also eliminates the debate over what material to use in the screw access channels. I am excited about the benefits that this technology will bring to fixed full-arch implant prosthetics. Figures 9.72 to 9.74 are photos documenting a dual-arch case with a monolithic zirconia definitive prosthesis that I restored using the Smileloc system.

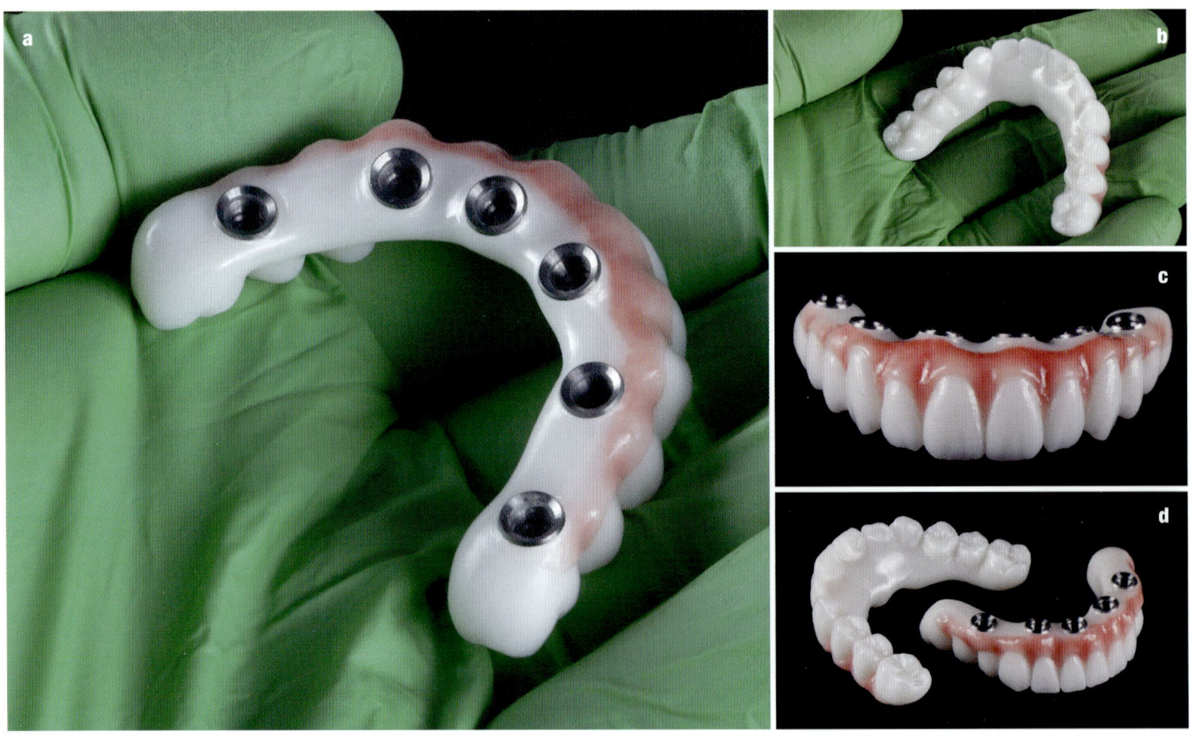

Figure 9.72 (a-d) Smileloc® system (RODO Medical) used in a full-arch monolithic zirconia prosthesis.

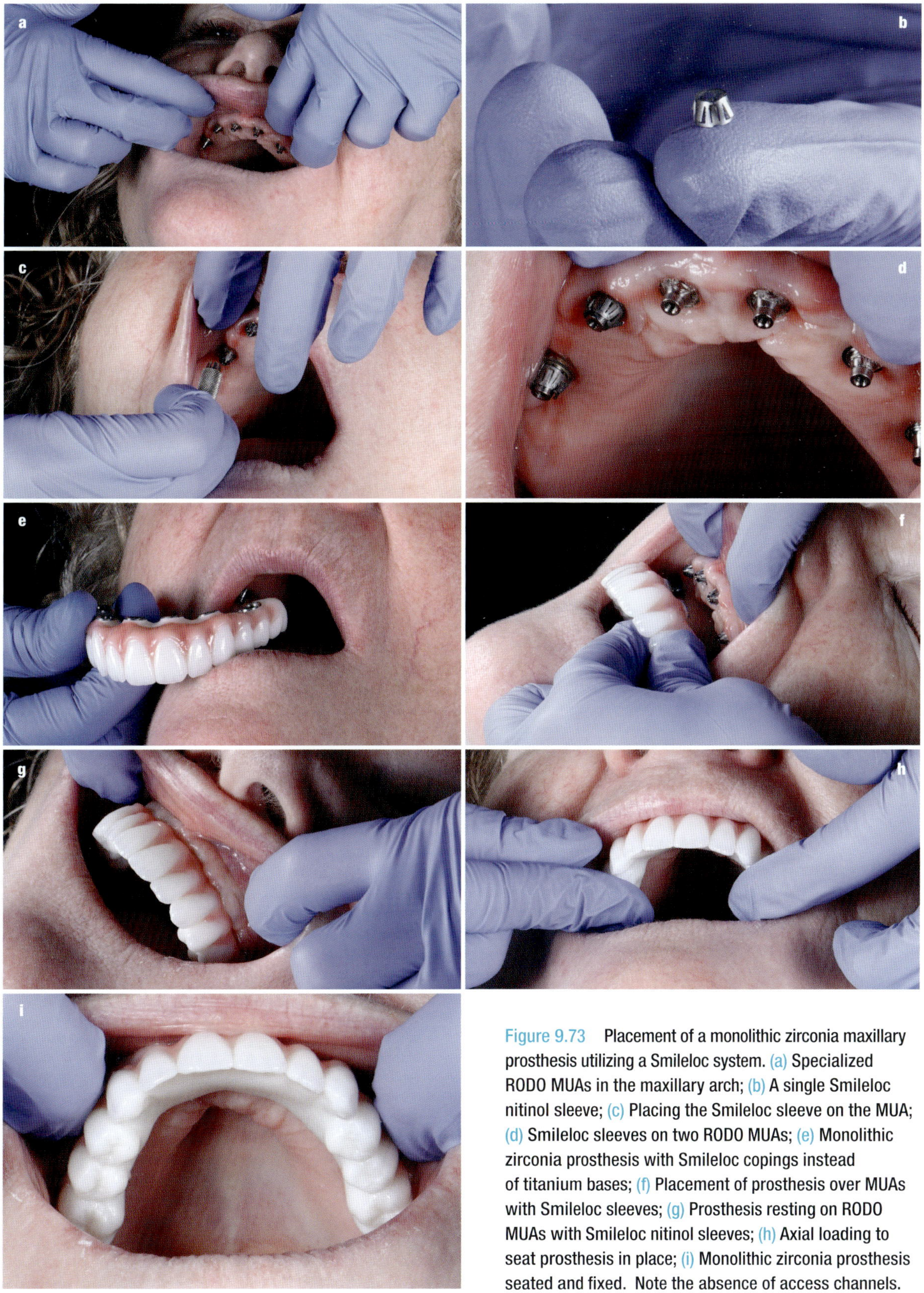

Figure 9.73 Placement of a monolithic zirconia maxillary prosthesis utilizing a Smileloc system. (a) Specialized RODO MUAs in the maxillary arch; (b) A single Smileloc nitinol sleeve; (c) Placing the Smileloc sleeve on the MUA; (d) Smileloc sleeves on two RODO MUAs; (e) Monolithic zirconia prosthesis with Smileloc copings instead of titanium bases; (f) Placement of prosthesis over MUAs with Smileloc sleeves; (g) Prosthesis resting on RODO MUAs with Smileloc nitinol sleeves; (h) Axial loading to seat prosthesis in place; (i) Monolithic zirconia prosthesis seated and fixed. Note the absence of access channels.

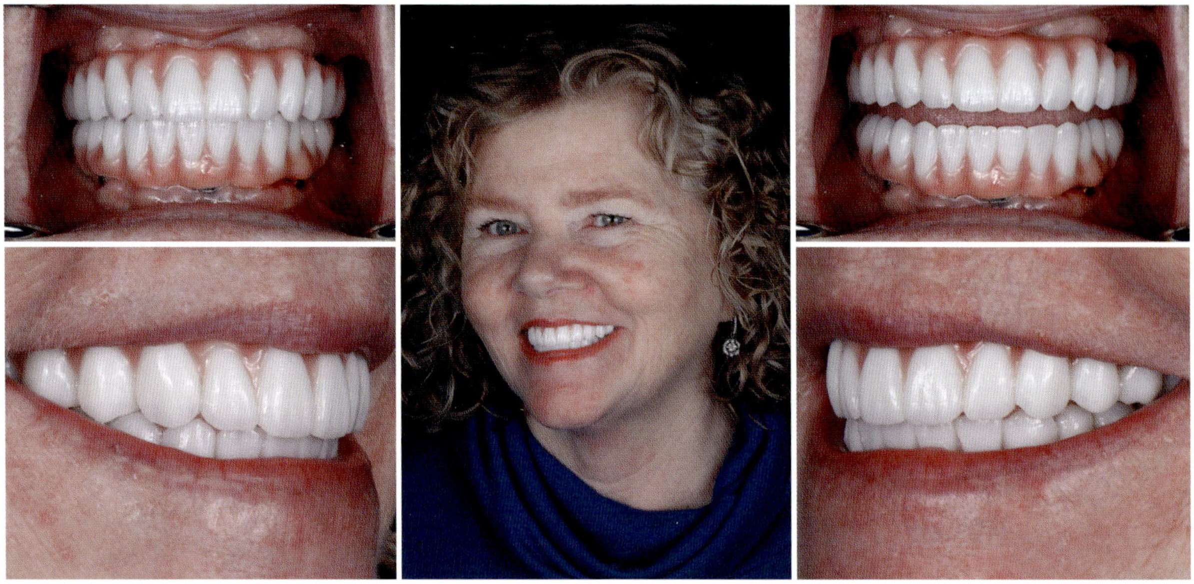

Figure 9.74 **Completed Smileloc fixed full-arch case.**

Another recent development in technology has shown great promise as a method to digitize processes I currently do in a mostly analog fashion using the verification or replica appliance techniques. Proprietary scan bodies that attach to MUAs can accurately record the locations of implants placed in the arch and a digital impression of these can be taken before or after tissue healing. Although techniques such as photogrammetry and other complete digital processes can also be used to capture the locations of implants with great precision, they require practitioners to purchase additional expensive equipment and undergo special training. For the average dental clinician in the early stages of offering fixed full-arch implant treatment to their patients, such upfront investments may not make good business sense for their practice. This is especially true if the clinician is only providing such treatment on a limited basis and to a limited number of patients. However, intraoral scanners that are used in the digital data collection process have become more precise and accurate over the past few years.

Recently I have begun working with dental labs to find ways of implementing a completely digital workflow by using these proprietary scan bodies at surgery and/or during the prosthetic workflow. Currently, I am not prepared to officially introduce this method into the prosthetic workflow, but the results are very promising. Figures 9.75 to 9.77 present several techniques that offer a preview of what is coming soon.

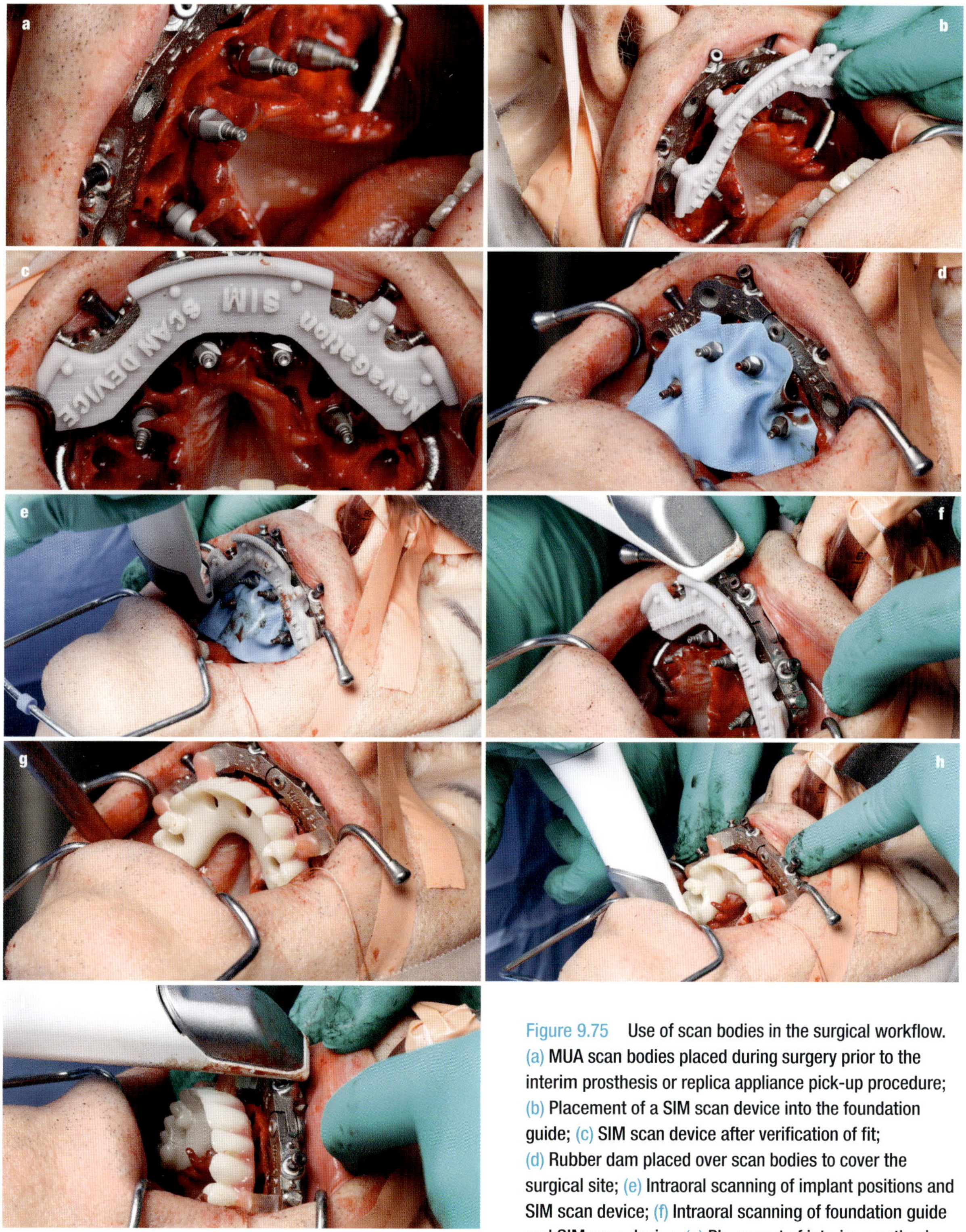

Figure 9.75 Use of scan bodies in the surgical workflow. (a) MUA scan bodies placed during surgery prior to the interim prosthesis or replica appliance pick-up procedure; (b) Placement of a SIM scan device into the foundation guide; (c) SIM scan device after verification of fit; (d) Rubber dam placed over scan bodies to cover the surgical site; (e) Intraoral scanning of implant positions and SIM scan device; (f) Intraoral scanning of foundation guide and SIM scan device; (g) Placement of interim prosthesis after removal of SIM scan device; (h) Intraoral scanning of interim prosthesis on foundation guide; (i) Intraoral scanning of interim prosthesis with foundation guide to index and merge into software with SIM device scan.

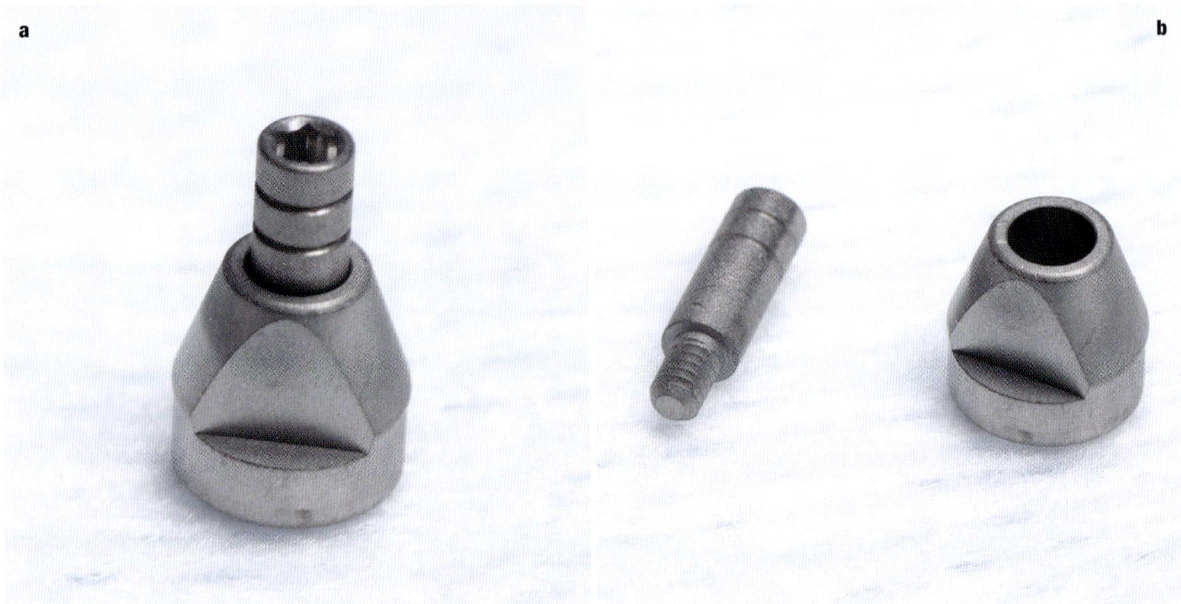

Figure 9.76 (a, b) Specialized MUA scan body components used during surgery.

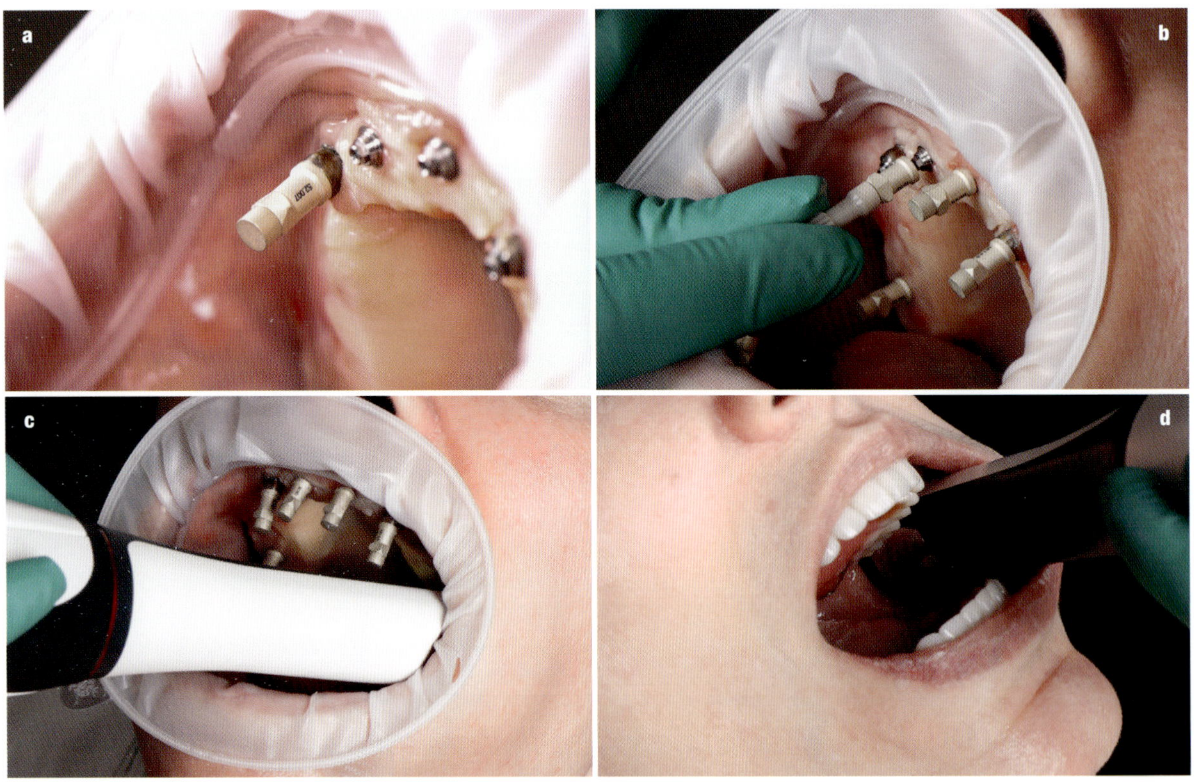

Figure 9.77 (a) Proprietary scan body used for verification in the prosthetic workflow; (b) Proprietary scan bodies placed throughout the maxillary arch; (c) Taking a digital impression of scan bodies prior to development of a prototype prosthesis; (d) Intraoral scanning of the interim prostheses and maxillomandibular relationship to obtain data for making a prototype prosthesis without the need for a verification or replica appliance.

References

1. Misch CE, Bidez MW. Implant-protected occlusion: A biomechanical rationale. Compendium 1994 Nov;15:1330, 1332, 1334 passim; quiz 1344.
2. Beumer J, Faulkner RF, Shah KC, Wu BM. Fundamentals of Implant Dentistry, Vol 1: Prosthodontic Principles. 2nd ed. Chicago: Quintessence, 2022.

CONCEPTS AND REASONING

- Research and literature
- Considerations and debate regarding prosthesis removal
- Risk assessment for dental implants
- Hygiene/Maintenance contract
- Maintenance and hygiene protocol

WORKFLOW

- Review medical history
- Occlusion/Nightguard
- Prosthesis removal
- Radiographs

→

- Examination
- Stability determination
- Probing/Palpation

↓

- Guided biofilm therapy

↓

- Inspection/Cleaning of prosthesis
- Doctor check

↓

- Replacement of prosthesis
- Oral hygiene instructions
- Reappointment

CASE STUDY

FIXED FULL-ARCH DENTISTRY MAINTENANCE AND HYGIENE

SECTION VI

STEP-BY-STEP MAINTENANCE AND HYGIENE PROTOCOL

CHAPTER **10**

Commitment: Treat yourself and others with respect.
To be respected, you must respect others. Respect is earned, and giving it is one of the greatest expressions of love.

HYGIENE AND MAINTENANCE CONCEPTS AND RATIONALE

The question of what role the dentist and dental hygienist should take in helping patients maintain a fixed full-arch prosthesis has been variously debated, questioned, and ignored. I see new patients with fixed full-arch implant prostheses that are several years old and have never been removed or cleaned under or around, as well as those who have had their prostheses removed religiously every 6 months. When I ask doctors who perform fixed full-arch implant dentistry to describe the hygiene protocols they follow for their patients, I get a variety of answers. I recently did a Google search using the key words *dental hygiene* and *fixed full-arch implants* and got a list of private dental practice websites and blog posts offering a range of often conflicting content that in some cases was difficult to understand. All of this can be partly explained by the fact that general dentists lack guidance on the subject of what adequate hygiene around a fixed full-arch implant prosthesis looks like. For example, the American Academy of Periodontology website states that dental implants require at-home care and regular dental visits to prevent implant disease, and yet offers nothing more than a vague assertion that the patient's periodontist will work closely with the patient and their dentist to develop the best care plan[1].

Several years ago, a nine-member scientific panel was convened by the American College of Prosthodontists (ACP) to develop a set of clinical practice guidelines (CPG) related to recall and maintenance of tooth- and implant-borne dental restorations, including patients in full-arch implant prostheses[2]. In addition to members of the ACP, the panel included experts from the American Dental Association, the Academy of General Dentistry, and the American Dental Hygienists Association, and in January 2016 the guidelines they developed were published in the *Journal of the American Dental Association* (JADA). Recommendations related to fixed full-arch implant-supported prostheses included the following:

- Patients with fixed full-arch implant-supported prostheses should be seen in the dental office at least every 6 months for their lifetime.
- Extraoral and intraoral examinations should be performed as well as prophylaxis/cleaning of the prosthesis/abutments, and oral hygiene instructions should be given.
- In patients with implant-supported fixed prostheses, the decision to remove the prosthesis for biological maintenance should be based on the patient's demonstrated inability to perform adequate oral hygiene.

The reader should note that not all recommendations made in the CPGs were supported by scientific evidence. Specifically, the recommendations for fixed full-arch implant-supported prostheses relied heavily on evidence from committee reports, opinions, or clinical experience from respected authorities.

Following publication of the CPGs, the ACP prepared a formal position statement on maintenance of fixed full-arch implant restorations that was approved by the ACP board in October 2016. In part, it states the following:

> Removal of a fixed, screw-retained implant prosthesis for evaluation is not needed unless there are signs of peri-implantitis, a demonstrated inability to maintain adequate oral hygiene, or there are mechanical complications that require removal... Based upon the present literature... removal of full-arch, implant-supported restorations at regular maintenance intervals is discouraged *unless* adequate professional hygiene is not possible with the superstructure in place *or* the restoration presents with mechanical complications[3].

Based on the ACP guidelines, my understanding of this statement is that patients in fixed full-arch prostheses should be visiting their dentist for an examination at least every 6 months. These patients should have professional hygiene performed on this visit as well. However, these patients should have their fixed full-arch implant prosthesis removed only if:

- The patient cannot demonstrate good hygiene at home
- It is not possible for the dental hygienist or a dentist to perform adequate hygiene with the prosthesis in place

- The patient displays peri-implantitis
- The restoration presents mechanical complications

There is clearly room here for more clinical and evidence-based research, as many questions remain. How do we define good or adequate at-home hygiene? What does adequate hygiene around a fixed full-arch prosthesis look like? Can peri-implantitis be diagnosed in all cases without removing a fixed full-arch implant prosthesis? Can a dentist or dental hygienist fully evaluate whether a prosthesis or the underlying implant components have a mechanical weakness or failure unless the prosthesis is removed? These are all questions that may be answered more definitively in the future.

It is important to acknowledge that fixed full-arch implant prostheses are not all the same. Different implant models and methods (e.g., FP1, FP2, FP3) are used, and there is wide variation in how the implants engage with the prostheses. (None of this is discussed in the recommendations and guidelines cited above.) Other factors to consider include the relatively recent introduction and adoption of MUAs in full- and partial-arch rehabilitation on dental implants and the differences in the maintenance needs for a prosthesis on a fixture that is designed for ease of removal versus one that is direct-to-implant.

Following is a summary of four points I reflected on and that informed my thinking during the period I was developing a hygiene and maintenance protocol for fixed full-arch implant patients in my practice.

1. Design and materials of the prosthesis

In the past, many types of prosthesis designs were considered acceptable. I readily concede that several of the prostheses my lab designed with me years ago resembled dentures attached to implants. Today we know that prostheses with concave intaglio surfaces, flanges, roughened areas, and inadequate space between the intaglio of the prosthesis and the edentulous ridge are not conducive to excellent soft tissue health and easy home care.

Whereas dentures and overdentures can be removed by patients to have all surfaces cleaned thoroughly, fixed full-arch implant prosthetics cannot. It is obvious to any clinician who has removed more than a few of these prostheses that all surfaces do not receive equal attention when it comes to patient home care. The intaglio surface—the area closest in proximity to the patient's implants—is generally at greatest risk of accumulating plaque, tartar, and biofilm. It seems logical that if the design of the patient's prosthesis is not ideal, it might need to be evaluated and cleaned at some frequency.

In terms of material, acrylic denture material wrapped over titanium, and even cobalt-chrome, was used in early designs for fixed full-arch implant prostheses. This style of prosthesis is still available and in use today. Recently, newer milled and printed polymethylmethacrylate (PMMA) has become available as well. Even with ideal designs, these acrylic materials accumulate stains and odors and absorb contaminants and bacteria[4]. If a patient's prosthesis was fabricated from acrylic or even milled/printed PMMA, it may be more likely to harbor bacteria. This might be another consideration for removal at hygiene visits.

2. Dental implants and abutments

When implants have been placed too close together, patients and hygienists may have trouble cleaning between them without removing the prosthesis. This is more commonly seen in cases where implants were placed in a manual or free-handed approach and that were not prosthetically driven.

Before the widespread use of MUAs, clinicians and labs would often design prosthetics that were direct-to-implant—that is, the substructures would engage the implants without the use of MUA abutments. In such a design, the abutment screws that engage the implant must be removed every time the prosthesis is removed, and this can negatively affect the implants. Abutment screws are torqued with significantly more force than MUA prosthetic screws and are not designed to be removed multiple times. Broken implant abutment screws are more complicated to manage than damaged MUA prosthetic screws, and the latter are much easier to replace. When an abutment is repeatedly removed from an implant, as required in a direct-to-implant connection, there is injury to the peri-implant mucosa. Over time, this can cause problems at the implant-abutment interface. When a prosthesis is supported by MUAs, however, the MUA prosthetic screws are easily removed and replaced, and there is considerably less risk of damaging the dental implant or replacing implant-specific abutment screws.

Nevertheless, clinicians sometimes hesitate to change MUA prosthetic screws because of the expense, but if patients are informed ahead of time that this is part of the maintenance of their prosthesis, they are more accepting of the process. Ultimately it hinges on patient expectations.

Manufacturers of implant systems usually offer guidance on how many times an MUA prosthetic screw can be torqued before it needs to be replaced. The danger of not replacing the screws on a consistent or planned basis is that loose or fractured screws can create complications and unstable conditions within the system. Over time, prosthetic screws may also become more easily deformed, and the head may become stripped.

3. Patient home care

Patients with poor dexterity, disabilities, poor compliance, or other limitations may not be able to provide "adequate" home care for themselves. In my practice, adequate home care means that the patient can remove the debris and biofilm around their implant abutments, appliance, and the surrounding tissues, leaving little or no presence of peri-mucositis or peri-implantitis. In my opinion, assessing this is virtually impossible unless a patient's prosthesis is removed at regular intervals.

4. Access for professional in-office maintenance

I am deeply skeptical of the idea that a dental hygienist can adequately remove all tartar, debris, and biofilm and probe around dental implant abutments under a fixed full-arch prosthesis without removing it. This is especially true when it comes to probing, which is another topic under debate. I have my own opinions about probing around dental implants and abutments, and I recommend that others read through the literature and make their own determinations. (If you decide to implement implant probing in your maintenance protocol, be aware that it is not recommended until at least 1 year postloading to avoid the risk of introducing pathogens through the perimucosal seal.)

Risk assessment for dental implants

A tool to assess the risk of peri-implantitis was developed by a research group led by Dr. Miguel de Araújo Nobre and validated in 2019[5]. This assessment tool, which can be accessed free of charge on the Foundation for Oral Rehabilitation (FOR) website (http://for.org), helps clinicians predict the risk of peri-implant pathology in their patients for up to 5 years after surgery and offers recommendations for recall regimens. I have used this tool to develop recall plans for hygiene and maintenance for my patients and to help them understand any potential risks they should be aware of. Having a means of objective assessment can be helpful for both you and your patients.

Hygiene and maintenance contract for patients

It is important to obtain consent from your patients and educate them about the benefits and risks of treatment before it commences. It is equally important to help them understand the value of maintaining their fixed full-arch implant prostheses and the potential problems that may result if they do not. Patients should have a clear picture of what to expect after they have gone through their surgical and prosthetic experiences. Part of these expectations will depend on how their prosthesis and implants are maintained.

When I explain hygiene and maintenance to our patients undergoing fixed full-arch implant rehabilitation, I try to use analogies they can relate to. Our patients invest in many products that require routine maintenance to operate at their best—vehicles, major appliances, heating and air conditioning systems, and so forth—and those products last longer and work better when they are properly maintained. Most people understand that their house is a significant investment and that its foundation—though not something they dwell on unless a problem arises—is one of the keys to its longevity. By having a customized hygiene and maintenance program designed for patients, we can help them avoid many of the pitfalls they might encounter if their dental foundation was ignored.

To create expectations early on, we developed a hygiene and maintenance "contract" for patients to read and sign. The contract gives them an understanding of what is expected on their part and what we will provide to help them get as much value out of their investment as possible. The implementation of this contract has helped us build a thriving hygiene department. It gives our patients an understanding of why hygiene and maintenance are important and how it works.

Please note that this contract is not a legal document nor intended to bind patients to any suggested recommendations.

Hygiene and Maintenance Program for Patients with Implant-Supported Full-Arch Prosthesis

Patient Name ____ Date _________________

Long-term implant success comes from the interaction of many variables, one of which focuses on implant maintenance protocols in our hygiene department. Implant maintenance is crucial to the longevity of your dental implants and your prosthesis. The frequency of appointments recommended for you depends on your individual condition. Compliance with the following recommendations is critical to any warranty or guarantee of your prosthesis.

After conversion to your definitive prosthesis, the following care is recommended:

1. Your first maintenance visit will be 4–6 months after delivery of your prosthesis. At this appointment the dental hygienist will remove, clean, and inspect your prosthesis. The multi-unit abutments on your implants will be checked, cleaned, and decontaminated. Generally, we will remove your prosthesis every 9–12 months if you are doing well with your home care. The fee for this appointment is $ ______ per arch. *Note: If you have your own natural teeth in an opposing arch, the regular prophylaxis or periodontal maintenance fee will be assessed for that.*
2. On alternating visits, where your prosthesis is not removed, the hygienist will clean around the prosthesis, remove stains, and check for any unusual wear patterns. The doctor may or may not examine you at this visit. The fee for this appointment is $ ______ .
3. Depending on your individual needs, the doctor will recommend removal of the prosthesis and replacement of the prosthetic screws every 18–24 months. Each titanium screw has a cost of $ ______. This is done to keep your prosthesis from becoming loose over time and to prevent the implants and components from becoming damaged.
4. The doctor will come in once a year to do an exam for oral cancer as well as a general overview of your prosthesis, bite, etc. The charge for this is an exam fee.
5. Dental x-rays may be taken at your hygiene maintenance visits and a CBCT scan may also be taken every 5 years. This is to check bone levels and the overall health of the implants.
6. Strict compliance with your implant and prosthesis maintenance is important for the health and longevity of your implants and your prosthesis. It is important that you call if you sense any looseness or issues with your prosthesis.

I understand the above and that compliance with these recommendations is critical to any warranty of my dental implants, components, and prosthesis.

Patient signature ____

MAINTENANCE AND HYGIENE PROTOCOL

As discussed previously, we know there is little research and scientific evidence about recall regimens related to fixed full-arch implant dentistry. However, it has been confirmed that implant-borne fixed restorations require lifelong professional recall regimens that should be customized to each patient. In addition, the use of hygiene aids can improve your patient's and hygienist's ability to take care of their prostheses[6]. Adopting a systematic hygiene protocol for your patients with fixed full-arch implant prostheses is one of the most effective ways you can help them avoid complications with their dental implants[7].

Following is a hygiene and maintenance workflow that I developed—with the help of my hygienists and other well-respected clinicians—for patients with fixed full-arch implant prostheses fastened to MUAs[6-9]. We base much of our early individualized protocols on four identifiers in the beginning and then use the FOR risk assessment after the first year. The four identifiers are:

1. Is the patient a smoker?
2. Does the patient have a history of periodontal disease?
3. Does the patient have any systemic health/medical conditions that could create complications over time?
4. Does the patient have limited dexterity, vision, or access to care?

In our hygiene department, there are two types of visits: one in which their prosthesis/es is removed, and one in which their prosthesis/es is left in place. The steps outlined in the workflow can be followed at either appointment depending on the customized plan for the individual patient. Some of these steps are completed at each visit and some may only be necessary at alternate appointments. However, every patient who has undergone treatment based on the processes outlined in this book will have all these steps completed at least once a year.

Note: *The following workflow is intended particularly for patients that have gone through the process where their treatment has included the workflow and protocols addressed in this book. This workflow and protocol is a guideline and is not necessarily intended to cover all the scenarios for every type of prosthetic situation or design. As a dentist, it is best to review this workflow yourself and determine if you are confident having your team follow it.*
Having a hygienist complete the vast majority of the workflow is most efficient and profitable. However, you may want to make changes and customize it based on your own comfort level, guidelines set forth by your state and/or local dental licensing boards, and your hygienist's experience and training.

FIXED FULL-ARCH IMPLANT DENTISTRY WORKFLOW FOR THE HYGIENIST

A. Review the patient's medical history

Most clinicians would agree that we should be reviewing our dental patients' medical and health conditions on a routine basis. A review of your patient's medical history will be one of the factors that helps you determine the best protocol for maintenance and hygiene as well as any new risk factors that may have evolved regarding their dental implants (Fig. 10.1). Also, it may be helpful to discuss any questions or concerns the patient has at this point in the visit. It is most important to confirm that the patient is not having pain or experiencing anything abnormal with their prosthesis. Advise the dentist of any reported issues before removing the patient's prosthesis.

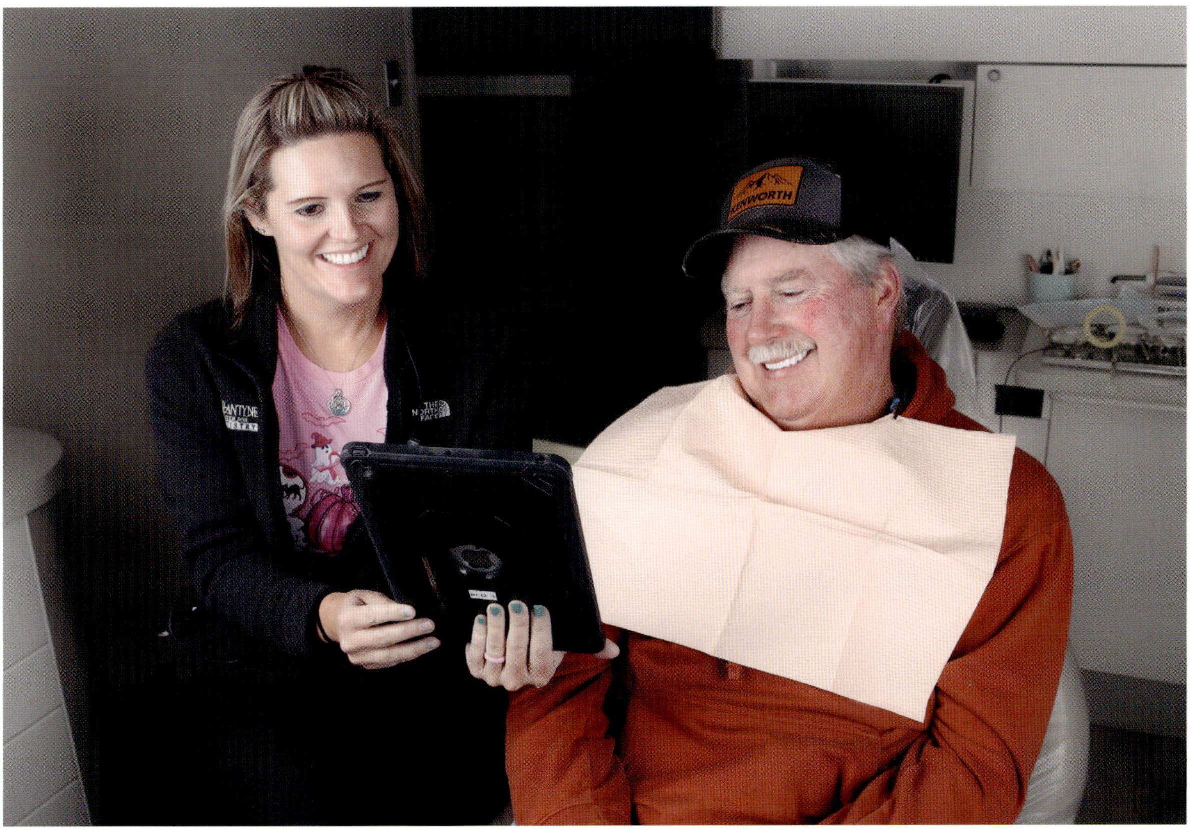

Figure 10.1 **Patient and hygienist reviewing and updating the patient's medical and health history on a handheld tablet at the beginning of the hygiene appointment.**

B. Check the occlusion and examine the nightguard for any signs of wear

Evaluating a patient's occlusion objectively with a T-Scan Novus™ (TekScan) or OccluSense® (Bausch) device may not be necessary at each hygiene and maintenance visit, but it could be helpful. At the very least, ask the patient for subjective feedback on how their bite feels. You may also want to use full-arch articulating paper to disclose any areas of contact and make note of any changes reported by the patient (Fig. 10.2). At times, it may be appropriate to have the dentist come to the operatory and examine the patient's occlusion prior to prosthesis removal.

If the patient is wearing a nightguard, examine it for wear and evaluate whether it needs to be modified, adjusted, or replaced.

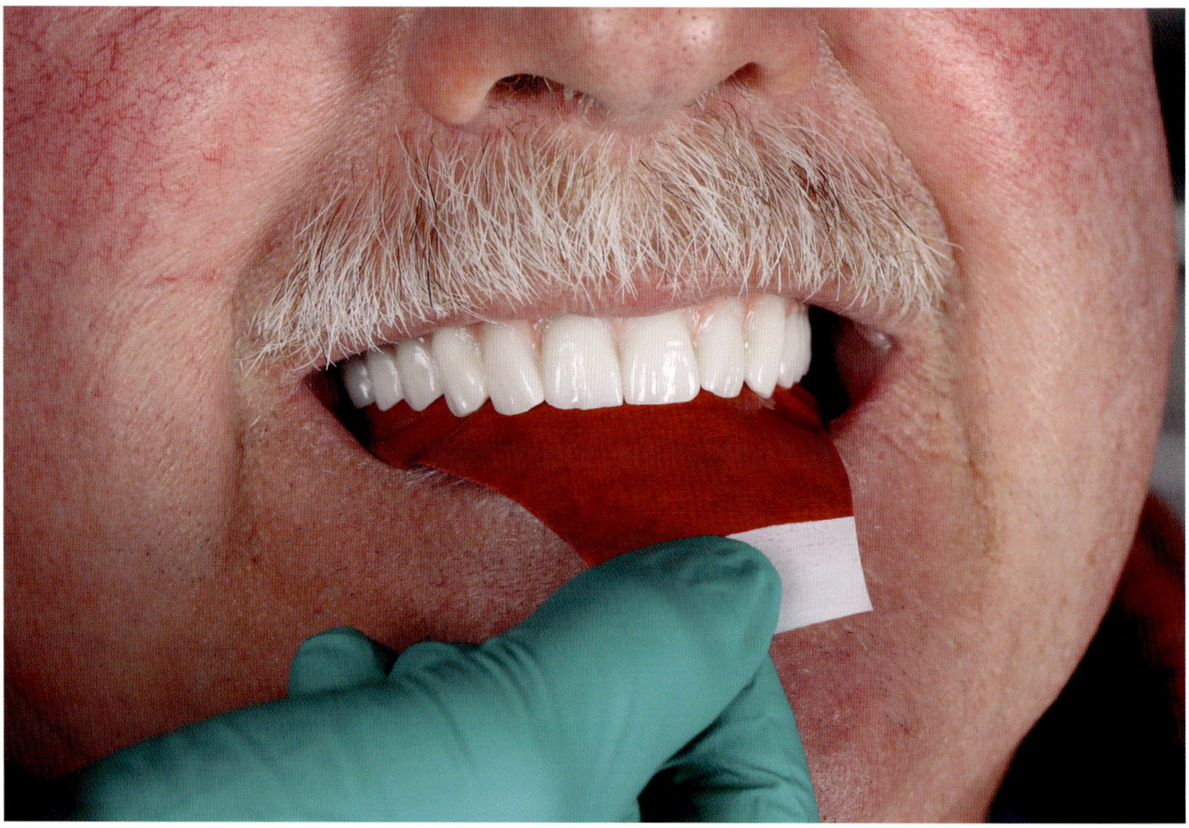

Figure 10.2 **Evaluation of patient's maxillomandibular relationship with horseshoe-shaped articulating paper.**

C. Remove the prosthesis

In most cases, you should begin by removing the screw access hole material in the prosthesis, unless the material is composite resin or some other substance that is too difficult to remove without the use of a high-speed handpiece and bur (Figs. 10.3, 10.4). For those cases, it may be appropriate to have the dentist remove the material to avoid the possibility of damaging the prosthesis or underlying structures.

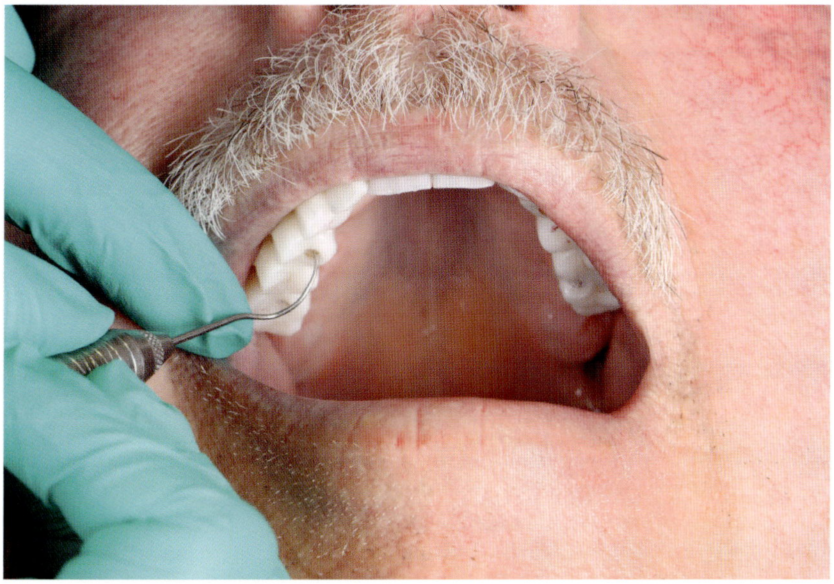

Figure 10.3 Removal of block-out material from a screw access channel with a dental explorer.

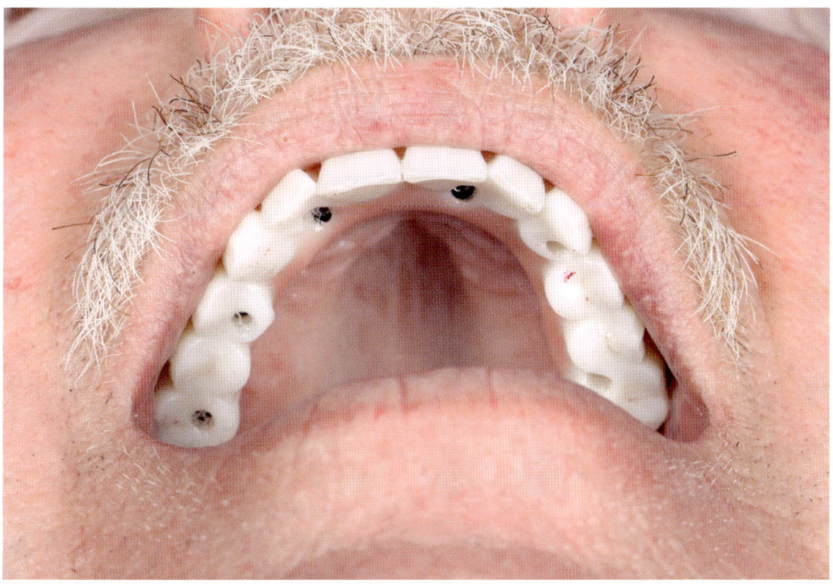

Figure 10.4 Appearance of the prosthesis with all block-out material removed from the screw access channels.

Once the screw access channels are clear, remove the prosthetic screws by turning them counterclockwise with a hand driver or torque wrench (Fig. 10.5). It is beneficial to remove all the screws in the prosthesis and place them in a small cup or dappen dish filled with an antimicrobial rinse[9] (Fig. 10.6a). We prefer to soak the prosthetic screws in OraCare® Health Rinse (Fig. 10.6b). If you have trouble removing a screw from the access channel, make sure it is completely loose and wait until after the prosthesis has been taken out of the patient's mouth to remove it. While removing the patient's prosthesis, look at the tissues and make a general assessment of the patient's home care based on what you see (Fig. 10.7).

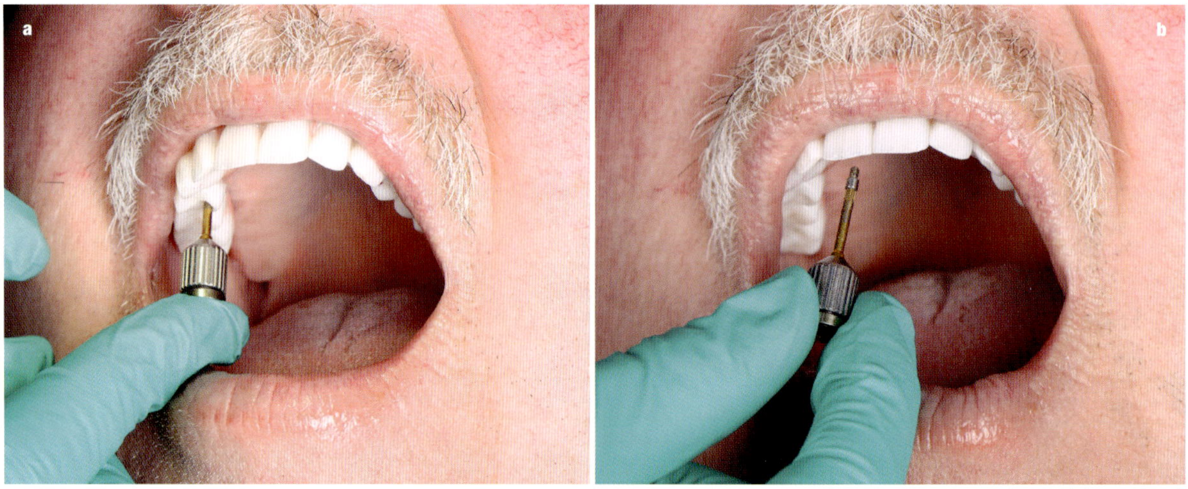

Figure 10.5 (a, b) Use of an implant driver to remove a prosthetic screw from an access channel.

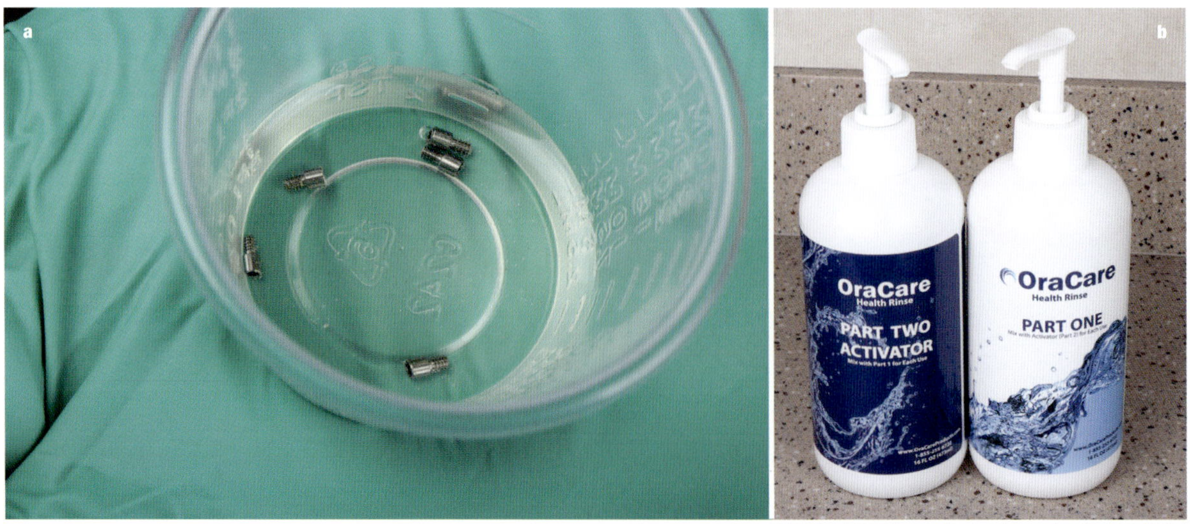

Figure 10.6 (a) Prosthetic screws placed in a dish containing (b) OraCare® chlorine dioxide health rinse.

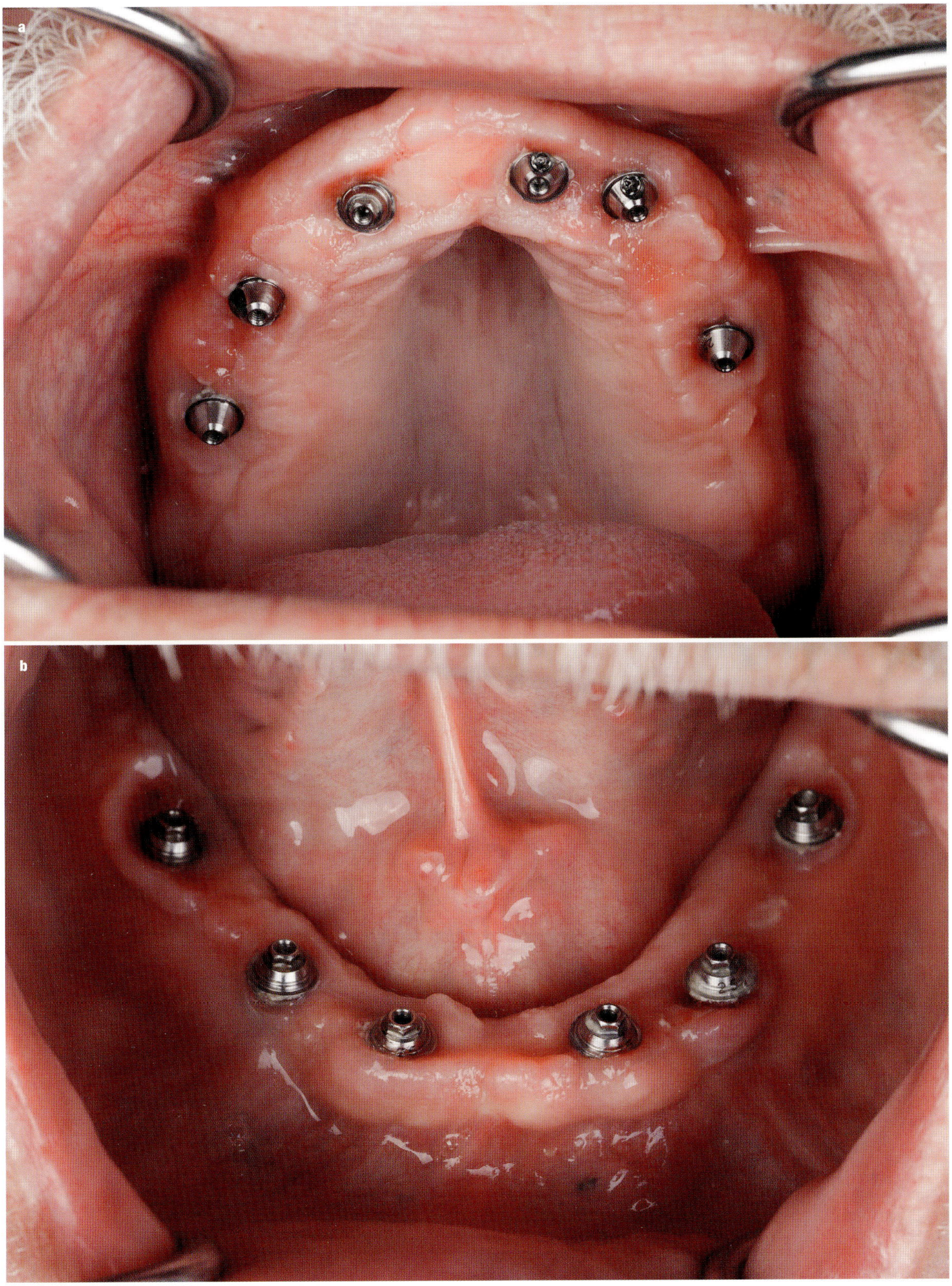

Figure 10.7 Appearance of the (a) maxillary and (b) mandibular arches after removal of the monolithic zirconia prostheses.

Once you have the screws and prosthesis removed, place the prosthesis in a zip-closure bag containing a Polident® tablet (Haleon) and tartar/stain remover and place it in an ultrasonic cleaner or shaker for 10 to 15 minutes (Figs. 10.8, 10.9). Upon removing the prosthesis, rinse the patient's mouth thoroughly to remove any loose debris and have the patient use an antimicrobial mouth rinse (such as OraCare Health Rinse) if necessary.

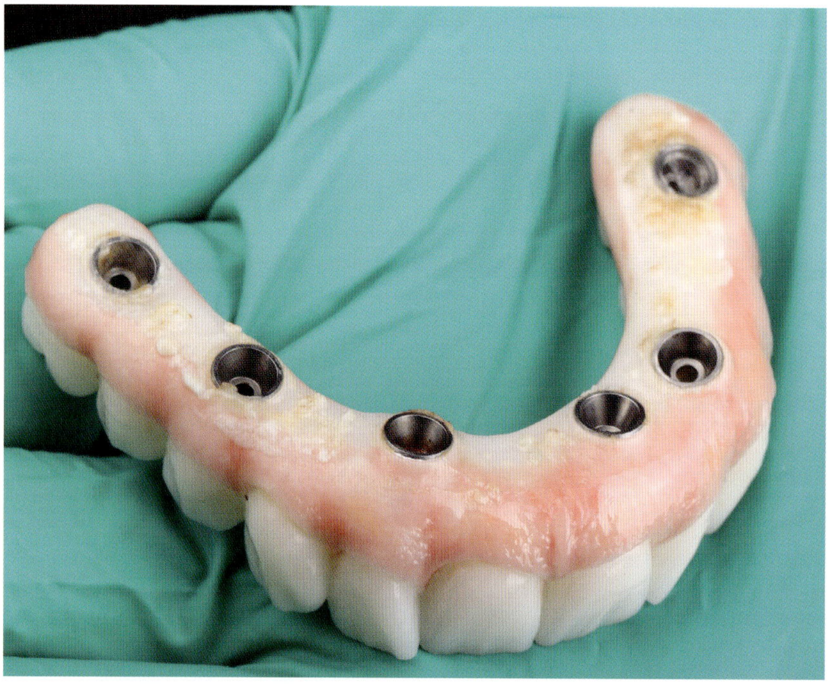

Figure 10.8 Appearance of the intaglio surface of the maxillary monolithic zirconia prosthesis after removal.

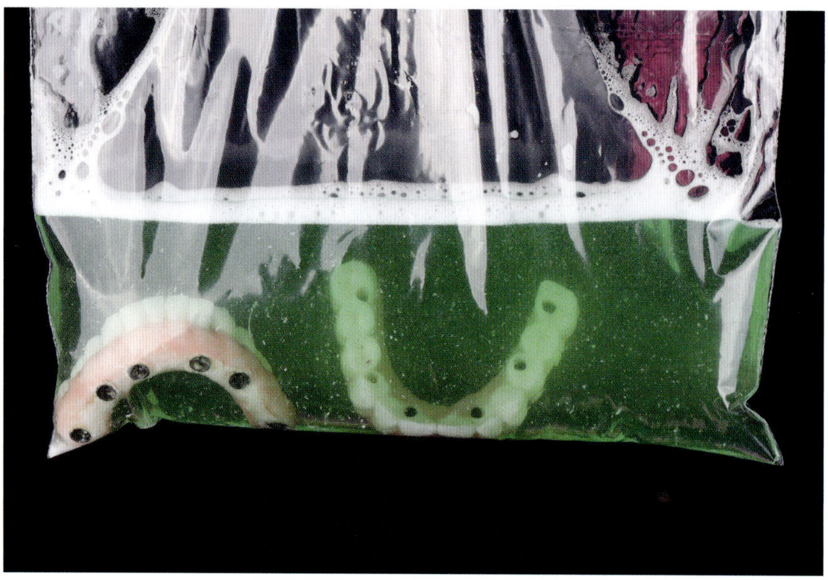

Figure 10.9 Prostheses placed in zip-closure bag containing tartar and stain remover.

D. Take radiographs of the implants and the multiunit abutments (MUAs)

After the patient's first year of wearing the prosthesis, take periapical radiographs of each implant at an angle that will reveal any bone loss around the implant or change in the position of the MUA (Fig. 10.10). In some cases, it may be easier to position the x-ray device as you would when taking a bitewing to capture the bone height around the implant collar. After the first year, these radiographs may be taken every 1 to 3 years depending on the patient's risk levels.

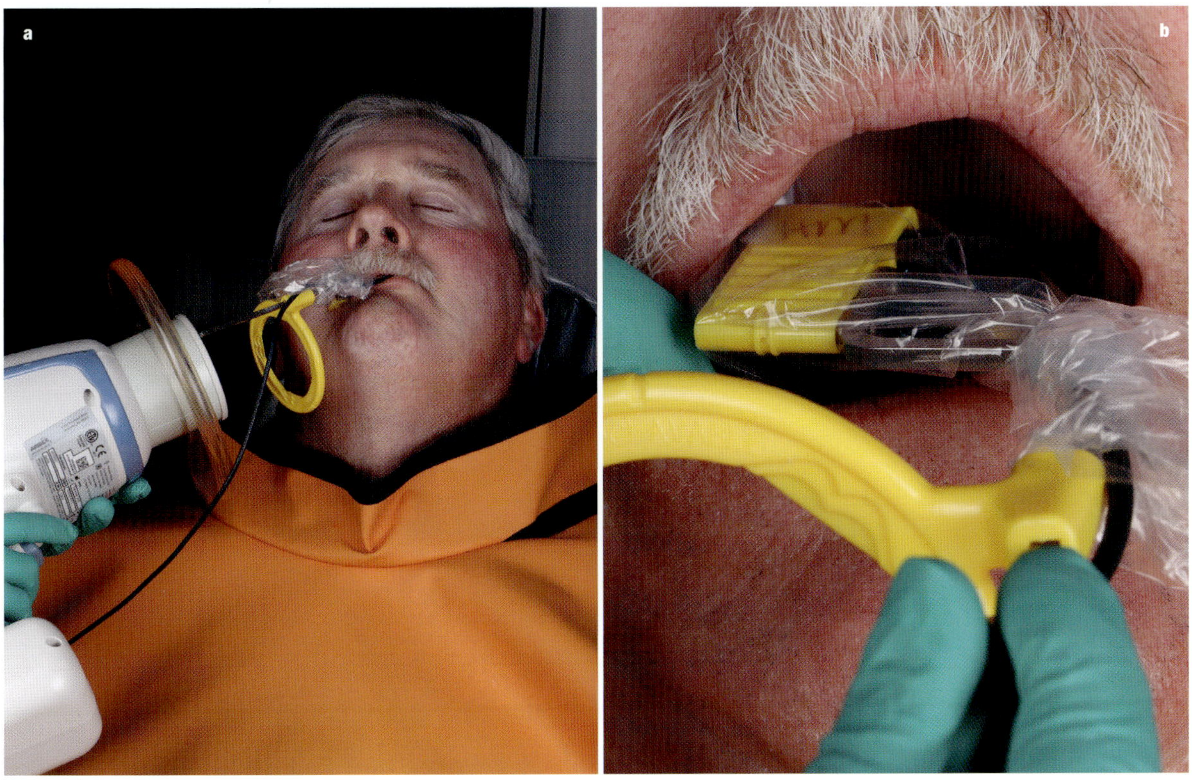

Figure 10.10 Taking a digital radiograph of dental implants using the (a) NOMAD™ Handheld X-ray System (DEXIS) with a (b) dental radiograph positioner.

E. Perform a full intraoral and extraoral examination, including cancer screening

Examine the fixed full-arch implant rehabilitation patient as you would any other dental patient, with a full intra- and extraoral exam and cancer screening. In our office, all the hygienists use magnification and headlamps, which allow for close inspection and more thorough visualization. You will want to inspect the mucosa, the edentulous areas, and the tissue around the implants and MUAs. Look for evidence of and chart:

- Inflammation and signs of swelling
- Signs of peri-implantitis and peri-mucositis
- The volume and quality of keratinized tissue around the MUAs and implants
- Tissue recession around implants and/or MUAs
- The presence of suppuration around implants when the tissues are being pressed
- Plaque and calculus around the implants and MUAs

F. Assess the stability of the MUAs and confirm osseointegration of the implants

One of the easiest ways to confirm a problem with an MUA is to take the end of a metal intraoral mirror or other metal device and gently tap on it (Fig. 10.11). If you hear a crisp audible tone, there is a good chance that the MUA and implant are stable and healthy. If the tone is dull- or hollow-sounding and/or it differs from the sound you hear from other MUAs in the arch, take note: The MUA may be loose and need to be tightened or retorqued or, in a worst-case scenario, the implant may be failing. If the patient experiences no pain during percussion, consider using the implant driver or torque wrench to tighten the abutment (Fig. 10.12). If the patient is uncomfortable at any time during percussion testing or manipulation of the MUA, you may want to have the abutment evaluated by the dentist during their examination of the patient. Assessing the osseointegration of the patient's dental implants is reasonably straightforward if all the MUAs provide a crisp tone during percussion. Use a Periotest M® (Medizintechnik Gulden) or a similar device in the manner described in previous chapters of this book to measure the stability of each implant and then record the readings in the patient's chart (Fig. 10.13). This may not be necessary every time the prosthesis is removed, but it can be helpful if any questions arise as to whether the implants are stable.

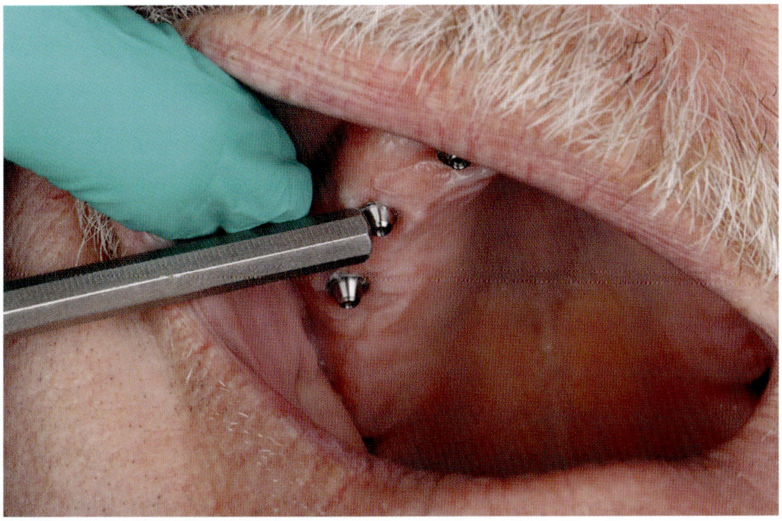

Figure 10.11 Tapping an MUA with the end of a metal intraoral mirror to assess health and stability.

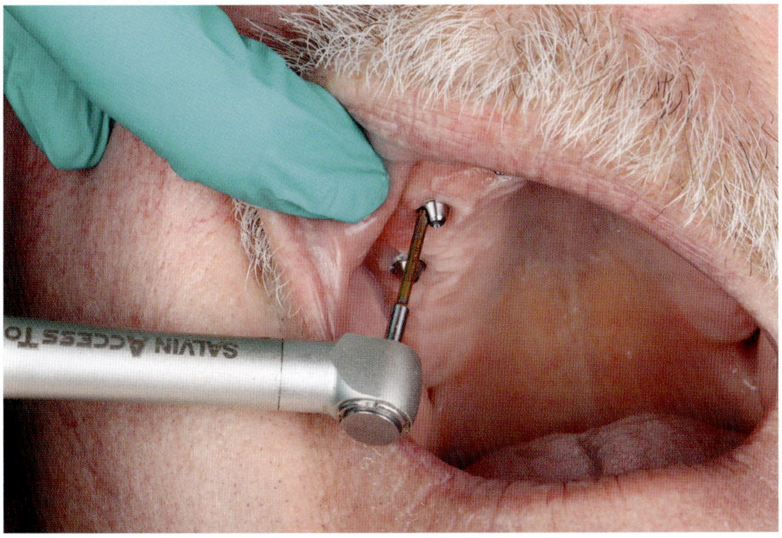

Figure 10.12 Using a torque driver to assess the torque level of an MUA.

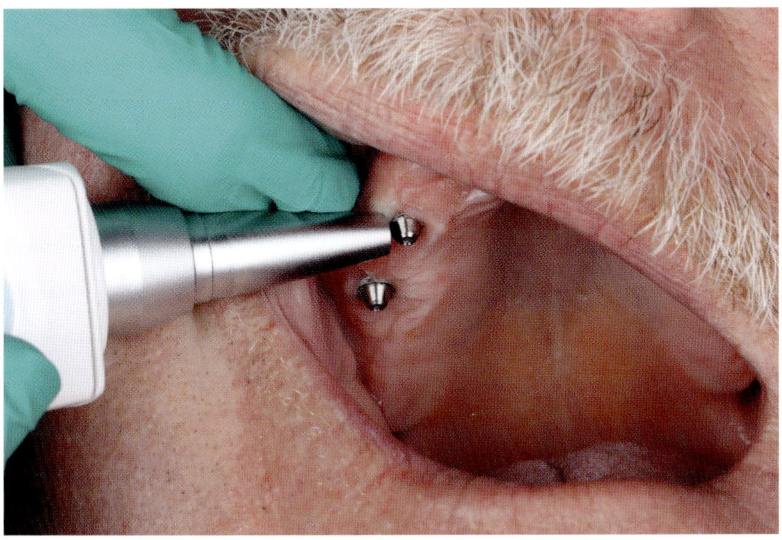

Figure 10.13 Using a Periotest M® device to confirm osseointegration of a dental implant.

G. Probe and palpate the peri-implant tissues

If you choose to probe around the MUAs, you can do so now. (You should not do so until at least 1 year after the implants have been loaded.) There are several types of dental implant probes on the market that are designed specifically for probing around dental implants[9]. Record your findings in the patient's chart and monitor for changes each time the prosthesis is removed. You should also palpate around each implant in the arch, using your fingers to gently apply pressure around the tissues of the ridge and move them in a motion toward the MUA (Fig. 10.14). Look for signs of bleeding or exudate that extrudes around the MUA and advise the doctor of any abnormal findings.

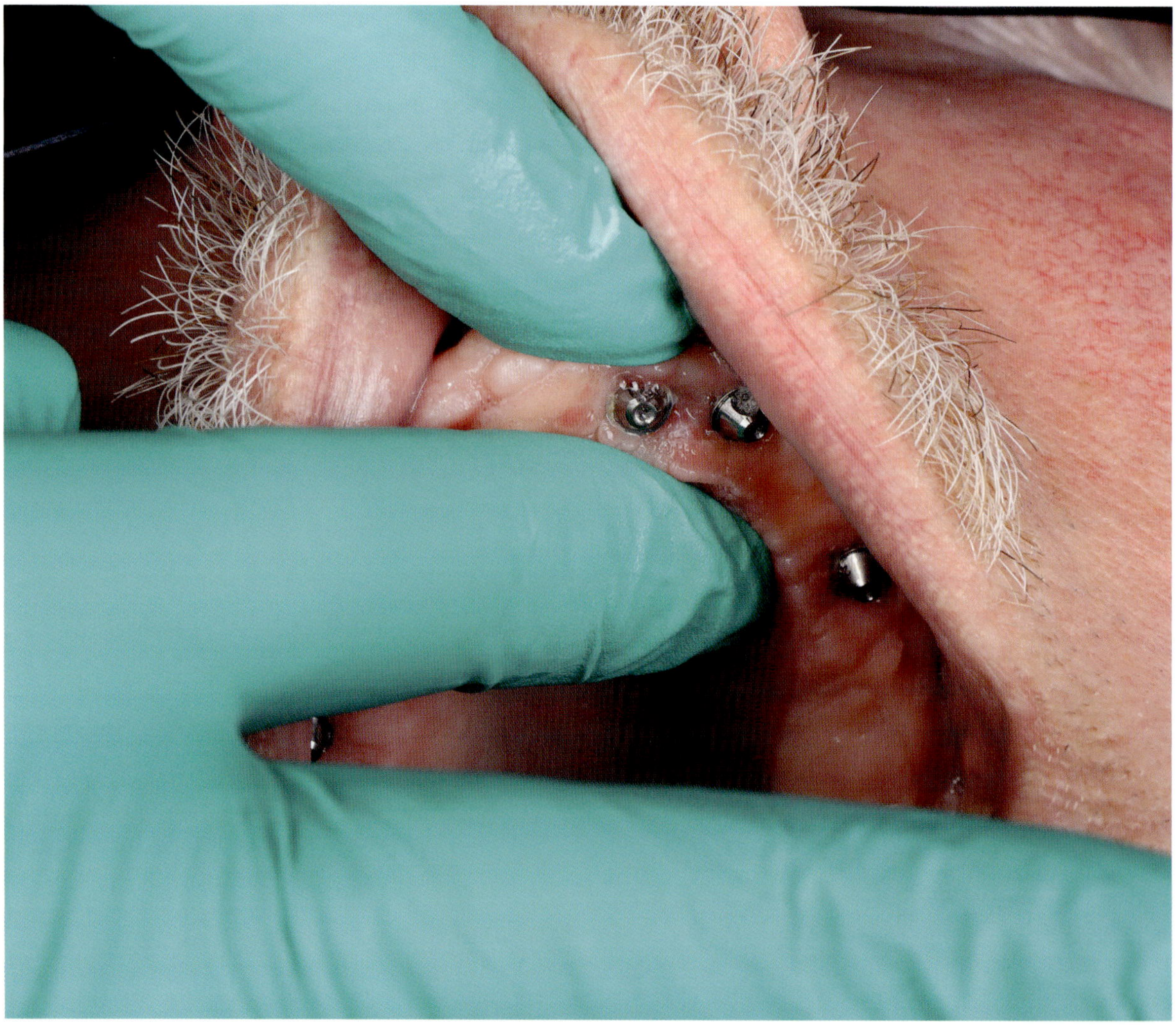

Figure 10.14 Palpating the tissue surrounding an implant for signs of bleeding or exudate.

H. Perform guided biofilm therapy

Guided biofilm therapy (GBT) is a clinical treatment protocol introduced in 2019 by the Swiss company Electro Medical Systems (EMS) to remove biofilm and plaque around teeth and implant structures. In this protocol, a disclosing agent is used to make biofilm visible, and plaque and stains are then removed with an air abrasive powder[10]. The treatment may also require the use of scaling instrumentation and ultrasonics. GBT is becoming widely accepted for dental implant maintenance. EMS manufactures and distributes several devices, instruments, and powders that can be utilized during GBT.

We have used this technique in our practice over the last few years and have found it effective for maintaining our patients' implant foundations. For more information and specific instructions on how to use GBT in your practice, see the EMS website (www.ems-dental.com).

The steps we use when applying GBT in our practice are as follows:

1. Place a lip and cheek retraction device in the patient's mouth. In our practice, we use the OptraGate® (Ivoclar Vivadent) latex-free lip and cheek retractor (Fig. 10.15).
2. Use a disclosing solution to make biofilm visible and show patient with a handheld mirror the areas where they may not be achieving adequate hygiene results with their home care.
3. Use the Airflow Max® device with Airflow Plus powder to remove supragingival and subgingival biofilm and plaque and an implant-safe ultrasonic or hand instrument to debride around the MUAs and remove any remaining calculus (Figs. 10.16, 10.17).
4. After cleaning, apply an antimicrobial varnish or gel around the MUAs (Fig. 10.18).

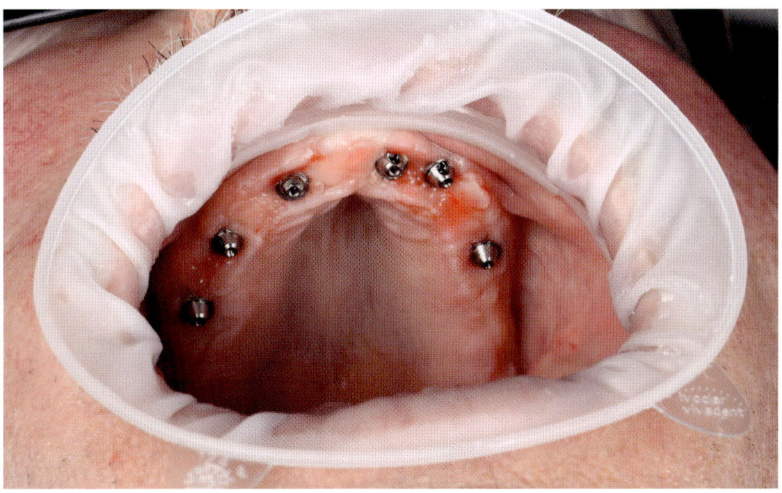

Figure 10.15 **Placement of OptraGate® latex-free cheek and lip retractor (Ivoclar Vivadent).**

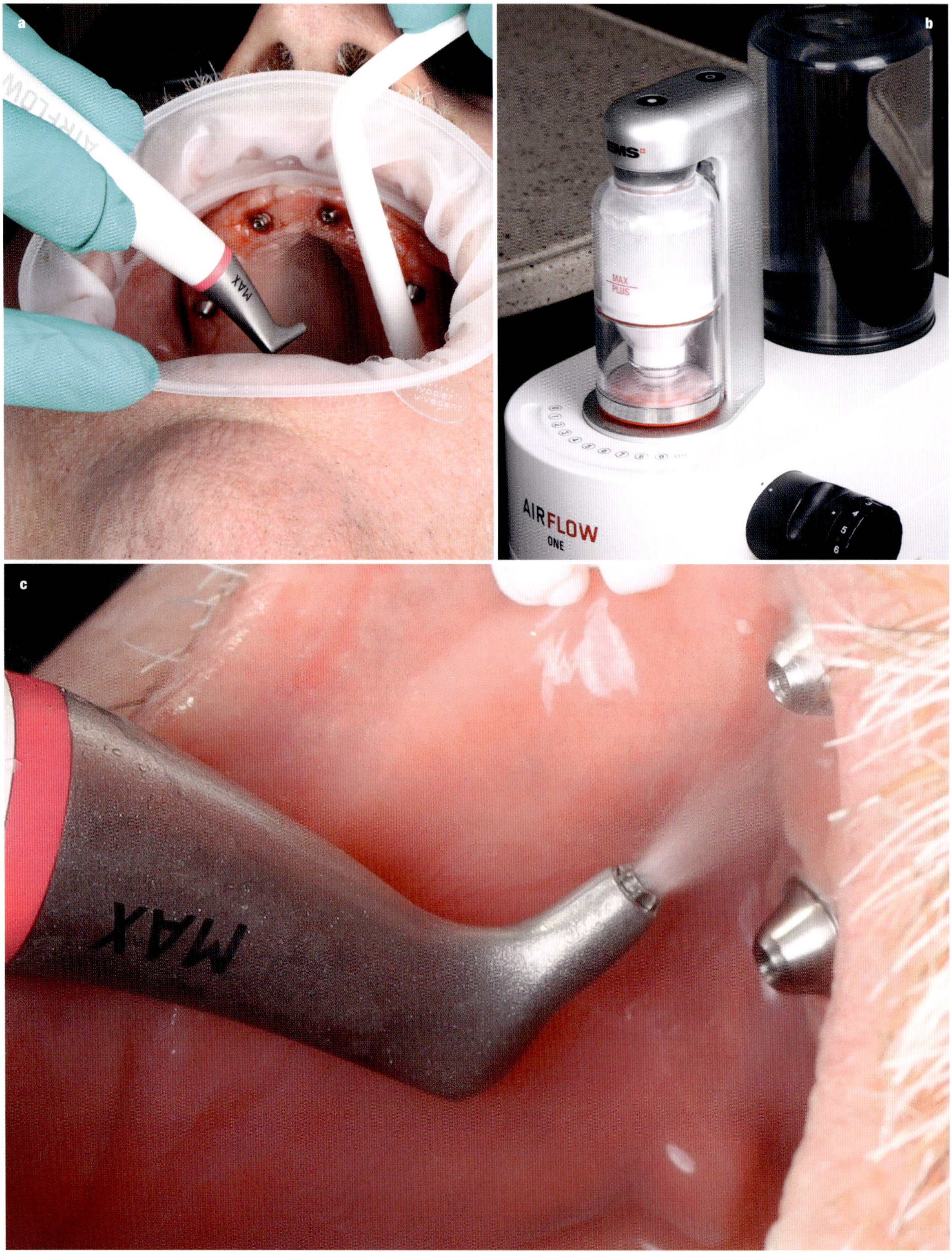

Figure 10.16 (a-c) Use of an Airflow Max® device (Electro Medical Systems) to remove supragingival plaque and biofilm from MUAs.

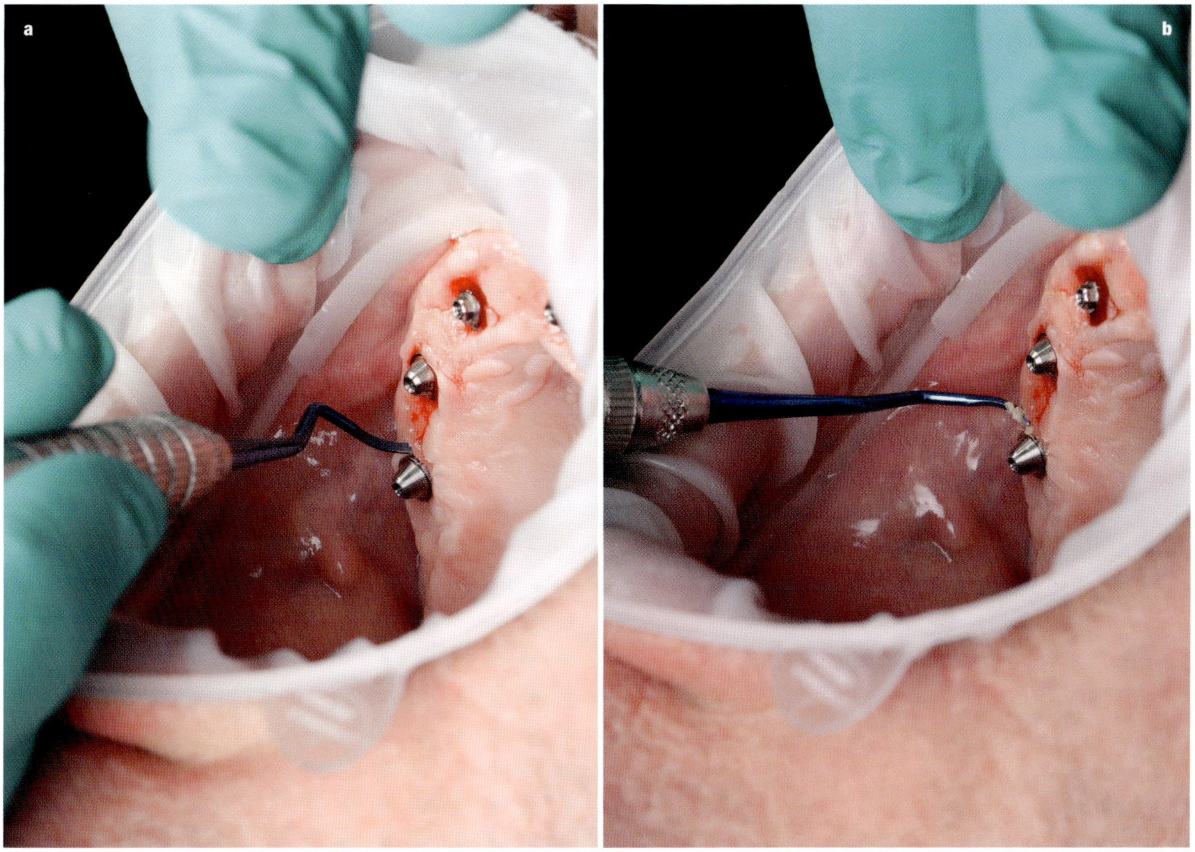

Figure 10.17 (a, b) Hand scaling to remove subgingival debris.

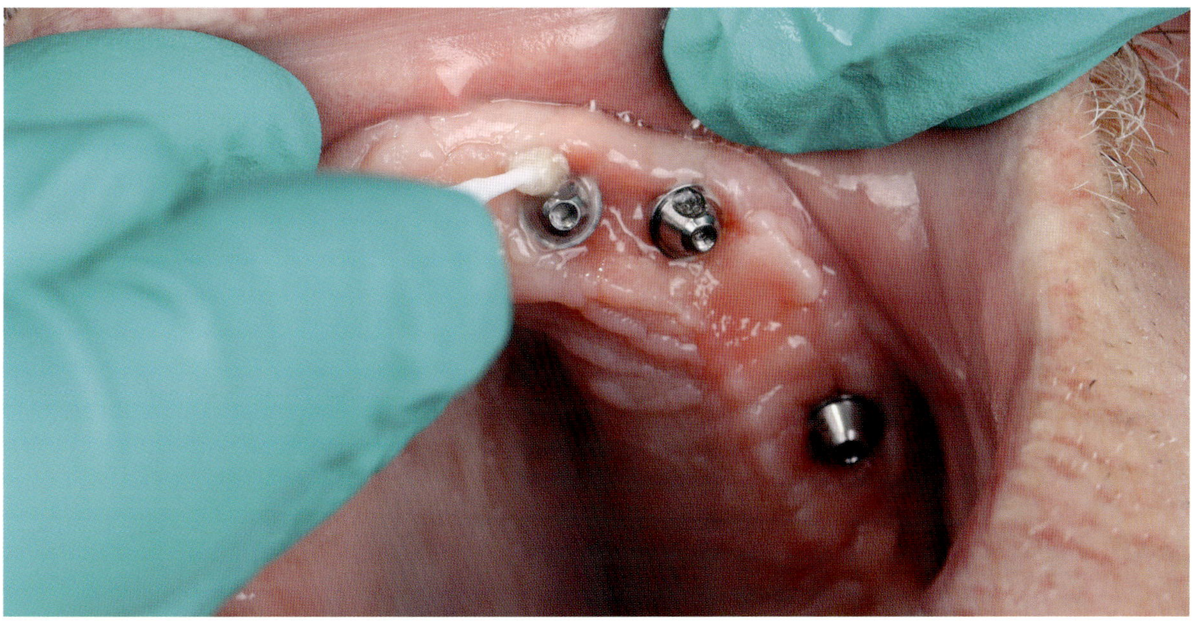

Figure 10.18 Application of antimicrobial varnish around an MUA.

I. Inspect and clean the prosthesis

Once the foundation for the prosthesis is free of debris, plaque, tartar, and biofilm, retrieve the patient's prosthesis from the ultrasonic and examine it carefully. Check for any loose parts, such as the titanium bases on the intaglio surface of the prosthesis, using an explorer or hand scaler. Also, check the screw access channels for any MUA screws and either remove them or make a note of them to avoid creating a future "second screw" phenomenon. Inspect the prosthesis for any cracks or craze lines, especially near the cantilevers of the prosthesis, and note any wear that may be present.

Some materials used in the fabrication of fixed full-arch implant prostheses are more susceptible to staining, plaque, and tartar accumulation. Prostheses made from PMMA can be more difficult to clean than prostheses fabricated from zirconia. Use a denture brush to remove loose debris from the prosthesis and carefully and gently remove any harder material with hand or ultrasonic scalers that are safe to use on the material (Fig. 10.19). Be sure to do this over a surface that is forgiving in case you accidentally drop the prosthesis. Although these prostheses are designed to be strong and resist breakage and fracture, they can be damaged if dropped on a hard floor or countertop. Finish by cleansing the prosthesis in an antimicrobial rinse.

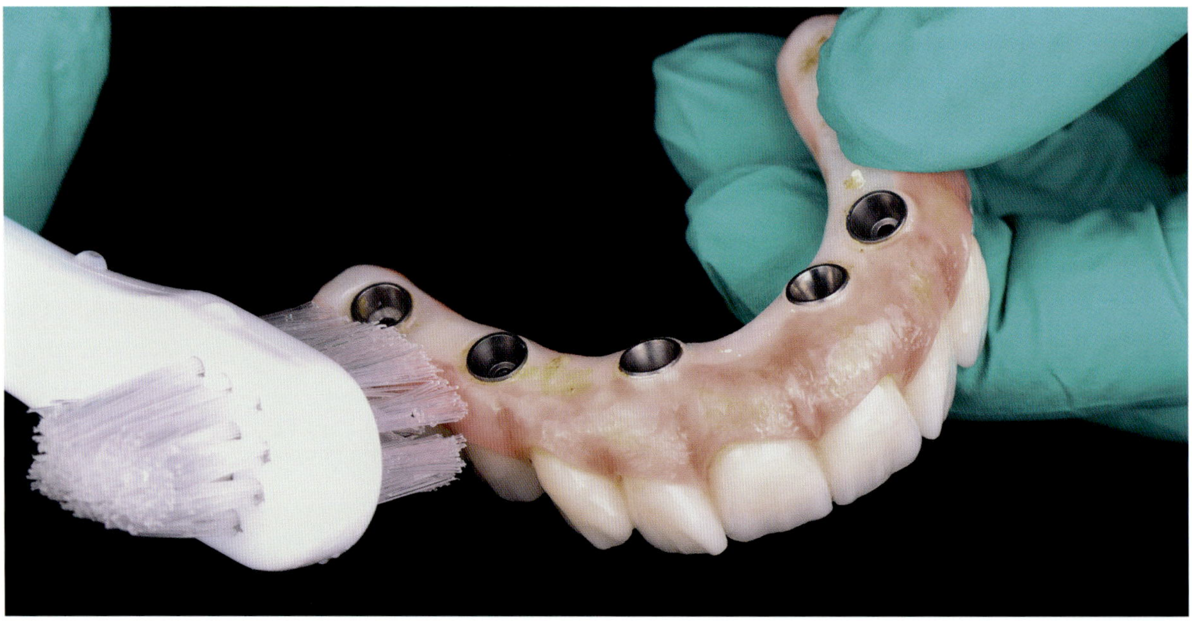

Figure 10.19 **Use of a denture brush to remove loose debris from a maxillary monolithic zirconia prosthesis.**

J. Notify the doctor that the patient is ready to be examined (alternate visits only)

Once the prosthesis and the patient's intraoral fixtures are cleaned, the dentist should be notified, and he or she should perform a periodic exam. In our practice, this may only occur on visits when the prosthesis is removed and/or at least once per year. However, if the patient is experiencing any issues or there are findings that compel you to have the dentist see them, do not hesitate to ask the dentist to do so. I prefer to visit with patients briefly before their hygiene appointment begins, when their prosthesis is still in place, and then return for the exam after it has been removed. Patients generally feel more comfortable having conversations with their smile in place (Fig. 10.20a).

During the dentist's examination, share your findings and notes with them, including a synopsis of any changes in the patient's medical history. The dentist may repeat the oral cancer screening and examine the same areas you did during your examination (Fig. 10.20b). Once the dentist finishes, make sure to note in the chart a clear diagnosis of any problems that may exist and any recommendations that were made. You may also remove the OptraGate or other retraction devices at this time.

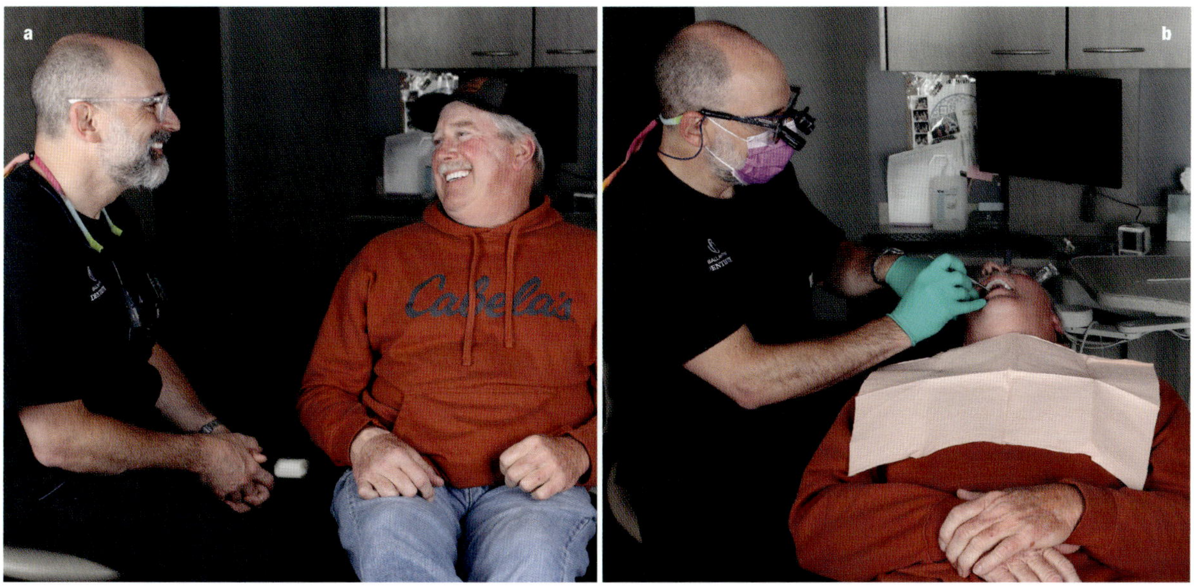

Figure 10.20 **The author (a) visiting with the patient before beginning (b) the hygiene examination.**

K. Replace the prosthesis

Replacing the patient's prosthesis is essentially the reverse of removing it. You should keep track of how many times the prosthesis has been removed and whether the MUA screws have been replaced. Implant systems vary regarding the number of times the MUA screws can be torqued before they need to be replaced and the amount of torque that should be applied to the screw. After this determination has been made, you can place the prosthesis back in the mouth over the MUAs (Fig. 10.21). Begin replacing the prosthetic screws into the screw access channels one at a time, confirming that there is no screw already in the access channel (Fig. 10.22a). The screws should go in passively and without resistance. Following a cross-arch pattern (rather than moving along the arch), lightly hand-tighten each screw. Once the prosthesis is aligned and the screws are hand tight, have the patient lightly tap their teeth together to see if it feels comfortable. If there is any area that is pinching or if they feel their occlusion has changed, remove the prosthesis and start over. Likewise, if there is any resistance or you are unable to tighten the screws, let the dentist know immediately. It is much better to determine what is causing the problem now and avoid possible complications that could develop later. Assuming the prosthesis is comfortably in place, the patient feels their bite is acceptable, and the MUA screws are hand tight, begin torquing each screw to the manufacturer's recommended specifications (Fig. 10.22b). Do this in a cross-arch pattern just as you did when you hand-tightened the screws.

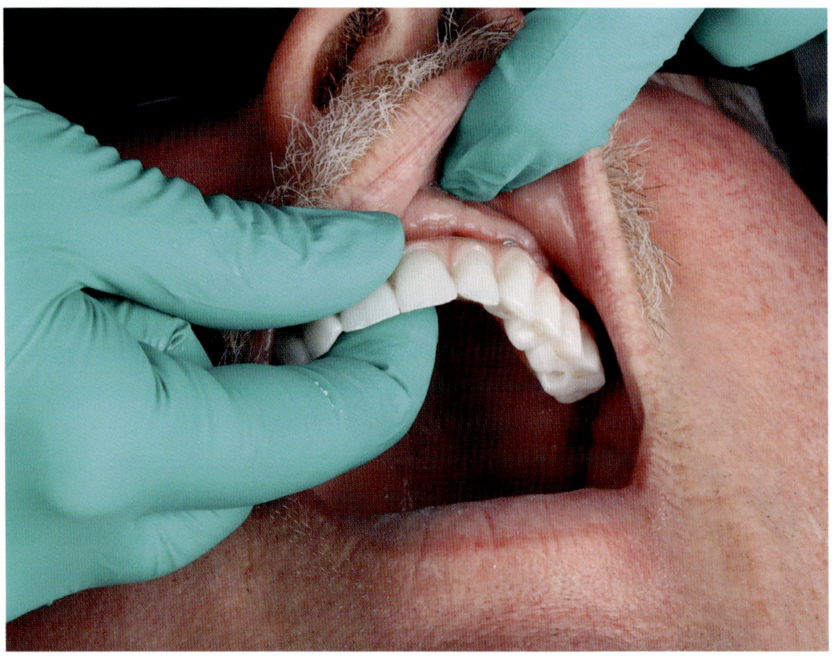

Figure 10.21 **Replacing the prosthesis in the maxillary arch.**

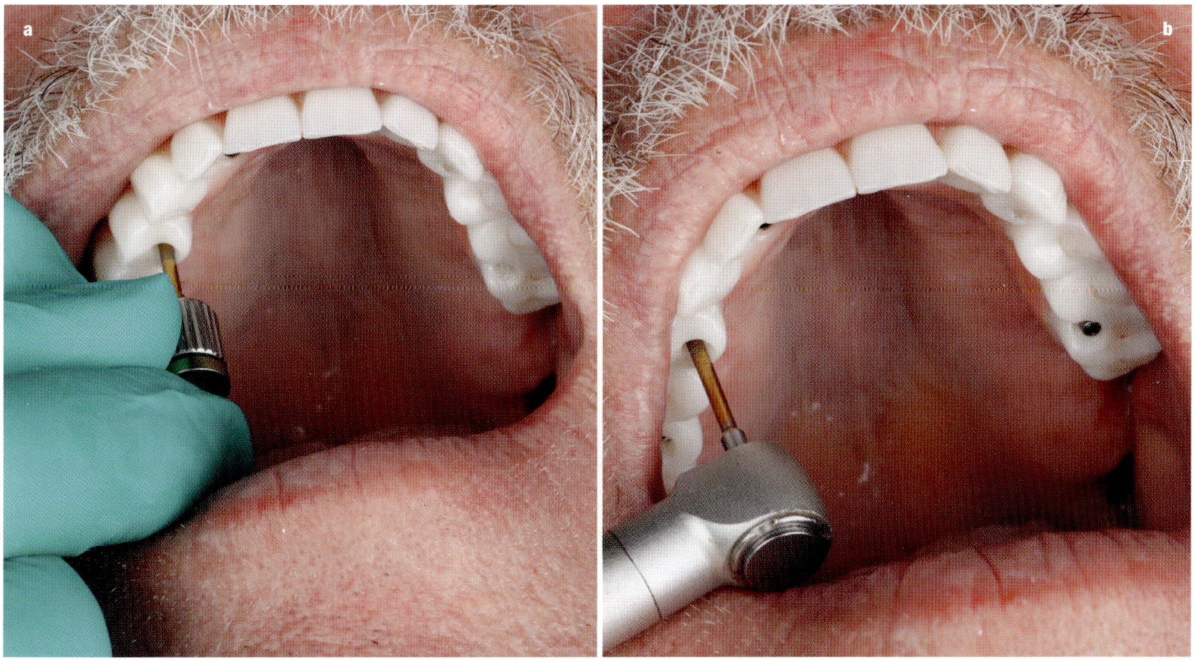

Figure 10.22 (a) Replacing a prosthetic screw through the access channel in the prosthesis and (b) torquing it to the correct value.

Filling the MUA screw access channels in the prosthesis should be done carefully and precisely. What you choose to fill these screw access channels with is up to the dentist and merits a discussion, but I recommend using a material that can be removed efficiently by the hygienist. Teflon tape with a flowable temporary composite such as Clip Flow® (VOCO GmbH) works well. Always use a Teflon-type tape or a similar material to protect the screw head before placing the final filling material. Fill the screw access channel two-thirds of the way with the Teflon tape and the remainder with the final filling product (Figs. 10.23, 10.24).

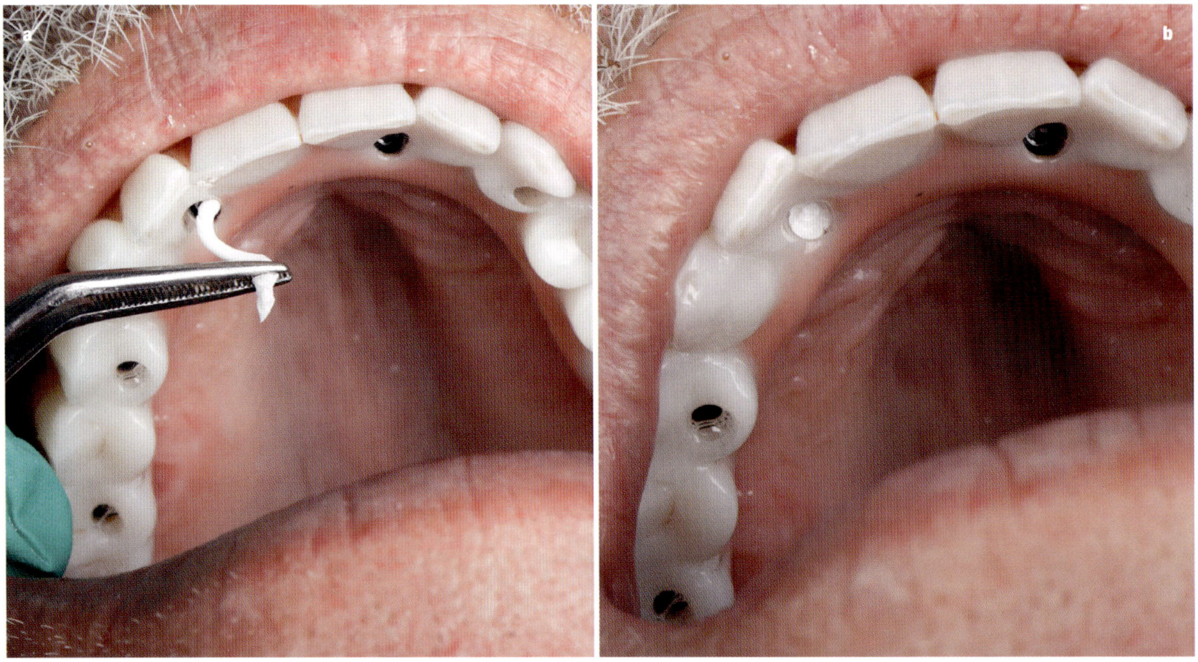

Figure 10.23 (a) Placing Teflon tape into an access channel after all the prosthetic screws have been torqued and (b) condensing it to about 2 mm below the surface of the prosthesis.

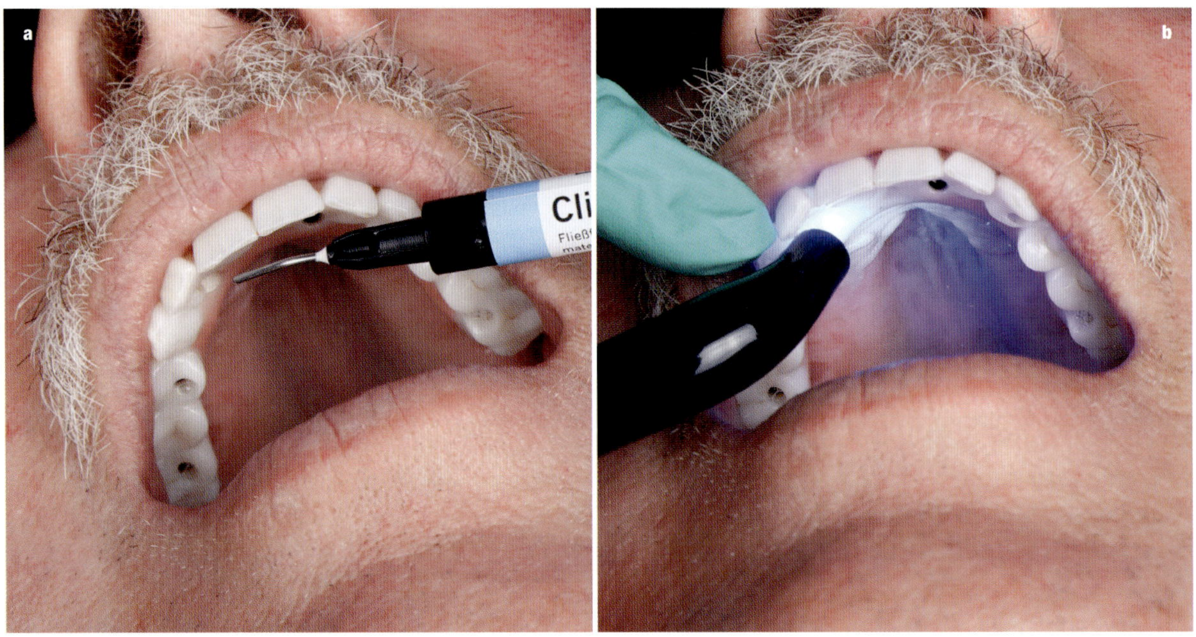

Figure 10.24 (a) Applying Clip Flow® (VOCO) over the Teflon tape to fill the remaining space and (b) using an LED dental curing light to harden it, thus finalizing the replacement of the prosthesis.

L. Give oral hygiene instructions and recommendations to the patient

Home-care instructions and recommendations for specific types of products may vary slightly from clinician to clinician and also depend on the patient. Some patients are meticulous about their oral hygiene and others are not. Our hygienists recommend the following protocol to most of our patients as the minimal requirement for keeping the tissues around their MUAs healthy.

- Brush around the implants and prosthesis at least twice daily using an electronic toothbrush (preferred) or a soft manual toothbrush.
- Use a water flosser once or twice daily, preferably in the evening before bed.
- Rinse at least twice daily for 1 minute with OraCare activated chlorine dioxide or other antimicrobial rinse. The best times to do this are after brushing and/or water flossing, in the morning before eating, and at night before bed.

Patients who are struggling with peri-implant mucositis are instructed to use rubber tip stimulators and interdental brushes around the MUAs twice a day, in the morning and before bed, in combination with the antimicrobial VEGA® Oral Care Gel (StellaLife).

M. Schedule the patient's next appointment

Reschedule your patient for another hygiene appointment after each visit. By doing this, you will at least have your patient on the schedule, which greatly reduces the chances of them not returning. The recall interval will be up to you and the dentist based on each patient's particular needs. We generally reschedule healthy patients to return in 6 months. At that appointment, a similar workflow is followed using GBT, although the prostheses are not removed and some of the other steps may not be necessary. We have adopted a hygiene recall for most healthy patients with good oral hygiene that only requires us to remove their prostheses and do all the steps in this workflow once per year.

FULL-ARCH IMPLANT REHABILITATION CASE STUDY

In 2009, a patient presented in my office complaining of pain and a complete lack of confidence in her smile. She had a highly restored maxillary dentition with many failing restorations and moderate periodontal disease. Her chief concern was her long-span fixed partial denture, which was loose. She was only interested in a fixed option that would provide long-term predictability. At that time I was working closely with an oral surgeon. After careful consideration and taking into account the amount of caries, infection, tooth mobility, failing dentistry, and other patient factors, we determined that a fixed full-arch implant prosthesis in combination with a Le Fort I procedure was the best option. The patient was presented with several options and ultimately chose to move forward with the proposed treatment (Fig. 10.25). At that point, the oral surgeon I referred to took over the patient's treatment and advised me that once the surgeries were completed and the implants were placed, I would be able to prosthetically restore the case.

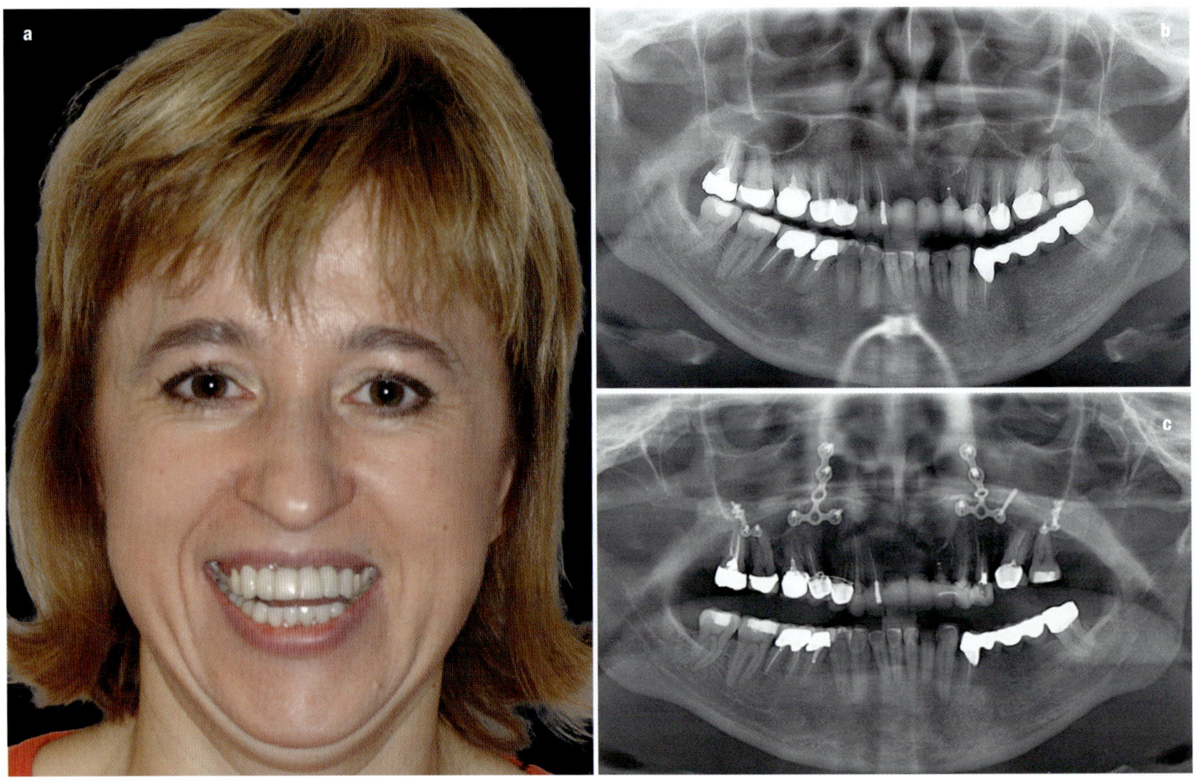

Figure 10.25 (a) Preoperative portrait photo and (b) panoramic radiograph of the patient at the initial visit; (c) Postoperative panoramic radiograph of the patient after a Le Fort I procedure.

The patient returned to my office after her surgeries, having been in an interim prosthesis for quite some time. I began the arduous task of working with the lab to develop a definitive fixed full-arch implant prosthesis, which took several months and 8 to 10 appointments. When it was finally completed, the prosthesis provided an acceptable esthetic result (Figs. 10.26, 10.27).

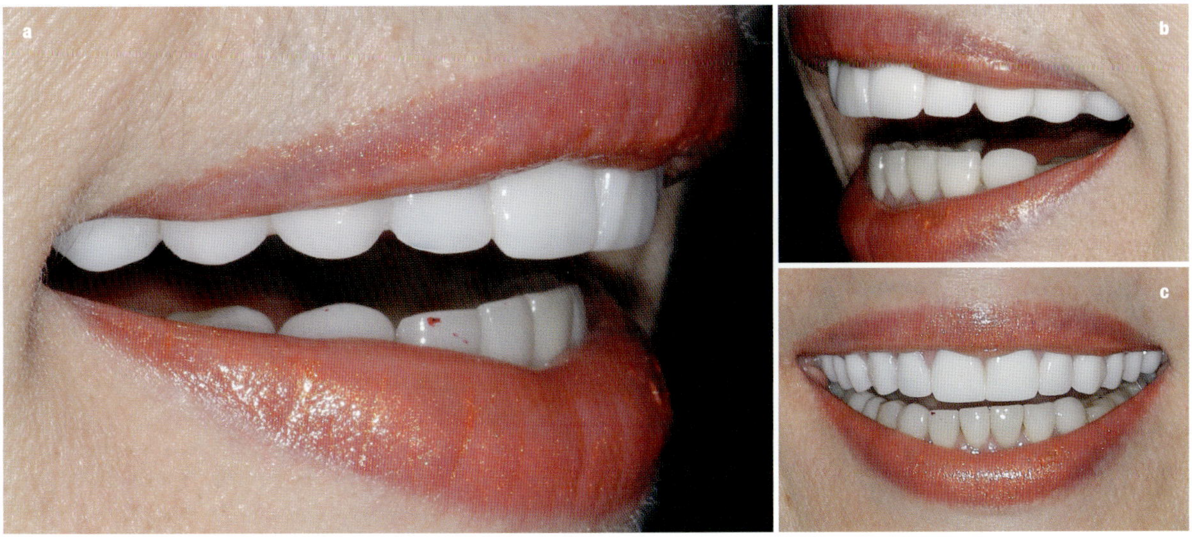

Figure 10.26 (a-c) Postoperative close-up photos of patient smiling from various angles. The definitive prosthesis is a traditional full-arch acrylic hybrid prosthesis with a titanium substructure.

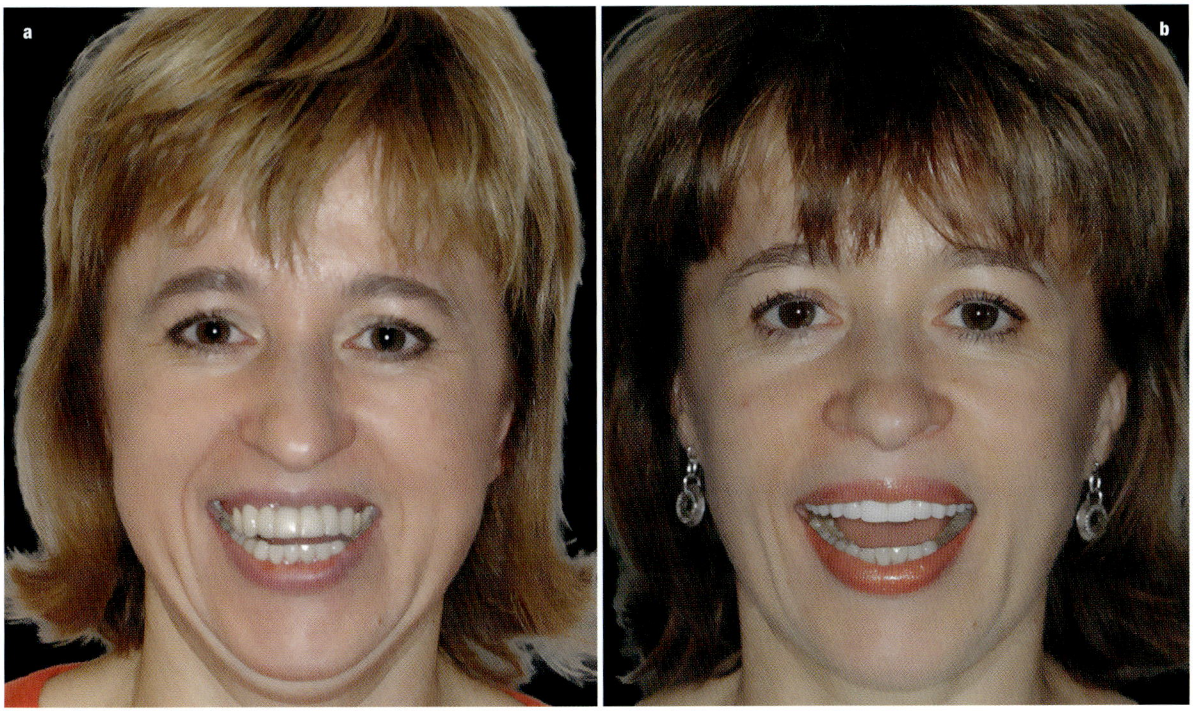

Figure 10.27 Portrait photos of the patient (a) before and (b) after treatment.

The patient subsequently moved to Europe, and I lost track of her for many years. Recently, she reappeared in our practice complaining of some mild discomfort under the prosthesis as well as noticeable wear and staining. While overseas, she had sporadic dental care but did have the prosthesis removed once. Her home care was better than average and she was doing her best to keep the prosthesis and surrounding tissues clean. I examined the patient and took a CBCT to establish the new baseline (Fig. 10.28).

After removing the prosthesis, I found—to my disappointment—the conditions shown in Figures 10.29-10.31. Note that the prosthesis has considerable wear and was not designed to be easily cleaned by the patient. The less-than-hygienic design is my fault and reveals the lack of knowledge and understanding I and my dental lab had at the time it was fabricated.

Besides the less-than-satisfactory results I achieved prosthetically, the tissues under the prosthesis were not in spectacular condition either. Purulence was not present, but there was considerable peri-mucositis and peri-implantitis as well as notable tissue hypertrophy. Each implant was tested for stability and osseointegration. Fortunately, all the implants were still osseointegrated and, despite the less-than-favorable condition of the tissues, we decided to treat the patient's peri-implant disease and see if we could salvage all the implants.

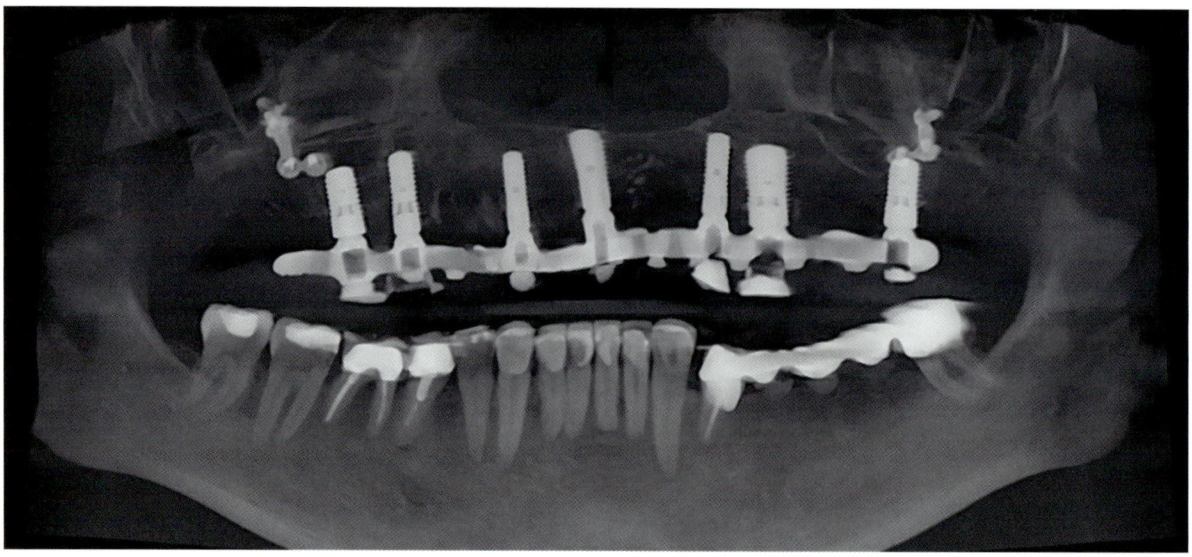

Figure 10.28 **CBCT scan 11 years after completion of treatment.**

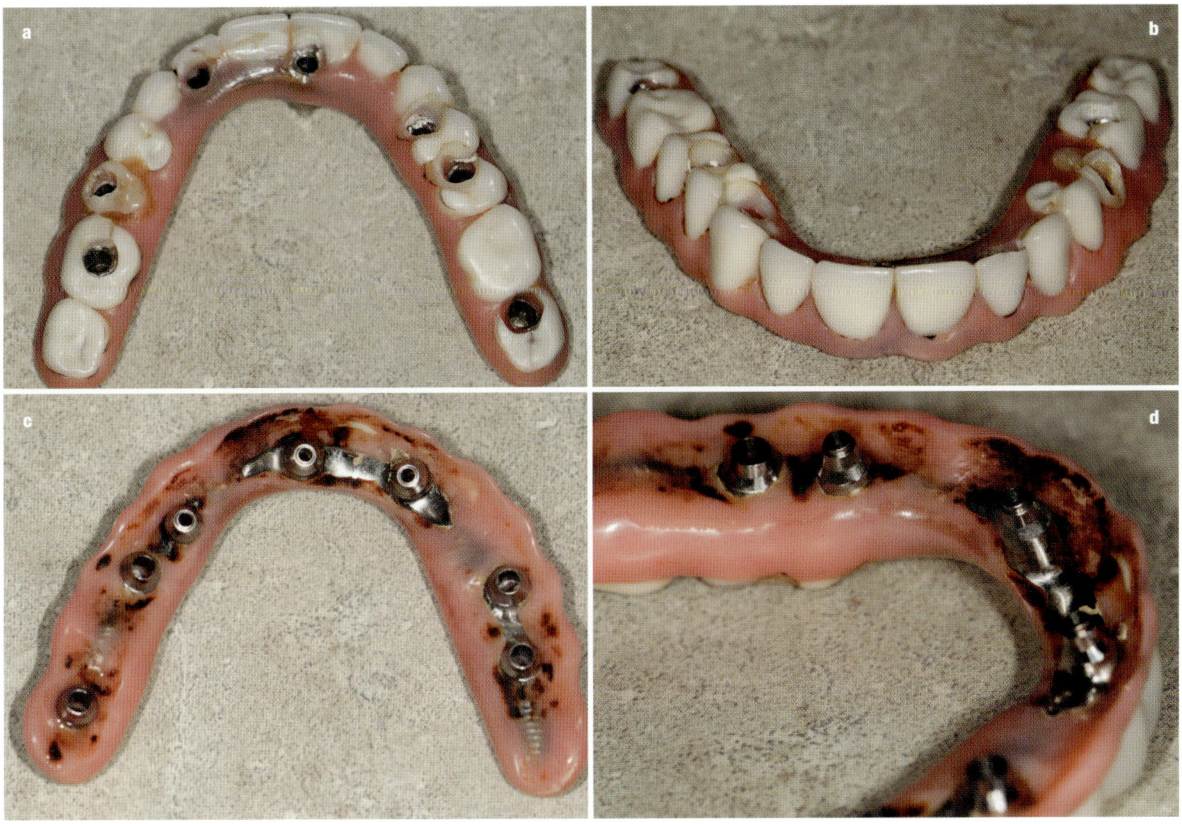

Figure 10.29 Appearance of the maxillary prosthesis 11 years after completion of treatment: (a, b) Antagonist surface; (c, d) Intaglio surface exhibiting significant stain. Note the buccal flange and nonhygienic contours.

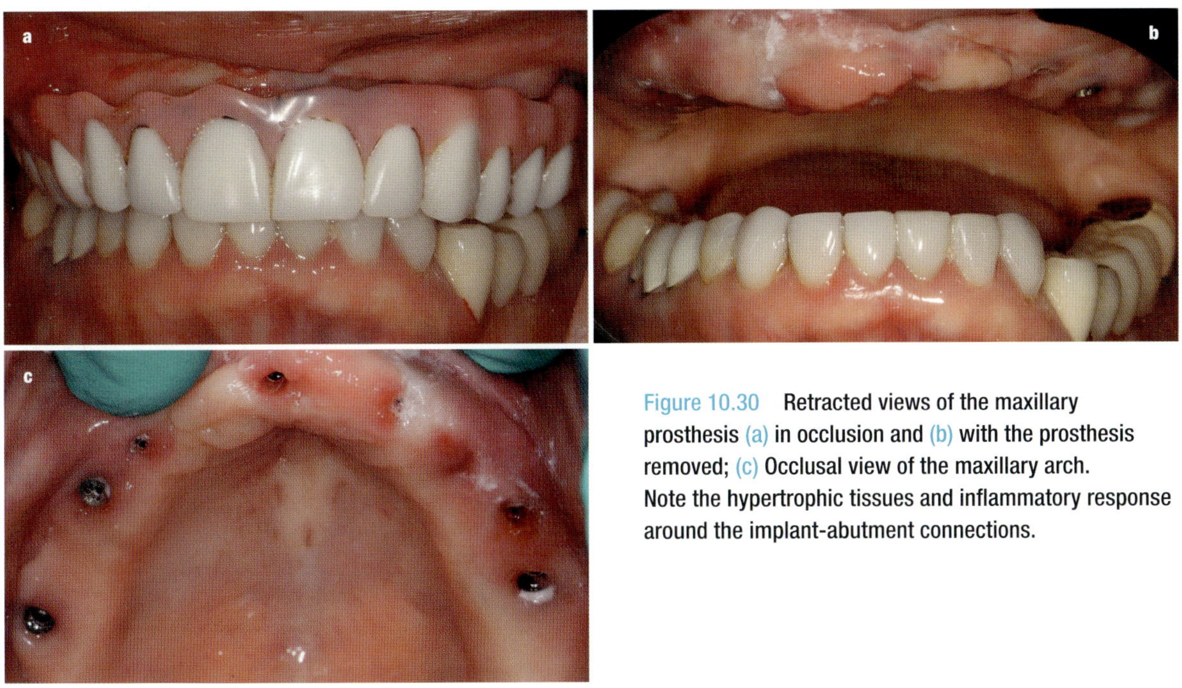

Figure 10.30 Retracted views of the maxillary prosthesis (a) in occlusion and (b) with the prosthesis removed; (c) Occlusal view of the maxillary arch. Note the hypertrophic tissues and inflammatory response around the implant-abutment connections.

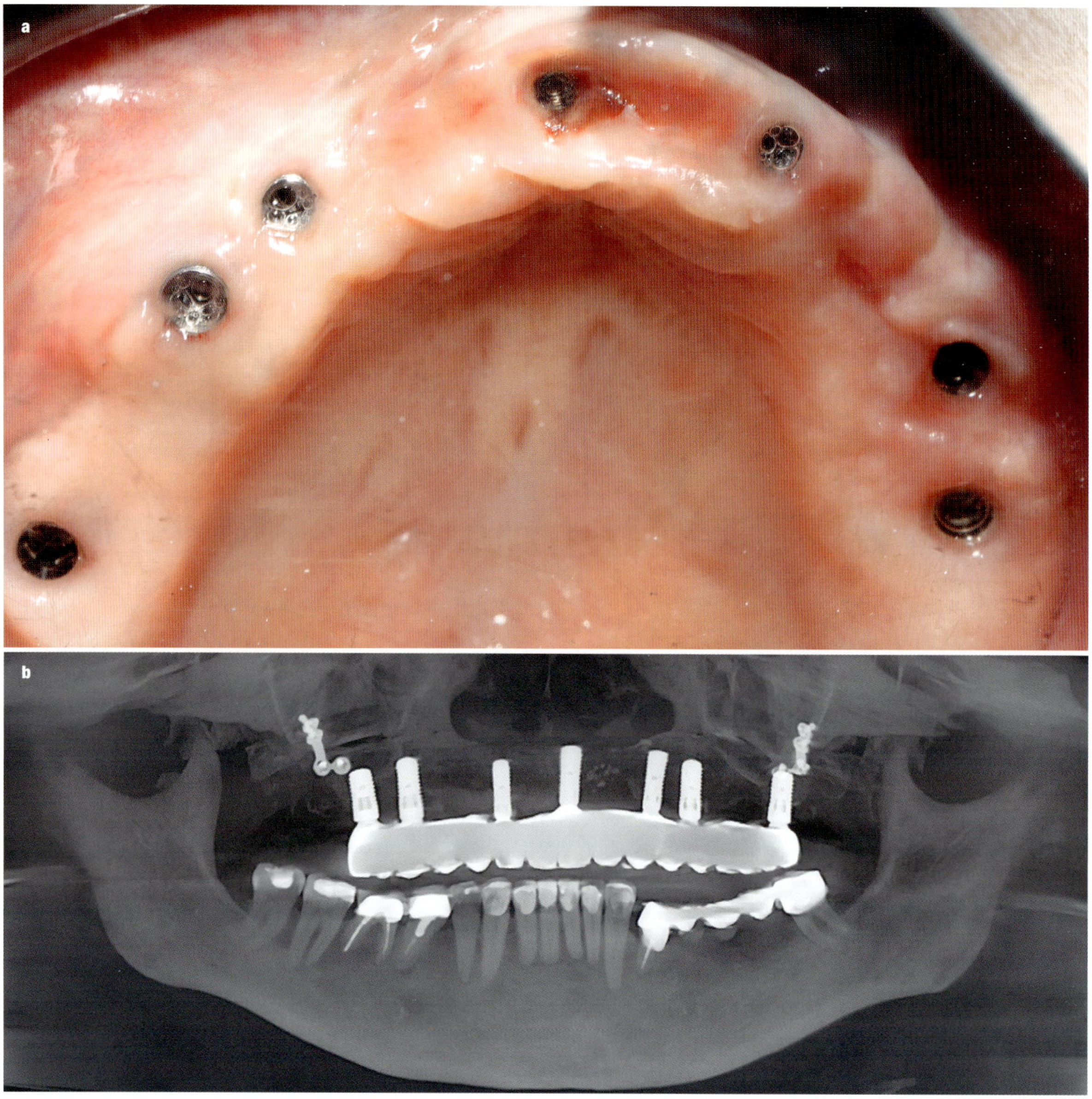

Figure 10.31 (a) **Appearance of the soft tissue and implants in the maxillary arch 4 months after surgical intervention;** (b) **Postoperative CBCT scan with a monolithic zirconia fixed full-arch prosthesis in place.**

I treated this patient's implant and tissue complications using localized surgical procedures and then developed an interim prosthesis that the patient could wear during the healing phase after surgery. Once the patient's tissues showed greater stability, we developed a new prosthesis using the prosthetic workflow outlined in this book. As you can see, a much more clinically acceptable and hygienic prosthesis was fabricated and even better esthetic results were achieved **(Figs. 10.32-10.34)**.

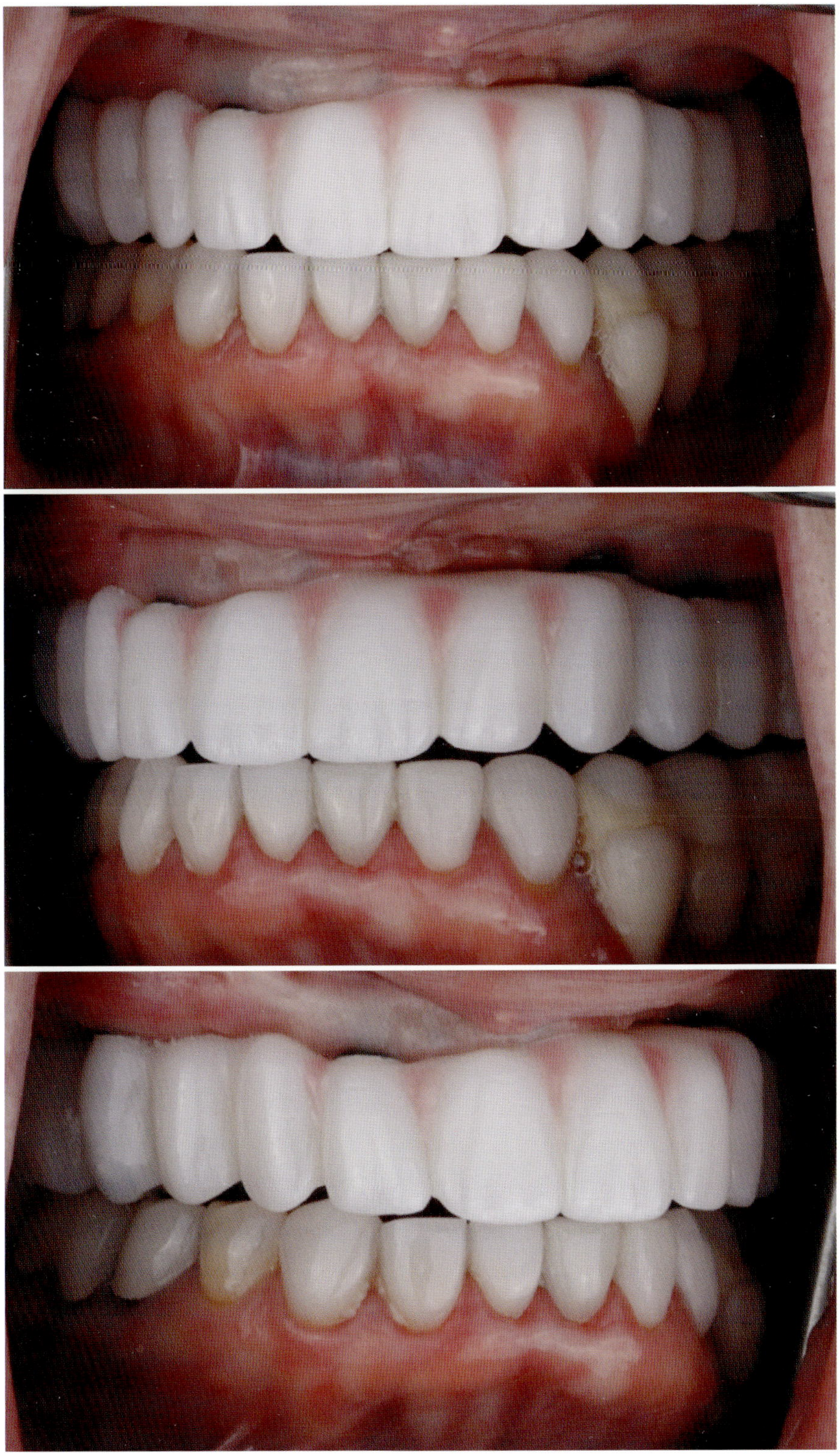

Figure 10.32 Retracted frontal and lateral views of the definitive monolithic zirconia maxillary prosthesis. The patient's occlusion was corrected with a provisional prosthesis over the bridge on the left side of the posterior mandible, and a plan was developed for rehabilitation of the mandibular arch.

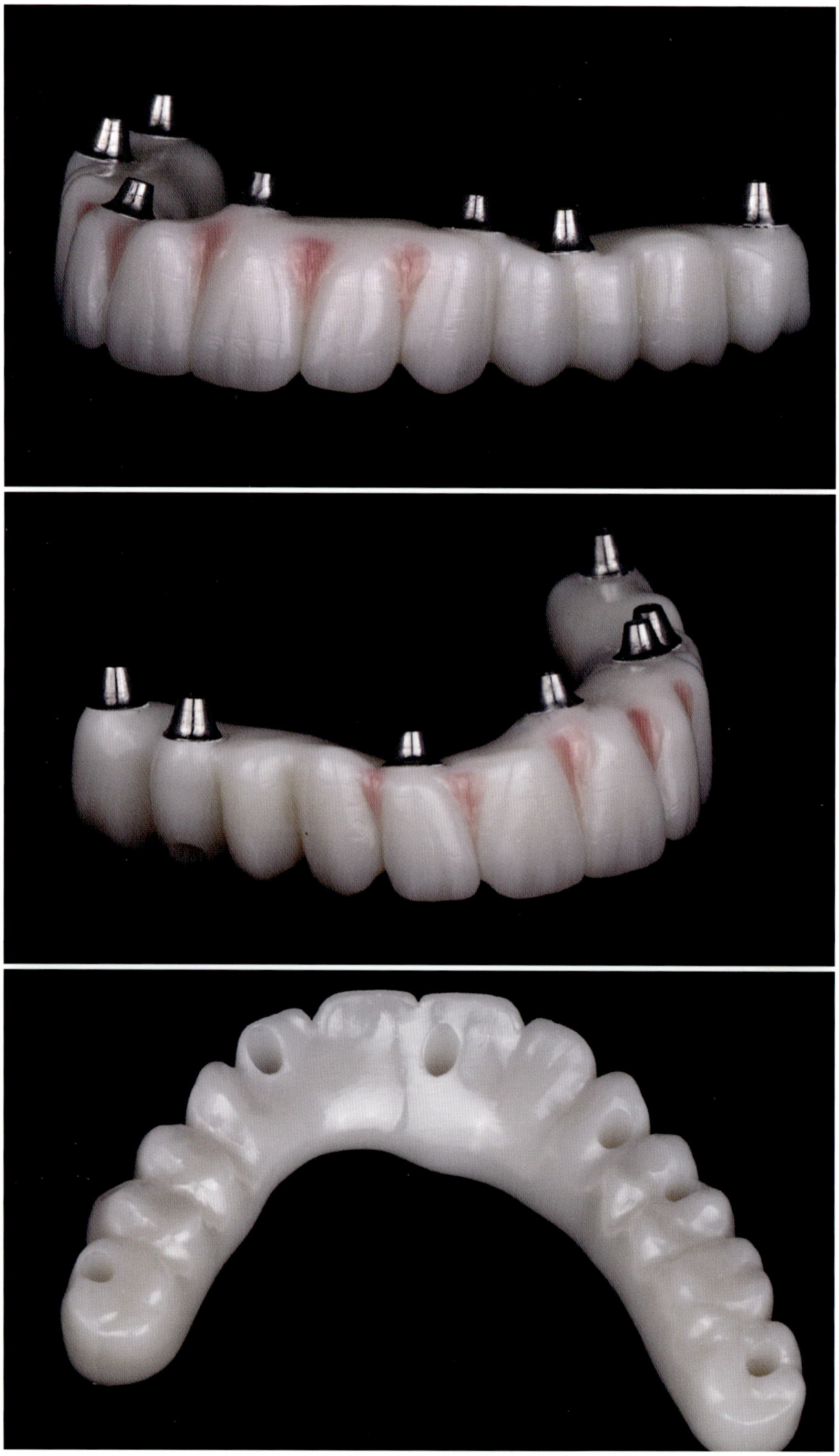

Figure 10.32 (*cont'd*) **Contrasting extraoral views of the definitive monolithic zirconia prosthesis.**

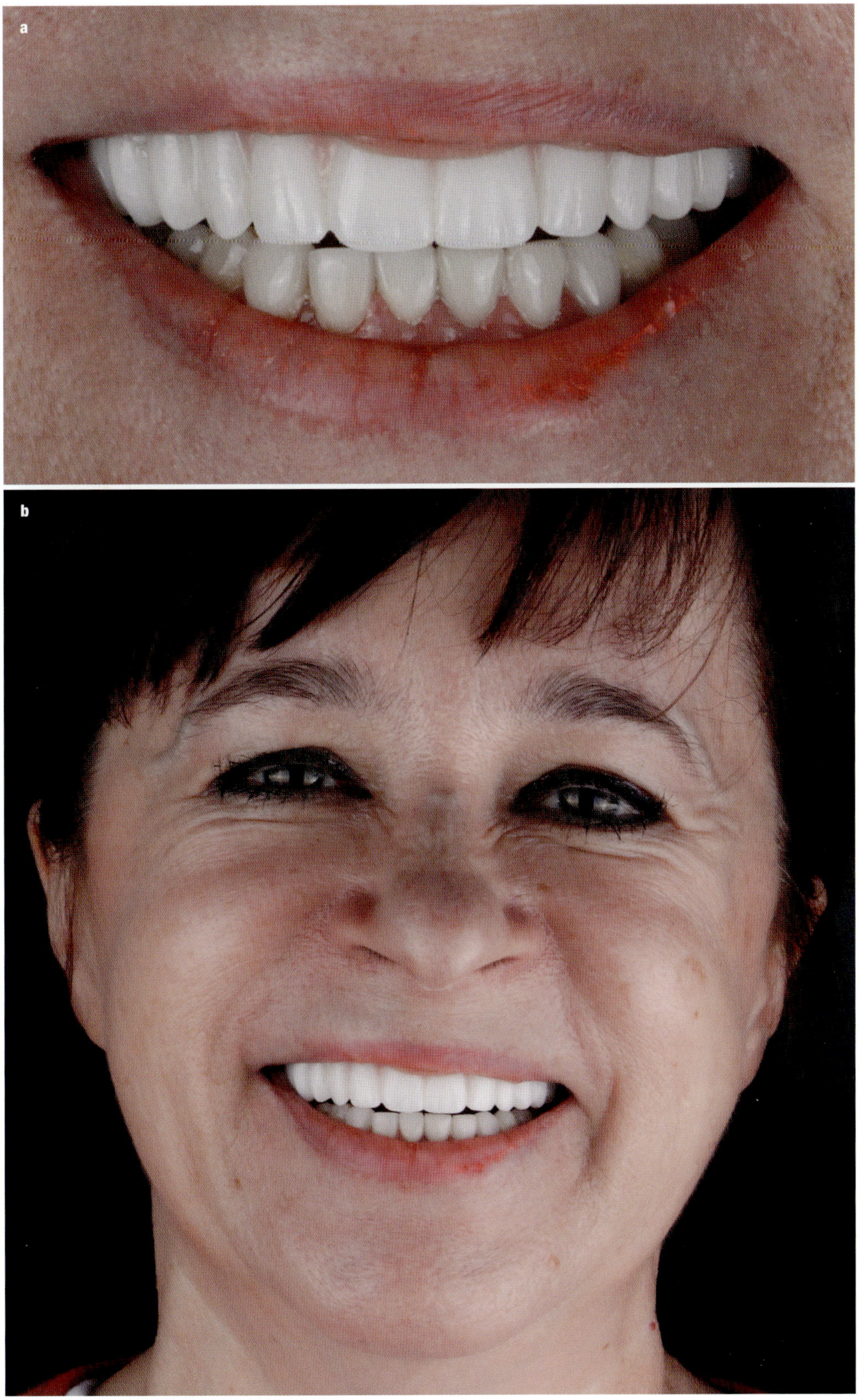

Figure 10.33 (a) Close-up smile and (b) portrait photos of patient after delivery of the definitive prosthesis.

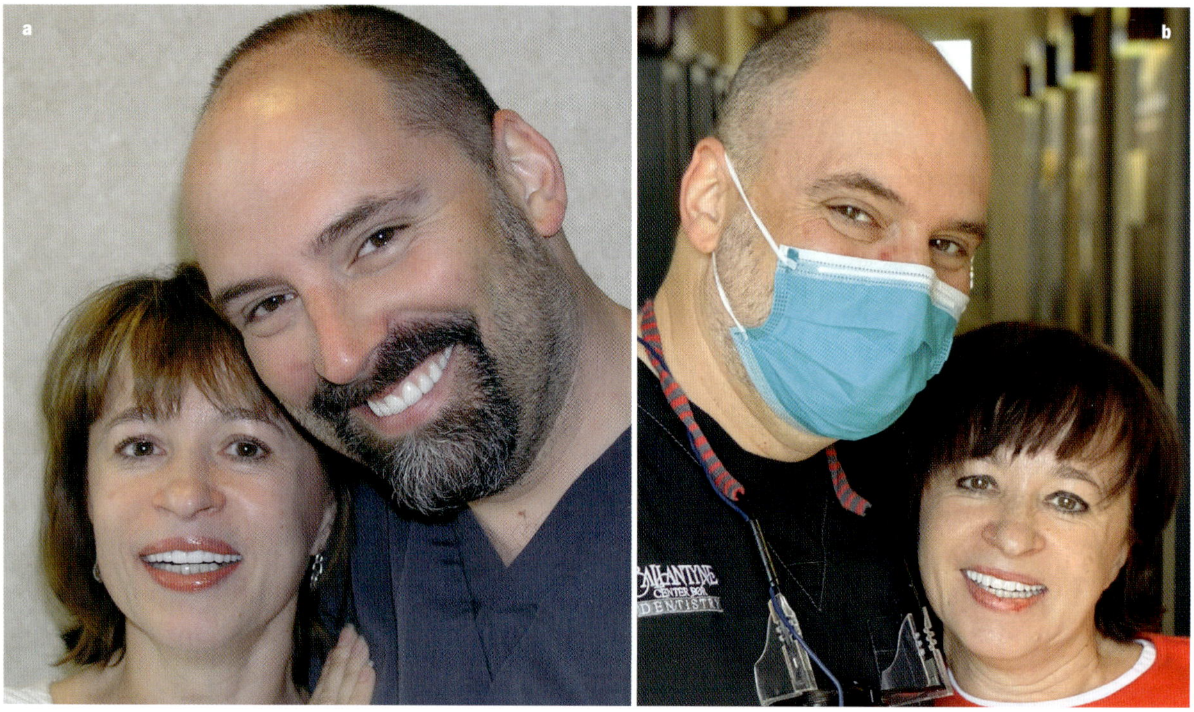

Figure 10.34 **The author and the patient (a) at her original delivery appointment and (b) 12 years later (with COVID-19 protocols in place).**

The best thing about this case study is that it has a happy ending, which is not always the outcome in these situations. If this patient came to my office today as she had presented originally, I would handle this case much differently. Digital planning and engineering would have been implemented at the very beginning and it would be prosthetically rather than surgically driven. The Le Fort I surgery may have been unnecessary. Fewer implants would have been needed, they would have been placed in more ideal positions using guided surgery, and MUAs would have been part of the foundation. The definitive prosthesis would be hygienic as well as esthetic and made from monolithic zirconia instead of denture acrylic wrapped over a milled titanium bar. In addition, the workflow would have been simpler, it would have taken fewer appointments, and the case would have been more cost effective for the patient and for me.

This case demonstrates several important points, the most obvious being how much has changed in fixed full-arch implant dentistry over the last decade or so. We are fortunate to have developed a better understanding of how to achieve better and more predictable results for our patients. We can do this because of advancements in technology and the collaborative experiences and ideas from clinicians, lab technicians, and other industry professionals throughout the world.

References

1. American Academy of Periodontology [Internet]. Chicago, IL: AAP; 2023. Dental Implant Procedures; 2023; [about 1 screen]. Available from: https://www.perio.org/for-patients/periodontal-treatments-and-procedures/dental-implant-procedures/
2. Bidra AS, Daubert DM, Garcia LT, Kosinski TF, Nenn CA, Olsen JA, Platt JA, Wingrove SS, Chandler ND, Curtis DA. Clinical practice guidelines for recall and maintenance of patients with tooth-borne and implant-borne dental restorations. J Am Dent Assoc 2016 Jan;147(1):67-74.
3. American College of Prosthodontists [Internet]. Chicago, IL: ACP; 2023. Maintenance of Full-Arch Implant Restorations: Position Statement of the American College of Prosthodontists; 4 Oct 2016; [about 1 screen]. Available from: https://www.prosthodontics.org/about-acp/position-statement-maintenance-of-full-arch-implant-restorations/
4. Takeuchi Y, Nakajo K, Sato T, Koyama S, Sasaki K, Takahashi N. Quantification and identification of bacteria in acrylic resin dentures and dento-maxillary obturator-prostheses. Am J Dent 2012 Jun;25:171-175.
5. de Araújo Nobre M, Salvado F, Nogueira P, Rocha E, Ilg P, Maló P. A peri-implant disease risk score for patients with dental implants: Validation and the influence of the interval between maintenance appointments. J Clin Med 2019;8:252.
6. Bidra AS, Daubert DM, Garcia LT, Gauthier MF, Kosinski TF, Nenn CA, Olsen JA, Platt JA, Wingrove SS, Chandler ND, Curtis DA. A systematic review of recall regimen and maintenance regimen of patients with dental restorations. Part 2: Implant-borne restorations. J Prosthodont 2016;25 Suppl 1:S16-S31.
7. Corbella S, Del Fabbro M, Taschieri S, De Siena F, Francetti L. Clinical evaluation of an implant maintenance protocol for the prevention of peri-implant diseases in patients treated with immediately loaded full-arch rehabilitations. Int J Dent Hyg 2011;9:216-222.
8. Gulati M, Govila V, Anand V, Anand B. Implant maintenance: A clinical update. Int Sch Res Notices 2014 Jul 9;2014:908534.
9. Wingrove SS. Peri-Implant Therapy for the Dental Hygienist, 2nd ed. Hoboken, NJ: Wiley-Blackwell, 2022.
10. Shrivastava D, Natoli V, Srivastava KC, Alzoubi IA, Nagy AI, Hamza MO, Al-Johani K, Alam MK, Khurshid Z. Novel approach to dental biofilm management through guided biofilm therapy (GBT): A review. Microorganisms 2021;9:1966-1982.

ACKNOWLEDGEMENTS

First and foremost, I thank God for leading and guiding me throughout my life and professional journey; I am grateful for his timing in my experiences and placing opportunities and individuals in my path. Without the insight, determination, and passion granted me by my creator, I would never have been able to author this book.

Secondly, I am enormously thankful to Mark Ferber, who challenged and inspired me to share my knowledge and experience with you. It was by his influence and introduction that I was able to establish a relationship with Edra Publishing. Throughout the process of writing this book, Mark provided the fostering and relentless accountability that I needed to complete the task. He has steered me through the complexities of losing my friend and late partner, Dr. Joseph Hufanda, and has become a trusted advisor and friend.

I am indebted to the accomplished dentists and specialists who took the time to help me review and edit this volume of work: Dr. Nick Fahey, Dr. Joe McEnhill, Dr. Emmanuelle Zennie, Dr. Pamela Ray, and Dr. David Little. I also am very appreciative of the team of doctors I have the pleasure of working with in my practice: Dr. Devon Binns, Dr. Grant Tesmer, and Dr. Eric Davis. I consider it an honor to have the pleasure of working alongside these talented friends and clinicians.

I would be remiss if I did not mention the outstanding professionals on the dental laboratory side who collaborated with me to test and develop better ways of providing stackable surgical guide solutions and prosthetics to my patients: Dr. Bushra Immam, Thomas Kuun, MDT, Joe Ambrose, CDT and Technical Director at Roe Dental Laboratory, Matt Vrhovac, Jack Marrano, CDT, and Conrad Rensburg of Absolute Dental Services in Durham NC, USA.

I would like to recognize Jay Watson, the inventor of CHROME™ Guided Smile Pat. #11576755, #11589963 and #11806209B2, who first encouraged me to pursue guided full-arch dental implant surgery in my practice. He inspired my curiosity and shifted my paradigm.

I owe much of the professional success I have achieved to my coaches and mentors: Dr. Tony Feck and Dr. Matt VanderMolen. My admiration for these two men is hard to measure. I would also like to acknowledge all my friends and brilliant colleagues at Sunrise Dental Solutions, who have taught me, over the last 15 years, to carve out my niche in the dental industry, become a stronger clinician, be a better businessman, and the importance of servant leadership.

I would like to express my gratitude to my friends at Edra Publishing. Giorgio Albonetti, President and CEO, and Tommaso Albonetti, General Manager at Edra Publishing, saw the value of sharing with you, the reader, the ideas and concepts explored in this text and invested their resources to bring it to fruition. I greatly appreciate the hard work done by Paola Sammaritano, Sandra Calarota, and the editors and designers of this textbook.

I want to give a big thank you to my parents, Tom and Michelle, who raised me to understand that serving God is the highest purpose in this life, and patiently waited for me to figure it out. They taught me by example to have integrity, be humble and generous, the value of hard work, and the joy that is found in serving others.

Last, but surely not least, I want to recognize and thank my beautiful wife Gabriela, who has selflessly accepted my professional pursuits throughout our 27 years of marriage, and my two awesome children, Alexander and Isabella. For 3 years I have spent hours at a time tucked away on my computer, combing through thousands of photographs and tapping out my thoughts on a keyboard. Not once did my family complain about my wild obsession with completing the task at hand. I have been blessed with an incredible family and am eternally grateful. I love you all.

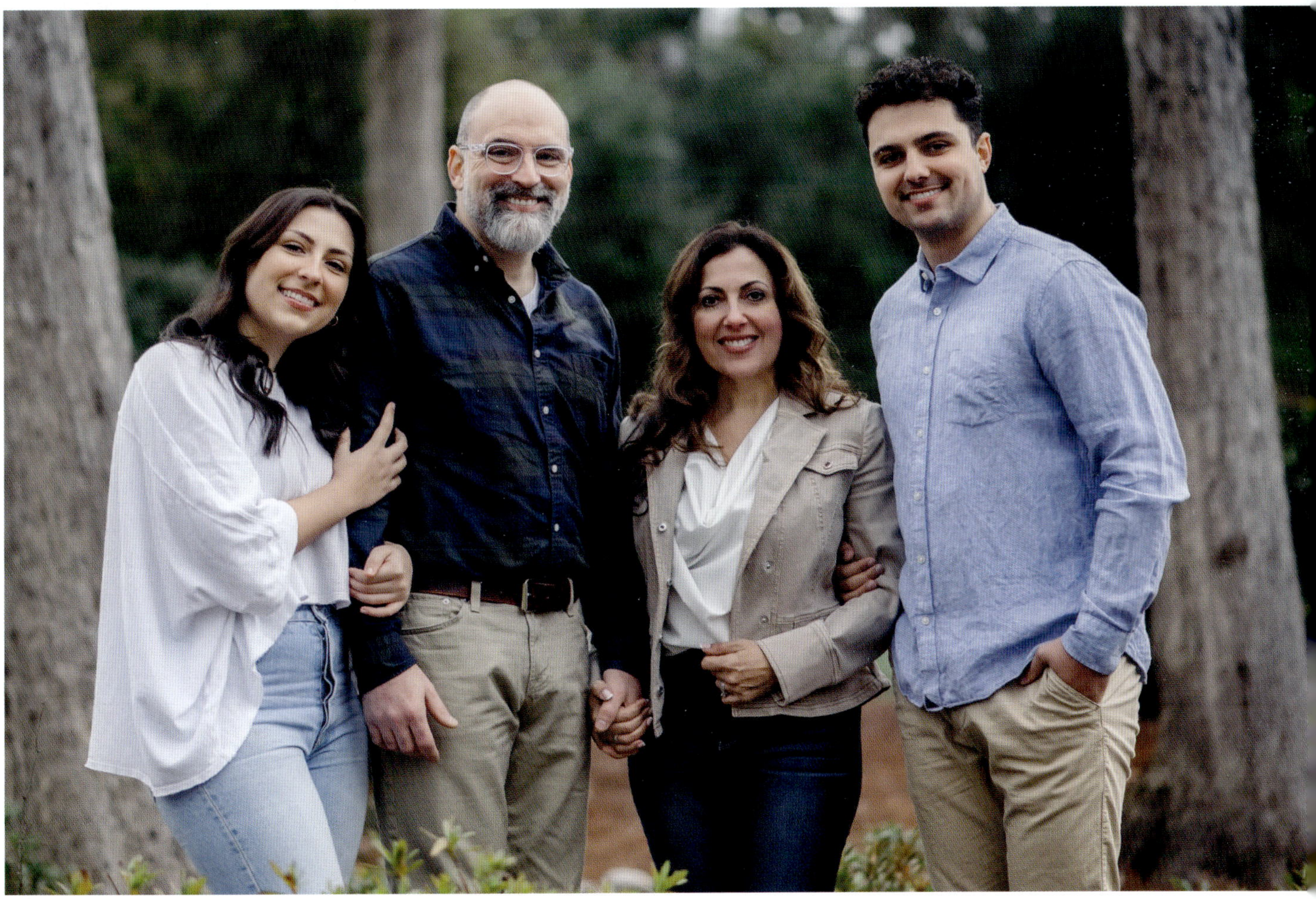

My wife Gabriela and my two children, Alexander and Isabella.